Diuretics

Chemistry, Pharmacology, and Clinical Applications

Diuretics

Chemistry, Pharmacology, and Clinical Applications

Proceedings of the First International Conference on Diuretics, held March 4–9, 1984, in Miami Beach, Florida, U.S.A.

Editor:

Jules B. Puschett, M.D.

Professor of Medicine, Director, Renal-Electrolyte Division, University of Pittsburgh School of Medicine, Pennsylvania, U.S.A.

Associate Editor:

Arthur Greenberg, M.D.

Assistant Professor of Medicine, Member, Renal-Electrolyte Division, University of Pittsburgh School of Medicine, Pennsylvania, U.S.A.

Elsevier

New York • Amsterdam • Oxford

Published by:

Elsevier Science Publishing Company, Inc.
52 Vanderbilt Avenue, New York, New York 10017

Sole distributors outside the United States and Canada:

Elsevier Science Publishers B.V.
P.O. Box 211, 1000 AE Amsterdam, The Netherlands

Library of Congress Cataloging in Publication Data

Diuretics: chemistry, pharmacology, and clinical applications.
International Conference on Diuretics (1st: 1984: Miami Beach, Fla.)
Sponsored by Bayer A.G. and other firms, co-sponsored, American Society for Clinical Pharmacology and Therapeutics, held Mar. 5-9, 1984, at Miami Beach, Fla.

Includes bibliographies and indexes.
1. Diuretics—Congresses. I. Puschett, Jules B. II. Greenberg, Arthur.
III. Farbenfabriken Bayer Aktiengesellschaft. IV. American Society for Clinical Pharmacology and Therapeutics. V. Title. [DNLM: 1. Diuretics—congresses.
W3 IN172M 1st 1984m / QV 160 1984m]
RM377.I36 1984 615'.761 84-18778
ISBN 0-444-00950-7

Manufactured in the United States of America

TABLE OF CONTENTS

Section I: Discovery and Development of Diuretic Agents.

Section II
Diuretics: Antihypertensive and Hemodynamic Actions.

Section VII: Diuretic Pharmacology and Pharmacokinetics.

Section VIII: Diuretics: In Vivo and In Vitro Studies.

Section IX: Diuretic Effects on the Kidney.

Section X: Extra-renal Effects of Diuretics.

Section XI: Use of Diuretics in Acute and Chronic Renal Failure.

Section XII: Diuretics: Metabolic and Hormonal Effects.

Sponsors

The Organizing Committee expresses its deep appreciation for the very generous support of this meeting by the following sponsors:

Bayer A.G.

Eisai Ltd.

Hoechst A.G.

Hoffman-La Roche, Inc.

Merck, Sharp and Dohme

Smith, Kline, Beckman

Contributors

We are grateful for the support provided by the following contributors:

Boehringer-Ingelheim Ltd.

Miles Laboratories

Pennwalt Pharmaceuticals

Sandoz, Inc.

U.S. Vitamin Pharmaceuticals

Co-Sponsor

American Society for Clinical Pharmacology and Therapeutics

Organizing Committee

Jules B. Puschett, M.D., *Chairman*
Professor of Medicine
Director, Renal-Electrolyte Division
University of Pittsburgh
School of Medicine
Pittsburgh, PA, U.S.A.

Vittorio E. Andreucci, M.D.
Professor of Nephrology and Chairman
Second Faculty of Medicine
University of Naples
Naples, Italy

Ezequiel Bellorin-Font, M.D.
Agregate Professor of Medicine
School of Medicine
Universidad de Oriente
Center for Dialysis and Transplantation
Hospital Universitario de Caracas
Caracas, Venezuela

William M. Bennett, M.D.
Professor of Medicine and Pharmacology
Head, Division of Nephrology
The Oregon Health Sciences University
Portland, OR, U.S.A.

Edward J. Cragoe, Ph.D.
Distinguished Senior Scientist
Medicinal Chemistry
Merck, Sharp & Dohme Research Laboratories
West Point, PA, U.S.A.

Peter Deetjen, M.D.
Professor of Physiology
Institut für Physiologie und Balneologie
der Universität Innsbruck
Innsbruck, Austria

Professor A. Fernandez-Cruz
Facultad de Medicina
Cuidad Universitaria
Madrid, Spain

Bernardo Rodriquez-Iturbé, M.D.
Professor of Medicine
Chief, Renal Service and Laboratory
Hospital Universitario de Maracaibo
Maracaibo, Venezuela

Professor Dr. J. Greven
Abteilung Pharmakologie
der Medizinischen Fakultät
an der Rhein-Westf. Techn. Hochschule
Aachen, West Germany

Nishio Honda, M.D.
Professor
First Department of Medicine
Hamamatsu University
Hamamatsu, Japan

Max Hropot, M.D.
Department of Pharmacology
Hoechst A.G.
Frankfurt, West Germany

Professor Ariel Lant
Department of Therapeutics
Westminster Medical School
University of London
Westminster Hospital
London, England

Barry Materson, M.D.
Assistant Chief, Medical Services
VA Medical Center
Professor of Medicine
University of Miami Medical School
Miami, FL, U.S.A.

Gaddo Onesti, M.D.
Professor of Medicine and Pharmacology
Hahnemann Medical College
Philadelphia, PA, U.S.A.

José Carlos Peña, M.D.
Professor of Medicine
Head, Department of Nephrology
and Mineral Metabolism
Instituto Nácional de la Nutricion
Salvador Zubiran
Mexico City, Mexico

John F. Seely, M.D.
Chairman, Department of Medicine
University of Ottawa
Ottawa General Hospital
Ottawa, Ontario, Canada

SECTION I

DISCOVERY AND DEVELOPMENT OF DIURETIC AGENTS

DISCOVERY OF CHLOROTHIAZIDE

John E. Baer, Ph.D., Staff Executive,
Merck Sharp & Dohme Research Laboratories,
West Point, PA 19486

An early landmark in our understanding of electrolyte transport was the remarkable micropuncture research in the frog conducted by A. N. Richards, Phyllis Bott and their colleagues at the University of Pennsylvania. It is almost inconceivable that their analytical work involved gravimetric methods for measuring sodium and potassium. Flame photometers had not been invented. Later, the mechanistic basis for mercurial diuretics was strongly influenced by the ease with which chloride could be measured directly by titration, the sodium excretion being inferred therefrom. In the late 1940's, when the flame photometer became available, electrolyte physiology developed rapidly.

A solid basis for understanding renal transport, secretion and reabsorption of organic compounds (urea, inulin, organic acids) was laid in the 1940's by Homer Smith and his colleagues at New York University, notably J. A. Shannon who later directed the growth of the National Institutes of Health. R. F. Pitts, at Cornell, was performing exquisite physiological studies on the renal transport of inorganic substances (phosphate, bicarbonate).

In 1949, the physiological research on ion transport intersected with biochemical work that had been proceeding, principally in England, on the enzyme carbonic anhydrase. Sulfanilamide, an inhibitor of the enzyme, blocked urinary acidification and enhanced the excretion of sodium, the first instance of a sulfonamide diuretic in man [3].

An enzymologically-oriented research group might have chosen to set up an <u>in vitro</u> screening program and try to synthesize the most potent inhibitor. R. O. Roblin and his colleagues at American Cyanamid did just this; from among the most potent, T. M. Maren selected acetazolamide on the basis of its stability and lack of toxicity. In contrast, K. H. Beyer chose the physiological -- whole animal -- approach that had served well in the Sharp and Dohme penicillin blocker program.

J. M. Sprague, director of medicinal chemistry at Sharp and Dohme, had successfully developed several sulfonamide antibacterial agents during World War II. K. H. Beyer, physiologist and physician, had investigated the renal transport of sulfonamides and of penicillin, which had just come into clinical use. Together, starting from p-aminohippurate, the Sharp and Dohme team discovered the penicillin-sparing action of analogs of the sulfonamide type: carinamide and probenecid. The latter has been used widely to investigate, and therapeutically to regulate, renal tubular transport of organic acids, notably the net renal secretion of urate.

Using their experience in sulfonamide chemistry and renal pharmacology, Sprague and Beyer set out to discover a natriuretic molecule that would enhance sodium excretion, but would act selectively along the nephron so as to minimize acid retention (bicarbonate loss). The history of the early chemical efforts has been described. [4] [13] (In 1953, Merck Sharp and Dohme Research Laboratories was formed when the two firms merged.)

Based on the competitive inhibition of organic acids for renal transport (for which no enzymic mechanism was or is evident), we presumed that inhibition of inorganic ion transport might be modulated by organic compounds. Two renal enzyme systems for ion transport were recognized as reasonable in 1950: carbonic anhydrase and an unidentified sulfydryl-con-

<u>Diuretics</u>, Jules B. Puschett, Editor

taining enzyme that was attacked by mercurial diuretics. Pursuing the former led to acetazolamide and the thiazides. Pursuing the latter led to the 'loop' diuretic ethacrynic acid. (Though probably incorrect, both putative enzymic mechanisms led to fruitful research. This is not unusual in science.)

One of the first leads synthesized was p-carboxybenzene-sulfonamide. Later, Sprague and Novello found that aromatic disulfonamides had considerable natriuretic acitvity. Bicarbonate excretion and the HCO_3^-/Cl^- excretion ratio, reflecting H^+ retention, was strongly influenced by other substituents on the ring. Dichlorphenamide resembled acetazolamide, whereas 4-chloro-6-amino-1,3-disulfonamide had significant chloruretic activity. Novello, who was investigating N-acylated analogs, found that ring closure to the benzothiadiazine was readily accomplished. The first dog experiment with chlorothiazide convinced me that this molecule had the properties we were seeking. Synthesized by Novello in 1955, clinical trials were reported in 1957 [2] [14], and the drug was approved by the Food and Drug Administration and marketed in 1958. Hydrochlorothiazide followed a year later.

The biochemical basis for the actions of thiazides is not yet established. We found that the potency of several thiazides to inhibit glycolysis at 10^{-3} to 10^{-5} molar in renal medulla homogenates was parallel to their saluretic activity in the rat. Thiazides are not inhibitors of Na^+/K^+ -ATPase. [5]

Were we surprised that chlorothiazide was effective in the treatment of hypertension? No. Contemporary data suggested that an inappropriate glomerulo-tubular balance of sodium occurred, at least in some types of hypertension. Further, salt-free diets, and even periodic injections of organomercurial diuretics were effective in some cases, though not pleasant for the patient. At the least, the saluretic drug would allow a more pleasant regime with some ingestion of salt, augmented by an enhanced pathway of salt elimination. Fries [1] and Hollander [2] soon demonstrated the utility of the drug in hypertension. The precise mechanisms whereby chlorothiazide enhances the action of other classes of antihypertensive drugs are not understood.

We have earlier addressed the relative potency of thiazides in terms of inherent carbonic anhydrase inhibitory activity, pKa, lipid partition ratio, etc. [6] Data from recent studies on the bioavailability of chlorothiazide and hydrochlorothiazide suggest that the tenfold difference in potency of these two drugs in man may relate primarily to their absorption and hepatobiliary circulation.

Chlorothiazide is excreted rapidly and nearly quantitatively in the urine of humans after intravenous administration. Absorption of orally administered solutions is dose-dependent. Food enhances absorption, as does proprantheline, suggesting that absorption is improved by decreased gastrointestinal motility. About 20% of a clinically effective dose (250 mg.) is absorbed. [7] [8] Absorption of chlorothiazide appears to be saturable and site-specific.

Only 72% of an intravenous dose of hydrochlorothiazide appears in 12 hours in human urine; additional drug is excreted slowly for up to 4 days. The pattern strongly suggests enterohepatic recycling, and in fact radioactivity has been found in aspirated intestinal contents following an intravenous dose of labeled hydrochlorothiazide. [9] [10]

K. C. Kwan (unpublished observations), of our laboratories, has examined plasma and urinary hydrochlorothiazide for volunteers that had received intravenous and tablet formulations (50 mg.) in a crossover design study. Following the intravenous dose, plasma levels fell exponentially at first. Divergence with time from the initial exponential plasma curves was used to estimate enterohepatic recirculation. When expressed as a cumulative amount of drug entering the systemic circulation as a function of time, the total amount having re-entered the circulation ranged from 200 to 700 percent of the intravenous dose in four subjects. That is, one molecule of hydrochlorothiazide may be recycled one to seven times.

Bioavailability of the tablet forms, relative to the bioavailability of the intravenous case, was nearly quantitative. Furthermore, enterohepatic recycling would be expected to obscure even relatively large differences among formulations, and indeed apparent bioequivalence has been reported for thirteen tablet forms of hydrochlorothiazide. [11] [12]

The nearly quantitative absorption of hydrochlorothiazide (vs. 20% for chlorothiazide) and its more efficient (200 to 700%) recycling may suffice to account for the difference in apparent potency of the two drugs in man.

REFERENCES

1. E.D. Fries and I.M. Wilson, Med. Ann. D.C. 26, 468 (1957).
2. W. Hollander and R.W. Wilkins, Boston Med. Quarterly 8, 69-75 (1957).
3. W.B. Schwartz, New Eng. J. Med. 240, 173 (1949).
4. J.M. Sprague, Ann. N.Y. Acad. Med. 71, 328-343 (1958).
5. J.E. Baer and K.H. Beyer in Drugs Affecting Kidney Function and Metabolism, K.D.G. Edwards, ed., Karger, Basel (1972), pp. 71-76.
6. K.H. Beyer and J.E. Baer, Pharmacol. Rev. 13, 517-562 (1961).
7. M.A. Osman and P.G. Welling, Curr. Therap. Res. 34, 404-408 (1983).
8. M.A. Osman, R.B. Patel, D.S. Irwin, W.A. Craig and P.G. Welling, Biopharm. Drug Disp. 3, 89-94 (1982).
9. R.H. Barbhaiya, T.A. Phillips and P.G. Welling, J. Pharm. Sci. 70, 291 (1981).
10. B. Beermann, M. Groschinsky-Grind and A. Rosen, Clin. Pharm. Therap. 19, 531-537 (1976).
11. M.C. Meyer, A.P. Melikian, P.L. Whyatt and G.W.A. Slywka, Curr. Therap. Res. 17, 570-577 (1975).
12. B. Beermann, M. Groschinsky-Grind and B. Lindstrom, Europ. J. Clin. Pharmacol. 11, 203-205 (1977).
13. K.H. Beyer, Discovery, Development and Delivery of New Drugs, Spectrum Publications, New York 1978.
14. R.V. Ford, J.H. Moyer and C.L. Spurr, Arch. Int. Med. 100, 582-596 (1957).

DISCOVERY AND DEVELOPMENT OF FUROSEMIDE; HISTORICAL REMARKS

ROMAN MUSCHAWECK
Hoechst AG, Postfach 80 03 20, 6230 Frankfurt/M. 80, FRG

ABSTRACT

A historical retrospective will be provided on the discovery of the loop diuretic furosemide 25 years ago, and its introduction into therapy 20 years ago. The understanding of tubular transport processes within the nephron for the development of new compounds will be emphasized. Furosemide was the start of a new era in experimental and clinical nephrology.

The subject of this talk is "The history of the discovery and development of high-ceiling diuretics, in particular of furosemide". High-ceiling diuretics have always been a domain of Hoechst research. It is now almost sixty years since Hoechst's mercurial diuretic mersalyl was included in therapy. Hoechst took another big step forward in nephrology with 4-chloro-N-furfuryl-5-sulfamoyl anthranilic acid, a compound which celebrates its 25th (or 20th) jubilee this year (This has nothing either directly or indirectly to do with Orwell's futuristic novel "1984"). Furosemide was discovered in 1959 and launched as a medicament in 1964.

I am now going to give a short survey of diuretics and saluretics, presenting them in the order they come in medical history.

In the history of man, the most disparate methods have been used to treat edema. Starting with cantharidin from the Spanish fly, which stimulates the kidneys, and proceeding to volatile oils, etc., contained in diuretics (of, for example, the juniper berry, lovage, licorice juice, senna leaves, birch leaves, bean blossoms and pansies), the most diverse plants have been used as diuretics. Osmotic and urea diuresis, as well as alcohol diuresis, were also used therapeutically. Eventually, the diuretics of the xanthine category - caffeine and theophylline - appeared on the scene. The diuretic effect of coffee, tea and pure caffeine had already been used in early years to treat edema. Some physicians like Riegler 1884, for example, believed they had to assume that the effect was through the medium of the circulation - as with digitalis. Others, like Curschmann 1885 and Brenner 1886, detected an effect on the kidney quite independent of the circulation. F. Schröder was the first to carry out comparative studies with theobromine and caffeine in rabbits in Schmiedeberg's laboratories.

Theophylline proved to be superior in dogs and in man. Even today, derivatives of theophylline or caffeine are still being investigated for a diuretic effect.

After this short excursion into the pharmacology of natural substances, or rather of plants, I will proceed to the development of mercurial diuretics.

Metallic mercury has been known since the 15th or 16th century B.C. and was used by Hippocrates as a drug as early as around 400 B.C. "Mercurius praecipitatus" or calomel was introduced as a diuretic by Theoprastus Bombastus von Hohenheim - called Paracelsus. He thus became the first physician in renal therapeutics to treat patients with chemical agents.

Diuretics, Jules B. Puschett, Editor

In England, calomel seems to have remained in use for a long time. In 1854, W. Stokes, in his book: "The diseases of the heart and the aorta", recommended this salt for the treatment of edema: "The exhibition of mercury will, as if by enchantment, remove the edema". A pill containing digitalis, squill and 1 to 3 grains of calomel is officially listed in the British Pharmacopoeia of 1871. This pill was known as "Guy's Hospital pill", but was also commonly called Bailey's or Niemeyer's pill. In German-speaking regions, Jendrassik (1886) rediscovered the diuretic effect of calomel, which had been completely forgotten, and made use of this in practice. For edema, he administered 0.2 g of calomel daily and reported side effects such as stomatitis and diarrhoea.

In animals experimental investigations with organic mercurial compounds using a compound in a 5 % aspartic acid solution which had stood for 24 hours over yellow mercuric oxide and thus contained 2 - 3 % mercury, Rosenheim (1888) observed considerable diuretic effect on the isolated dog's kidney perfused with blood. Blumenthal and Oppenheim (1913) reported on the good diuretic effect of mercury salicylate and acetylaminomercuribenzoic acid sodium, i.e. Asurol, in rabbits. Novasurol was eventually referred to in 1917 (Zieler) as the best tolerated mercurial compound. Alfred Vogl, a third year student in the Wenckebach Clinic in Vienna, became aware in 1919 of the diuretic effect of Novasurol. On the temperature chart of a non-edematous 19-year-old female patient with congenital syphilis, a nurse who had just joined the clinic had namely recorded the daily urine volume in the form of columns.

The ward physician, Dr. Saxl, subsequently used Novasurol [1, 2] on an edematous syphilitic patient and for the first time reported the diuretic effect of this substance to the Society of Physicians in Vienna in February 1920. One year later, i.e. in 1921, Brunn wrote on the excretion of sodium chloride in the urine. With the introduction of further less toxic mercurial compounds such as Salyrgan(R) (mersalyl by Hoechst), which remained in use for a long time, or less known Neptal (mercuderamide), Novurit (mercurophylline) and Mercuhydrin (meralluride), widespread use of mercurial diuretics set in. Between 1920 and 1950, thousands of organic mercurial compounds were synthesized and investigated for diuretic activity. In these investigations, importance was placed particularly on low toxicity and oral absorbability. The last mercurial compound developed in Hoechst AG was Dr. Leditschke's meluginan (1959) [1, 2]. The era of the mercurial diuretics was also terminated with this.

As a result of the discovery of new orally effective categories of diuretics, there was a distinct drop in the therapeutic use of mercurial diuretics. Labelled mersalyl is only used nowadays for renal diagnostic purposes. For thousands of years, natural substances dominated the field of diuretic therapy and, for approximately 400 years, mercurial compounds were used.

About 30 years ago, sulfonamide diuretics finally began their triumphant advance. The great J. Baer and his colleagues are the most famous pioneers of thiazide-like diuretics in medicine. These sulfonamide diuretics introduced the era of modern chemotherapeutic diuretics free of heavy metals. First of all came the acetazolamide-type CAH-inhibitors, followed by thiazides such as chlorothiazide, hydrochlorothiazide, etc. Then came ultimately the high-ceiling diuretics such as furosemide, bumetanide, the non-sulfonamide diuretic ethacrynic acid and others [1, 2].

The thiazide diuretics were a major step forward in edema and hypertension therapy and, except in acute cases, largely replaced mercurial diuretics. Although thiazides induced an excretion of only 5 % of the sodium filtered glomerularly - which is about one quarter of the maximum effect attainable with mercurial compounds -, they are particularly valuable on account of their low toxicity and oral efficacy [3].

Following the discovery of hydrochlorothiazide, a great many diuretics similar in effect to thiazide were found. The potency and duration of effect could be extended, yet the maximum diuretic and saluretic effect remained the same.

To go into the differences in potency here would take us too far off-course. For the physician, it is unimportant whether a compound is potent at a dose of 100 mg or 5 - 10 mg or less, provided that the effect and the side effects are the same. Even when used over a rather long period of time, no outstanding advantages were observed with the sulfonamide range. These compounds have experienced the most multifarious modifications. Just when the thiazide diuretics had reached their peak, it seemed as if no further or better properties could be found for diuretics. It was felt that the scientific zenith in nephrology had been reached and nothing new could be expected. Nevertheless, new synthesis and my personal conviction confirmed that there must also be other chemical compounds and physiological points of attack for new diuretics.

The pharmaceutical-chemical synthesis group around Sturm, Siedel, Weyer and others in Hoechst have therefore nonetheless concentrated their particular interest on other structures in the sulfonamides, especially on metadisulfonamides of thiophene or benzene. These, however, showed no therapeutic value at first [2].

In the course of these studies, the chemists succeeded in introducing a basic radical into the chlorodisulfonamide. Starting from 1,3-dichlorobenzene-4,6-disulfonamide, 1-chloro-3-benzylaminobenzene-4,6-disulfonamide was synthesized in sufficient yield. These new reactions were eventually also successfully applied to 2,4-dihalogen-5-sulfamoylbenzoic acid, whereby, surprisingly, halogen could be selectively treated in substitution 2 [4].

By reacting 2,4-dichloro-5-sulfamoylbenzoic acid with various amines such as benzylamine, 2-thenylamine or furfurylamine and others, various substitutions were ultimately obtained [4].

The belief that carbonic anhydrase-inhibiting compounds alone would produce a diuretic or saluretic effect was dropped. Instead, it was assumed that genuine diuretics should act as saluretics.

The hypothesis that, in a real saluretic, the ion excretion ratio Cl^-: $(Na^+ + K^+)$ should be in the vicinity of 1.0 served this assumption. The direct state of dependency between CAH-inhibition and this ratio is of importance, as emphasized by Muschaweck in a symposium on: "La diuresi ed i diuretic nella clinica e nella terapia" (1963) and in "Osservazioni sul compartemento degli ioni durante la sperimentazione di sostanze ad effetto salidiuretico" (1965) [5, 6].

The first compound which met the requirements I wanted was the 2-amino-4-chloro-5-sulfamoylbenzoic acid. The compound had hardly any saluretic or diuretic efficacy, however. Up to this point, only the saluretic efficacy had been to the fore and insufficient attention had been paid to the diuretic effect. With the development of furosemide, the term "salidiuretic" came into being and both a new therapeutic principle and new trends were created in the clinic and in general practice. Since 1959, additional knowledge in the field of experimental pharmacology and physiology has also been uncovered.

Until furosemide was finally developed, a long rugged path paved with a great many obstacles had to be mastered. At the time, the difficulties and requirements to be fulfilled in testing a new drug, as imposed today by national and international legislation, could only be guessed at. Furosemide - or Lasix(R), as it was called - was developed. At this time, the drug market had also been shaken by a few pharmaceutical catastrophes - I am thinking of Thalidomide and others. I am therefore grateful to my teacher, Fritz Eichholtz, for the fact that, in my youth, I was confronted with a multitude of toxicological problems in pharmacology and that, through him, I was able to get to know the work of the former head of FDA, A.J. Lehmann, a friend of my boss !

In agreement with our toxicologists and in particular with Dr. Schütz, I elaborated a schedule for long-term administration of the new compound furosemide. The clinical chemistry tests carried out by Dr. Hajdù were incorporated into our study programme. Single-dose studies had already mostly been concluded. Groups of four dogs were given oral doses of 6, 60 or 360 mg of furosemide per kg. One group served as control.

Our repeated-dose studies began in the summer of 1962 and were to run until the end of July or beginning of August, 1963. I would like to add that, at the time, I had no experience with dogs under long-term treatment with high-ceiling diuretics.

Following clinical trials, furosemide was introduced generally into practice in 1964. In what respects did furosemide differ from the thiazides? The thiazide curves exhibit an S-shaped course, i.e. the effect reaches a plateau and cannot be intensified by the dose being increased. The dose-effect curves of furosemide are linear in a much larger dose range. The overall effect attainable can be increased by increasing the furosemide dose. One speaks of a reserve of effect which is valuable in the treatment of edematous disorders. Fig. 1 shows the diuretic effect after oral administration of hydrochlorothiazide, furosemide and chlorothiazide to the rat.

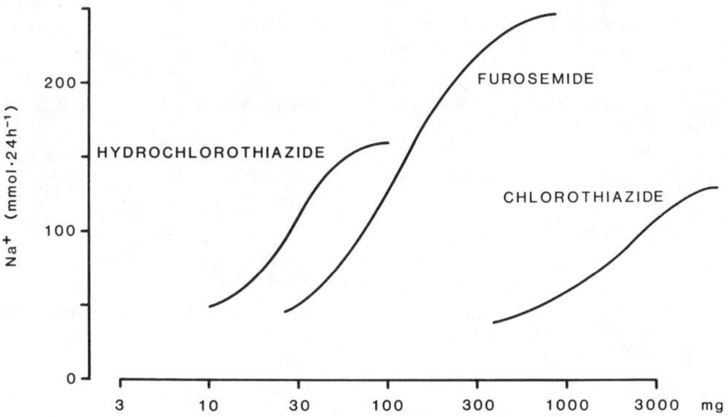

Fig. 1. Dose-response curves of low-ceiling and high-ceiling diuretics after oral administration in rats.

The dose-effect curve of hydrochlorothiazide e.g. given orally in doses between 8 and 16 mg/kg reaches a plateau, and the diuretic effect cannot be further increased by increasing the dose. When furosemide is administered with hydrochlorothiazide, a further increase in diuresis is obtained (Fig. 2). One speaks of superposition of the thiazide effect as a result of furosemide [1, 2, 5]. On the basis of this mode of action, the terms "low-ceiling diuretics" for thiazides and "high-ceiling" or "loop diuretics" for furosemide and ethacrynic acid were introduced. Through furosemide, new trends and new therapeutic principles were created. Due to its excellent tolerance and rapid onset of effect, furosemide became the tool of two generations of researchers.

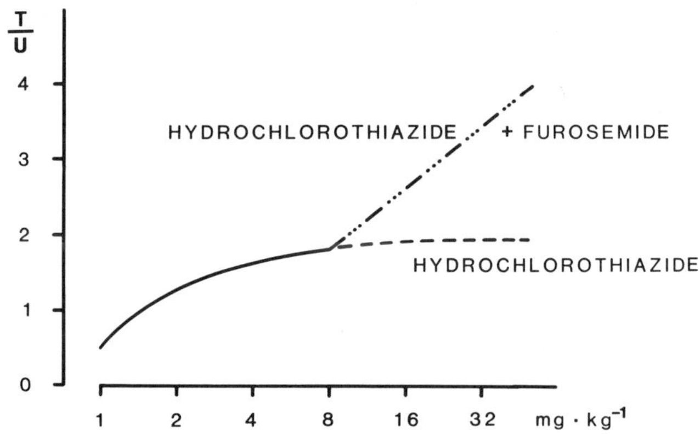

Fig. 2. Aumgentation of maximum thiazide diuresis after addition of furosemide in rats

Under the influence of furosemide, clearance and micropuncture studies were speeded up and perfected. Consequently, on the occasion of the furosemide symposium in Bad Homburg [1, 7, 8] at the end of 1963, Deetjen was able to report on the exact site of action of furosemide. By micropuncture technique on the isolated kidney in situ, he found the main site of action of furosemide in Henle's loop and an additional effect in the proximal tubule. A large number of studies were performed on isolated organs: isolated rabbit colon (Heintze) or shark rectal gland (Kinne), frog skin, isolated aorta or vein strips and isolated renal tubules, the latter being a very sophisticated method introduced by Burg and others [9, 10, 11, 12, 13]. Ehrlich ascitic cells (Geck), erythrocytes and leukocytes and other models, have contributed decisively to understanding the mode of action of diuretics. The Na^+ $2Cl^-$ K^+ co-transport localised in the luminal cell membrane is sensitive to furosemide. Inhibition of this transport by furosemide leads to electrolyte and water excretion which reduces the intracellular Na^+ concentrations. The co-transport carrier is stimulated by the electrochemical gradient for Na^+ which is directed towards the interior of the cell. The electrochemical gradient, for this part, is maintained by the sodium pump located in the peritubular cell membrane. The carrier, however, is also inhibited when, for example, the tubules are perfused with solution containing no Na^+ or Cl^-. The transepithelial potential difference (PD), which is lumen-positive, then drops to zero. The potassium is transported upwards on both sides of the cell. Suppression of Na^+/Cl^- transport induces, on the one hand, potassium secretion. The potassium is not absorbed into the cells. On the other hand, the presence of K^+ is, however, the prerequisite for the carrier-induced co-transport of Na^+/Cl^-. This co-transport system is even equated to a furosemide receptor which occurs both in the kidneys and in other organs of the body with transporting epithelia.

Furosemide has not only proved successful as a potent loop diuretic in the treatment of edema, but has also taken its place in the treatment of hypertension. The positive effect of furosemide in treating chronic and, above all, acute left ventricular failure was explained by its potent diuretic effect.

Biamino and others, however, observed that, in patients with acute left ventricular failure, furosemide administered in high doses led to a significant drop in left ventricular filling pressure and in right atrial pressure before significant diuresis was obtained, whereupon this diuretic was assumed to have primary vascular effects. In occlusion plethysmographical tests on the forearm of healthy volunteers, Biamino showed that 40 mg of furosemide administered intravenously did not affect the arterial blood flow, while a significant increase of 15 % in vein capacity was observed. The variations in volume of the forearm, which were measured with a strain gauge, reflected the filling state of the venous vessels. In vitro tests in isolated portal veins confirmed the afore-mentioned findings. Namely, furosemide brought about a dose-dependent reduction of up to 65 % in the isometric tension of portal veins [14].

In all vertebrate animal species and birds tested to date, furosemide showed its great efficacy. This has ultimately contributed to the transport processes in the proximal tubule being better understood. The proximal tubule in fact possesses amongst other things a transport mechanism for weak organic acids, an anion transport system. As a result of this transport mechanism, furosemide, like other organic compounds, is excreted proximally into the lumen. This active transport process enables furosemide not to reach the necessary effective concentration before Henle's loop and then to develop its main action.

It would be incomplete if the further developments in the field of loop diuretics in our laboratories were not mentioned. Hence, in 1974 - ten years ago -, the vasoactive diuretic piretanide was developed and was introduced in the therapy in 1982 [15].

Fig. 3 shows the essential difference between furosemide and piretanide. The dose-response curve of piretanide in dogs exhibits a slight rise in Na^+ excretion, which ultimately signifies a more moderate saluretic effect. The potassium excretion after piretanide is, if anything, favourable. Numerous clinical studies in hypertensive patients have demonstrated that piretanide can distinctly lower the systolic and diastolic blood pressure. The potassium balance is influenced only in a small percentage of cases. Piretanide became useful for the treatment of hypertension. Compared to furosemide, the action on the resistance vessels is markedly intensified, consequently a vasoactive principle can be assumed for piretanide.

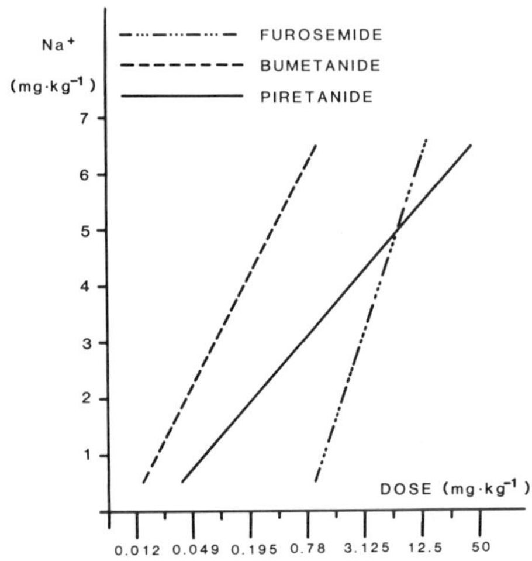

Fig. 3. Dose-response curve of piretanide in comparison with those of furosemide and bumetanide.

Piretanide clearly distinguishes itself by its relaxing effect on the pretreated rat aorta. Dr. Klaus will report on this issue.

Finally, I would now like to draw attention to a further new development of a loop diuretic, namely Hoe 365, a 3-aminomethyl-2-hydroxyphenyl sulfone from our work group. Dr. Hropot will report on this. In addition to its salidiuretic properties, the main effects of Hoe 365 consist in its influence on elevated blood pressure in experiments. A dose-dependent drop in blood pressure was observed both in rats with spontaneous hypertension and in dogs with chronic renal hypertension. Extrarenal sites of action were observed and admit of new possibilities in research with diuretics.

Let me now conclude. Particularly as a result of the introduction of loop (high-ceiling) diuretics, the development of modern diuretics has led to considerable advance in the field of experimental and clinical nephrology. With furosemide (Lasix(R)), which was synthesized in 1959 and originates from a group of about 300 systematically investigated compounds and the pharmacological effect of which was recognized by us as a new salidiuretic principle, scientific studies were initiated world-wide. As a crowning finish, I would particularly like to mention the publications of Greger and colleagues in recent years, which show the relevance of the Na^+ $2Cl^-$ K^+ co-transport [16, 17, 18]. Furosemide became the standard and a necessary tool in experimental nephrology. It was the drug of choice in treating disorders of the electrolyte and water balance. It is consequently justifiable to look back on a quarter century of furosemide. In doing so, thanks and recognition have to be given to those who helped with scientific élan to search for new ways of coming across new knowledge. As mentioned in the case of piretanide and Hoe 365, by structural changes and by establishing and developing new categories of chemical compounds, new activity profiles and sites of action in the nephron and in the organism will undoubtedly be found in the future.

I would finally like to express my thanks to the chemists, biochemists, biologists, pathologists and pharmacologists responsible for the era of the loop diuretics. My particular thanks goes to my successor and colleague of many years, Dr. Max Hropot.

REFERENCES

1. H. Herken, Handbook of Experimental Pharmacology, Vol. XXII, Springer Verlag, Berlin-Heidelberg-New York (1969)
2. R. Muschaweck and K. Sturm, Diuretika in G. Ehrhart and H. Ruschig, Arzneimittel Entwicklung, Darstellung, Vol. 2, p. 318 (sec. ed.), Verlag Chemie GmbH, Weinheim/Bergstr. (1972)
3. K. Meng and D. Loew, Diuretika, Gg. Thieme Verlag, Stuttgart (1974)
4. W. Siedel, K. Sturm, and R. Muschaweck, Prod. et Prob. Pharm. 22, 867 (1967)
5. R. Muschaweck, Atti della Academia Med. Lombarda (Ed. Minerva Medica) 18, 1289 (1963)
6. R. Muschaweck, Atti del Symposium Internazionale sul Pottassio in Bologna ed in Medicina, Siena, May 22 - 23 (1965), p. 565, Istituto Sclavo-Sez., Ed. Siena
7. R. Muschaweck and P. Hajdù, Arzneim.-Forsch. (Drug Res.) 14, 44 (1964)
8. P. Deetjen, Am. N.Y. Acad. Sci. 139, 408 (1966)
9. K. Heintze et al., Naunyn-Schmiedeberg's Arch. Pharmacol. 318, 363 (1982)
10. R. Kinne and E. Kinne-Saffran, Mar. Ecol. Progr. Ser. 1, 129 (1979)
11. M.B. Burg, Kidney Intern. 22, 417 (1982)
12. H.R. Jacobson and J.P. Kokko, Kidney Intern. 22, 415 (1982)
13. F. Krück and A. Schrey, II. Diuretika Symposium, Paris 1981
14. G. Biamino et al., Int. J. Clin. Pharmacol. 12, 356 (1975)
15. W. Merkel, D. Bormann, D. Mania, R. Muschaweck, and M. Hropot, J. Med. Ch.-Chimica Therapeutica 11, 399 (1976)
16. R. Greger and E. Schlatter, Pflügers Arch. 396, 325 (1983)
17. R. Greger, E. Schlatter, and F. Lang, Pflügers Arch. 396, 308 (1983)
18. E. Schlatter, R. Greger, and C. Weidtke, Pflügers Arch. 396, 210 (1983)

RECENT EVENTS IN THE DEVELOPMENT OF NEWER DIURETICS

EDWARD J. CRAGOE, JR.
Merck Sharp and Dohme Research Laboratories, West Point, PA 19486

It is well-known that the discovery of diuretics was one of the most significant advances in modern medicine. These were not only among the first synthetic drugs to be used in medicine, but they are among the safest and most sophisticated therapeutic agents. Nevertheless, currently available diuretics have deficiencies which impart to them an obsolescence liability. Common side effects include elevated blood levels of uric acid, glucose and lipids and decreased blood levels of potassium and magnesium ions. Fundamental renal and ion transport research has permitted the generation of new concepts that have led to the design and synthesis of a cascade of new diuretics including those with unique structures and novel mechanisms and sites of action.

To chronicle the significant recent advances in the diuretic field will require describing those drugs that are in one of three stages of development: (1) those that have entered the market somewhere in the world, (2) those in some stage of clinical evaluation and (3) a select few that are still under preclinical study. The sources of information regarding many of the newest diuretics are limited and the reliability of

3-SULFAMOYLBENZOIC ACIDS AND ANALOGS

BUMETANIDE

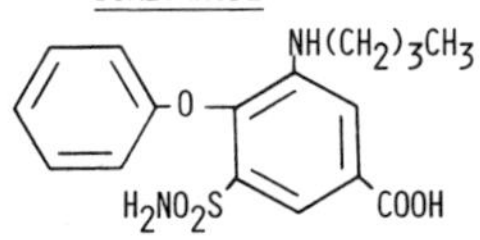

BESUNIDE

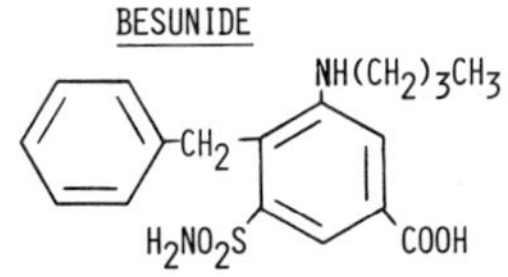

PIRETANIDE

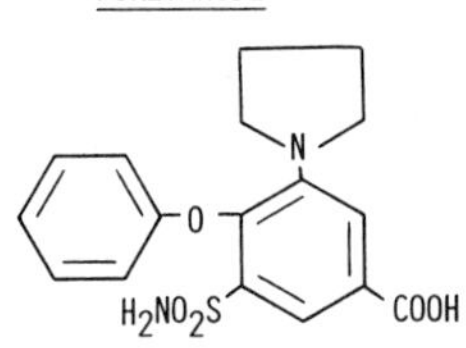

AZOSEMIDE

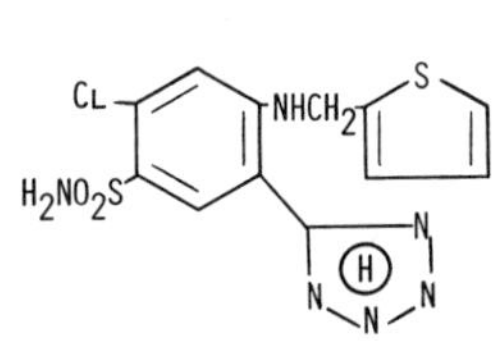

3-SULFAMOYL-4-CHLOROBENZOIC ACID HYDRAZIDES

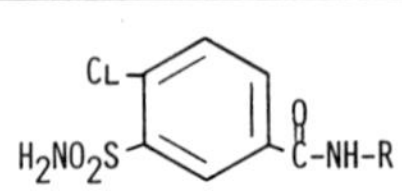

R= R=

CLOPAMIDE

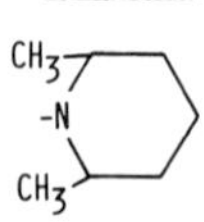

INDAPAMIDE

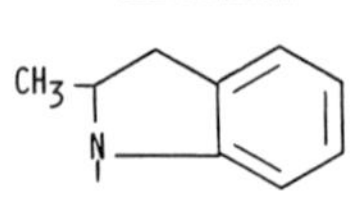

ISODAPAMIDE

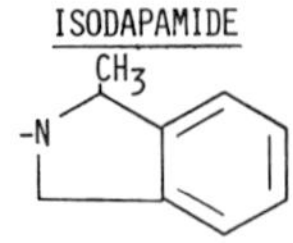

TRIPAMIDE

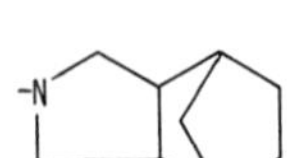

Diuretics, Jules B. Puschett, Editor

the information is not always optimal. Also, a drug under study may be abandoned for reasons which may not be disclosed, whether due to insufficient activity, toxicity, marketing strategies or other economic considerations.

The newer diuretics will be discussed in groups according to structural types since this is a fairly rigid criterion and other classification methods are more vague, tentative and sometimes uncertain. There are quite a number of significant new diuretics, so only a few details regarding each one can be considered. The first series consists of about a dozen sulfonamide diuretics. The initial group of four are 3-sulfamoylbenzoic acid analogs which are structurally and biologically related loop diuretics. These are bumetanide, besunide, piretanide and azosemide.

Bumetanide is biologically very similar to furosemide but it is about 20-fold more potent. It is clinically useful in congestive heart failure, chronic renal insufficiency and hypertension. The Na^+/K^+ excretion ratio is generally better than that seen with furosemide but greater hyperuricemia and phosphaturia are observed. Although besunide is at least five times as potent as bumetanide, making it one of the most potent loop diuretics, the lack of significant advantages make its future questionable.

Piretanide is about seven-fold more potent than furosemide and exhibits some proximal and distal tubular effects, in addition to its major site of action in the thick ascending limb of Henle's loop. Azosemide is structurally interesting in that it bears a 5-tetrazolyl moiety as a carboxy surrogate. It is equipotent to furosemide but its onset of action is somewhat slower. It exhibits some proximal tubular activity, as well as a major effect in Henle's loop. Patients on low sodium diets develop a striking hyperuricemia and metabolic acidosis when using this drug.

There are four 3-sulfamoylbenzoic acid hydrazides with very similar chemical structures and thiazide-like biological activity. These are clopamide, indapamide, isodapamide and tripamide. The first one, clopamide, is thiazide-like in both its diuretic effects and its side effects. It is clinically effective in doses of 20 to 100 mg. with a duration of

6-SULFAMOYLTETRAHYDROQUINAZOLIN-4-ONE DIURETICS

FENQUIZONE

(MAGGIONI)

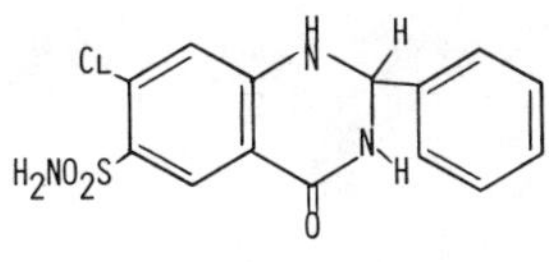

METOLAZONE

(PENWALT)

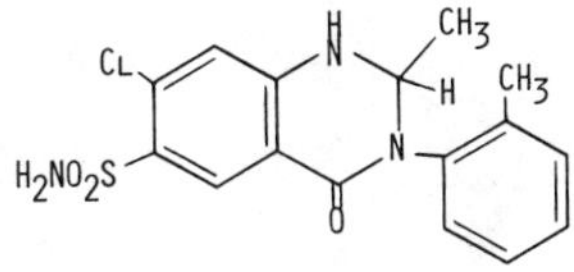

XIPAMIDE

(BEIRSDORF)

MJF10938, BEI1293, AQUAPHOR®, DIUREXAN®

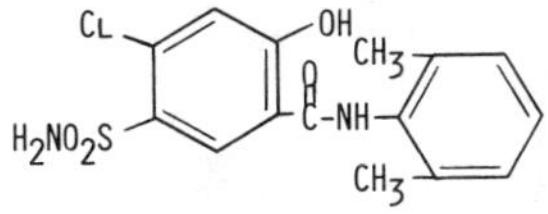

action of 16 to 24 hours. It is effective in the treatment of hypertension, edema due to congestive heart failure, cirrhosis and nephrotic syndrome.

Indapamide entered the U.S. market as LOZOL® in August of 1983. It's properties are much like that of clopamide but it is somewhat more potent and exhibits a longer duration of action. Recent data suggests the drug possesses direct renal vasodilator effects and calcium antagonistic-like activity. Isodapamide, now in the later stages of clinical trials, is a potent clopamide-like diuretic. Tripamide is another closely related diuretic agent which is reported to have a direct effect on smooth muscle similar to that of the calcium antagonists. This drug will be discussed in detail later in this symposium.

Fenquizone and metolazone are 6-sulfamoyltetrahydroquinazolin-4-ones with similar, thiazide-like properties. Fenquizone is effective in clinical doses of 10 to 20 mg. while metolazone is about five-fold more potent. Xipamide, although structurally a somewhat unique diuretic, is thiazide-like in diuretic profile with a potency five-times greater than hydrochlorothiazide. Diapamide, which has been known for some time, is reported to be currently under clinical trial. It is a loop diuretic with about 1/10 the potency of furosemide.

Tizolemide is a chemically and biologically unique sulfonamide diuretic. It's basic character makes it most unusual and, although it behaves biologically in most respects like a thiazide, its reported uricosuric activity gives it a noteworthy quality.

DIAPAMIDE

(WARNER-LAMBERT)

CL-456, CN-36337, D-1593, VECTRIN®

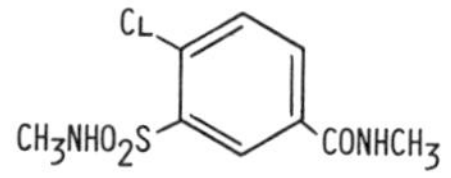

TIZOLEMIDE

(HOECHST)

HOE740, S-730, 704-B

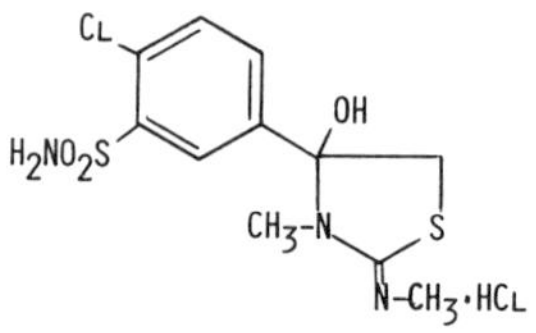

There are at least ten compounds that represent subclasses of the (acylaryloxy)acetic acid series of diuretics whose design emanated from a knowledge of the structure of ethacrynic acid. Significant contributions to the development of this class of diuretic agent came from five different laboratories. Although the development of furacrynic acid, tienilic acid, A-48722 and halocrinic acid have been discontinued, they played an important role in the evolution of this type of diuretic. The three compounds from this series that will be discussed - indacrinone, Abbott-53385 and Abbott-49816, are currently in various stages of clinical evaluation but they will be considered only briefly since each of them will be the subject of a paper in this symposium.

Indacrinone (MK-196) is a potent uricosuric, loop diuretic which, at a clinical dose of 10 mg., produces salidiuresis equivalent to 40 mg. of furosemide but elicits less kaliuresis and exhibits a longer duration of action. MK-196 is a racemate consisting of a 1:1 ratio of two enantiomers

THE (ARYLOXY)ACETIC ACID FAMILY

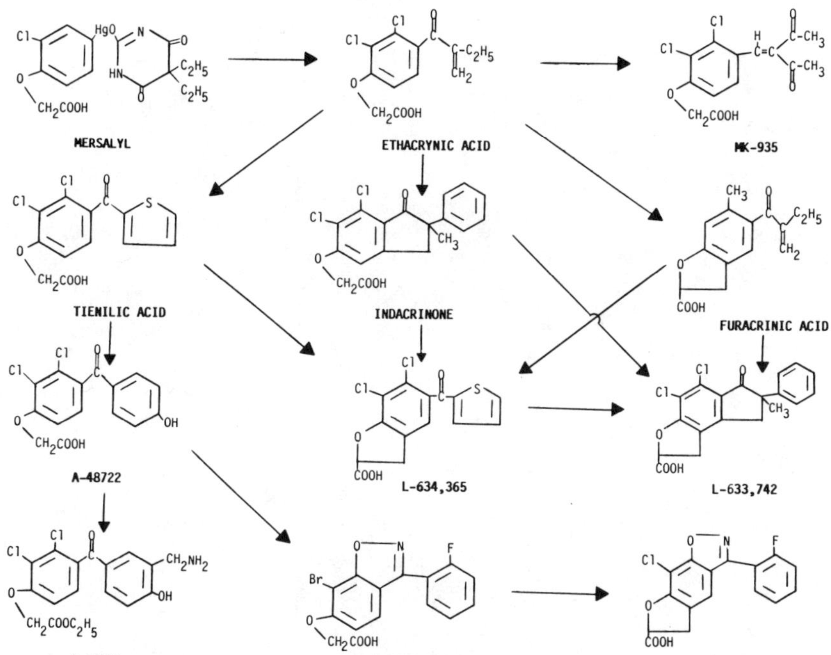

which have approximately equal uricosuric potency. However, the R(-)-enantiomer is a more potent salidiuretic and is metabolized faster than the S(+)-enantiomer. An enantiomeric ratio of 1:9 of R(-) to S(+) (MK-286) produces what is considered to be an optimal salidiuretic/uricosuric ratio.

Abbott-53385 is still in the early stages of study, but it appears to have biological properties similar to that of indacrinone. Both of its enantiomers are equally uricosuric but the S(+)-enantiomer possesses all of the salidiuretic activity exhibited by the racemate. Abbott-49816 bears structural similarities to both the (acylaryloxy)acetic acid and the salicylamine classes of diuretics. However, since it exhibits loop salidiuretic activity and uric acid retaining properties, it more closely resembles the salicylamines biologically.

Four salicylamines have entered the scene in recent years; these are MK-447, Ono-3122, HOE-365 and Abbott-49816. MK-447 is unique both structurally and by virtue of its basic character. It exhibits a triad of pharmacological properties - salidiuretic, antihypertensive and antiinflammatory activity. These effects appear to be associated, to some degree, with its effects on prostaglandin biosynthesis. Its salidiuretic effects in man were comparable to those seen with furosemide, both in regard to efficacy and potency, but its duration of action was longer. At diuretic doses, antihypertensive activity was observed in mild to moderately hypertensive patients.

Ono-3122, now under clinical investigation, appears to be much like

SALICYLAMINE DIURETICS

MK-447

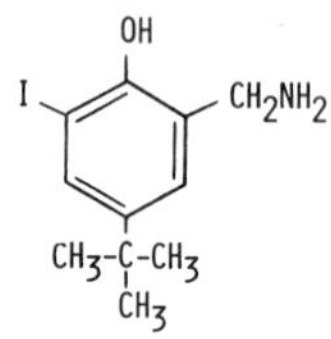

ONO-3122

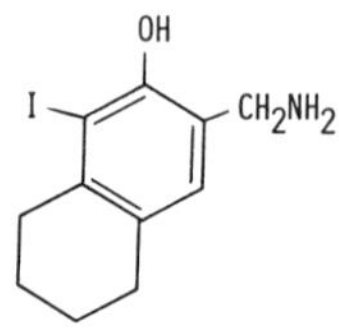

HOE-365

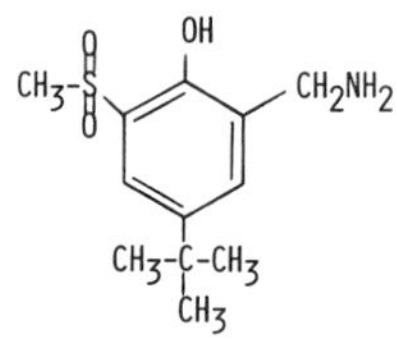

A-49816

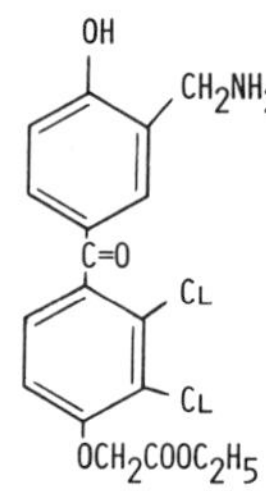

ETOZOLINE

(GÖDECKE, WARNER-LAMBERT)

W2900A, EKLAPIN®

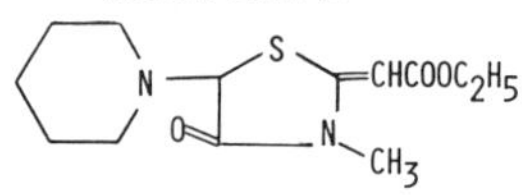

(+)-ENANTIOMER = DEXETOZOLINE

MK-447. It also seems to act as a tryptophane-like cofactor in PG-endoperoxide biosynthesis from arachidonate. A report on the status of the newest salicylamine diuretic, HOE-365, will be made later in this symposium. Abbott-49816 was discussed earlier in this lecture.

Etozoline is a structurally novel, low potency, loop diuretic requiring clinical doses of 400 to 1200 mg. It's therapeutic indications and side effects are similar to those of furosemide; however, it is said to be less kaliuretic. The R(-)-enantiomer possesses all of the salidiuretic activity exhibited by the racemate and has some antihypertensive activity. Surprisingly, the S(+)-enantiomer, dexetozoline, is devoid of diuretic activity but is considerably more antihypertensive than the R(-)-enantiomer. Etozoline is metabolized essentially to the corresponding carboxylic acid, ozolinone, which appears to be largely responsible for etozoline's biological effects.

Musolimine is a structurally novel loop diuretic presently under clinical investigation. It is similar in action to furosemide; however, it is slightly more potent and has a longer duration of action. Amazingly, there is no record of its optical resolution. Torasemide is an interesting, high ceiling diuretic. It is more potent than bumetanide in animals and shows salidiuretic activity in man in oral doses as low as 500 micrograms. Although this compound is a sulfonylurea, no report of any effect on glucose metabolism has been published.

MUSOLIMINE

(BAYER, SCHERING-PLOUGH)

BAY G2821, EDRUL®, NAUZOLIMINE®

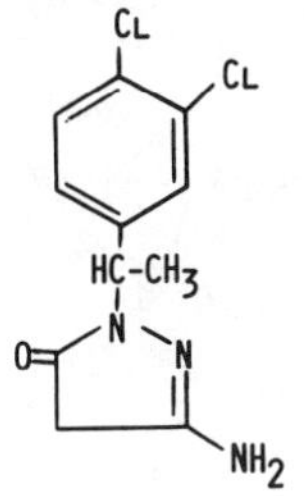

TORASEMIDE

(CHRISTIAENS)

JDL-464, AC4464

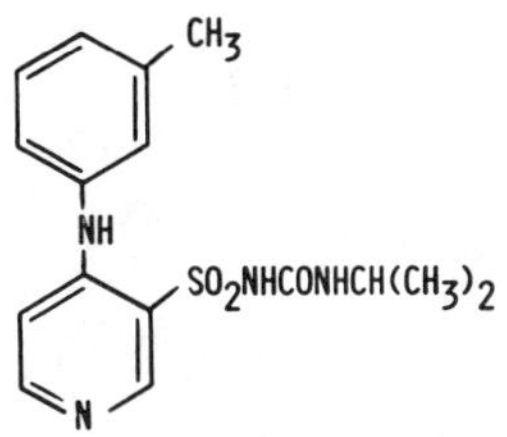

There are at least seven steroidal aldosterone antagonists that have reached the stage of clinical investigation. However, only potassium canrenoate has been marketed. This drug appears to be less potent than spironolactone but its biological properties appear to be quite similar.

Ibotamine is an orally active, dopamine-like prodrug of deoxyepinephrine which possesses diuretic and cardiostimulant activity. It exhibits a positive inotropic effect similar to, but of shorter duration than, digitalis. As a renal vasodilator, it may be useful in cardiac failure and impared renal function.

Fenoldopam is another orally active renal vasodilator now under clinical study. It is about three-fold more potent than dopamine with the S-enantiomer possessing all the activity exhibited by the racemate. Doses of 25, 50 and 100 mg. in man produced graded increases in urine flow rate, as well as electrolyte and uric acid excretion. Interestingly, ciproquazone and traxanox were initially developed for other therapeutic purposes but clinical reports indicate these drugs were found to be both salidiuretic and uricosuric.

Diuretics continue to be a major research objective. The significant break-throughs will be characterized by their novel structure and mecha-

POTASSIUM CANRENOATE

(SEARLE)

PHANURENE® (THERAPHIX), SOLUDACTONE®

SOLDACTONE®, VENACTONE®

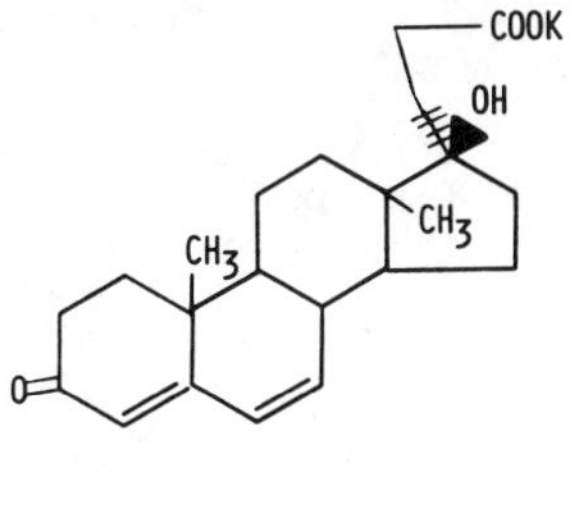

IBOTAMINE

(SIMES, SKF, YOSHITOMI)

SKF-100168, SB 7505, IBOPAMINA®

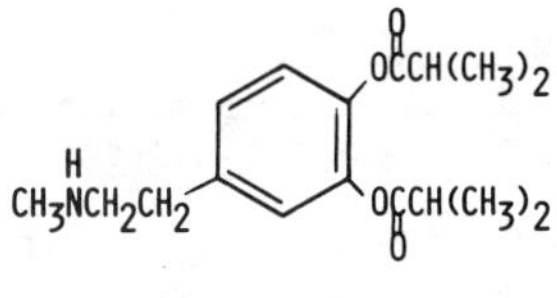

FENOLDOPAM

(SKF)

SKF-82526, SKF-82526-J

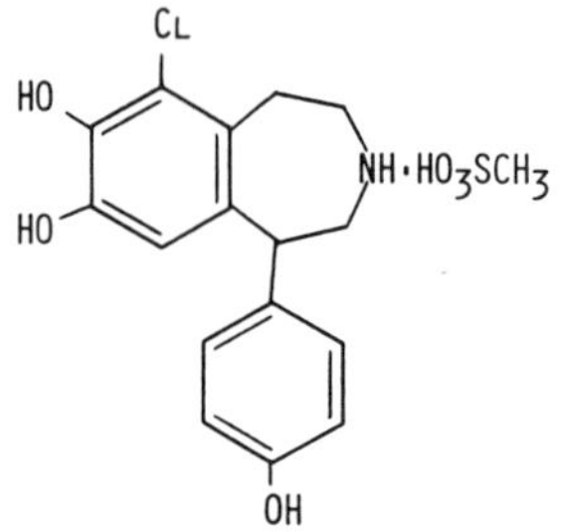

MEDICAL TARGETS FOR AGENTS THAT MODULATE ION TRANSPORT

1. BRAIN INJURY
   A. Traumatic Brain Injury
   B. Ischemic Stroke
   C. Cerebral Infection Edema
   D. Post-operative Brain Trauma
2. CYSTIC FIBROSIS
3. CANCER
   A. Antitumor
   B. Anti-leukemia
4. GUT
   A. Diarrhea
5. MUSCLE DYSTROPHY

nisms of action and fewer side effects. Efforts will be made to design polyvalent salidiuretics, i.e., those that possess adjunctive antihypertensive, β-adrenergic blocking or angiotensin converting enzyme blocking effects.

More importantly, there are a number of important diseases that involve aberrant water and electrolyte transport, many of which are in areas of medicine where no specific therapeutic agent exists. The concepts that have led to the design of the salidiuretic agents which function by modulation of electrolyte transport, can serve as a pattern for the design of new agents. These drugs will function similarly biochemically but with new organ and tissue targets. The investigation of compounds that regulate electrolyte transport should not only help define the biochemical lesion(s) that characterize these diseases but suggest new kinds of therapy.

Several examples of such disorders are worthy of mention. Various types of brain injury have been shown to involve a cascade of events which include a specific cellular edema. The edema is a target for drug intervention since it involves chloride transport in the astrocyte which suggests evaluating loop diuretics since they block chloride transport in the thick ascending limb of Henle's loop.

Cystic fibrosis is a disease characterized by abnormal electrolyte transport in various tissues, especially the respiratory system. Electrolyte transport modifying agents appear to normalize transmembrane potential and, at appropriate doses, normalize some aspects of the disease process in patients with cystic fibrosis.

An approach to cancer chemotherapy involves a theory that high intracellular sodium ion concentrations and the resulting depolarized transmembrane potential characterize the rapidly proliferating cells of many tumors. Agents that selectively inhibit elevated sodium ion concentration have been shown to suppress the growth of several transplanted tumors in animals. Also, ion flux changes induced by certain diuretics have been reported to promote differentiation in certain transformed cells, including those from erythroleukemic cell lines.

Electrolyte transport has been shown to play an important role in problems involving the gut, e.g., diarrhea, which can be normalized by diuretics and even their non-diuretic analogs. Basic studies on various blood cells have demonstrated the importance of ion transport, particularly of H^+ which regulates intracellular pH and, thus, controls enzyme activation. Muscular dystrophy is a disease involving increased cellular permeability to chloride, rendering a key chloride requiring enzyme, dipeptidylaminopepidase-I, inexcitable. Intervention with chloride transport blockers is suggested as an approach both to the understanding and the therapy of this disorder.

A major challenge is presented to the medicinal chemist as to how to modify a diuretic molecule to make it more specific to a particular tissue or transport system. An example of each type can be cited. MK-473 is a loop diuretic which by either of two structural maneuvers looses its renal effects and enhances its *in vitro* brain slice, chloride-transport inhibitory activity. Homologation of either the 2-methyl to 2-butyl or the side chain from 1 to 3 methylene units (to give DCPIB) achieves this objective. That this effect appears to carry over to an *in vivo* system is seen in a study in brain injured cats. Although not statistically significant, a 1 mg/kg intravenous dose of DCPIB reduces the mortality over controls by 26% as compared to 15% for ethacrynic acid.

Another example where structural modification of a diuretic changes the relative effects on the various systems involving Na^+ transport concerns analogs of amiloride. In most cell systems, certain substituents,

IN VITRO INHIBITION OF BRAIN SLICE SWELLING

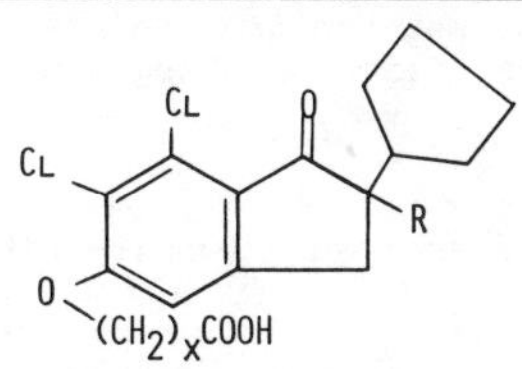

X	R	ENANTIOMER	SALIDIURESIS (DOG)	IN VITRO BRAIN INHIB. I_{50}(M)
1	$-CH_3$	± (MK-473)	+2	2×10^{-7}
1	$-(CH_2)_3CH_3$	±	0	3×10^{-9}
		+	0	3×10^{-10}
		-	0	5×10^{-5}
3	$-CH_3$	± (DCPIB)	±	2×10^{-8}
		+		10^{-8}
		-		2.5×10^{-7}
Ethacrynic Acid				5×10^{-7}

IN VIVO BRAIN INJURY ASSAY IN CATS

COMPOUND	MG/KG. DOSE	MORTALITY (%) CONTROL	TREAT	Δ
Ethacrynic Acid	1	51	36	15
DCPIB	1	51	25	26

NA^{+} TRANSPORT SYSTEMS

	STRUCTURAL FEATURES	
	R	5-R^{1}R^{2}N-
NA^{+}-CHANNEL BLOCKERS	X	
NA^{+}/CA^{++} EXCHANGER BLOCKERS	X	X
NA^{+}/H^{+} ANTIPORTER BLOCKERS		X

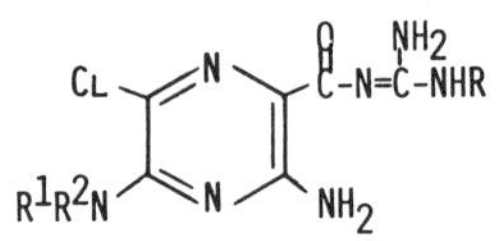

e.g., benzyl, on the terminal guanidino nitrogen atom (R) enhances its Na^{+}-channel blocking activity while decreasing or eliminating its effect on the Na^{+}/H^{+} antiporter. On the other hand, certain substituents, e.g., ethyl and isopropyl on the 5-amino nitrogen (R^1 and R^2), generally have an effect opposite to that just described. Substitutions of either type, especially those on the terminal guanidino nitrogen atom, generally enhance the Na^{+}/Ca^{++} exchanger blocking effects.

It does not require unusual vision to see that basic research involving electrolyte transport and the agents that modulate it have provided the foundation for ideas that can provide not only a cornucopia of novel diuretics but new classes of ion-blocking drugs in days to come.

REFERENCES

This review includes such an extensive bibliography that only a few key references are listed:

1. E. J. Cragoe, Jr., ed., Diuretics, Chemistry, Pharmacology and Medicine, (John Wiley and Sons, New York, 1983).
2. E. J. Cragoe, Jr., N. P. Gould, O. W. Woltersdorf, Jr., C. Ziegler, R. S. Bourke, L. R. Nelson, H. K. Kimelberg, J. B. Waldman, A. J. Popp and N. Sedranski, J. Med. Chem., 25, 567 (1982).
3. M. Knowles, J. Gatzy and R. Boucher, N. Engl. J. Med., 305, 1489 (1981).
4. R. L. Sparks, T. B. Pool, N. K. R. Smith and I. C. Cameron, in: Genetic Expression in the Cell, G. M. Padilla and K. S. McCarty, Sr., eds., (Academic Press, Inc., New York, 1982).
5. J. Carlson, F. Dorey, E. J. Cragoe, Jr. and H. P. Koeffler, J. Nat. Cancer Inst., in press (1984).
6. K. Bukhave and J. Rask-Madsen, Scand. J. Gastro., 16, 1100 (1981).
7. B. B. Gelman, M. H. Davis, R. E. Morris and E. Greunstein, J. Cell Biol., 88, 329 (1981).
8. M. S. Jurkowitz, R. A. Altschuld, G. P. Brierley and E. J. Cragoe, Jr., FEBS, 162(2), 202 (1983).
9. P. Vigne, C. Frelin, E. J. Cragoe, Jr. and M. Lazdunski, Biochem. Biophys. Res. Comm. 116(1), 86 (1983).
10. J. K. Dethmers, E. J. Cragoe, Jr. and G. J. Kaczorowski, Fed. Proc. Abstr., 42, 2245 (1983).
11. G. J. Kaczorowski, E. J. Cragoe, Jr. and J. M. Dethmers, Fed. Proc. Abstr., 42, 2245 (1983).

DISCOVERY AND DEVELOPMENT OF THE (AMINOMETHYLARYLOXY)ACETIC ACID DIURETICS.

J. J. PLATTNER,* C. M. LEE,* B. W. HORROM,* A. K. L. FUNG,* P. R. BUNNELL,* B. A. BOPP,* M. J. FIELD** AND G. H. GIEBISCH**
*Abbott Laboratories, North Chicago, IL 60064; **Department of Physiology, Yale University School of Medicine, New Haven, CT 06510

Since the discovery of ethacrynic acid more than 20 years ago, many (aryloxy)acetic acid derivatives have been synthesized and evaluated for their diuretic properties. The high level of interest in this class of compounds has been stimulated by the ability of medicinal chemists to dramatically alter the diuretic profile of these agents by structural manipulation of the phenoxyacetic acid pharmacophore. Thus, the uric acid retention caused by ethacrynic acid **I** is sharply contrasted to the uricosuric nature of indacrinone **II** [1] and the dihydrobenzofuran derivative **III** [2]. Still further differences in profile are found with tienilic acid **IV**, which elicits a low ceiling uricosuric effect [3] and, more recently **V** (HP-522), which has been described [4] as a high ceiling moderate uricosuric. In our own laboratories we have discovered yet a new addition to the class of (aryloxy)acetic acid diuretics which differs from all previous derivatives in that a basic nitrogen functionality is essential to their high ceiling profile. These latter compounds are represented generically by structure **VI.**

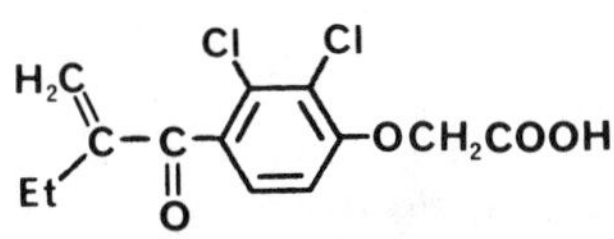

I

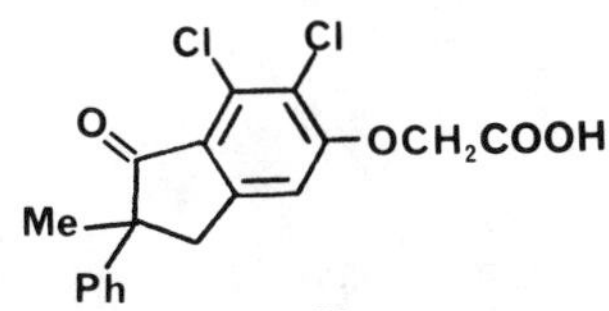

II

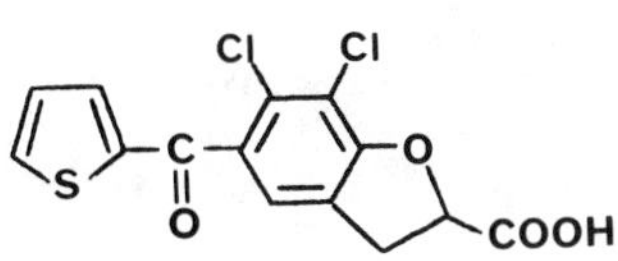

III

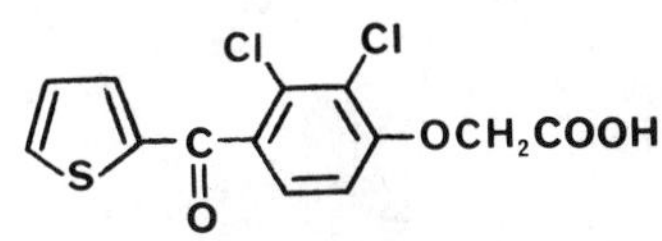

IV

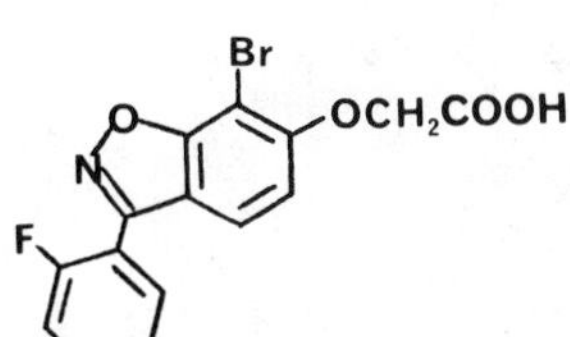

V

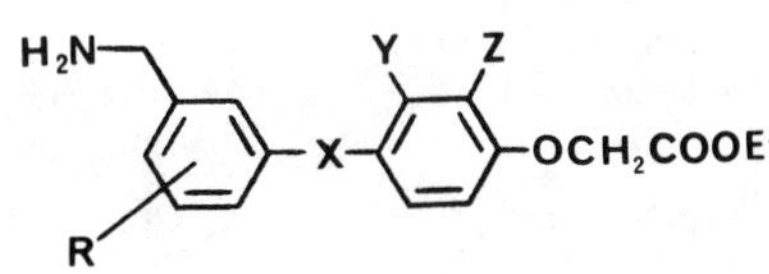

VI

Our involvement with the chemistry of (aryloxy)acetic acids began in the mid-1970's when we found 2,3-dichloro-4-(p-hydroxybenzoyl)phenoxyacetic acid **VII** to be a low ceiling, uricosuric diuretic [5]. Systematic structure-activity studies around this compound led to the synthesis of the corresponding bis-Mannich base adduct **VIII.** Although this analog proved to be devoid of oral diuretic activity, the corresponding ethyl ester **IX** caused a profound salidiuresis in rats and dogs, which was comparable to that of furosemide. This unexpected change in profile upon introduction of the N,N-dimethylaminomethyl and ethyl ester substituents stimulated an intensive program to evaluate this new diuretic series. From this effort we have identified A-49816 as the prototype structure possessing the essential

Diuretics, Jules B. Puschett, Editor

features of the (aminomethylaryloxy)acetic acids. Herein we describe the SAR's and pharmacologic properties for these high ceiling diuretics.

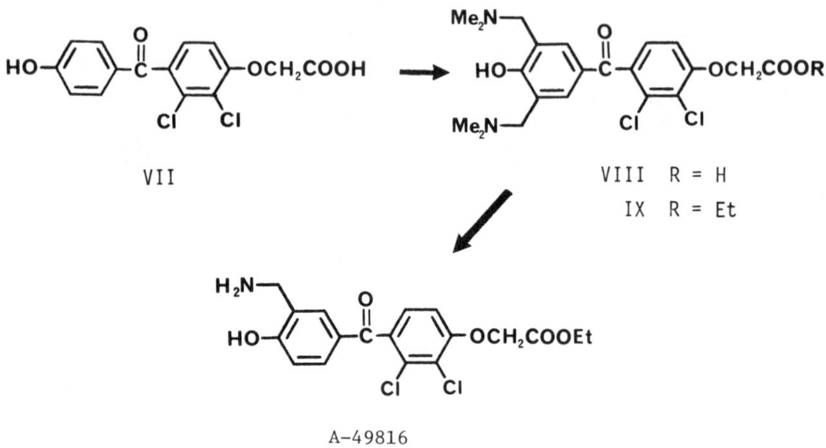

SALIDIURETIC ACTIVITY ASSAYS

Diuretic screening of the compounds described in this study was conducted in normotensive, female rats [6]. Dose-response experiments measuring the urine volume, Na^+, K^+, and Cl^- concentrations were used to establish the salidiuretic excretion profile of the target compounds. In order to compare the relative potencies of these derivatives, we have established the use of ED_2 values as presented in the Tables I-IV. An ED_2 is defined as the oral dose (mg/kg) required to produce an excretion of 2 milliequivalents (mEq) of Na^+ per kilogram of body weight during the 4 hr collection period. These values were obtained by plotting the linear regression of the response curve of Na^+ excretion versus the log of the dose. The specific value of 2 mEq/kg for the Na^+ excretion was chosen since this amount corresponds to doses that cause a statistically significant natriuresis relative to the control level for both low and high ceiling diuretic classes. Although only the Na^+ excretion was used to determine the ED_2 values, the urine volume and Cl^- excretion generally paralleled that of the Na^+, and thus either of these parameters could also be used for relative potency comparisons.

STRUCTURE-ACTIVITY RELATIONSHIPS

Structurally, A-49816 and its congeners incorporate the essential, pharmacophoric elements of two separate diuretic classes, the dichlorophenoxyacetic acids [7] and the 2-aminomethylphenols [8]. It is not readily apparent, however, that molecular hybridization of the dichlorophenoxyacetic acid structure with that of a salicylamine nucleus should lead to a new high ceiling diuretic series. Since compounds derived from each of these respective diuretic classes are themselves capable of producing potent salidiuresis (e.g., ethacrynic acid and MK-447), the high ceiling profile observed for A-49816 and its analogs can be rationalized in terms of a contributing effect from each pharmacophoric component. We sought to evaluate this concept during our SAR studies and chose to approach the task in the following manner. The prototype structure A-49816 was divided into four discrete portions as indicated below. Each portion was then separately modified while keeping the remainder of the molecule constant in order to ascertain the relative contribution of each of these four structural components to the observed biological effect.

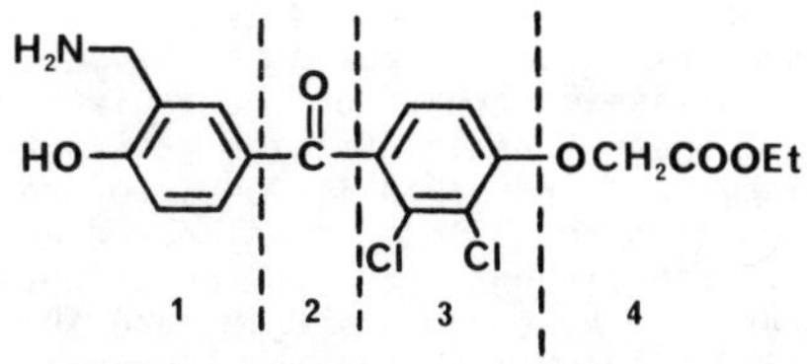

The initial phase of the SAR investigation was directed towards the aminomethylphenol portion of the A-49816 structure, and the results of this study are tabulated for a representative series of compounds in Table I.

TABLE I. Effect of Substituents on the Phenyl Group.

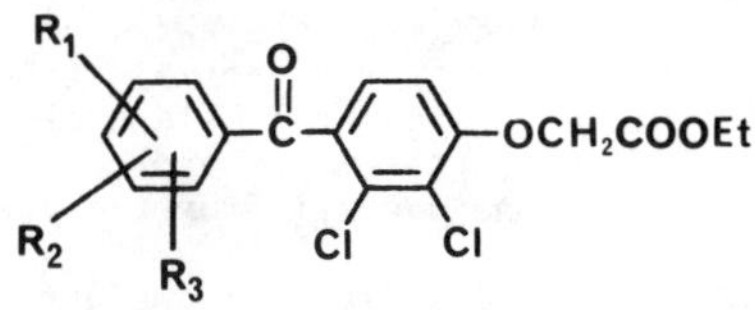

Compound	R_1	R_2	R_3	Rat ED_2 (mg/kg)
1	3-$CH_2N(Me)_2$	4-OH	5-$CH_2N(Me)_2$	7
2	3-$CH_2N(Me)_2$	4-OH	H	16
3	3-CH_2NH_2	4-OH	5-CH_2NH_2	11
4[a]	3-CH_2NH_2	4-OH	H	3
5	3-CH_2NH_2	2-OH	H	Inactive
6	5-CH_2NH_2	2-OH	H	3
7	4-CH_2NH_2	3-OH	H	Inactive
8	3-CH_2NH_2	4-OH	5-CH_3	1
9	3-CH_2NH_2	4-OH	5-Cl	1
10	3-CH_2NH_2	4-OH	5-I	1
11	3-CH_2NH_2	H	H	12
12	3-CH_2NH_2	4-Cl	H	50
13	3-CH_2NH_2	4-OCH_3	H	Inactive
14	3-$CH(CH_3)NH_2$	4-OH	H	1.2
15	3-$CH_2CH_2NH_2$	4-OH	H	Inactive
16	3-CH_2NHAc	4-OH	H	Inactive
17	3-CH_2OH	4-OH	H	Inactive
18	3-CO_2H	4-OH	H	Inactive
19	3-$CONH_2$	4-OH	H	Inactive

[a] Compound **4** = A-49816

As seen from the data, the mono-Mannich adduct **2** displayed significant saluretic activity, but was somewhat less potent than bis-adduct **1**. This pattern was reversed, however, with the primary aminomethyl congeners as seen by the enhanced potency of compound **4** over that of **3**. The relative position of the aminomethyl group compared to that of the hydroxyl group in the benzoyl ring nucleus is important for the activity. In the 2-hydroxy derivatives, the 5-aminomethyl analog **6** is as active as **4**. Transposition of the hydroxyl and aminomethyl groups in **4**, i.e., to provide the isomeric derivative **7**, resulted in a total loss of saluretic activity. Introduction of a halogen or methyl substituent ortho to the phenol in **4** led to a slight increase in potency as seen by compounds **8**, **9**, and **10**. Replacement of the phenolic hydroxyl group by either a hydrogen (Compound **11**) or a chlorine atom (Compound **12**) decreases saluretic effects while methylation of the hydroxyl group (Compound **13**) completely eliminates activity. Alteration of the aminomethyl group, e.g., by α-substitution (Compound **14**) preserves potent diuretic activity whereas homologation (Compound **15**), acylation (Compound **16**), and replacement of the amine with non-basic functions (Compounds **17-19**) results in a total loss of activity. The structure-activity patterns described above for the salicylamine ring of A-49816 serve to distinguish this class of compounds from the 2-aminomethylphenols, which require a phenolic hydroxyl function as an essential structural feature. The less demanding requirements of the salicylamine nucleus of A-49816 may reflect incorporation of the dichlorophenoxyacetate component into the structure which serves to augment the overall diuretic potency.

The effect of varying the group linking the two aromatic rings was explored next, and the results are presented in Table II.

TABLE II. Effect of Varying the Group Linking the two Aromatic Rings

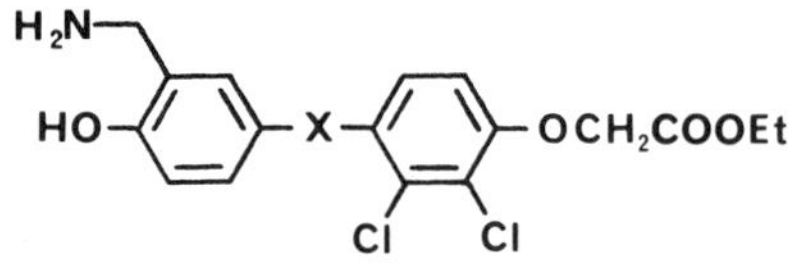

Compound	X	Rat ED_2 (mg/kg)
4	CO	3
20	CH_2	16
21	O	1
22	S	3
23	SO	23
24	SO_2	Inactive
25	COCO	Inactive
26	OCH_2	Inactive
27	NHCO	Inactive
28	bond	Inactive
29	$COCH_2CH_2$	100
30	$COCH{=}CH_2$	140
31	$H_2C{=}CHCO$	Inactive

As can be seen from the data, the keto group can be effectively replaced with an ether or thioether function with a slight increase in potency, whereas the methylene and sulfoxide linking groups lead to diminished saluretic activity. Replacement with either a sulfone, diketone, methyleneoxy, amide function or direct bond, however, results in a loss of activity. Increasing the distance between the two aryl rings leads to either greatly diminished activity (Compounds **29** and **30**) or no activity (Compound **31**). An attempt was made to correlate these pharmacological results with the pK_a's for the various phenols in this series, but no useful correlation could be obtained. The variation in saluretic activity seen within this series of compounds may be a reflection of the relative spatial orientation of the two aryl rings, which then affects the distance between the aminomethyl and oxyacetate side chain substituents.

A consideration of the role of nuclear substitution on the phenoxyacetate ring is presented in Table III. As the data indicate, the 2,3-dichloro, 2,3-dimethyl, and both monochloro analogs show appreciable diuretic activity, whereas the 3,5-dichloro, benzo, and unsubstituted congener exhibit somewhat reduced activity. In general, substituent variations at this part of the structure did not cause a dramatic change in saluretic activity.

TABLE III. Effect of Varying Substituents on the Aromatic Ring Bearing the Oxyacetic Side Chain.

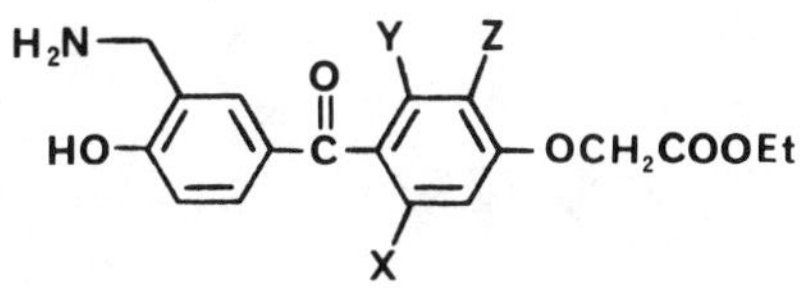

Compound	X	Y	Z	Rat ED_2 (mg/kg)
4	H	Cl	Cl	3
32	H	Me	Me	6
33	Cl	Cl	H	18
34	H	H	H	10
35	H	Cl	H	5
36	H	H	Cl	5
37	H	BENZO		11

To complete the SAR studies, the effects of varying the oxyacetic side chain were determined; these results are summarized in Table IV. Alteration of the ester group to a carboxylic acid totally abolished oral diuretic activity. The result most likely reflects the poor absorption of the carboxylic acid since both analogs displayed about equal activity when administered intravenously. Conversion of the ester function to a carboxamide (Compound **38**) caused a moderate decrease in activity whereas the corresponding nitrile analog (Compound **40**) was devoid of saluretic activity. Reduction of the ester group in the side chain to the corresponding alcohol (Compound **43**) bestowed a slight increase in diuretic activity. Conversion to the amine **44**, on the other hand, led to a moderate decrease in activity.

TABLE IV. Effect of Varying the Oxyacetic Side Chain.

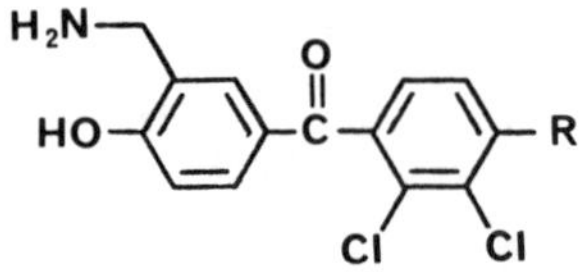

Compound	R	Rat ED_2 (mg/kg)
4	OCH_2COOEt	3
38	OCH_2CONH_2	19
39	OCH_2COOH	Inactive
40	OCH_2CN	Inactive
41	OCH(Me)COOEt	30
42	$OC(Me)_2COOEt$	Inactive
43	OCH_2CH_2OH	1.5
44	$OCH_2CH_2NH_2$	18
45	OMe	Inactive
46	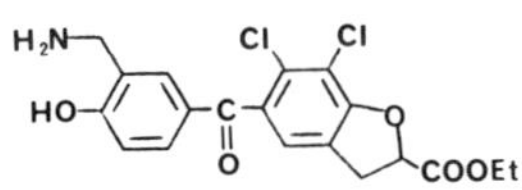	0.12

The effect of introducing alkyl substituents on the oxyacetate side chain is seen with compounds **41, 42** and **46** (Table IV). Successive incorporation of methyl groups leads first to a reduction and then to a total elimination of saluretic activity. However, introduction of the alkyl substituent by ring annelation (Compound **46**) resulted in a significant increase in natriuretic potency. These results parallel previous findings reported for the 2,3-dihydro-5-acyl-2-benzofurancarboxylic acids [9] and the indeno-[5,4-b]furan-2-carboxylic acids [10], where ring annelation to a dihydrobenzofuran also caused a substantial increase in saluretic potency. This large increase in potency upon ring annelation of the phenoxyacetic acids to the corresponding dihydrobenzofuran carboxylic acids most likely results from a highly favorable positioning of the side chain carboxylic ester function.

PHARMACOLOGY AND METABOLISM OF A-49816

The diuretic and saluretic activities of A-49816 were compared to that of furosemide in rats, dogs and cynomolgus monkeys. The onset of activity for A-49816 and furosemide was less than 1 hr in all species tested, and the duration of action for both compounds was approximately 4 hr in rats, 6 hr or more in dogs and 4 hr in monkeys. Two hr after oral administration of comparable natriuretic doses, A-49816 was approximately 4 times more potent than furosemide in NaCl/KCl-loaded female rats and 4-5 times more potent than furosemide in conscious female dogs and water-loaded male and female cynomolgus monkeys. At doses of A-49816 and furosemide that produced equal natriuretic responses, both compounds had similar effects on the excretion of K^+ and Cl^- ions. A comparison of the salidiuretic activities of A-49816 and reference diuretics in female dogs is presented in Figure 1.

Orally administered A-49816 was rapidly, but not extensively (24-74%), absorbed from the gastrointestinal tract of several animal species. The parent drug, an ethyl ester, was quickly hydrolyzed to the carboxylic acid in blood or plasma, and the acid was the predominant circulating compound. After a single oral dose of A-49816, the terminal half-life of the acid was about 2 hr in both rats and dogs, but it was increased to 5 hr in dogs given 7 daily oral doses of the drug. The plasma protein binding of the acid averaged 80% in man, 96% in the rat and 70% in the dog. Tissue distribution studies conducted in rats given A-49816-^{14}C, orally, indicated that the kidneys contained the highest levels of radioactivity. After oral administration of A-49816-^{14}C, about 20-40% of the ^{14}C-dose was excreted in the urine of rats, dogs, mice and monkeys; the rest of the dose was eliminated in the feces. After intravenous administration, approximately 60-70% was excreted in the urine while 25-35% was eliminated in the feces, thus indicating the importance of biliary excretion in the disposition of the compound. The carboxylic acid was the major metabolite in both urine and feces.

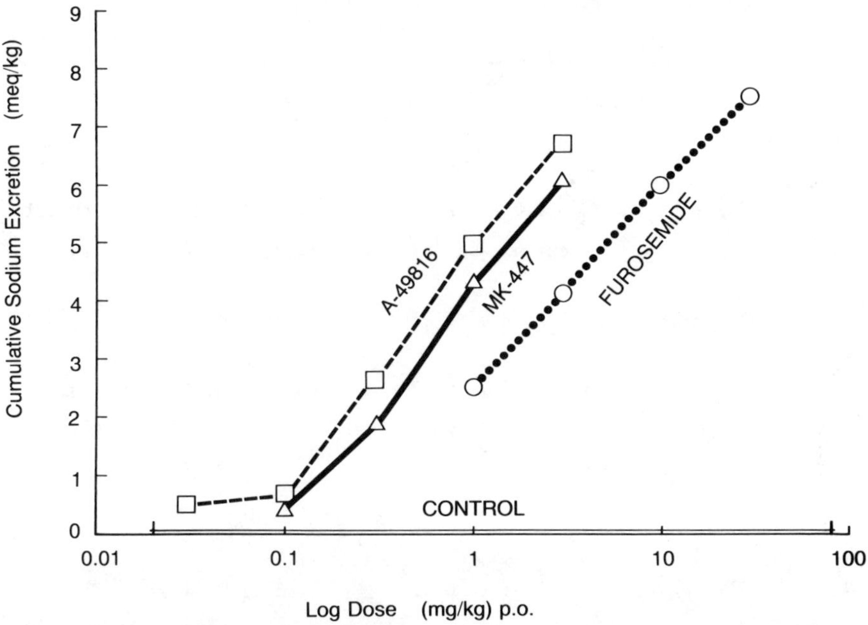

FIG. 1. Sodium excretion during 6 hr period after oral administration of A-49816 and reference diuretics to conscious female dogs. Each point is the mean of 6 dogs/dose.

CLEARANCE AND MICROPUNCTURE STUDIES

Structure-activity studies described earlier in this report identified compound **46** (Table IV) as the most potent derivative from the class of (aminomethylaryloxy)acetic acids. In order to further characterize the pharmacologic properties of this new diuretic series, **46** (A-52773) was selected for clearance and micropuncture studies. Male adult Sprague-Dawley rats were used in all experiments and were prepared for standard free-flow micropuncture as previously described [11]. Clearance studies involved the collection of two 30-minute urine samples ("control" period), together with blood samples at the midpoint of each. A-52773 was then injected as a single i.v. bolus of 0.1 mg/kg, given over 20-30 sec. Thirty minutes later, two more 30-minute clearance periods were observed during which time supplementary i.v. fluid was administered to replace that lost by the diuretic. From the measurement of urine volumes, Na^+ and K^+ concentrations, and radioactive inulin counts in plasma and urine samples, GFR as well as absolute and fractional electrolyte excretion before and after diuretic treatment could be calculated, using standard formulae. Free-flow distal tubular micropuncture studies were conducted on the exposed kidney during the same "control" and "diuretic" periods described above. Selected results from these experiments are summarized in Table V. The data indicate the powerful diuretic action of A-52773, manifesting itself as an increase in urine flow rate, a fall in U/P inulin and a striking increase in fractional Na^+ and K^+ excretion. A "loop" effect is apparent by significantly augmented fractional delivery rates of both Na^+ and K^+ into the early distal tubule.

TABLE V. Summary of Clearance and Micropuncture Data for A-52773.

	Control	Diuretic	P
Clearance			
Urine Flow Rate (μl/min/kidney)	6.01 ± 2.45	67.57 ± 7.91	<0.001
U/P Inulin	407.84 ± 84.97	19.73 ± 2.75	<0.01
GFR (ml/min/100 g rat)	0.56 ± 0.04	0.46 ± 0.03	<0.05
FE_{Na} (%)	0.44 ± 0.23	6.30 ± 0.83	<0.001
FE_K (%)	23.33 ± 3.21	54.61 ± 3.80	<0.01
Micropuncture			
FD_{Na} (%, Early Distal)	5.61 ± 0.52	13.64 ± 0.74	<0.001
FD_K (%, Early Distal)	10.82 ± 1.65	22.96 ± 2.16	<0.01

HUMAN PHARMACOLOGY

The safety and the salidiuretic efficacy of A-49816 were evaluated in a placebo-controlled, single-blind study involving 18 normal male volunteers [12]. In this study single, oral doses of A-49816 or placebo were administered to the subjects, and urine was collected during specific intervals following drug administration. Urine volume and urinary excretion of sodium, chloride and potassium increased following the 5, 10 and 20 mg doses of A-49816. The data shown in Table VI indicate that A-49816 possesses diuretic and saluretic activity in man. An additional study comparing the effects of A-49816 and furosemide in normal volunteers will be reported elsewhere.

TABLE VI. Diuretic Response in Humans to A-49816.

	N	Mean cumulative response after 12 hr Diuresis (ml)	Natriuresis (meq)	Kaliuresis (meq)
Placebo	6	1165	101	38.2
A-49816				
5 mg	4	1188	139	51.0
10 mg	4	1244	155	50.2
20 mg	4	3208	272	60.3

REFERENCES

1. B.A. Brooks, E. M. Blair, R. Finch, and A.F. Lant, Br. J. Clin. Pharmac., 10, 249 (1980).
2. G. M. Fanelli, Jr., L.S. Watson, D.L. Bohn and H.F. Russo, J. Pharmacol. Exp. Ther., 212, 190 (1980).
3. E.D. Frohlich, New England J. Med., 301, 1378 (1979).
4. J.M. Kitzen, M.A. Schwenkler, P.R. Bixby, S.J. Wilson, G. Shutske, L. Setescak, R.C. Allen and I. Rosenblum, Life Sci., 27, 2547 (1980).
5. P.H. Jones, D.S. Bariana, A.K.L. Fung, Y.C. Martin, J. Kyncl, and A. Lall, U.S. Patent 4,058,559 (1979).
6. J.J. Plattner, A.K.L. Fung, J.A. Parks, R.J. Pariza, S.R. Crowley, A.G. Pernet, P.R. Bunnell, and P.W. Dodge, J. Med. Chem., in press.
7. E.J. Cragoe, Jr. in: Diuretics. Chemistry, Pharmacology and Medicine, E.J. Cragoe, Jr., Ed. (Wiley-Interscience, New York, 1983) Chapter 4.
8. R.L. Smith in: Diuretics. Chemistry, Pharmacology and Medicine, E.J. Cragoe, Jr., Ed. (Wiley-Interscience, New York, 1983) Chapter 5.
9. W.F. Hoffman, O.W. Woltersdorf, Jr., F.C. Novello, E.J. Cragoe, Jr., J.P. Springer, L.S. Watson, and G.M. Fanelli, Jr., J. Med. Chem., 24, 865 (1981).
10. O.W. Woltersdorf, Jr., S.J. deSolms and E.J. Cragoe, Jr., J. Med. Chem., 24, 874 (1981).
11. E.E. Windhager and G. Giebisch, Am. J. Physiol., 200, 581 (1961).
12. Personal communication from Drs. K.G. Tolman and D.E. Rolling, Drug Research Center, University of Utah.

Chemistry of HOE 365

H. C. Englert, H.J. Lang, D. Mania,
Hoechst AG, Postfach 80 03 20
6230 Frankfurt 80, West-Germany

INTRODUCTION

To a large extent, diuretic research at the Hoechst company has been closely connected with the investigation of sulfamoylbenzoic acids. Two important contributions in the field of high ceiling diuretics emerged from those studies. In 1959 furosemide was synthezised, soon becoming the standard drug in the treatment of edemas and cardiac diseases. 16 years later Piretanide followed. Both agents have proven their utility in clinical practice and are said to be safe, non toxic drugs which are well tolerated. It is part of our philosophy to think that mainly the sulfonamide moiety contributes to these properties.

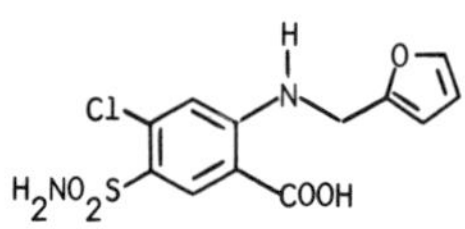

1

furosemide

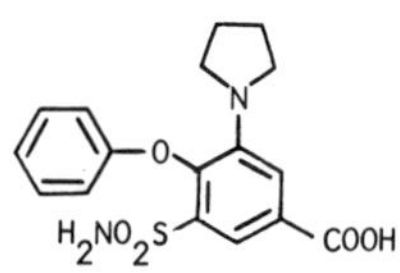

2

piretanide

Apart from the known sulfamoylbenzoic acid pattern, diuretics with unusual structural features have always attracted our attention. Already in 1971 a synthetic program in the field of benzylamine diuretics was started at Hoechst. These studies had been influenced by the discovery of diuretic Mannichbases (compound 3) derived from isoeugenol [1]. However the

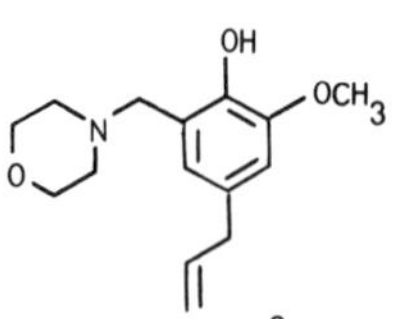

3

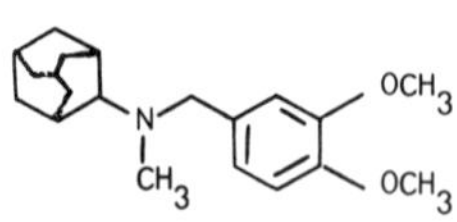

4

Diuretics, Jules B. Puschett, Editor

compound (4) chosen for further investigations at that time could not compete with furosemide with regard to toxicity datas, despite an excellent diuretic profile.

On the other hand, more recent developements like Merck Sharp and Dohme's antihypertensive diuretic MK 447 (compound 5) or Ono's antiinflammatory Ono-3144 (compound 6) have proven that benzylamines are indeed a valuable source of diuretics with novel pharmacological profiles. Influence on ion-transport systems outside the kidney may account for some of the additional activities not observed among sulfonamide diuretics up to now.

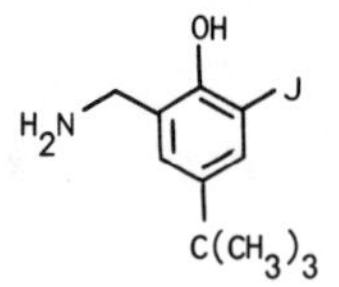

5

MK 447

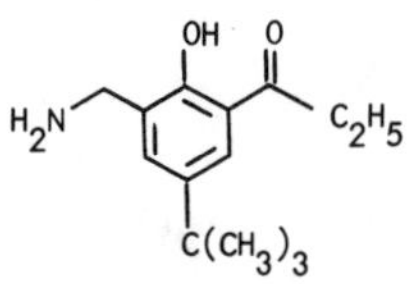

6

Ono 3144

The present report will show that the sulfonamide group and related moieties with all their beneficial influence on toxicity properties may be successfully included in the design of new benzylamine diuretics with improved antihypertensive activities. This approach makes use of the o-hydroxybenzylamine framework and combines it with various oxidized sulfur substituents.

STRUCTURE ACTIVITY RELATIONSHIPS

Structure activity relationships of MK 447 revealed that many substituents in the 6-position account for diuretic activity. Among them, halogen derivatives proved to be the most potent agents. MK 447's unusual antihypertensive activities however were shown to be closely associated with the iodine substituent[2].

One important synthetic objective of our research program was the replacement of this iodine by a sulfonamide moiety. It led to a potent high ceiling diuretic (compound 7) in rats and dogs comparable with piretanide. Dose response curves that were routinely established in rats up to doses of 1g/kg revealed, contrary to MK 447, no acute toxic side effects. But this favourable profile was not associated with MK 447's pronounced antihypertensive activities. At the strongly saluretic dose of 16 mg/kg no influence on the blood pressure of spontaneous hypertensive rats (SHR) could be demonstrated.

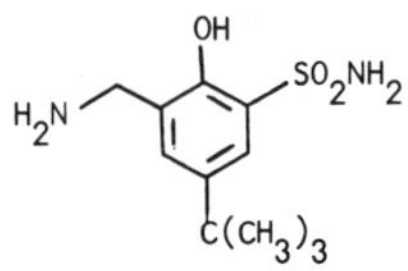

7

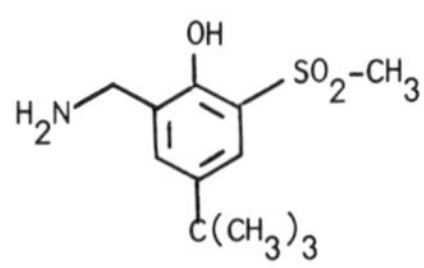

8 (HOE 365)

A breakthrough in this matter was achieved when we replaced the sulfonamide by the methylsulfonyl group. In general, interchange of these moieties is known from the sulfamoylbenzoic acid series to decrease saluretic potency[3]. The methylsulfonyl derivative (compound 8) displayed indeed a reduced salidiuretic activity: It was shown to be as potent as furosemide in the rat and dog assay. But this was more than outweighed by the strong antihypertensive activities displayed in the SHR assay even at the threshold dose of saluresis. In addition it was found to be effective against ethanol induced gastric damage. In comparison to MK 447 it is 8 times more potent as a cytoprotective. On account of this favourable pharmacological profile associated with a furosemide-like low toxicity it was selected for further investigations (HOE 365) and is currently undergoing clinical evaluations.

In crder to elucidate the outstanding antihypertensive activities of HOE 365 in the SHR-assay, we compared it with MK 447 and piretanide in relation to equipotent doses of saluresis. Figure 1 shows dose response curves (interrupted lines) of antihypertensive activity based on a relative dose scale. Dose unit "1" indicates the highest non-saluretic dose. All higher doses are manyfolds of this saluretic threshold dose. As a consequence the saluretic dose response curves (plain lines) are superposed. However, curves of the blood pressure are separated now according to the amount of saluresis associated with the antihypertensive effect.

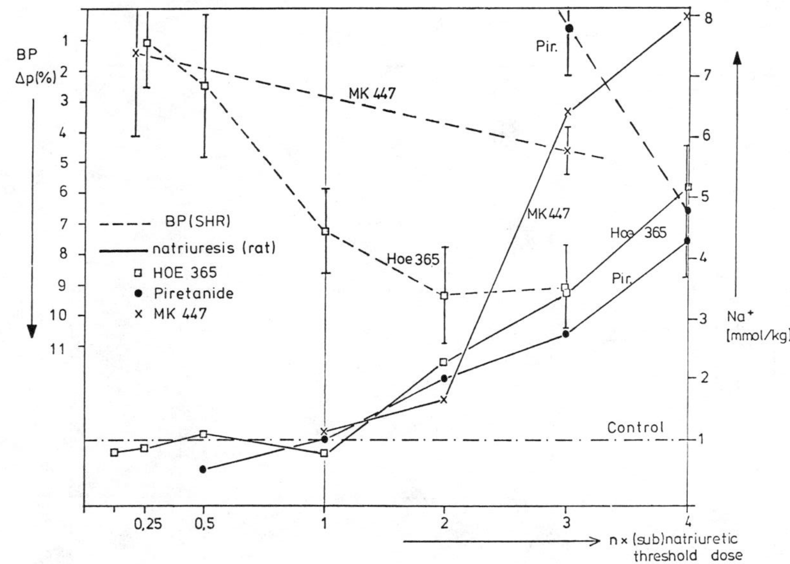

Figure 1. Comparative dose response curves of natriuresis (1-5h) and antihypertensive activity (24h) - HOE 365 vs. MK 447 vs. piretanide. All activities are related to the (sub) natriuretic threshold dose.

They reveal that HOE 365 is superior to MK 447 in the non-diuretic dose range and that piretanide's antihypertensive activities are inherent to doses connected with strong saluretic effects. Up to the dose "4" many well-known diuretics like furosemide, hydrochlorothiazide or even indapamide are devoid of any antihypertensive activity in our SHR-assay. We think that this model is a stringent criterion for an additional antihypertensive mode of action beside those activities which are due to saluresis. (Further pharmacological details are given in "Pharmacology of HOE 365").

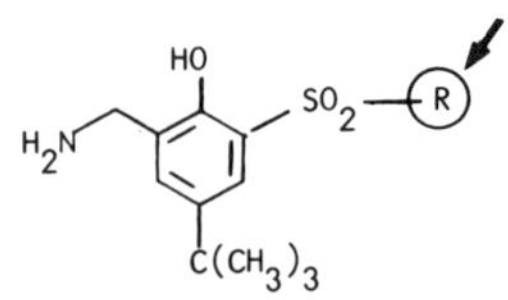

	R	Saluretic Score Rat	Saluretic Score Dog	Subdiuretic antihypertensive act.
8	Me (HOE 365)	+++	+++	+++
9	CH_2Cl	++++	+	0
10	Et	++++	+	0
11	Prop	++		0
12	iProp	++	+	0
13	Allyl	++	+	0
14	iBut	++		
7	NH_2	+++	++++	0
15	C_6H_5	+		
16	p-tolyl	+		0
1	Furosemide	+++	+++	0
2	Piretanide	+++	++++	0
5	MK 447	++++	++++	+

Figure 2. Structural variations of HOE 365 - effects of the sulfur substituent.

Figure 2 surveys the most important variations of HOE 365 concerning the sulfur substituents. As already outlined for the NH_2-substituent (compound 7) there are further variations resulting in an increased saluretic activity. Replacement of the CH_3-moiety by C_2H_5 or CH_2Cl (compounds 9 and 10) provided diuretics which were superior to HOE 365 in the rat but were devoid of any antihypertensive effects at subdiuretic doses. Their piretanide-like activities in the SHR-assay are scored with "0". Substituents with increasing chain length such as propyl, isobutyl or allyl (compounds 11, 13, 14) led to diminution of activity in all test species. Phenyl and p-tolyl (compounds 15 and 16) showed marginal effects but with the latter compound cytoprotection reappeared to a certain extent.

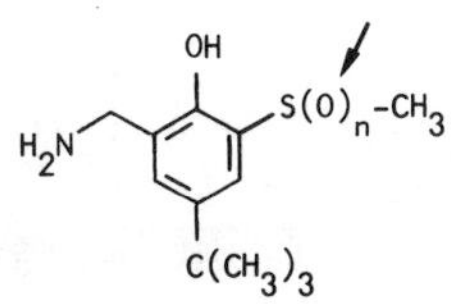

	$S(O)_n$	saluretic score rat	dog	subdiuretic anti-hypertensive act.
8	SO_2 (HOE 365)	+++	+++	+++
17	SO	+++	++	0
18	S *1)	+++	++++	0

*1) published by Merck, Sharp & Dohme, toxic $\geq$ 512mg/kg (rat, p.o.)

Figure 3. Structural variations of HOE 365 - effects of oxidation state.

Other interesting structural variations concern the oxidation state of the sulfur-atom. Figure 3 compares HOE 365 with the sulfoxide and methylthioether derivative (compounds 17 and 18). Strong salidiuretic properties were found for all compounds but evaluated in the SH-rat, the unique antihypertensive activities of HOE 365 were confirmed once again. The synthesis of the thioether analogue was reported by Merck Sharp and Dohme [2]. This compound differed from Hoe 365 by the removal of two oxygen atoms. It was shown to be toxic at 500 mg/kg in the rat (p.o.). and to be devoid of any cytoprotective activity.

Summarizing our results, we can say that subdiuretic antihypertensive activities of HOE 365 are highly sensitive even to small steric and electronic variations of the mesyl moiety whereas salidiuretic properties are insensitive to a large extent. Structure activity relationships as well as pharmacolgical datas reveal a new antihpyertensive mode of action. Finally our studies demonstrate that detoxifying properties are attached to oxidized sulfur substituents.

CHEMISTRY

Figure 4 demonstrates two important synthetic routes frequently used to prepare the new m-sulfonyl-o-hydroxybenzylamines. Tert. butylanisol is chlorosulfonated at temperatures below 0° C to give 2-Methoxy-5-tert.-butylbenzenesulfochloride (compound 20). One route involves treatment of this sulfochloride with ammonia, protection of the SO_2NH_2-moiety by formation of its dimethylformamidine derivative followed by an other cleavage. The protected o-sulfamoylphenol (compound 21) thus obtained readily undergoes amidomethylation. Acidic hydrolysis removes all protecting groups. Alkylsulfones are obtained in a similar manner starting with mild reduction of the sulfochloride (compound 20) and subsequent methylation of the intermediate sulfinic acid. Ether cleavage of the alkylsulfonylanisol, amidcmethylation and saponification are carried out as described above.

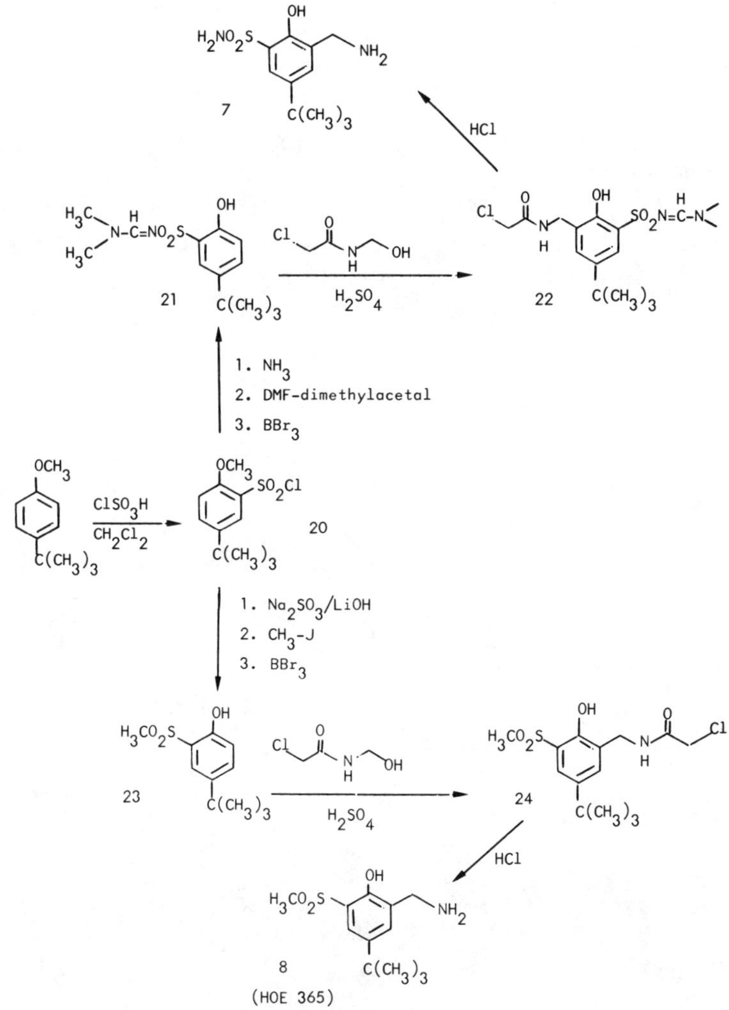

Figure 4. Synthetic routes to m-sulfonyl-o-hydroxybenzylamines

ACKNOWLEDGEMENT

We wish to thank Dr. M. Bickel for cytoprotective evaluations.

REFERENCES

1. Meadow, J.; Berger, J.; and Schert, R.; Chim. Therap. (1968), 3, 253
2. Stokker, G.E.; Deana, A.A.; de Solms, S.J.; Schultz, E.M.; Smith, R.L.; Cragoe, E.J., Jr.; Baer, J.E.; Ludden, C.T.; Russo, H.F.; Scriabine, A.; Sweet, C.S.; Watson, L.S.; J. Med. Chem., 1980, 23, 1414
3. Tvaermose Nielsen, O.B.; Feit, P.W. in "diuretic agents", ACS Symposium series 83, 1978, 12 - 13

PHARMACOLOGICAL PROFILE OF HOE 365, A NEW DIURETIC WITH ANTIHYPERTENSIVE EFFECT

MAX HROPOT, ERIK KLAUS, and ROMAN MUSCHAWECK
Hoechst AG, Postfach 80 03 20, 6230 Frankfurt/M. 80, FRG

ABSTRACT

The agent Hoe 365 (2-aminomethyl-4-(1,1-dimethylethyl)-6-methylsulfonylphenol-hydrochloride) is a derivative of the new 3-aminomethyl-2-hydroxyphenylsulfone category of compounds with diuretic activity. Dose-response studies in rats demonstrate that oral and intravenous administration of Hoe 365 exert a highly potent salidiuretic effect in the dose range from 1 to 1024 mg/kg. The threshold oral dose for salidiuretic activity lies between 4 - 8 mg/kg. In dogs, the salidiuretic effect starts with the oral dose of 1.56 mg/kg. The main effect of Hoe 365 occurs within 6 hrs after dosing. The experiments in Rhesus monkeys also produce a dose-dependent salidiuretic response to Hoe 365. The micropuncture studies reveal the main site of action in Henle's loop and an additional effect in the proximal tubules. In spontaneously hypertensive rats, Hoe 365 in oral doses from 2 to 16 mg/kg decreases the blood pressure dose-dependently. The threshold dose which lowers blood pressure is about 4 mg/kg p.o. In isolated rat thoracic aorta, Hoe 365 inhibits the norepinephrine (10^{-6} mol/l) and KCl-induced contractions with an IC_{50} of 2.4 and 1.5 mmol/l respectively, indicating an extrarenal site of antihypertensive activity of Hoe 365.

INTRODUCTION

Numerous clinical, epidemiological and experimental studies indicate that NaCl has an important role in the pathogenesis of essential hypertension. The intracellular sodium concentration, and in particular the sodium and calcium transport processes between extracellular and intracellular compartment, seem to be closely associated with the development and persistance of essential hypertension. Essential hypertension could be regarded as a disorder of the cell membrane [1]. Consequently, on account of their effect on the cell membrane, saluretics, in addition to specific antihypertensive agents, are becoming more and more important in the treatment of hypertension. Besides having a saluretic effect, Hoe 365, a new development from the m-sulfonylbenzylamine category of compounds, exhibits a marked antihypertensive effect in the spontaneously hypertensive rat. Although Hoe 365 is a high-ceiling-type diuretic, compared to other high-ceiling diuretics it already significantly reduces blood pressure in the spontaneously hypertensive rat at a subdiuretic dose. In human therapy, this would mean an absence of the undesired peak diuresis and relatively small compensatory effects whereby the diuretic's antihypertensive effect comes to the fore.

METHODS

The diuretic and saluretic effect of Hoe 365 was studied in Wistar rats weighing 100 - 150 g according to the Lipschitz test and by means of the saluresis test described previously [2, 3, 4].

Diuretics, Jules B. Puschett, Editor

Salidiuretic studies were carried out on male beagle dogs with a mean body weight of 17.2 ± 2.5 kg. Food was withdrawn 24 hours prior to the experiment and the animals received only tap water ad libitum. On the morning of the first day of the study, the urinary bladder of the animals was emptied by means of a catheter. This urine was discarded. Subsequently, the animals received 20 ml/kg tap water by gastric tube. Following this, the dogs were catheterized hourly up to 8 hours. After each catheterisation, the dogs received 4 ml/kg tap water orally. The urine samples of the first two hours were used as control values. After the second catheterisation, the dogs were orally administered the test compound. The volume of 6 subsequent urine samples was measured and the Na^+, K^+ and Cl^- content was determined. The data were accumulated to give results for the collection periods 1 - 6 and 1 - 24 hours. After the last catheterisation 6 hours after administration, the dogs were then placed in metabolism cages overnight. Twenty-four hours after the start of the test, the animals were once more catheterized. The urine excreted during the night plus that withdrawn by catheterisation represented the collection period 7 - 24 hours. Sodium and potassium were determined by flame photometry with an Eppendorf flame photometer and chloride was determined with an Eppendorf chloridometer. The dose response curves for the excretion values of water, ions and osmolality were calculated by the method of least squares. Regression lines and correlation coefficients are plotted in the figures.

Salidiuretic experiments with Hoe 365 were also carried out on conscious male Rhesus Macaca monkeys with a mean body weight of 4.8 ± 1.5 kg. The experimental design was almost the same as in the dogs, the only difference being that urine was collected spontaneously [5].

Clearance and micropuncture experiments were performed in male Wistar rats with a mean body weight of 250 ± 10 g as described previously [4, 6].

The effect of Hoe 365 on blood pressure was evaluated in spontaneously hypertensive male rats (body weights from 240 - 400 g) obtained from Boehringer Mannheim. For a period of 5 days, blood pressure was measured once daily by a tail-cuff method. Measurements were done with Technilab Instruments Equipment (Technilab Instruments, Pequannock, New Jersey, USA). Recordings were made with a Hellige Multiscriptor EK 21 (Hellige & Co., Freiburg, Germany). The rats were then treated with the test substance for another 5-day period, whereby blood pressure measurements were performed before administration of the drug. Calculations were done with the values 24 hours after the first to fourth treatment. The mean blood pressure of each rat before treatment on days 4 and 5 of the first week and on day 1 of the second week (average 208 ± 17 (SD) mmHg) was used as the initial value. Calculation of the blood pressure was performed and listed as a time effect relationship of the estimates $\bar{x} \pm$ SEM separately for each time and each dose. In additional, the areas under the curves over 4 days were expressed as mean percent differences from the initial values.

The effect of Hoe 365 on norepinephrine- and KCl-induced contractility was studied in the rat thoracic aorta strip. Strips from the thoracic aorta of male Sprague-Dawley rats were cut at an angle of 20 to 30° (25 x 2 mm). Each preparation was incubated under 300 mg tension in a 25 ml bath with modified Tyrode solution according to Biamino and Kruckenberg [7] at 37° C and oxygenated with carbogen (95 % O and 5 % CO_2). Isometric recordings were made with a Gould Statham UC2 transducer and Hellige recorder. After equilibration for approximately 2 hrs, cumulative concentration response curves were obtained using norepinephrine (NE, 1.18×10^{-9} to 1.18×10^{-6} mol/l) and KCl (10 - 40 mmol/l). After washout, the dose response curve was repeated twice. The strips were preincubated with increasing concentrations of Hoe 365 (0.5 to 3.0 mmol/l) for 4 min and the NE- and KCl-induced contractions repeated. The 50 % relaxing concentration (IC_{50}) was calculated by regression analysis.

RESULTS

In the Lipschitz test model, Hoe 365 exhibited a very good diuretic effect with a Lipschitz value of 4.52 when administered in a single oral dose of 50 mg/kg to rats (table 1).

TABLE I. Diuresis in male rats after oral administration of Hoe 365, 5-hour values according to the Lipschitz test (T, test compound; U, urea).

Compound	Body weight of groups	Diuresis in ml/100 g over 5 hours	T/U
Urea 1 g/kg orally	1) 270 g 2) 290 g	2.59 3.10 $\bar{x}$ = 2.85	
Hoe 365 50 mg/kg orally	1) 250 g 2) 270 g	12.80 12.96 $\bar{x}$ = 12.88	4.52

Dose response studies in rats demonstrate that oral administration of Hoe 365 caused a potent natriuretic effect (Fig. 1).

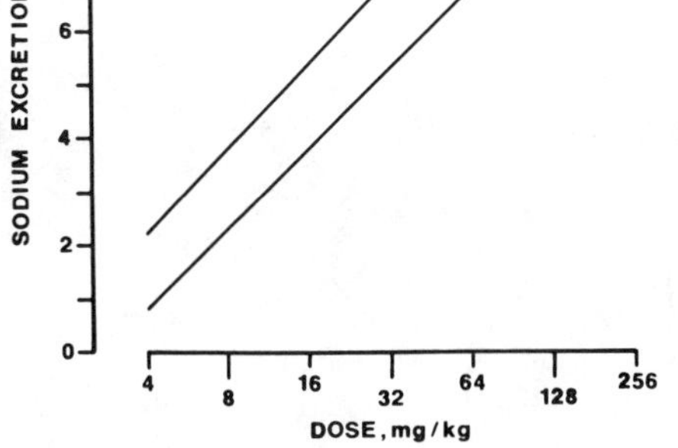

Fig. 1. Dose-dependent natriuretic activity of Hoe 365 in rats ($Y_{5\ h}$, 1 - 5 and $Y_{24\ h}$, 1 - 24 hours collection periods).

The threshold dose for salidiuretic activity lies between 4 - 8 mg/kg orally. The maximum of the activity of Hoe 365 was observed with a dose of 256 mg/kg. The relationship between log. dose and saluretic effect is linear and steep (Fig. 1), whereas the regression line for potassium is flat, indicating a low potassium excretion (Fig. 2). The ratio Na^+/K^+ increased up to four.

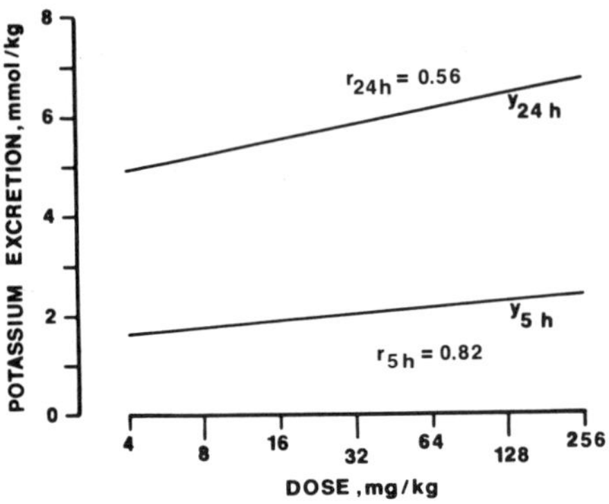

Fig. 2. Dose-dependent kaliuretic activity of Hoe 365 after oral administration to rats ($Y_{5\ h}$, 1 - 5 and $Y_{24\ h}$, 1 - 24 hours collection periods).

Hoe 365 was also very effective in dogs. The regression lines show dose-dependent increase of sodium in Fig. 3.

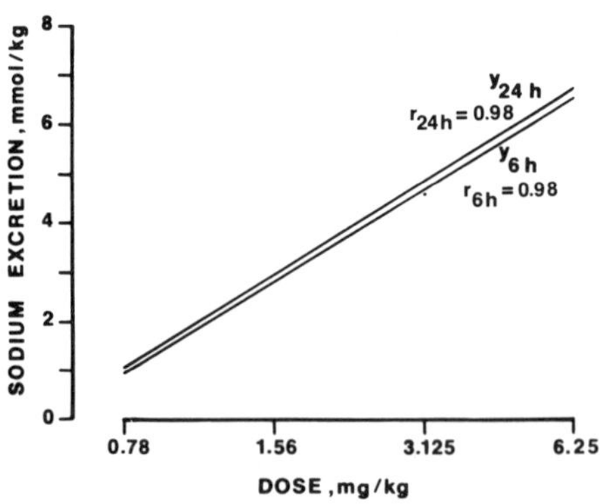

Fig. 3. Dose-dependent natriuretic activity of Hoe 365 after oral administration to dogs ($Y_{6\ h}$, 1 - 6 and $Y_{24\ h}$, 1 - 24 hours collection periods).

The salidiuretic efficacy of Hoe 365 started with an oral dose of 1.56 mg/kg. Up to the maximum effective oral dose of 6.25 mg/kg, the excretion of urine and electrolyte increased progressively. As shown by the regression lines in Fig. 3 the main activity of Hoe 365 occurs within the first six hours after administration. Fig. 4 shows the comparison of 24 hour sodium excretion in dogs after oral and intravenous administration of Hoe 365.

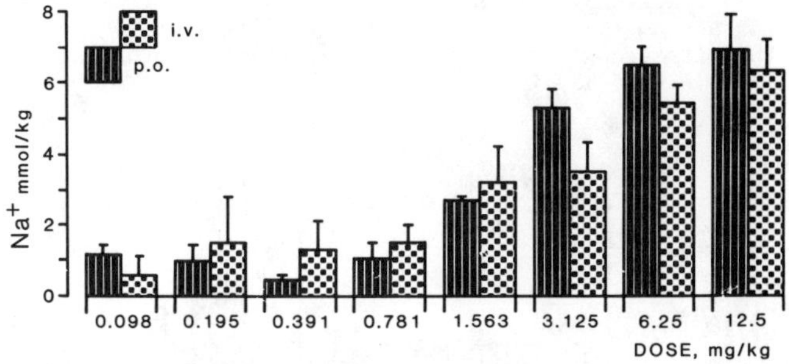

Fig. 4. Comparison of 24 hour sodium excretion in dogs after oral and intravenous administration of Hoe 365 ($\bar{x} \pm$ SD, n = 4).

It is obvious that with respect to pharmacodynamic effect there are no major differences between the two routes of administration.

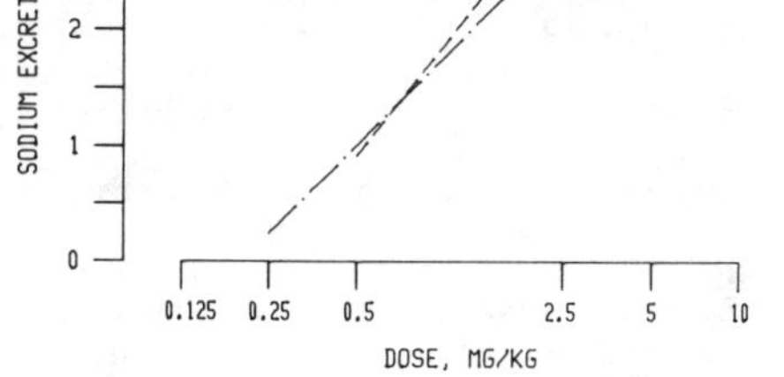

Fig. 5. Dose-dependent natriuretic activity of Hoe 365 after oral (Y_1, r = 0.92) and intravenous (Y_2, r = 0.89) administration (1 - 6 hour collection period) in monkeys.

Hoe 365 was even more effective in Rhesus monkeys than in dogs. The regression lines in Fig. 5 show a steep dose-dependent increase in sodium excretion. The threshold dose was about 0.5 mg/kg orally, whereas the maximum natriuretic effect was observed at 10 mg/kg. The potassium excretion was moderate.

Clearance- and micropuncture studies were performed in anaesthetized Wistar rats to determine the site of action of Hoe 365 and fractional excretion of electrolytes. After intravenous infusion of 5 mg/kg per hour of Hoe 365, the fractional excretion of water, sodium and potassium amounted to 12.7 %, 14 %,and 33 % respectively. Fractional delivery of sodium at the early-distal site increased from 6 % in the controls to 26 % after Hoe 365; at the same time fractional potassium delivery increased from 5 % to 19 % of the filtered potassium load (Fig. 6). Proximal effects of Hoe 365 were less pronounced, thus fractional sodium delivery at the late-proximal site increased from 43 $\pm$ 6 % to 53 $\pm$ 7 %.

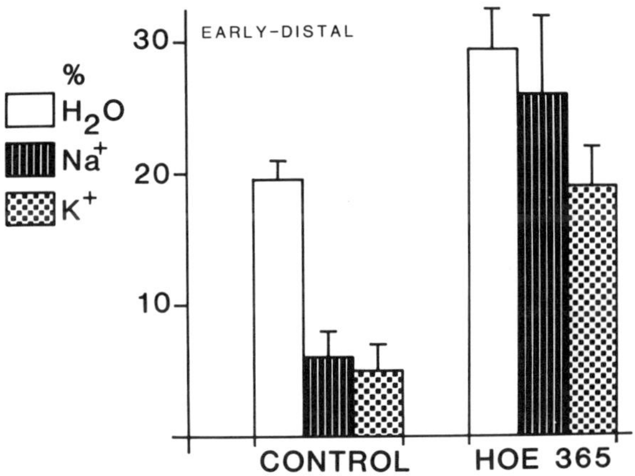

Fig. 6. Fractional delivery of fluid, sodium and potassium at the early-distal site of renal tubules in rats ($\bar{x} \pm$ SD, n = 28).

The antihypertensive effect of Hoe 365 was studied in spontaneously hypertensive rats over a 4 day period. As shown in Fig. 7, Hoe 365 lowered the blood pressure dose-dependently from 2 to 16 mg/kg orally. The threshold dose of Hoe 365 for blood pressure lowering activity was about 4 mg/kg p.o., thus distinctly under the threshold dose for diuretic activity. At doses higher than 16 mg/kg orally, the blood pressure lowering activity did not increase further. At the lower dose level a clear dissociation between salidiuretic and antihypertensive activity could be established.

The concentration-response curves of Hoe 365 in either norepinephrine- or KCl-contracted rat aorta strips are shown in Fig. 8. The contractions induced by norepinephrine and KCl were inhibited dose-dependently, with an IC_{50} of 2.4 mmol/l and 1.5 mmol/l respectively. Although Hoe 365 dose-dependently attenuated the vascular reactivity to vasoconstrictor agents in both experimental models, a clear-cut explanation for its mechanism of action cannot be deduced from this experiment, since Hoe 365 did not show any calcium antagonistic activity in isolated K^+ depolarized pulmonary artery of the guinea pig (own observation).

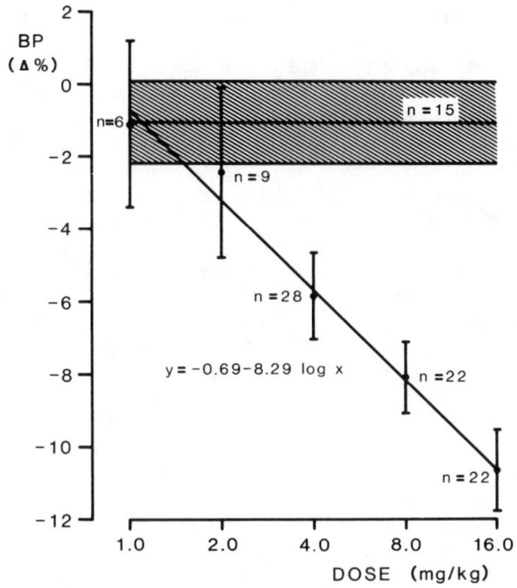

Fig. 7. Effect of Hoe 365 on blood pressure in spontaneously hypertensive rats, expressed as mean percent difference from initial values of the areas under the curves over 4 days ($\bar{x} \pm$ SEM).

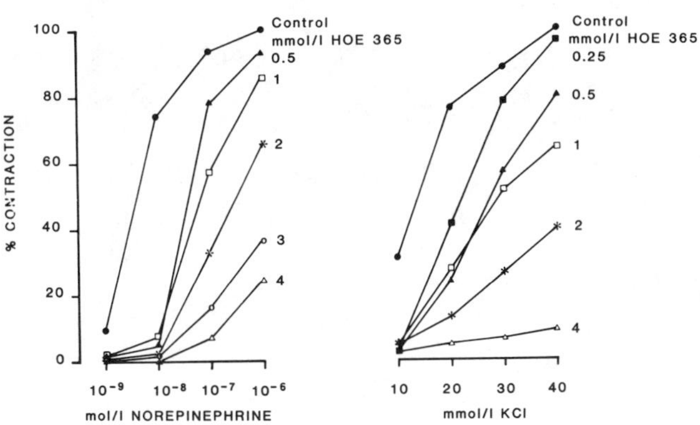

Fig. 8. Effect of Hoe 365 on norepinephrine- and KCl-induced contractions in rat aorta strips ($\bar{x}$, n = 4 - 11).

DISCUSSION

In rats, dogs,and in monkeys, the compound Hoe 365 revealed a potent dose-dependent salidiuretic effect. The salidiuretic potency of Hoe 365 in rats is higher than that of furosemide, whereas in dogs the potency of both drugs is comparable [3, 4, 6]. The salidiuretic effect of Hoe 365 is short-lived and was almost completed 6 hours after administration of the drug.

Oral and intravenous administration of Hoe 365 in dogs has shown a comparable pharmacodynamic response indicating a high bioavailability of the compound. The micropuncture study in rats revealed the main site of action of Hoe 365 in Henle's loop and an additional effect in the proximal tubules. In spontaneously hypertensive rats, Hoe 365 caused a dose-dependent decrease in blood pressure. It is obvious that this compound already diminished the blood pressure in rats at an oral dose of 4 mg/kg, whereas its salidiuretic activity first started in a dose range of 4 to 8 mg/kg orally. Some other mechanisms (not only salidiuresis) might be additionally responsible for the antihypertensive effect. Changes in the intracellular concentration of ions and decreased contractility of the resistance vessels to norepinephrine after diuretics have been postulated [1, 7]. In rat aorta strips, Hoe 365 dose-dependently decreased norepinephrine- and KCl-induced contractions with an IC_{50} of 2.4 and 1.5 mmol/l respectively, indicating an extrarenal site of action of this drug. In summary it can be said that Hoe 365 is a salidiuretic agent with a potent antihypertensive effect in rats, whereby both effects can be dissociated at lower dose levels. In the subdiuretic dose of Hoe 365 in rats, the direct effect on vessels might be responsible for its antihypertensive activity.

REFERENCES

1. Ph. Meyer and R.P. Garay, Eur. J. Clin. Invest. 11, pp. 337-339 (1981).
2. W.L. Lipschitz, Z. Hadidian,and A. Kerpcsar, J. Pharmacol. Exp. Ther. 85, 97 (1943).
3. R. Muschaweck and K. Sturm, Diuretika in Ehrhart, G. and Ruschig H., Arzneimittel-Entwicklung-Wirkung-Darstellung, Vol. 2, pp. 322-325, Verlag Chemie, Weinheim Bergstr. (1972).
4. W. Merkel, D. Bormann, D. Mania, R. Muschaweck,and M. Hropot, Eur. J. Med. Chem. Chimica Therapeutica 11, No. 5, pp. 399-406 (1976).
5. F. Roch-Rammel and I.M. Weiner, Am. J. Physiol. 224, No. 6 (1973).
6. K. Meng, Naunyn-Schmiedeberg's Arch. Pharmacol. Exp. Path. 257, pp. 355-371 (1967)
7. G. Biamino and P. Kruckenberg, Am. J. Physiol. 79, pp. 376 (1969).

PHARMACOLOGY OF TRIPAMIDE, A NEW ANTIHYPERTENSIVE DRUG

T. IGARASHI
Department of Pharmacology, Tsukuba Research Laboratories, Eisai Co., Ltd., Toyosatomachi, Ibaraki, Japan.

Tripamide is a new chlorosulfamoylbenzamide derivative which has been shown to have antihypertensive and diuretic actions in animals and man. Tripamide was introduced to clinical study in 1974 and launched in 1982 in Japan. Tripamide was selected from more than 300 compounds designed and synthesized in Eisai Research Laboratories during 1968 - 1970. In those days, the antihypertensive effect of diazoxide, a non-diuretic thiazide, was still a hot topic of conversation. A new class of extremely potent diuretics such as furosemide and the congeners also attracted a good deal of attention among medicinal chemists. We aimed for a development of a new antihypertensive agent with a mild but long-lasting diuretic action. Fig. 1 shows the chemical structure of tripamide : 4-chloro-N-(endo-hexahydro-4,7-methanoisoindolin-2-yl)-3-sulfamoylbenzamide (E-614; ADR-033; Normonal).

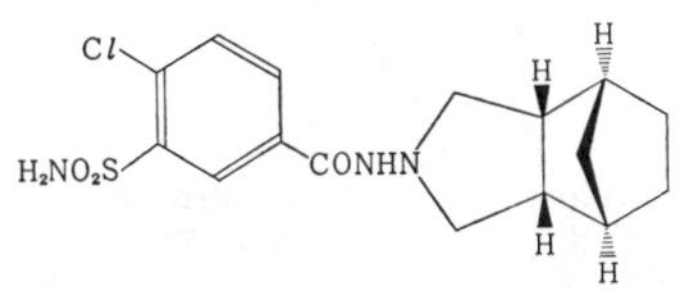

Fig.1. The chemical structure of tripamide

1. TOXICOLOGY

Tripamide had low acute toxicity [1, 2]. It did not cause death in mice, rats and dogs at oral doses of 5000, 8000 and 2000 mg/kg, respectively. The LD50 values for tripamide by intraperitoneal and intramuscular injections were greater than 2000 mg/kg in mice and rats.

Tripamide was well tolerated in chronic toxicity studies (6 months) at oral doses of 20 - 2000 mg/kg in rats and 8 - 800 mg/kg in dogs. A mild hypokalemia occured at doses higher than 1000 and 400 mg/kg in rats and dogs, respectively. Neither teratogenicity nor embryotoxicity were observed in rats and rabbits at doses 40 - 200 mg/kg.

2. DIURETIC PROPERTIES

The renal effect of tripamide has been studied in rats, dogs and man [3-5]. The effects of tripamide on urine volume and urinary sodium, potassium and chloride excretions in rats are summarized in Fig. 2. The animals were loaded with 25 ml/kg of 0.9% saline by stomach tube before the administration of test drugs. Tripamide increased urine volume and sodium and chloride excretions dose-dependently at a wide dose range (0.13 - 160 mg/kg, p.o.). The slope of the dose-response curve for diuretic action of tripamide was remarkably less steep when compared with those of furosemide, acetazolamide and hydrochlorothiazide. The increase in potassium excretion caused by tripamide was dependent on the experimental conditions, but was definitely less than those of the refference drugs. The increase in urine volume caused by tripamide was also less remarkable than the increases in sodium and chloride excretions. For example, in an acute toxicity study in beagle dogs which were given extremely high doses of tripamide (200 - 2000 mg/kg, p.o.), urine volume per 24 hours increased two fold, sodium

Diuretics, Jules B. Puschett, Editor

eight fold, potassium 1.3 fold and chloride five fold [2].

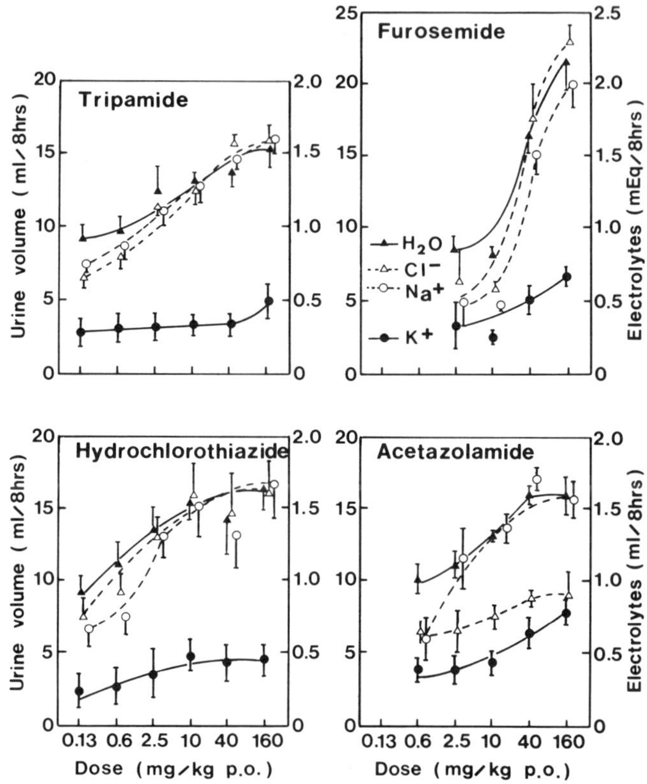

Fig. 2. Dose-response curves for the effects of tripamide, hydrochlorothiazide, acetazolamide, and furosemide on urine volume (-▲-), urinary excretion of Cl (- △ -), Na (- ○ -) and K (-●-) in rats. Each point with a vertical bar represents the mean and S.E. of 6 animals. Control values obtained from 24 untreated animals are shown in the column of furosemide. (From Kobayashi et al. [3], with permission)

The effects of tripamide on renal blood flow and osmolar- and water-clearances were studied in anesthetized dogs [2]. Tripamide was dissolved in NaOH solution (pH 10 - 11) and injected intravenously. Tripamide at doses 30, 100 and 300 µg/kg, had no influence on systemic blood pressure, heart rate or renal blood flow (measured with a magnetic flow meter). GFR and RPF determined by clearance methods were not affected by tripamide. Fig. 3 shows changes in urine volume, electrolyte excretion, osmolar- and free-water clearances after injection of 100 µg/kg of tripamide. The increase in chloride excretion was the most prominent change followed by increases in magnesium and sodium excretions, in that order. The effects of hydrochlorothiazide were similar to those of tripamide, although it increased calcium and potassium excretions to a considerable degree. Furosemide caused prompt and prominent increases in urinary excretions of calcium, magnesium, chloride, sodium and potassium.

To investigate the duration of the diuretic action of tripamide, diuretic tests after a saline-loading were performed in rats which were given an oral dose of tripamide 24 - 72 hours before the test. The diuretic effect of tripamide at 200 mg/kg was detected even 48 hours after the administration.

As shown in Fig. 3, tripamide markedly increased both osmolar clearance and free-water reabsorption. The ratio of osmolar clearance to free-water reabsorption was decreased slightly by tripamide. These changes were similar to those induced by hydrochlorothiazide, and definitely different from those caused by furosemide. Furosemide prominently increased osmolar clearance but rather decreased free-water reabsorption, resulting in a marked decrease in the ratio. These data may suggest that the sites of the renal action of tripamide resemble those of hydrochlorothiazide, at least in dogs.

Regarding the sites of action of tripamide, Brater and Anderson [5] have recently reported that tripamide behaved as a loop diuretic and might have an additional effect at more proximal part of nephron. In contrast to thiazide diuretics, tripamide increased fractional free-water clearance during water loading in normal subjects.

The carbonic anhydrase activity of rat's erythrocytes and the Na-K-ATPase activity of rat's renal homogenate were inhibited by tripamide at 1 - 10 μM (1/62 of acetazolamide in potency) and at 0.1 - 1 mM (equipotent to ethacrynic acid) [6]. However, it remains unclear whether these inhibitory activities on enzymes are related to the mechanism of renal action of tripamide or not.

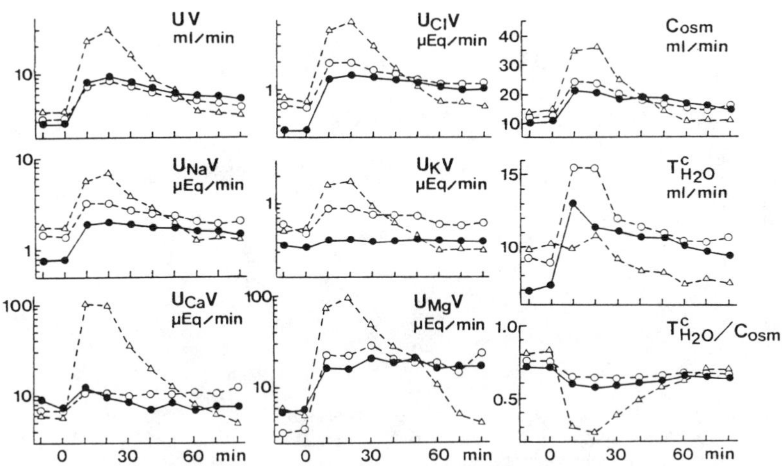

Fig. 3. Changes in electrolyte excretion, osmolar clearance and free-water reabsorption after 100 μg/kg (i.v.) of tripamide (n=7, -●-), hydrochlorothiazide (n=3, -○-) and furosemide (n=2, -△-) in anesthetized dogs. (From Kobayashi et al. [3], with permission)

3. EFFECTS ON GLUCOSE TOLERANCE

The induction of hyperglycemia or the aggravation of pre-existing diabetes mellitus is known to be one of the side effects of thiazides and loop diuretics.

Noguchi et al. [7] studied the effect of tripamide on blood glucose level and glucose tolerance in alloxan diabetic rats. The animals were hyperglycemic and the blood glucose level ranged from 300 to 700 mg/dl on feeding, but the level decreased to 160 - 185 mg/dl after 16 hours of fasting when tripamide and reference drugs were administered. As shown in Fig. 4, furosemide and hydrochlorothiazide elevated the plasma glucose level by about 30% and aggravated the response to glucose-loading. Tripamide and acetazolamide (not shown in the figure) had no significant effect on the tolerance.

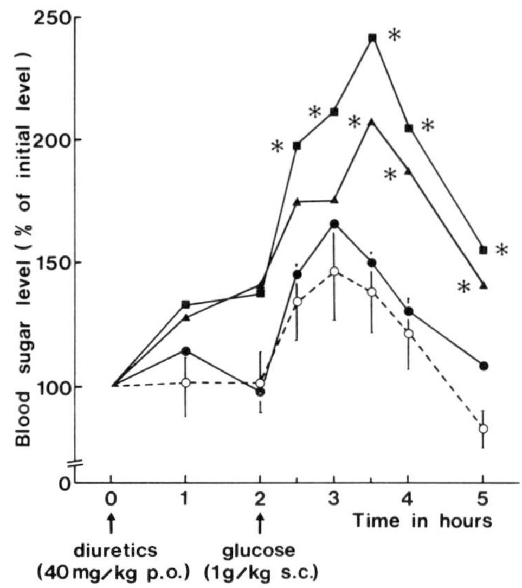

Fig. 4. The effects of 40 mg/kg (p.o.) of tripamide (—●—), hydrochlorothiazide (—▲—) and furosemide (—■—) on blood glucose tolerance test in alloxan diabetic rats fasted for 16 hours. Control animals (- - ○ - -) received 5% gum arabic solution instead of diuretics. Each point is the mean of 6-8 animals. S.E. is shown only in the control curve. *: $P < 0.05$ (From Noguchi et al. [7], with permission)

4. EFFECTS ON BLOOD PRESSURE

Igarashi et al. [4] studied the antihypertensive effect of tripamide in rats and dogs. Systolic blood pressure was measured indirectly by a tail cuff method, unless otherwise stated. In some experiments, the effects of tripamide on blood pressure and urinary electrolyte excretion were compared in the same animals.

Blood pressure and heart rate of normotensive rats (male, 15 weeks old) were not affected by tripamide (1 - 100 mg/kg, p.o.). In DOCA-salt hypertensive rats (blood pressure: 155 - 185 mmHg) a single oral dose of 1 or 10 mg/kg of tripamide reduced the pressure by 15 - 25 mmHg at 3, 6 and 9 hours, whereas heart rate remained unchanged. A lower dose of 0.1 mg/kg had no effect. The antihypertensive effect of tripamide was compared with hydrochlorothiazide and furosemide in aged SHR (male, 67 - 77 weeks after birth, blood pressure: 230 - 250 mmHg). The mean reductions in blood pressure determined at 2 and 4 hours after oral administrations at 1, 10 and 100 mg/kg were 12, 25 and 28 mmHg for tripamide and 0, 13 and 23 mmHg for hydrochlorthiazide, respectively. The mean fall in blood pressure after the administration of furosemide at 10 and 100 mg/kg were 3 and 18 mmHg, respectively. Heart rate was not affected by any of the drugs.

The blood pressure which had been reduced by a single dose of tripamide returned nearly to the level of pre-dosing value within 24 hours. However, when DOCA-salt hypertensive rats were given 5 mg/kg (p.o.) of tripamide once a day for consecutive 10 days, the blood pressure at 24 hours after each dosing decreased stepwise from 185 to 150 mmHg, on average. Also, in dogs with one-kidney one-clip renal hypertension the initial blood pressure (150 - 200 mmHg) decreased gradually to 140 - 160 mmHg with a daily dose of 5 mg/kg (p.o.) of tripamide for 10 days. The higher was the blood pressure, the more remarkable was the antihypertensive action of tripamide.

Fig. 5 compares the renal and antihypertensive actions of a chronic administration of tripamide in SHR. Tripamide was administered by stomach tube at doses of 1 and 10 mg/kg once a day for four weeks. Changes in blood pressure and electrolyte excretion were determined once a week.

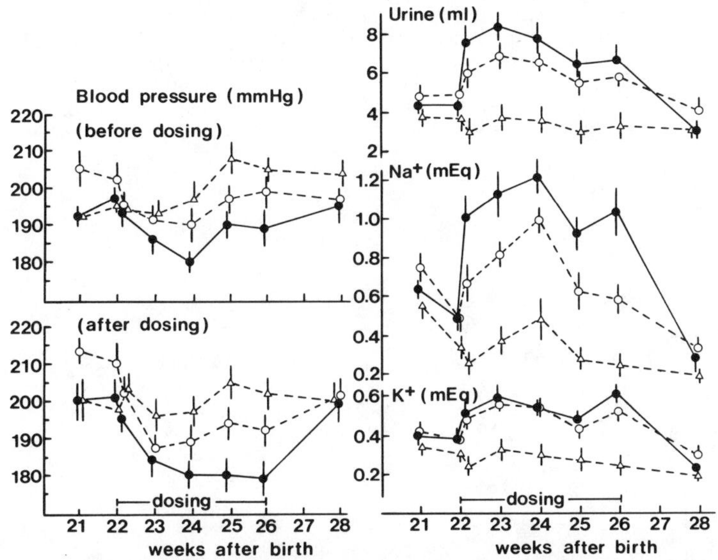

Fig. 5. The effects of chronic administration of tripamide on blood pressure, urine volume and electrolyte excretion in male SHR. The animals were given by stomach tube 1 mg/kg (-○-), 10 mg/kg (-●-) of tripamide or vehicle alone (-△-) once a day for four weeks. Blood pressure was determined before and three hours after the dosing and urine was collected for three hours after the dosing. Each point represents the mean of 15 animals with S.E. (From Igarashi et al [4], with permission)

Blood pressure was determined before and at three hours after the administration of tripamide for the day. Urine was collected for three hours after the administration. Blood pressure of the control animals which received gum arabic alone still tended to increase during the period 21 - 28 weeks after birth. The antihypertensive action of tripamide was more evident when blood pressure was determined after the administration for the day. It was considered noteworthy that there was no definite difference between blood pressure reduction (difference from the control period) caused by 1 and 10 mg/kg of tripamide, while urine volume and sodium excretion were dose-relatedly increased.

To investigate the contribution of the diuretic effect to the antihypertensive action of tripamide, an experiment was carried out in SHR loaded with saline (Fig. 6). Male SHR 10 weeks after birth were divided into two groups. The animals in group A and B were allowed to drink freely tap water and 1% saline, respectively. As shown in Fig. 6B, the progress of hypertension in SHR during the 10th to 30th week after birth was much accelerated by the salt loading. In this experiment, the initial dose for the first 10 weeks was doubled every two weeks thereafter. Tripamide at an initial dose of 5 mg/kg and multiplied doses clearly delayed the progress of hypertension in SHR given tap water. On the other hand, the antihypertensive action of tripamide was not evident at doses of 0.5 mg/kg and 5 mg/kg (not shown in the figure) in the SHR given saline. Furosemide at doses starting from 5 mg/kg and increased finally up to 40 mg/kg did not reduce blood pressure at all in the saline-loaded SHR. Urine volume and electrolyte (Na and K) excretion were monitored throughout this study. In the salt-loaded rats, salt excretion amounted to about three times of that in the SHR given tap water. Tripamide at all doses examined and furosemide at doses less than 20 mg/kg did not significantly increase sodium excretion.

The antihypertensive action of tripamide in SHR was also studied by direct determination of blood pressure with an indwelling aortic catheter [8]. Tripamide at doses 4 and 40 mg/kg (p.o.) reduced blood pressure by about 10 mmHg within the few hours after the first dosing and by 20 - 30 mmHg after the dosing on the second and third days. Cardiac output remained unchanged throughout this study. Therefore, the reduction in blood pressure caused by tripamide was accounted for by a reduction in peripheral vascular resistance.

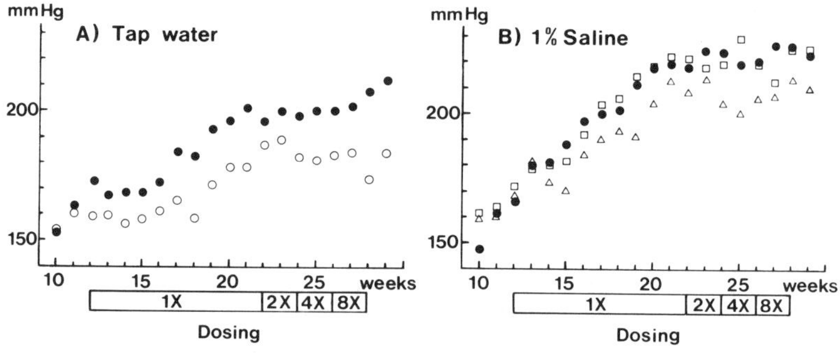

Fig. 6. The effects of tripamide and furosemide on the development of hypertension in SHR given tap water (A) and 1% saline (B). Animals were administered a drug by stomach tube once a day for 16 weeks. The initial doses were, (A) ○ : 5 mg/kg of tripamide, (B) △ : 0.5 mg/kg of tripamide and □ : 5 mg/kg of furosemide. Control animals (●) were given gum arabic. Each point represents the mean of n=14 or 15 SHR in A and n=9 or 10 SHR in B.

5. EFFECTS ON VASCULAR SMOOTH MUSCLES

Ogawa et al. [9] studied the vasoreactivity of the mesenteric vessels isolated from rats pretreated with a repeated dose of tripamide. Age matched rats (18 weeks after birth) of normotensive Wistar (blood pressure 125 - 150 mmHg) and SHR (180 - 200 mmHg) were given tripamide daily for more than 7 days. The mesenteric vessel preparations were prepared according to the method described by McGregor [10]. The preparations were perfused with Krebs-Henseleit solution at a constant rate. Vasoreactivities to noradrenaline and KCl were assessed by an increase in perfusion pressure. The mesenteric vessels isolated from SHR had a higher vasoreactivity to both noradrenaline and KCl. In the preparations isolated from normotensive rats, there was no difference in vasoreactivity to noradrenaline or KCl between control and tripamide-treated groups. Pretreatment of SHR with tripamide at a daily dose of 2 mg/kg did not affect the increased vasoreactivity to noradrenaline but reduced significantly that to KCl.

Asada et al. [11] investigated the effects of tripamide on the membrane potentials and contractile properties of guinea-pig mesenteric artery. Tripamide at a concentration higher than 0.1 ng/ml, suppressed the contractions evoked by KCl and noradrenaline. Tripamide did not modify the membrane potential or membrane resistance, but suppressed spikes which were evoked by outward current pulses in the presence of 3 - 5 mM TEA. Tripamide (0.1 µg/ml) also suppressed the amplitude of excitatory junction potentials (e.j.ps) evoked by perivascular nerve stimulation. The facillitation process produced by repetitive stimulation was less affected.

6. BIOLOGICAL DISPOSITION

Horie et al. [12 - 15] studied pharmacokinetics, metabolism and excretion of tripamide in rats, rabbits and man. Both in rats and rabbits, oral absorption of tripamide was rapid and essentially complete. When [14C]-labeled tripamide was administered orally at a dose of 5 mg/kg, blood levels of radioactivity reached a maximum within one hour. The maximum levels of radioactivity in rats and rabbits were equivalent to 4.96 and 2.88 µg/ml of tripamide, respectively. The half-life of the initial phase was 2.6 hours and that of the second phase was 12.8 hours in rats, and those in rabbits were 44 minutes and 5.31 hours, respectively [12]. In man, the concentrations of tripamide in biological fluids were determined by high-performance liquid chromatography. The maximum level for tripamide in whole blood was reached four hours after an oral administration of 90 mg. The peak level in plasma and erythrocytes were 0.12 and 4.98 µg/ml, respectively. The concentration of tripamide in erythrocytes declined monophasically. The half-life was 9.5 hours [13]. Binding of tripamide to plasma proteins was studied in vitro by an ultrafiltration method and found to be 65%.

The radiolabeled tripamide distributed highly in the liver and kidney and scarecely in tissues such as brain, nerve, testis and muscle. The radioactivity retained in the body 7 days after the administration was less than 0.05% in rats and 0.3% in rabbits. Tripamide did not accumulate in any specific tissue even after repeated administration [12]. The placental transfer rate of tripamide was low. Only 0.01 - 0.04% of the total radioactivity given as labeled tripamide to pregnant rats was found in the fetuses. The concentration of radioactivity in the fetus was 15% of that in mother animal's blood [12].

Fig. 7 shows postulated metabolic pathways of tripamide. Five metabolites were isolated from rat urine and identified as 3-hydroxy- and 8-hydroxy- tripamide, CSBA, CSBH and CSBM [14]. Tripamide was rapidly metabolized by liver microsomal enzymes. The main enzymes responsible for the metabolism were hepatic arylamidase and microsomal monooxygenase [15]. Tripamide was rapidly hydrolyzed by arylamidase in rats and rabbits, but slowly in man. The main metabolites detected in human urine were 3- and 8-hydroxy tripamide [13].

Of the total radioactivity after an oral administration of labeled tripamide to rats, 41.6 and 47.0% were recovered from urine and feces, respectively. In rabbits, 80% was recovered from urine and the rest was found in feces [12]. In man, less than 2% was excreted unchanged and 8 - 12% as either 3- or 8-hydroxylated metabolite in urine [13].

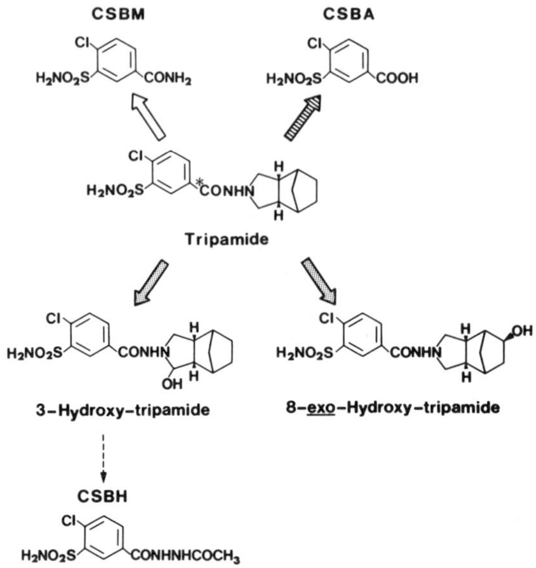

Fig. 7. Postulated metabolic pathways of tripamide. Enzymes responsible for the metabolism of tripamide are arylamidase (⇨) and monooxygenase (⇨). The position of [14C] in the radio-labeled molecule is marked with *.

7. CLINICAL STUDIES

The second-phase studies were carried out during 1974 - 1976 in Japan. Of the total of 228 patients investigated, 218 were with essential hypertension. They received a daily dose ranging from 10 to 200 mg for 1 - 75 weeks. The antihypertensive effect was recognized in 112 of 135 (83%) of patients who were treated with a daily dose ranging from 10 to 30 mg. Daily doses higher than 40 mg caused additional increases in urine volume and electrolyte excretion. However, the increase in dose was not accompanied by a further decrease in blood pressure.

Tripamide was compared with methyclothiazide in the multicenter double blind study carried out during 1976 - 1978 [16]. Blood pressure reduction of more than 10 mmHg in systole and 5 mmHg in diastole at the 6th and 12th weeks of treatment was found in 77% and 83% of patients treated with a daily dose of 30 mg of tripamide, and in 70% and 74% of the patients treated with 5 mg of methyclothiazide. Hypokalemia occured in 8 of 92 patients treated with tripamide and in 14 of 87 patients administered with methyclothiazide. Hyperuricemia occured in 4 patients treated with tripamide and 9 patients administered with methyclothiazide. Aggravation of glucose tolerance was found in neither the tripamide- nor the methyclothiazide-treated group.

DISCUSSION

In general, thiazides and related diuretics show low toxicity in animal studies. In acute toxicity studies, tripamide did not cause any demonstrable toxic signs even at extremely high doses such as 1000-fold of those required for its pharmacological action. Tripamide appears to be an antihypertensive drug which causes few adverse effects such as hypokalemia and disturbances in carbohydrate metabolism, as expected from the preclinical studies.

Tripamide does not reduce blood pressure in normotensive animals and its antihypertensive action was mild and comparable with those of thiazides.

However, as mentioned above (e.g. Fig. 5), the maximal antihypertensive action of tripamide was manifested at much smaller doses than needed for the diuretic action. This finding could be accounted for by the characteristically shallow slope in the dose-response (diuretic) curve of tripamide, if we assume that the diuretics induce their maximal antihypertensive action at a small dose which causes a mild salt-loss. The shallow dose-response curve for the diuretic action of tripamide (Fig. 2) and also the long duration of action may be related to the finding that tripamide is taken up rapidly by erythrocytes and then released gradually as the plasma level declines.

Data shown in Fig. 6 indicated that the antihypertensive action of tripamide decreased markedly in SHR when the animals drank 1% saline freely. These data may suggest that the antihypertensive action should be accounted for by its diuretic action. On the other hand, the finding that tripamide partially retained its antihypertensive action even under the condition of salt-loading, while furosemide did not, may suggest the existence of an additional mechanism for the antihypertensive action. It might be a direct effect on the vascular smooth muscles or an indirect effect through suppression of transmitter release from sympathetic nerve endings as shown by Asada et al. [11].

REFERENCES

1. I. Ohsumi, O. Tagaya, H. Shiojiri, and K. Nakao, Yakubutsu-ryoho 12, 651-698 (1979), (in Japanese).
2. T. Chimoto, M. Okada, F. Sagami, and M. Noguchi, Yakubutsu-ryoho 12, 559-589 (1979), (in Japanese).
3. M. Kobayashi, N. Mori, T. Tomiuga and T. Igarashi, Shinryo to Shinyaku 16, 1001-1010 (1979), (in Japanese).
4. T. Igarashi, Y. Nakajima and M. Kobayashi, Shinryo to Shinyaku 16, 1253-1261 (1979), (in Japanese).
5. D. C. Brater and S. Anderson, Clin. Pharmacol. Ther. 34, 79-85 (1983).
6. T. Tomiuga, I. Ohkawa and M. Tanaka, Shinryo to Shinyaku 16, 1263-1278 (1979), (in Japanese).
7. M. Noguchi, N. Mori and T. Ohgo, Yakubutsu-ryoho 12, 549-558 (1979), (in Japanese).
8. T. Igarashi, This proceeding.
9. T. Ogawa, T. Yamanaka and T. Igarashi, Folia Pharmacol. Japonica 79, 84P (1982), (in Japanese).
10. D. D. McGregor, J. Physiol. (Lond.) 177, 21-30 (1965).
11. H. Asada, T. Itoh, H. Suzuki, Y. Ito and H. Kuriyama, Gen. Pharmacol. 13, 215-223 (1982).
12. T. Horie, T. Ohno and K. Kinoshita, Japan. J. Pharmacol. 32, 1041-1049 (1982).
13. T. Horie, T. Ohno and K. Kinoshita, J. Chromatography 231, 111-119 (1982).
14. T. Horie, T. Ohno and K. Kinoshita, Xenobiotica 11, 197-206 (1981).
15. T. Horie, T. Ohno and K. Kinoshita, Xenobiotica 11, 693-699 (1981).
16. Y. Masuyama, Igaku no ayumi 113, 928-942 (1980), (in Japanese).

VASOPRESSIN ANTAGONISTS

ROBERT W. SCHRIER, AND JIN K. KIM
Department of Medicine, University of Colorado Health Sciences Center, 4200 E. 9th Ave., Denver, CO 80262, USA

INTRODUCTION

In the search for ideal vasopressin antagonists, there has been a great deal of effort focused on synthesizing analogues of vasopressin for the past 20 years. Since vasopressin has been shown to have a role in several pathological states with water retention such as thyroid disease [1,2], cirrhosis [3-5], mineralocorticoid deficiency [6], glucocorticoid deficiency [7,8], and cardiac failure [9], the development for clinical use of specific vasopressin antagonists of the hormone's antidiuretic action would provide important therapeutic applications.

Recently Manning, Sawyer and associates [10-15] synthesized specific antagonists against the vasopressor or antidiuretic action of vasopressin by producing analogues of arginine vasopressin (AVP). The structure of AVP (Fig. 1) and the analogues involved in various amino acid substitutions are shown in Table I. The detailed description of the changes in the amino acids for the analogues of AVP have been described in the papers by Manning, Sawyer and colleagues [10-15].

```
1     2     3     4     5     6    7     8     9

Cy - Tyr - Phe - Gln - Asn - Cy - Pro - Arg - Gly - NH2
|                            |
|                            |
S -------------------------- S
```

FIG. 1. Structure of arginine vasopressin.

TABLE I. Some potent antagonists for vasopressor or antidiuretic activity of arginine vasopressin.

Antivasopressor Antagonists	Effective Dose (nmol/kg)	pA_2	References
$d(CH_2)_5$VDAVP	1.5	7.68	11
dPTyr(Me)AVP	0.8	7.96	10,17
$d(CH_2)_5$AVP	0.6	8.35	12,16
$d(CH_2)_5$Tyr(Me)AVP	0.16	8.62	12,16,18,26
Antiantidiuretic Antagonists			
$d(CH_2)_5$Tyr(Et)VAVP	1.9	7.57	14,19,21,23
$d(CH_2)_5$D-Tyr(Et)VAVP	1.1	7.81	19,21
$d(CH_2)_5$Tyr(Me)VAVP	3.1	7.35	19

Abbreviations: $d(CH_2)_5$ = 1-(β-mercapto-β,β-cyclopentamethylene propionic acid); VDAVP = 4-valine, 8-D-arginine vasopressin; dPTyr(Me) = 1-deamino penicillamine, 2-(O-methyl) tyrosine
pA_2 = negative logarithms of the "effective dose" divided by the estimated volume of distribution (67 ml/kg)

Diuretics, Jules B. Puschett, Editor

Some antagonists that have been studied using in vitro tissue preparations and experimental animals in vivo are shown in Table I. All four antagonists against vasopressor action of AVP were reported to contain potent antioxytocic activity and negligible antidiuretic activity [10-12]. Antagonists of the antidiuretic response caused a transient antidiruetic effect in the early stage of administration [13,23]. Other potentially, more potent and specific antagonists have recently been reported [15,24], however, the antagonistic effects of these agents need to be documented in additional physiological and biochemical studies.

ANTAGONISTS AGAINST VASOPRESSOR ACTION OF AVP

The pressor property of AVP has been known since the late 1800s and the baroreceptor-mediated nonosmotic release of AVP has been suggested to be an integral part of the response to maintain circulatory homeostasis [25]. The development of vasopressor antagonists not only provided exciting therapeutic implications but also supplied an important experimental approach to study the vascular role of AVP and its interaction with the renin-angiotensin system, circulating catecholamines, and the sympathetic nervous system. In our laboratory dPTyr(Me)AVP was found to completely block the increase in mean arterial pressure caused by large doses of AVP in conscious rats (Fig. 2). No effect of dPTyr(Me)AVP was demonstrated in the water-diuresing rats without detectable vasopressin levels (Fig. 3). When the endogenous AVP were increased to approximately 20 pg/ml by 24 hours of fluid deprivation in the conscious rat, dPTyr(Me)AVP significantly decreased mean arterial pressure (Fig. 3). These results suggest that AVP exerts an important role in circulatory homeostasis during fluid deprivation in the conscious rat. The pressor role of AVP in blood pressure regulation has also been studied during hemorrhage in dogs using AVP antagonists. The AVP antagonists, $d(CH_2)_5AVP$ or $d(CH_2)_5Tyr(Me)AVP$ decreased mean arterial pressure during the non-hypotensive hemorrhage in conscious dogs [16], and the blood pressure regulation by endogenous AVP during hypotensive hemorrhage was impaired in the presence of the AVP antagonists in the anesthetized dogs [26]. There is also important evidence for a vascular interaction between AVP, renin-angiotensin and norepinephrine. Recently a study using $d(CH_2)_5Tyr(Me)AVP$ demonstrated an effect of elevated endogenous AVP to maintain blood pressure in the mineralocorticoid and glucocorticoid deficient rats [27]. In addition to the high endogenous AVP, elevated plasma renin activity and norepinephrine were present in the mineralocorticoid deficient rats. The duration of the hypotensive effect of AVP was dependent on whether compensatory vasoconstrictor pathways were blocked. Specifically, angiotensin antagonist and alpha-adrenergic blocking agents substantially prolonged the hypotensive effect of the AVP antagonists in the conscious rats with adrenal insufficiency [27]. Another study with $d(CH_2)_5Tyr(Me)AVP$ also demonstrated that both vasopressin and the renin-angiotensin systems are involved in the control of mean arterial pressure and peripheral vascular resistance following hypotensive hemorrhage in anesthetized rats [18]. Taken together, these studies with AVP vascular antagonists have advanced to the understanding of the role AVP has in the blood pressure regulation in hypotensive states and the vascular interaction between AVP with the renin-angiotensin and the adrenergic systems in the circulatory homeostasis. The role of vasopressin in various hypertensive disorders is not as yet so clearly defined.

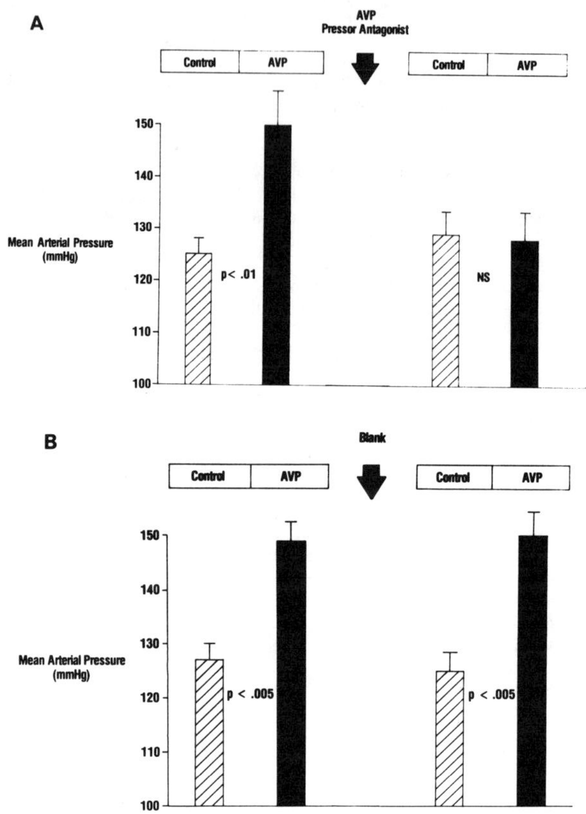

FIG. 2. Comparison of AVP pressor antagonist (A) and blank (B) on sequential pressor responses to AVP in the conscious rat. (Reproduced with permission of G. A. Aisenbrey, et al. [17])

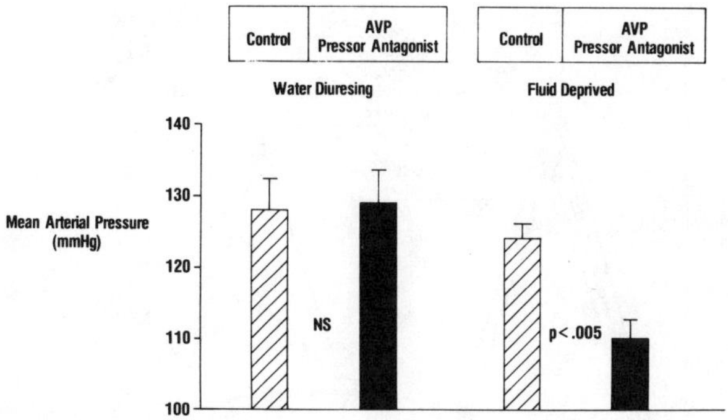

FIG. 3. Effect of AVP pressor antagonist on blood pressure in water diuresing (left two bars) and fluid deprived (right two bars) rats. (Reproduced with permission of G. A. Aisenbrey, et al. [17])

ANTAGONISTS AGAINST ANTIDIURETIC ACTION OF AVP

The antagonists of the antidiuretic effect of AVP have even more important therapeutic implications, since at present there is no specific treatment for the various pathological states of water retention. The development of the various AVP analogues initiated physiological and biochemical studies of these agents to understand better their mechanisms of action $d(CH_2)_5$Tyr(Et)VAVP was found to block completely the antidiuretic effect of exogenous AVP (Fig. 4) and endogenous AVP in the conscious rats (Fig. 5). This antagonistic effect of the antidiuretic action of AVP was not accompanied by changes in glomerular filtration rate, urinary solute excretion, and mean arterial pressure [23]. The antagonist also showed a short lived (10 min) agonist effect and urinary osmolality initially increased [23].

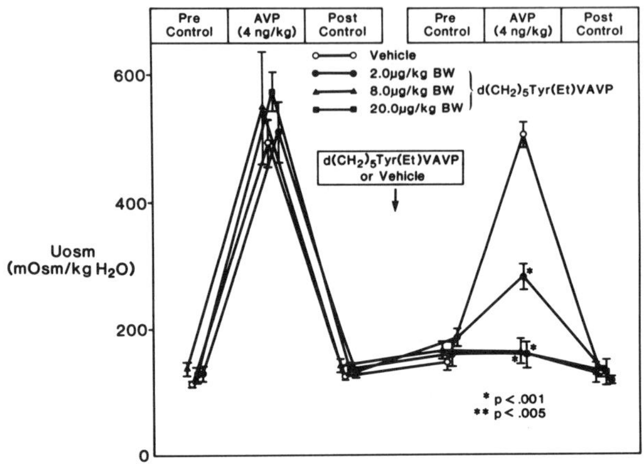

FIG. 4. The response of urinary osmolality (Uosm) to exogenous AVP in the presence and absence of $d(CH_2)_5)Tyr(Et)VAVP$. Values plotted for AVP periods represent means of the highest Uosm observed in 4 minute urine collections (n=6 in each group). (Reproduced with permission of S. Ishikawa, et al. [23])

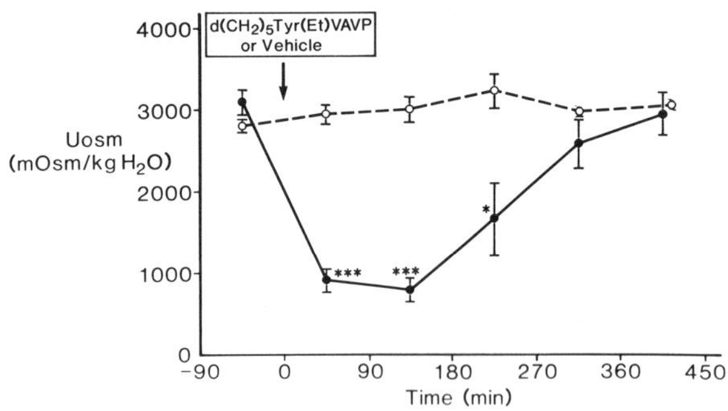

FIG. 5. The response of urinary osmolality (Uosm) to the intraperiotoneal administration of $d(CH_2)_5Tyr(Et)VAVP$ in rats after 24 hours of fluid deprivation (n=6 in experimental group and n=8 in control group). o---o Vehicle, •——• 30.0 μg/kg $d(CH_2)_5Tyr(Et)VAVP$; * p<.01, *** p<.001 (Reproduced with permission of S. Ishikawa, et al. [23])

There appears to be a species difference in the action of some of the antagonists. $d(CH_2)_5Tyr(Et)VAVP$ was found not to inhibit the antidiuretic action of AVP in dogs, however, $d(CH_2)_5D\text{-}Tyr(Et)VAVP$ completely blocked the hydroosmotic response to AVP in conscious dogs [22]. In the in vitro studies, the effect of $d(CH_2)_5Tyr(Et)VAVP$ was examined on adenylate cyclase stimulation by AVP in the isolated tubules from rats. The antagonist inhibited the stimulation of adenylate cyclase by AVP but not by any other hormones, thus suggesting the antagonist is a specific inhibitor of AVP action [21]. Further studies in the isolated, perfused rabbit cortical collecting tubule demonstrated that the enhanced net water flux induced by AVP was completely blocked by this AVP antagonist [21]. $d(CH_2)_5D\text{-}Tyr(Et)VAVP$ also has been shown to diminish adenylate cyclase activation by AVP in the renal membranes from several different species [19]. In spite of the species differences in the action of the various AVP antagonists, the recent observation that $d(CH_2)_5Tyr(Et)VAVP$ inhibited the adenylate cyclase activation by AVP in the isolated papillary collecting tubules from human is encouraging [28]. Thus, the potential clinical application of thes antagonists against the hydroosmotic response of AVP is promising. In this regard, it has been recently demonstrated that $d(CH_2)_5Tyr(Et)VAVP$ significantly reverses the water retention associated with glucocorticoid (Fig. 6) and mineralocorticoid (Fig. 7) deficiency in rats [20].

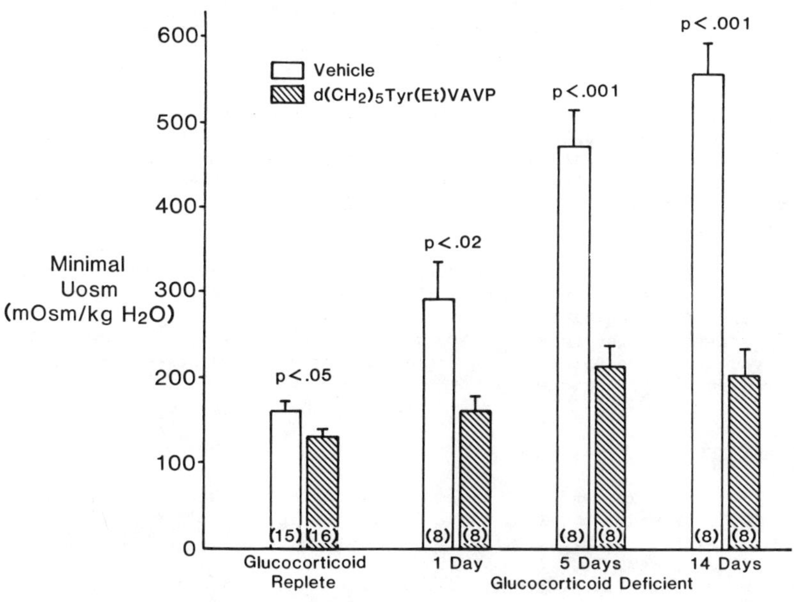

FIG. 6. Effect of the AVP antagonist (hatched bars) and vehicle (open bars) on urinary dilution as assessed by minimal urinary osmolality (Uosm) in response to an acute oral water load in glucocorticoid replete rats and after 1, 5, and 14 days of glucocorticoid deficiency. Values indicate mean ± SEM. (Reproduced with permission of S. Ishikawa, et al. [20])

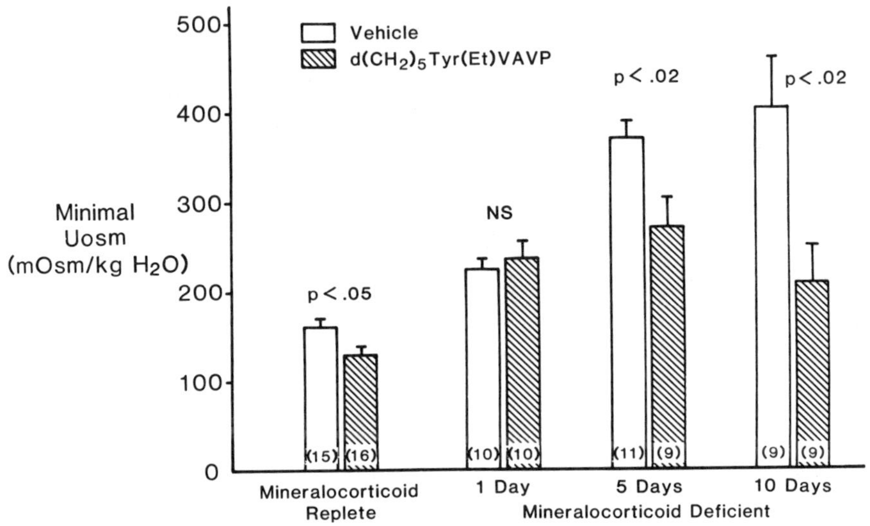

FIG. 7. Effect of the AVP antagonist (hatched bars) and vehicle (open bars) on urinary dilution as assessed by minimal urinary osmolality (Uosm) in response to an acute oral water load in mineralocorticoid replete rats and after 1, 5, and 10 days of mineralocorticoid deficiency. Values indicate mean ± SEM. (Reproduced with permission of J. Boykin, et al. [7])

In summary, the recent development of specific vasopressin antagonists for the vasopressor and antidiuretic actions of vasopressin has provided further understanding of vascular role of vasopressin in the circulatory homeostasis and the role of vasopressin in water retaining states. Both the vascular antagonists and hydroosmotic antagonists have promising therapeutic implications.

REFERENCES

1. W.R. Skowsky, and D.A. Fisher. Endocrinology 100, 1022-1026 (1977).
2. W.R. Skowsky, and T.A. Kikuchi. Am. J. Med. 64, 613-621 (1978).
3. D. Bichet, V. Szatalowicz, C. Chaimovitz, and R.W. Schrier. Ann. Intern. Med. 96, 413-417 (1982).
4. D. Bichet, V.J. Van Putten, and R.W. Schrier. N. Engl. J. Med. 307, 1552-1557 (1982).
5. S.L. Linas, R.J. Anderson, S.J. Guggenheim, G.L. Robertson, and T. Berl. Kidney Int. 20, 173-180 (1981).
6. J. Boykin, A. de Torrente, G. Robertson, A. Erickson and R.W. Schrier. Mineral Electrolyte Metab. 2, 310-315 (1979).
7. J. Boykin, A. de Torrente, A. Erickson, G. Robertson, and R.W. Schrier. J. Clin. Invest. 62, 738-744 (1978).

8. S.L. Linas, T. Berl, G.L. Robertson, G.A. Aisenbrey, R.W. Schrier, and R.J. Anderson. Kidney Int. 18, 58-67 (1980).
9. V.L. Szatalowicz, P.A. Arnold, C. Chaimovitz, D. Bichet, T. Berl, and R.W. Schrier. N. Engl. J. Med. 305, 263-266 (1981).
10. K. Bankowski, and M. Manning. J. Med. Chem. 21, 850-853 (1978).
11. J. Lowbridge, and M. Manning. J. Med. Chem. 21, 313-315 (1978).
12. M. Kruszynski, B. Lammek, M. Manning, J. Seto, J. Haldar, and W.H. Sawyer. J. Med. Chem. 23, 364-368 (1980).
13. M. Manning, A. Olma, W.A. Klis, A.M. Kolodziejczyk, J. Seto, and W.H. Sawyer. J. Med. Chem. 25, 45-50 (1982).
14. W.H. Sawyer, P.K.T. Pang, J. Seto, M. McEnroe, B. Lammek, and M. Manning. Science 212, 49-51 (1981).
15. M. Manning, B. Lammek, A.M. Kolodziezczyk, J. Seto, and W.H. Sawyer. J. Med. Chem. 24, 701-706 (1981).
16. J. Schwartz, and I.A. Reid. Endocrinology 109, 1778-1780 (1981).
17. G.A. Aisenbrey, W.A. Handelman, P. Arnold, M. Manning, and R.W. Schrier. J. Clin. Invest. 67, 961-968 (1981).
18. C.C.Y. Pang. Am. J. Physiol. 245, H749-H755 (1983).
19. F.L. Stassen, R.W. Erickson, W.F. Huffman, J. Stefankiewicz, L. Sulat, and V.D. Wiebelhaus. J. Pharmacol. Exp. Ther. 223, 50-54 (1982).
20. S. Ishikawa, and R.W. Schrier. Kidney Int. 22, 587-598 (1982).
21. J.K. Kim, M. Dillingham, S. Summer, and R.W. Schrier. Proc. Am. Soc. Nephrol. (1983) pp. 167A.
22. L.B. Kinter, W. Mann, G. Heckman, W. Huffman, M. Gross, and F. Stassen. Proc. Am. Soc. Nephrol. (1983) pp. 167A.
23. S. Ishikawa, J.K. Kim, and R.W. Schrier. Am. J. Physiol. in press, (1984).
24. W.H. Sawyer, and M. Manning. Fed. Proc. 43, 87-90 (1984).
25. R.W. Schrier, T. Berl, and R.J. Anderson. Am. J. Physiol. 236, F321-F332 (1979).
26. A.W. Cowley, Jr., S.J. Switzer, and M.M. Quinn. Circ. Res. 46, 58-65 (1980).
27. S. Ishikawa, and R.W. Schrier. Am. J. Physiol. 246, H104-H113 (1984).
28. J.K. Kim, S.N. Summer, and R.W. Schrier. (unpublished observation).

MOLECULAR PHARMACOLOGY AND MECHANISMS OF ACTION OF AQUARETIC AGENTS

FRANS L. STASSEN,* BARRY B. BERKOWITZ,** WILLIAM F. HUFFMAN,***
VIRGIL D. WIEBELHAUS,** AND LEWIS B. KINTER**
Departments of Molecular Pharmacology,* Pharmacology,** and Medicinal Chemistry,*** Smith Kline & French Laboratories, Philadelphia, PA 19101

ABSTRACT

We have previously reported that the novel water diuretic ("aquaretic") vasopressin analogs discovered by Manning and Sawyer [1,2] are potent competitive inhibitors of activation of renal adenylate cyclase by vasopressin. The antagonists appear to act only at the vasopressin receptor. Other components of the adenylate cyclase system are not affected [3]. In the present study we evaluated the relationship between the *in vivo* aquaretic potency and the *in vitro* antagonism at the renal vasopressin receptors. We found that the aquaretic potency of a series of vasopressin antagonists in conscious hydropenic rats directly correlated with antagonism of adenylate cyclase activation in medullary membranes of rat kidney. There was no correlation between the aquaretic potency and antagonism of vasopressin-induced contraction of rat thoracic aorta (antipressor activity). We conclude that in hydropenic rats the aquaretic activity of vasopressin analogs was primarily due to antagonism of vasopressin at the renal epithelial receptors. Antagonism of vasopressin at the vascular receptors appears to play no major role in the aquaretic effect. In addition, the rank order of *in vitro* potency of vasopressin antagonists differed among species, indicating different recognition patterns of the renal vasopressin receptors for antagonists. This observation points to the importance of the study of human renal tissue in the discovery of aquaretic agents.

INTRODUCTION

Excessive body water is currently being treated with diuretic agents. Conventional diuretics (saluretics) promote the excretion of water indirectly by stimulating renal salt excretion. Such treatment can cause potentially dangerous salt depletion (hyponatremia and hypokalemia). Another class of diuretic agents (including demeclocycline and Li salts) have been used to selectively enhance water excretion (water diuretics or aquaretic agents). These agents interfere with the action of the antidiuretic hormone, vasopressin. While having serious side effects, demeclocycline and Li salts illustrate the potential therapeutic utility of drugs which selectively block vasopressin-stimulated renal water reabsorption.

In the kidney, vasopressin is thought to work by increasing the water permeability of the collecting ducts through interaction with specific receptors in the baso-lateral plasma membranes of the epithelial cells [5]. The binding leads to activation of adenylate cyclase, resulting in

Diuretics, Jules B. Puschett, Editor

increased formation and accumulation of intracellular cyclic AMP [cAMP; 5,6,7,8]. The elevated level of cAMP induces increased water permeability of the apical membranes [9,10], thus allowing water to move along the osmotic gradient from the lumen of the collecting duct to the renal interstitium and back into the circulation.

Recently, Manning _et al_. [1] and Sawyer _et al_. [2] discovered several vasopressin analogs which antagonize vasopressin-stimulated antidiuresis _in vivo_. These analogs are modifications primarily at position 2 of the vasopressin analog $d(CH_2)_5$VDAVP. We have previously shown that the new aquaretic agents have a high affinity for renal vasopressin binding sites and specifically inhibit vasopressin-stimulated adenylate cyclase in plasma membranes prepared from renal medulla [3]. We have also demonstrated that blockade of the vasopressin receptor with the analogs does not impair the other components of the adenylate cyclase system, including the cyclase unit and the putative regulatory protein. We have also characterized the pharmacological activity of several vasopressin analogs in rats, dogs, and primates [4,17,18,19,21,22]. However, the linkage between analog-associated vasopressin antagonist activity _in vitro_ and aquaretic potency _in vivo_ has not been directly demonstrated. In this paper, we will describe the relationship between the affinity and antagonism at the renal vasopressin receptors _in vitro_ and the aquaretic activity _in vivo_, employing a series of vasopressin analogs. We report that in rats a close correlation existed between antagonist potency _in vitro_ and aquaretic potency _in vivo_. Analog-associated antipressor potency was not correlated with aquaretic potency. In addition, by comparing the _in vitro_ rank order of antagonist potency of vasopressin analogs for adenylate cyclase activation of pig, rat, and human kidney, we found marked species differences in the recognition patterns of the renal vasopressin receptors.

MATERIALS AND METHODS

Preparation of Renal Medullary Membranes

Plasma membranes were prepared from carefully dissected medullary tissue of pig, rat, and human kidney as described elsewhere [3]. Human renal medulla was obtained from unmatched transplant kidneys.

Vasopressin Binding and Adenylate Cyclase Activity

Binding of ^{3}H-lysine vasopressin (LVP) and adenylate cyclase activity were measured using renal medullary membranes according to the methods published previously [3]. The affinity of the compounds for the vasopressin receptor was determined in competitive radioligand binding assays and expressed as a K_{bind}. The antagonist potency for inhibition of adenylate cyclase activation by vasopressin was expressed as a K_i. K_i and K_{bind} were both calculated from the equations for competitive inhibition put forth by Cheng and Prusoff [11].

Aquaretic Activity

The aquaretic potency of vasopressin analogs administered intraperitoneally was determined in hydropenic rats [4,19]. The aquaretic activity was expressed as the ED_{300} or ED_{10}, where the ED_{10} is the dose required to increase urine flow to 10 ml/kg/4 hr, and the ED_{300} is the dose required to decrease the urine osmolality from hydropenic levels ($>$1200 mOsmoles/kg) to 300 mOsmoles/kg.

Antivasopressor Activity

Antagonism of vasopressin-induced vasoconstriction was measured *in vitro* using rings of rat thoracic aorta as described by Berkowitz *et al.* [12]. The antipressor potency was expressed as a pA2 value.

Protein Determination

Protein was measured with the Folin reagent [13] and bovine serum albumin was the standard.

Statistical Evaluation

Experimental values were reported as the mean ± S.E.M. Two means are considered different if $P < 0.05$ by nonpaired Student's *t* test.

Materials

The sources of the reagents, vasopressin, and the radioligand were described previously [3,4]. The structures of the vasopressin antagonists were $d(CH_2)_5$Tyr(Me)AVP, [1-ß-mercapto-ß,ß-cyclopentamethylenepropionic acid),2-(O-methyl)tyrosine,8-arginine]vasopressin, SK&F 100273; $d(CH)_2)_5$Tyr(Et)VAVP, [1-ß-mercapto-ß,ß-cyclopentamethylenepropionic acid),2-(O-ethyl)tyrosine,4-valine,8-arginine] vasopressin, SK&F 100398; $d(CH_2)_5$D-TyrVAVP, [1-(ß-mercapto-ß, ß-cyclopentamethylenepropionic acid,2-D-tyrosine,4-valine,8-arginine] vasopressin, SK&F 100885; $d(CH_2)_5$D-PheVAVP, [1-(ß-mercapto-ß, ß-cyclopentamethylenepropionic acid),2-D-phenylalanine,4-valine,8-arginine]vasopressin, SK&F 101071; $d(CH_2)_5$D-Tyr(Et)VAVP, [1-(ß-mercapto-ß,ß-cyclopentamethylenepropionic acid)2-D-(O-ethyl) tyrosine,4-valine,8-arginine]vasopressin, SK&F 101498.

RESULTS AND DISCUSSION

Identification of Renal Vasopressin Receptors

Typical competitive inhibition of specific ^{3}H-LVP binding to medullary membranes of pig kidney by vasopressin antagonists is shown in Fig. 1. The vasopressin analogs were also competitive inhibitors of vasopressin-stimulated adenylate cyclase as exemplified by the parallel displacement of the vasopressin dose-response curves and no change in maximal activity using pig and human renal membranes (Fig. 2).

The correlation of analog affinity (K_{bind}) for the renal vasopressin binding sites and antagonist potency (K_i) for inhibition of adenylate cyclase activation in pig renal tissue is presented in Fig. 3. Data of 35 vasopressin antagonists are shown. The close correlation between the K_{bind} and K_i (r=0.93) over a range of three orders of magnitude indicated that the specific binding sites identified with the radioligand are the vasopressin receptors which mediate stimulation of adenylate cyclase activity [V_2 receptors; 14].

The vasopressin antagonists were judged selective for vasopressin receptors because the analogs did not affect the activation of renal adenylate cyclase by ß-adrenergic agents and prostaglandins E_1, E_2, and I_2 [3]. We have also previously shown that the antagonists did not impair other components of the adenylate cyclase system such as the cyclase unit or the putative guanine nucleotide regulatory protein, because these compounds did not alter basal enzyme activity and the activity stimulated by guanyl-5'-yl imidiphosphate and NaF [3].

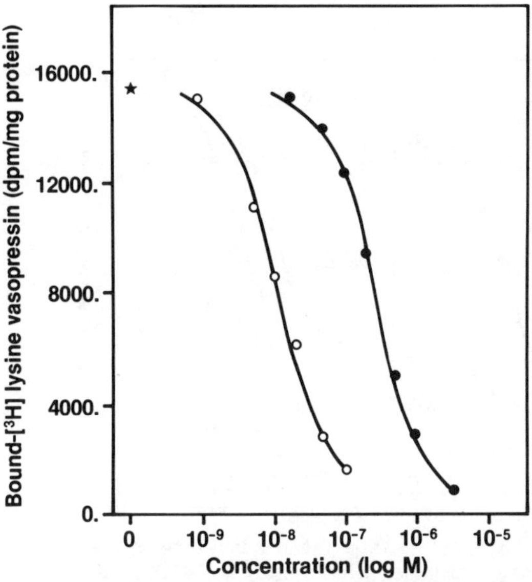

FIG. 1. Inhibition of ^{3}H-LVP binding to pig kidney membranes by SK&F 100398. Means of triplicate determinations are indicated. The individual values did not differ from the mean by more than 5%. ○, LVP; ●, SK&F 100398; ✱, bound ^{3}H-LVP in the absence of cold ligand. The concentration of ^{3}H-LVP was 7.0 x 10^{-9} M. K_{bind} LVP is 4.6 x 10^{-9}M; K_{bind} SK&F 100398 is 1.0 x 10^{-7}M. [From Stassen *et al*., 3]

Molecular Mechanisms of Aquaretic Activity

Vasopressin analogs have previously been reported by us [3] and others [2] to produce water diuresis (aquaresis) and to antagonize vasopressin-associated antidiuresis in experimental animals. The correlation of analog-associated *in vivo* aquaretic potency (expressed as the ED_{300}, Fig. 4A or the ED_{10}, Fig. 4B) in hydropenic rats and *in vitro* vasopressin antagonist potency (K_i) values in rat renal medullary membranes is presented in Fig. 4. Data of eight vasopressin analogs are shown. The close correlation (r=0.96 and 0.93 for ED_{300} and ED_{10}, respectively) between the *in vivo* and *in vitro* potencies supported the hypothesis that the analog-associated aquaretic activity was the result of inhibition of vasopressin at the renal epithelial receptor.

Antivasopressor Activity of Vasopressin Antagonists

Vasopressin analogs have also been reported to inhibit vasopressin-associated increases in arterial pressure [20]. Analog-associated relaxation of vasopressin-mediated contraction of vascular smooth muscle was studied *in vitro* using rat thoracic aortic rings (Table I). The rank orders of the antivasopressor potencies (pA2) and the aquaretic potencies were unrelated. These data confirmed that the vascular smooth muscle and renal epithelial activities of vasopressin were mediated by receptors of different subtypes (V1, vasopressor receptor; V2, antidiuretic hormone receptor; 14). The data show that the analog-associated antivasopressor activity is not likely to play a major role in the analog-induced aquaresis.

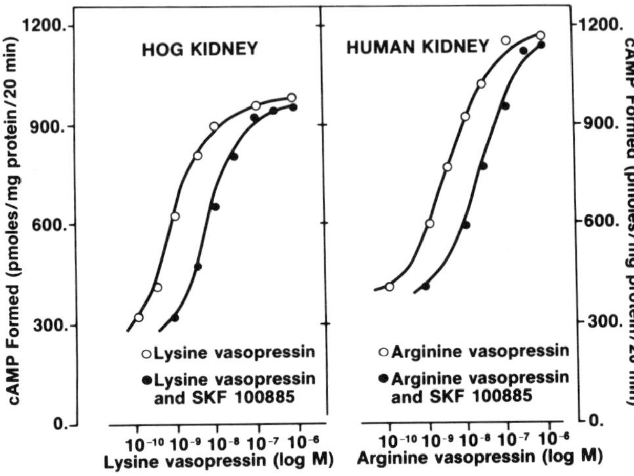

FIG. 2. Inhibition of vasopressin-stimulated adenylate cyclase of medullary membranes of pig and human kidney by 2 x 10^{-7}M SK&F 100885. Means of triplicate determinations are indicated. The individual values did not differ from the mean by more than 5%. K_{act} was 8.7 x 10^{-10}M and 3.4 x 10^{-9}M for LVP and AVP, respectively. K_i of SK&F 100885 was 3.0 x 10^{-8}M and 1.9 x 10^{-8}M for pig and human kidney, respectively.

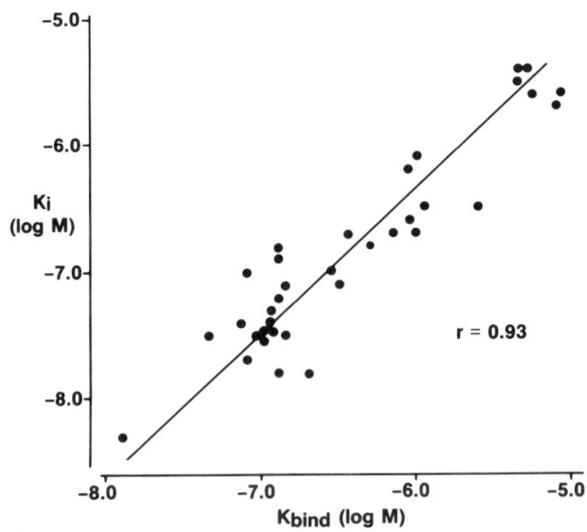

FIG. 3. Correlation between the affinity (K_{bind}) for vasopressin binding sites and the antagonist potency (K_i) for adenylate cyclase activation of 35 vasopressin antagonists using pig renal membranes. Means of triplicate determinations are presented.

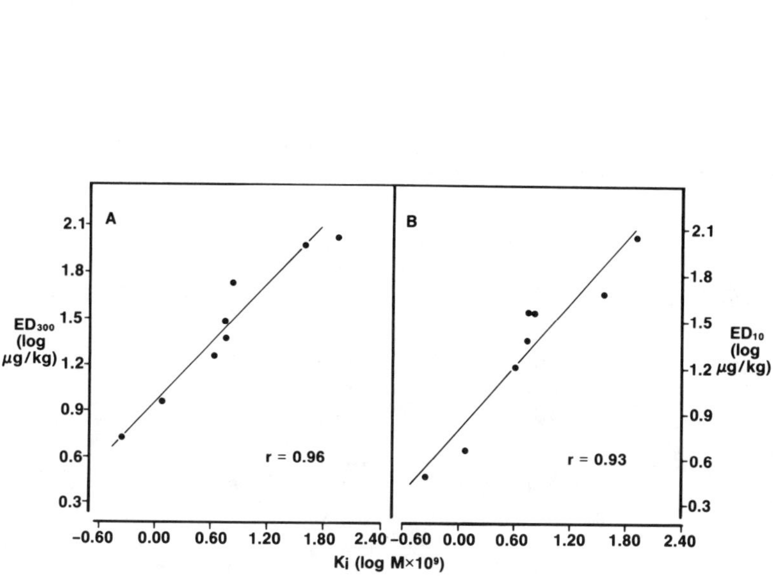

FIG. 4. Correlation between antagonist potency of vasopressin-stimulated adenylate cyclase of membranes of rat kidney and aquaretic potency in hydropenic rats of eight vasopressin antagonists. Aquaretic potency was expressed as the ED_{300} (A) or ED_{10} (B).

TABLE I. Aquaretic potency and antagonism of vasopressin-induced vasoconstriction by vasopressin analogs in rats.

SK&F #	Antivasopressor Activity[a] (pA_2)	Aquaretic Activity[b] (ED_{300})
100273	10.58	> 2600.
101926	9.40	4.7 ± 0.6 (9)
101498	9.12	7.7 ± 0.6 (8)
100885	8.81	48.8 ± 9.7 (2)
101071	8.58	18.3 ± 2.4 (15)

[a]Mean value of 4 observations. [b]Mean value ± S.E.M. (nmoles/kg, i.p.); ( ) number of determinations.

Species Differences in Antagonist Potency of Vasopressin Analogs

Manning *et al.* [15,16] identified $d(CH_2)_5$D-PheVAVP (SK&F 101071) as the most potent renal antagonist of vasopressin administered to ethanol-anesthetized, water-loaded rats. In our *in vitro* studies using rat, pig, and human kidney membranes, and in *in vivo* studies with conscious hydropenic rats, SK&F 101071 and $d(CH_2)_5$Tyr(Et)VAVP (SK&F 100398) exhibited similar potencies, while $d(CH_2)_5$D-Tyr(Et)VAVP (SK&F 101498) was 5- to 10-fold more potent [Table II; 17,18]. The analog SK&F 101926 was significantly more potent than SK&F 101498. The differences in potency might be related to altered responses in ethanol-anesthetized animals, where, in contrast to conscious hydropenic animals, the non-renal activities might play more prevalent roles. These activities could be the antivasopressor activity and possible effects on vasopressin secretion. It is notable that SK&F 101498 was also a more potent vasopressin antagonist and aquaretic agent than SK&F 101071 in dog renal medullary membranes *in vitro* [18], and in conscious dogs [18,21] and squirrel monkeys *in vivo*.

TABLE II. Rank order of vasopressin analogs according to antagonist potency of vasopressin-stimulated adenylate cyclase of rat, pig, and human kidney.

	Antagonist Potency (Ki x 10^9 M^{-1})		
SK&F #	Rat	Pig	Man
101926	0.4*	3.0*	2.3**
101498	1.2	5.9	4.4
100398	5.6	32.0	25.0
101071	5.9	47.0	23.0
100885	6.8	30.0	16.0
101216	55.0	1100.0	3200.0
101230	83.8	2260.0	1830.0
88864	91.0	230.0	ND
101505	100.0	4000.0	1100.0
100273	220.0	210.0	300.0

Mean values of at least two determinations in triplicate are presented. SK&F 101926 is significantly more potent than SK&F 101498 (*$p < 0.005$; **$p < 0.025$).

The rank order of potency of 10 vasopressin antagonists of adenylate cyclase activation was determined for rat, pig, and human kidney (Table II). At concentrations of up to 10^{-4} M, these analogs did not significantly stimulate basal enzyme activity (data not shown). The data show that each species rank-ordered the potency of the analogs differently. It is notable, however, that SK&F 101498 and 101926 are the most potent analogs in all species tested. We concluded that the recognition patterns of renal vasopressin receptors for vasopressin antagonists is different in different species. Therefore, analysis of the activity at human renal vasopressin receptors will be very helpful in the discovery of agents with aquaretic activity in man.

From these studies we conclude that the aquaretic activity of the vasopressin antagonists was primarily due to inhibition of the vasopressin-associated antidiuretic activity at the renal vasopressin receptors. The molecular mechanism involved inhibition of vasopressin-stimulated adenylate cyclase caused by blockade of vasopressin binding. The antagonists appeared selective for vasopressin receptors. They affected the binding site and no other components of the adenylate cyclase system. The recognition pattern of the renal vasopressin receptors for antagonists differed among species. Therefore, caution must be exercised in applying structure-activity data from one species to another.

ACKNOWLEDGEMENTS

We wish to thank G. Heckman, J. McDonald, D. Schmidt, D. Shue, J. Stefankiewicz, L. Sulat, and B. Zabko-Potapovich for their expert technical assistance and F. Ali, W. Bryan, J. Callahan, M. Moore, J. Silvestri, and N. Yim for the synthesis of the vasopressin analogs. Special thanks are due to S. Sammut and H. Nathan of the Delaware Valley Transplant Program for the procurement of outdated transplant kidneys. We are grateful to L. Steele for the professional preparation of this manuscript.

REFERENCES

1. M. Manning, B. Lammek, A.M. Kolodziejczyk, J. Seto, and W.H. Sawyer, J. Med. Chem. 24, 701-706 (1981).
2. W.H. Sawyer, P.K.T. Pang, J. Seto, M. McEnroe, B. Lammek, and M. Manning, Science 212, 49-51 (1981).
3. F.L. Stassen, R.W. Erickson, W.F. Huffman, J. Stefankiewicz, L. Sulat, and V.D. Wiebelhaus, J. Pharm. Exp. Ther. 223, 50-54 (1982).
4. F.L. Stassen, W. Bryan, M. Gross, B. Kavanagh, D. Shue, L. Sulat, V.D. Wiebelhaus, N. Yim, and L.B. Kinter, in: The Neurohypophsis Structure and Control, Progress in Brain Research, B.A. Cross and G.L. Leng, eds. (Elsevier, New York 1983) pp. 395-403.
5. J. Bockaert, C. Roy, R. Rajerison, and S. Jard, J. Biol. Chem. 248, 5922-5931 (1973).
6. W.A. Anderson Jr. and E. Brown, Biochim. Biophys. Acta 67, 674-676 (1963).
7. E. Brown, D.W. Clarke, V. Roux, and G.H. Sherman, J. Biol. Chem. 238, PC852-853 (1963).
8. F. Morel, D. Chabardès, and M. Imbert-Teboul, Proc. VII Int. Congr. Nephrol. pp. 209-216 (1978).
9. J. Orloff and J.S. Handler, J. Clin. Invest. 41, 702-709 (1962).
10. J.J. Grantham and M.B. Burg, Am. J. Physiol. 211, 255-259 (1966).
11. Y.C. Cheng and W.H. Prusoff, Biochem. Pharmacol. 22, 3099-3108 (1973).
12. B.B. Berkowitz, B. Zabko-Potapovich, and R. Valocik (in preparation).
13. O.H. Lowry, N.J. Rosebrough, A.L. Farr, and R.J. Randall, J. Biol. Chem. 193, 265-276 (1951).
14. R.H. Michel, C.J. Kirk, and M.J. Billah, Biochem. Soc. Trans. 7, 861 (1979).
15. M. Manning, A. Olma, W.A. Klis, A. Kolodziejczyk, J. Seto, and W.H. Sawyer, J. Med. Chem. 25, 45-50 (1982).
16. M. Manning, W.A. Klis, A. Olma, J. Seto, and W.H. Sawyer, J. Med. Chem. 25, 414-419 (1982).
17. F.L. Stassen, G. Heckman, W. Huffman, J. Stefankiewicz, L. Sulat, and S.T. Crooke, Fed. Proc. (1984, in press).
18. F.L. Stassen, G. Heckman, W.F. Huffman, and L.B. Kinter (in preparation).
19. L.B. Kinter, W.F. Huffman, V. Wiebelhaus, and F.L. Stassen, (1984) these proceedings.
20. M. Manning, B. Lammek, M. Kruszynski, J. Seto, and W.H. Sawyer, J. Med. Chem. 25, 408-414 (1982).
21. L.B. Kinter, W. Mann, G. Heckman, W. Huffman, M. Gross, and F.L. Stassen, Kidney Intl., 25 (1984; in press).
22. L.B. Kinter, F.L. Stassen, E. Horner, V.D. Wiebelhaus, and N. Yim, Kidney Intl., 23, 259 (1983).

RENAL EFFECTS OF AQUARETIC VASOPRESSIN ANALOGS *IN VIVO*

L.B. KINTER,* W.F. HUFFMAN,** V.D. WIEBELHAUS,* and F.L. STASSEN***
Departments of Pharmacology,* Molecular Pharmacology,*** and Medicinal Chemistry,** Smith Kline and French Laboratories, Philadelphia, PA 19101

ABSTRACT

Vasopressin is the primary physiological factor regulating renal water reabsorption. Inhibitors of vasopressin-stimulated water reabsorption have previously been used as water diuretic agents in both experimental animals and man. The present studies describe and characterize the pharmacological activities of specific vasopressin structural analogs on renal water and solute excretion in conscious rats. The analogs tested produced dose-dependent increases in renal water excretion in conscious hydropenic rats and antagonize in a competitive fashion exogenous vasopressin-stimulated antidiuresis in conscious water-loaded rats. The analogs tested diluted urine osmolality levels from >1600 mOsm/kg H_2O to levels <100 mOsm/kg H_2O. Only modest increases in analog-associated urinary solute excretion were observed. The most potent analogs were those having D-Tyr (alkyl) substitutions at position 2. We conclude that the analogs tested were potent water diuretic (aquaretic) agents. The mechanism of action is most probably antagonism of vasopressin at the renal epithelial receptor. Such vasopressin antagonists herald a new class of potent aquaretic agents potentially useful for the treatment of clinical conditions and pathologies characterized by excessive body water and/or inappropriate secretion of vasopressin.

INTRODUCTION

Diuretics form a large class of important therapeutic agents useful in the treatment of volume expanded states resulting from cardiovascular and renal pathologies or disease processes [1]. Conventional diuretic agents interfere with renal salt reabsorption, resulting in greatly increased renal salt loss [1]. Water lost as a result of these "saluretics" is that required to excrete the excess urinary solute. Loss of salt in excess of water can result in potentially dangerous hyponatremia.

Several groups have sought to describe new diuretic agents which would allow excretion of water, in excess of solute, as a treatment for hyponatremic states. Demeclocycline and lithium carbonate appear to interfere with vasopressin-stimulated renal water reabsorption and will produce a positive free-water clearance [2,3]. However, both agents have slow onsets of action, serious toxic liabilities, and poorly understood mechanisms of action [4].

Drs. Manning and Sawyer and their colleagues have recently reported vasopressin analogs having intrinsic vasopressin-antagonist activity in anesthetized rats [5-9]. We have previously shown that these diuretic analogs have high affinity for renal vasopressin binding sites and specifically antagonize renomedullary vasopressin-stimulated adenylate cyclase [10]. In this paper we will describe and characterize the activity of vasopressin antagonists on renal water and solute excretion in conscious

Diuretics, Jules B. Puschett, Editor

rats. The results show that vasopressin antagonist are potent and specific water-losing (aquaretic) agents in conscious rats. Only minimal effects on renal solute excretion were observed. Aquaresis associated with these agents can be used to selectively remove excess body water *in vivo*.

METHODS AND MATERIALS

General Methods

Male laboratory rats (Charles River CD strain, MA), and Brattleboro strain rats [11,12] heterozygous (+/-) and homozygous (-/-) for central diabetes insipidus (vasopressin-deficient rats, Blue Spruce Farms, NY) weighing 150-250 g were fasted (food and water) 18 hr prior to the experiment (hydropenia), or were allowed food and water *ad libitum* (control). On the morning of the experiment, rats were brought into the laboratory, weighed, and dosed with test substances. Vasopressin analogs were given intraperitoneally (0.1 to 100 ug/rat). Vasopressin was administered intramuscularly in a freshly prepared oil:water emulsion (50:1; 10 to 1000 ng/kg). Water loads were administered orally (5% bw). All rats were housed in stainless suspension-type metabolism cages that were scrupulously cleaned and rinsed to remove foreign solutes (4 rats/cage). Metabolism pans were treated with vegetable oil spray (PAM, Boyle-Midway, Inc., NY) to facilitate urine collection. Urine was collected at 30 to 60 min intervals for 4 hr. Samples of trunk blood were collected after decapitation in chilled tubes containing heparin (143 USP units/10 ml). Plasma was separated immediately by centrifugation at $4^{o}C$ and aliquots were analyzed for osmolality or stored frozen for subsequent measurement of vasopressin levels by specific radioimmunoassay.

Hydropenic Rats

The activity of vasopressin analogs against endogenous vasopressin was studied in conscious hydropenic rats. Groups of hydropenic rats were treated with vehicle or increasing doses of analog. Dose response relationships for diuresis and dilution of urine osmolality (Uosm) were developed. Potencies were expressed as effective doses (ED, nmoles/kg) required to increase urine flow (V) by 10 ml/kg in 4 hr (ED_{10}) and to dilute Uosm to 300 mOsm (ED_{300}), respectively.

Water-Loaded Rats

The activity of vasopressin analogs against exogenous vasopressin was studied in conscious water-loaded, vasopressin-loaded rats. Groups of hydropenic rats were given oral water loads (to suppress endogenous AVP), a fixed dose of vasopressin analog, and increasing doses of vasopressin. Agonist dose response relationships were developed in the absence and presence of antagonist. Antagonist potencies were evaluated as the apparent inhibition constant (Ki) according to methods developed by Cheng and Prusoff [13].

Experimental Hyponatremia

The activity of the vasopressin analog $d(CH_2)_5$D-TyrVAVP to reverse experimental hyponatremia was studied in conscious water-loaded, vasopressin-loaded rats. In these studies, groups of rats were given an oral water load, vehicle or vasopressin (150 ng, ip), and $d(CH_2)_5$D-TyrVAVP (200 ug/rat, ip). Groups of animals were sacrificed (decapitation) at 30 min intervals and samples of trunk blood were analyzed for osmolality.

Analytic Procedures

Plasma and urine osmolality were determined on fresh samples using the micro freezing point depression method (Precision Systems, Model 5004). Samples of urine were stored frozen for solute analysis. Na, K, creatinine and urea were determined on thawed well-mixed urine samples by standard autoanalyzer techniques. Plasma levels of vasopressin were determined according to methods described in [14].

Statistical Determinations

Mean values for multiple measurements are expressed ± standard error the mean (S.E.M.). Statistically significant differences ($p < .05$) between mean values have been assessed by application of the Student's *t* test.

Chemicals

Vasopressin was purchased from Bachem (Torrance, CA). The structures of the vasopressin antagonists were: d(CH_2)$_5$Tyr(Et)VAVP, [1-(ß-mercapto-ß,ß-cyclopentamethylenepropionic acid,2-(O-ethyl)tyrosine, 4-valine,8-arginine]vasopressin, SK&F 100398; d(CH_2)$_5$Tyr(Me)VAVP, [1-(ß-mercepto-ß,ß-cyclopentamethylenepropionic acid)2-(O-methyl)tyrosine, 4-valine,8-arginine]vasopressin, SK&F 100501; d(CH_2)$_5$D-TyrVAVP, [1-(ß-mercapto-ß,ß-cyclopentamethylenepropionic acid,2-D-tyrosine,4-valine, 8-arginine]vasopressin, SK&F 100885; d(CH_2)$_5$D-PheVAVP, [1-(ß-mercapto-ß-ß-cyclopentamethylenepropionic acid,2-D-phenylalanine,4-valine,8-arginine]vasopressin, SK&F 101071; d(CH_2)$_5$D-Tyr(Me)VAVP, [1-(ß-mercapto-ß-ß-cyclopentamethylenepropionic acid),2-D-(O-methyl)tyrosine, 4-valine,8-arginine]vasopressin, SK&F 101496; d(CH_2)$_5$D-Tyr(Et)VAVP, [1-(ß-mercapto-ß,ß-cyclopentamethylenepropionic acid)2-D-(O-ethyl)tyrosine, 4-valine,8-arginine]vasopressin, SK&F 101498; and d(CH_2)$_5$D-Tyr(n-Pr) VAVP, [1-(ß-mercapto-ß,ß-cyclopentamethylenepropionic acid)2-D-(O-n propyl)tyrosine,4-valine,8-argine]vasopressin, SK&F 101500. Samples of these analogs were obtained from Dr. M. Manning, and were prepared by SK&F Medicinal Chemists.

RESULTS

Endogenous Vasopressin Levels

The effect of hydropenia and water loading on endogenous plasma vasopressin levels was studied in control CD rats and Brattleboro strain rats heterozygous (+/-) and homozygous (-/-) for central diabetes insipidus (Fig. 1). Water-loading suppressed plasma vasopressin levels in both CD rats and +/- rats, compared to levels measured in the respective normally hydrated controls. Plasma vasopressin levels were undetectable in control and water-loaded vasopressin deficient (-/-) rats. Hydropenia stimulated plasma vasopressin levels in CD and +/- rats above levels measured in the respective controls. Hydropenia was also associated with a substantial level of immuno-reactive vasopressin-like material in the plasma of -/- rats. The nature of the material detected in -/- rat plasma was not determined.

Hydropenic Rats

The VP analogs tested increased urine flow in hydropenic rats in a dose-dependent fashion. Representative experiments are shown in Fig. 2. Onset was generally observed within 30 min. Maximal increases in urine flow (diuresis) occurred between 90 and 180 min following dosing. Urine flow rates during the 1st and 4th hr were always less than those during the 2nd and 3rd hr. The total urine excreted during the 4-hr test period in response to larger doses of analogs generally exceeded 25 ml/kg. Diuretic potency was estimated from the dose response relationships as the dose to increase urine flow rate 10 ml/kg above control vehicle-treated levels at the end of the 4-hr test period. Rank order of diuretic potency of VP analogs tested is listed in Table I. The most potent diuretic analogs were those with D-Tyr (alkyl) substitutions at position 2.

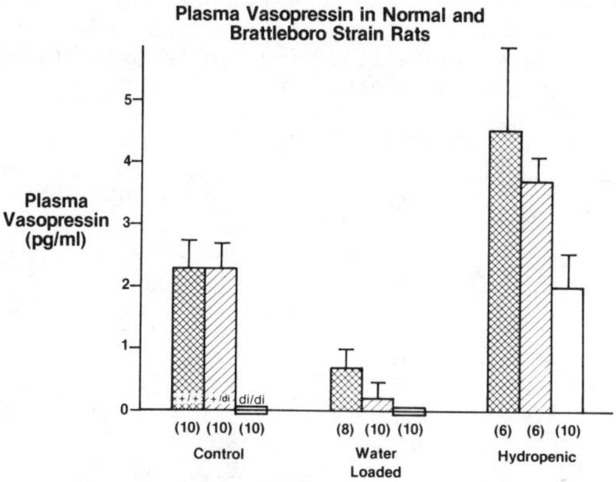

FIG. 1. Plasma vasopressin levels in normal and Brattleboro strain rats during water-loading and hydropenia.

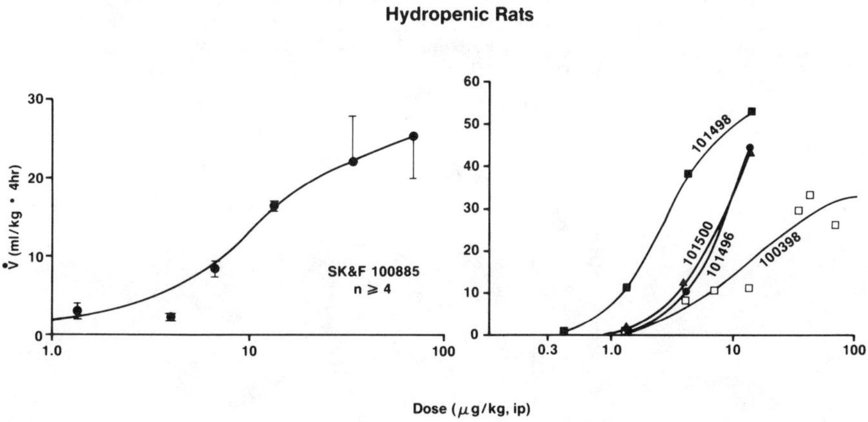

FIG. 2. Dose response of urine volume to vasopressin antagonists in hydropenic rats.

The VP analogs tested also decreased urine osmolality (Uosm) in a dose-dependent fashion (Fig. 3). Maximal dilution of urine occurred between 90 and 180 min following dosing and was associated with maximal increases in urine flow rate. Minimal levels of Uosm associated with larger doses of analogs were approximately 100 mOsm/kg H_2O. Potency to dilute urine in hydropenic rats was estimated from dose response relationships as the dose to dilute Uosm from hydropenic levels to a level of 300 mOsm/kg. The value of 300 mOsm was chosen because it approximates the value at which urine is isoosmotic to plasma and a net free-water clearance shifts from a net negative to net positive value. Rank order of aquaretic potency of tested analogs is presented in Table I. Aquaretic potency corresponded well with diuretic potency; the most potent analogs were again those with D-Tyr (alkyl) substitutions at position 2.

Urinary sodium, potassium, and urea excretion were slightly higher in hydropenic rats treated with antagonists as compared with either hydropenic or water-loaded controls (Table II). Creatinine excretion levels were not significantly affected by antagonist administration.

TABLE I. Summary of vasopressin antagonist potencies in the hydropenic rat.

Structure	n	Anti-ADH Activity: Urine Osmolality (ED_{300})	Anti-ADH Activity: Urine Volume (ED_{10})
		nmoles/kg	nmoles/kg
$d(CH_2)_5$D-Tyr(Et)VAVP	8	7.7 ± 0.6*	2.9 ± 0.3*
$d(CH_2)_5$D-Tyr(Me)VAVP	3	12.1 ± 3.9*	4.2 ± 1.0*
$d(CH_2)_5$D-PheVAVP	15	18.3 ± 2.4	10.7 ± 1.3
$d(CH_2)_5$Tyr(Et)VAVP	4	33.3 ± 13.0*	39.0 ± 5.0*
$d(CH_2)_5$D-TyrVAVP	4	50.1 ± 4.5*	23.8 ± 1.9*
$d(CH_2)_5$Tyr(Me)VAVP	2	123.0 ± 11.0*	76.0 ± 20.0*

Values are $\bar{X}$ ± S.E.M.; each determination (n) represents a full dose response relationship in hydropenic rats. ED_{300} and ED_{10} represent potencies to dilute Uosm from hydropenic levels to 300 mOsm/kg H_2O, and to increase urine flow by 10 ml/kg per 4 hr, respectively; *, $P < .01$ compared to $d(CH_2)_5$D-PheVAVP.

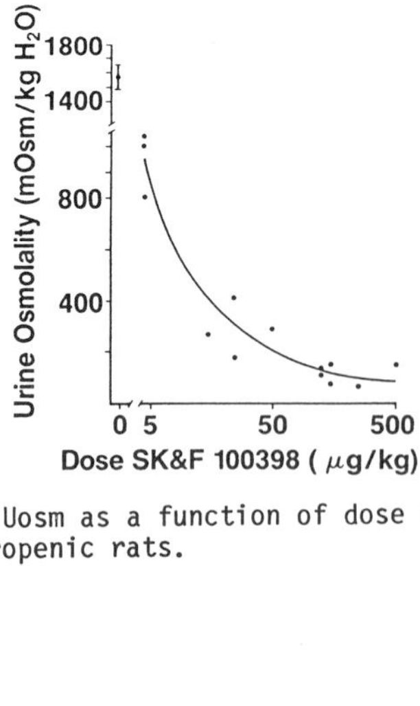

FIG. 3. Dilution of Uosm as a function of dose $d(CH_2)_5$Tyr(Et)VAVP (SK&F 100398) in hydropenic rats.

TABLE II: Summary of effects of vasopressin analogs or urinary solute excretion in conscious rats.

Structure	(n)	dose (ug/rat)	$U_{Na}V$	U_KV	$U_{urea}V$	$U_{Cr}V$
			(uEq/kg)		(mg/kg)	
Hydropenic Controls	(11)	0	0.78±.05	0.56±.03	207±16	4.4±.3
$d(CH_2)_5$D-Tyr(Et)VAVP	(5)	10	1.68±.25*+	1.09±.19*+	298±18*+	4.7±.5
$d(CH_2)_5$D-Tyr(Me)VAVP	(3)	10	1.16±.31*+	1.00±.12*+	258±19*	4.3±.5
$d(CH_2)_5$D-Phe-VAVP	(5)	10	1.56±.27*+	1.01±.14*+	250±14*	4.6±.4
$d(CH_2)_5$D-TyrVAVP	(5)	25	1.07±.15*+	0.72±.06*+	258±19*	4.3±.5
$d(CH_2)_5$Tyr(Et)VAVP	(5)	25	1.40±.17*+	0.65±.13*	234±36*	4.5±.6
$d(CH_2)_5$Tyr(Me)VAVP	(5)	25	1.47±.34*+	0.87±.16+	291±57*	4.7±.2
Water-loaded Controls	(11)	0	0.34±.06*	0.59±.04	240±14*	4.5±.3

Values are $\bar{x} \pm$ S.E.M.; doses selected to produce comparable high rates of urine flow; *, $p < .05$ compared to hydropenic controls; $^+$, $p < .05$ compared to water-loaded controls.

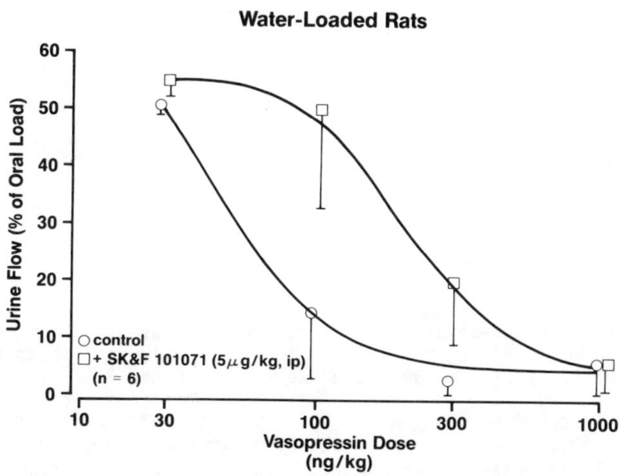

FIG. 4. Displacement of the vasopressin-stimulated antidiuresis dose response by $d(CH_2)_5$D-PheVAVP (SK&F 101071) in water-loaded rats.

Water-Loaded Rats

Analog antagonism of exogenously administered vasopressin was evaluated in groups of water-loaded rats given increasing doses of vasopressin (10-1000 ng/kg, im). In these studies, urine flow rate was expressed as the percentage of the water load excreted in 4 hr. A representative experiment is shown in Fig. 4. All analogs tested displaced the agonist dose response curve to the right in a parallel fashion. In some tests, analogs increased urine flow associated with sub-threshold vasopressin doses, suggesting that suppression of endogenous vasopressin in these studies was not complete.

Rank order of potency is presented in Table III. Potency of specific analogs to antagonize exogenously administered vasopressin corresponded well with the rank order of diuretic and aquaretic potency in hydropenic rats; the most potent analogs were again those with analogs D-Tyr (alkyl) substitutions at position 2.

Studies in Experimental Hyponatremia

The effect of $d(CH_2)_5$D-TyrVAVP to reverse hyponatremia associated with an experimental model of syndrome of inappropriate antidiuretic hormone (SIADH) was studied in conscious rats. Plasma osmolality was reduced from 312 to 297 mOsm/kg H_2O in rats given oral water loads plus exogenous vasopressin (150 ng/kg). $d(CH_2)_5$D-TyrVAVP administered to such hyponatremic rats rapidly produced the expected increase in excretion of urinary water and rapidly restored plasma osmolality toward control levels (Fig. 5).

TABLE III. Summary of vasopressin antagonist potencies in conscious water-loaded, vasopressin-infused rats.

SK&F #	n	Inhibition of AVP-Stimulated Antidiuresis (K_i)
		nmoles/kg
$d(CH_2)_5$D-Tyr(Et)VAVP	3	0.8 $\pm$ 0.2*
$d(CH_2)_5$D-Tyr(Me)VAVP	4	1.6 $\pm$ 0.4
$d(CH_2)_5$D-PheVAVP	4	3.1 $\pm$ 1.2
$d(CH_2)_5$D-TyrVAVP	4	9.9 $\pm$ 1.8*

Values are $\bar{x} \pm$ S.E.M.; each determination (n) represents duplicate dose response curves in the presence and absence of antagonist; *, $p < .01$ compared to $d(CH_2)_5$D-PheVAVP.

DISCUSSION

The present studies confirmed that rats deprived of food and water (hydropenic rats) have elevated plasma vasopressin levels, and excrete small amounts of concentrated urine. Rats given oral water loads have reduced plasma vasopressin levels and excrete the water load over several hr as dilute urine. Exogenous vasopressin, when administered to these rats, retards excretion of the water load. Agents which antagonize any aspect of renal vasopressin-stimulated water reabsorption or central vasopressin release will theoretically cause both increased urine flow and dilution of urine osmolality (Uosm). Agents which produce diuresis in the presence of exogenous vasopressin in water-loaded rats are likely *in vivo* antagonists specific for renal vasopressin receptors (as distinguished from hypothetical analog modulation of endogenous vasopressin release).

In the present studies, all the analogs tested increased urine volume and diluted urine osmolality in hydropenic rats. Minimal levels of urine osmolality associated with antagonist were 100 mOsm/kg H_2O or less, levels comparable to levels observed in water-loaded rats. 100 mOsm/kg in this species probably represents near-maximal dilution. The rank order of potency of the tested analogs correlates very well with the rank order of

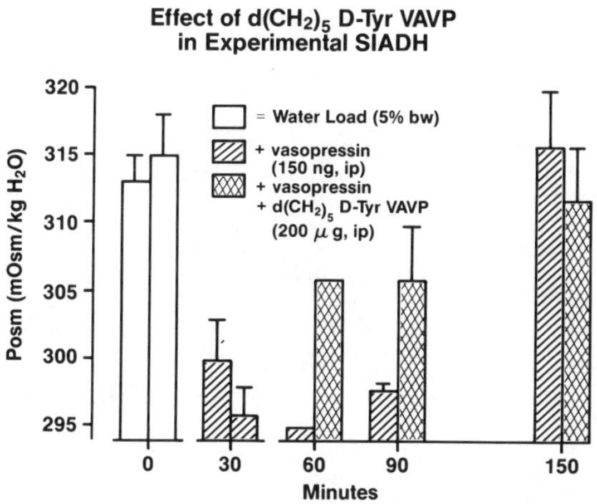

FIG. 5. Effect of $d(CH_2)_5$D-TyrVAVP on experimental SIADH in water-loaded rats.

the same antagonists as inhibitors of vasopressin-stimulated rat renal adenylate cyclase activity studied in vitro [15]. From these results it is reasonable to conclude that the in vivo diuretic activity of the tested analogs is due to antagonism of endogenous vasopressin at its renal epithelial receptor. However, analog inhibition of central vasopressin release can not be excluded.

To distinguish central and renal mechanisms of action, a second series of studies was performed in conscious water-loaded rats where central vasopressin release was suppressed by volume expansion and hemodilution. Radioimmunoassay of plasma vasopressin levels confirmed suppression of plasma vasopressin levels in this model. All the analogs tested displaced the dose response curve of exogenously administered vasopressin to the right in a parallel fashion. These results are compatible with analog-associated competitive inhibition of exogenous vasopressin at the renal epithelial vasopressin receptor. In addition, the rank order of potency of the tested analogs against exogenous vasopressin was identical to the rank order of the same analogs against endogenous vasopressin in conscious rats and the rank order for antagonism of vasopressin stimulation of rat renal adenylate cyclase [15]. These results support the hypothesis that the primary site of action of the tested analogs is at the renal vasopressin receptor.

The results of the present studies are in general agreement with previously published reports of diuretic and vasopressin antagonist activities associated with these analogs [6-9], with one prominent exception. The previous studies identified the D-Phe substitution at position 2 as more potent than the D-Tyr (alkyl) substitutions, whereas the present studies show the reverse. In vitro studies confirm that the D-Tyr (alkyl) substitutions bind with higher affinity to vasopressin receptors than the D-Phe analog and are more potent antagonists of vasopressin stimulation of rat renal adenylate cyclase [15]. The source of this discrepancy is not clear but may be related to ethanol anesthesia and/or surgical trauma associated with the previous studies [6-9].

Small but significant increases in urinary sodium, potassium, and urea excretion, but not creatinine excretion, were associated with several of the analogs tested. The increase may be due to elevated rates of urine flow in distal nephron segments [16] or alternatively may represent inhibition of vasopressin-stimulated salt reabsorption in thick ascending limb and/or salt and urea reabsorption collecting duct segments [17-19]. It is notable that diuresis associated with water loading alone was associated with a significant increase in urea excretion, but not electrolyte excretion, suggesting that multiple mechanisms may be involved. Lack of significant changes in endogenous creatinine excretion suggests that increases in Na, K, and urea excretion were not the result of changes in filtered loads.

The unique therapeutic utility of aquaretic vasopressin analogs is to selectively promote the excretion of excessive body water. An example of this is provided in Fig. 5. In this model of the syndrome of inappropriate antidiuretic hormone (SIADH), administration of the vasopressin analog rapidly promotes the excretion of the excess body water and restores plasma osmolality towards control levels.

The striking pharmacological feature of all the diuretic vasopressin analogs tested is the dilution of Uosm to levels substantially lower than plasma osmolality. This effect is independent of body fluid state and is accompanied by only a modest increase in electrolyte excretion. The analogs tested all produced net positive free-water clearances and are thus true water diuretic agents. We have previously reported similar effects of specific analogs in both dogs and primates [17,18]. We have previously proposed that these and other water diuretic agents be termed aquaretic agents to distinguish their pharmacology and potential therapeutic utility from conventional saluretic agents (Fig. 6). In contrast to previously described water diuretic agents, the onset of analog-associated water diuresis is rapid; the response and duration of the effect is both dose-dependent and predictable. The potential therapeutic utility of aquaretic vasopressin analogs may include SIADH, hyponatremia, surgical anuria and other conditions associated by either excessive vasopressin excretion or excessive water retention.

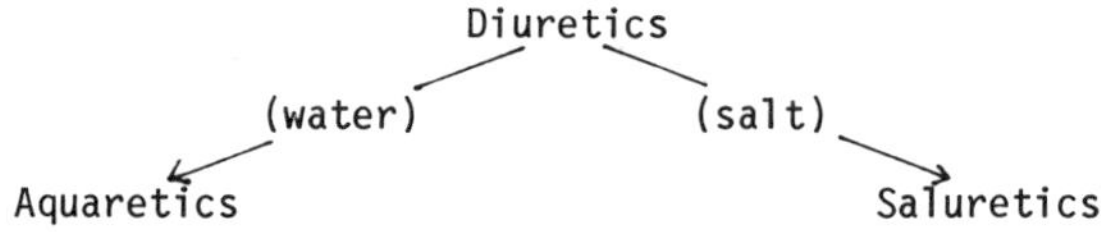

FIG. 6. Proposed nomenclature for diuretic agents.

ACKNOWLEDGMENTS

We wish to thank D. Shue and J. McDonald for their expert technical assistance; and F. Ali, W. Bryan, J. Callahan, M. Moore, J. Silvestri, H. Green, and N. Yim for the synthesis of the vasopressin analogs. We wish to thank Dr. W. Phyall for the radioimmunoassay of plasma vasopressin levels. We acknowledge continuing support and useful discussions with Drs. B. Berkowitz, M. Wasserman, and R. Beeuwkes. We are grateful to J. Koster and L. Steele for the professional preparation of this manuscript.

REFERENCES

1. G. Mudge in: The Pharmacological Basis of Therapeutics, A. G. Gilman, L. Goodman, and A. Gilman, ed. (Macmillan, New York, 1980) pp 885-915.
2. J. Forrest, M. Cox, C. Hong, G. Morrison, M. Bia, and I. Signer, N. Engl. J. Med 298, 173-177 (1978).
3. J. Oster, M. Epstein, H. Ulamo, Curr. Ther. Res. 20: 797-801 (1976).

4. R. Hays, in: The Pharmacological Basis of Therapeutics, A.G. Gilman, L.Goodman, A. Gilman, ed. (Macmillan, New York, 1980) pp. 916-928.
5. M. Bruszynski, D. Lammek, M. Manning, J. Seto, J. Haldoc, and W. Sawyer, J. Med. Chem. 23: 364-368 (1980).
6. M. Manning, W. Klis, A. Olma, J. Seto, and W. Sawyer, J. Med. Chem. 25: 414-419 (1981).
7. M. Manning, B. Lammek, A. Kolodziejczyk, J. Seto, and W. Sawyer, J. Med. Chem. 24, 701-706 (1981).
8. M. Manning, B. Lammek, A. Kolodziejczyk, J. Seto, and W. Sawyer, J. Med. Chem. 24, 408-414 (1981).
9. M. Manning, A. Olma, W. Klis, A. Kolodziejczyk, J. Seto, and W. Sawyer, J. Med. Chem. 25, 45-50 (1982).
10. F. Stassen, R. Erickson, W. Huffman, J. Stefankiewicz, L. Sulat, and V. Wiebelhaus, J. Pharmacol. Exp. Ther. 223, 50-54 (1982).
11. H. Valtin and H. Schroeder, Am. J. Physiol. 206, 425-430 (1984).
12. H. Sokol and H. Valtin, The Brattleboro Rat (Ann. N.Y. Acad. Sci. 394, New York, 1982).
13. Y. Cheng and W. Prusoff, Biochem. Pharmacol. 22, 3099-3108 (1973).
14. F. LaRochelle, W. North, and P. Stern, Flugers Arch. 387, 79-81 (1980).
15. F. Stassen, B. Berkowitz, W. Huffman, V. Wiebelhaus and L. Kinter (this volume).
16. F. Wright, Kidney Int. 11, 415-432 (1977).
17. F. Morel, D. Chabardes and M. Imbert-Teboul, Proc. VII Int. Congr. Nephrol. 209-216 (1978).
18. M. Reif and J. Schafer, Fed. Proc. 43, (in press, 1984).
19. K. Gardner and R. Maffly, in: Urea and the Kidney, B. Schmidt-Nielson, ed. (Excerpta Medica Foundation, Amsterdam, 1970) pp 159-168.
20. L. Kinter, F. Stassen, E. Horner, V. Wiebelhaus, and N. Yim, Kidney Int. 23, 259 (1983).
21. L. Kinter, W. Mann, G. Heckman, W. Huffman, M. Gross, and F. Stassen, Kidney Int. 25, 304 (1984).

SECTION II

ANTIHYPERTENSIVE AND HEMODYNAMIC ACTIONS

EXTRARENAL AND VASCULAR EFFECTS OF PIRETANIDE IN SEVERAL ANIMAL MODELS *)

E. KLAUS, H.G. ALPERMANN, G. CASPRITZ, M. HROPOT, W. LINZ, AND B. SCHÖLKENS
Hoechst AG, Postfach 80 03 20, 6230 Frankfurt/M. 80, FRG

ABSTRACT

The new diuretic piretanide (4-phenoxy-3-(1-pyrrolidinyl)-5-sulfamoyl benzoic acid, Arelix[R]) was studied for its vasoactive effects in several animal models. In rat, guinea pig and rabbit aorta strips, piretanide dose-dependently attenuated contractions induced either by norepinephrine or potassium or angiotensin II. Piretanide inhibited the vasoconstrictor response to norepinephrine and to KCl in the rat mesenteric vascular bed. Piretanide-superfused bovine coronary artery strips relaxed relative to the concentration. In both normotensive and spontaneously hypertensive bilaterally nephrectomized pithed rats, piretanide caused a significant reduction in diastolic blood pressure. A direct hypotensive effect of piretanide was also observed in a ganglion-blocked rat model with angiotensin II-supported blood pressure. Infusion of piretanide in the isolated guinea pig heart produced a reversible increase in coronary flow.
It can be concluded that the established antihypertensive effect of piretanide is at least partly due to its extrarenal action.

INTRODUCTION

Long-term treatment with diuretics can lower the blood pressure in patients with essential hypertension. The mechanisms for the antihypertensive activity seem to be independent of reduction of extracellular fluid by diuresis [2]. Thus, it is generally assumed that not only renal but also extrarenal effects are responsible for the antihypertensive action of diuretics. In micropuncture studies, the new diuretic piretanide (4-phenoxy-3-(1-pyrrolidinyl)-5-sulfamoyl benzoic acid, Arelix[R]; manufacturer: Hoechst AG, Frankfurt/M., FRG) reveals the main site of action in the ascending limb of Henle's loop with slight effects in the proximal tubules [3].

PIRETANIDE
MW 362.41

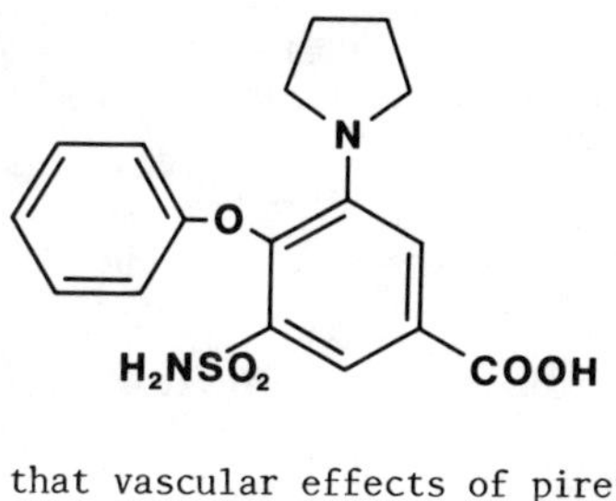

Clinical studies suggest that vascular effects of piretanide probably contribute to its cardiovascular [4, 5] and antihypertensive [6, 7] action.

*) In part previously published in [1]

Piretanide clearly lowers blood pressure in patients with essential hypertension treated over a long period and does not produce marked diuresis [7]. The aim of the present work was to study the extrarenal effects of piretanide on vascular smooth muscle in several animal models.

METHODS

Strips from the thoracic aorta of male Sprague-Dawley rats were helically cut at an angle of 20 to 30° (25 x 2 mm). They were incubated under 300 mg tension in a 25 ml bath with modified Tyrode solution according to Biamino and Kruckenberg [8] at 37° C and oxygenated with carbogen. Isometric recordings were made using Gould Statham UC2 transducers. After equilibration (2 h), cumulative concentration response curves were obtained using either norepinephrine (noradrenaline, NA, 10^{-9} - 10^{-6} mol/l; Arterenol[R], Hoechst AG, FRG) or KCl (12.7 - 42.7 mmol/l). After washout, the concentration response curve was repeated. Only strips with variations of less than 15 % were used. They were preincubated with piretanide (1 - 8 mmol/l) for 5 min and the NA- and KCl-induced contractions repeated.

Guinea pig thoracic aorta was cut at an angle of 45° (45 x 3 mm) and suspended under 0.5 g tension in a 10 ml organ bath at 37° C in Ringer solution. The solution was oxygenated with carbogen. Contractions were recorded with isotonic levers. Concentration response curves were obtained with angiotensin II (ANG II; 2.5 x 10^{-10} - 6.6 x 10^{-8} mol/l, Hypertensin-CIBA[R], Ciba-Geigy GmbH, FRG). Preincubation with piretanide (15 min) was conducted with concentrations from 1 to 2.5 mmol/l.

Strips from the thoracic aorta of rabbits (20 x 4 mm) were suspended under 2 g tension in a 15 ml bath at 37° in a modified Tyrode solution which was oxygenated with carbogen. Recordings were made using isotonic levers. Cumulative concentration response curves were obtained using NA (10^{-8} - 10^{-5} mol/l) or KCl (22.7 - 52.7 mmol/l). The strips were preincubated with piretanide (1 - 3 mmol/l) for 10 min.

The IC_{50} of piretanide were calculated according to the procedure described by Towart [9].

The superior mesenteric vascular bed was prepared as described by McGregor [10], modified by Manku and Horrobin [11]. Male rats of the Wistar strain were anaesthetized with ethylether. Krebs bicarbonate buffer (pH 7.4) containing glucose was oxygenated with carbogen and was used for perfusion of the mesenteric artery by a peristaltic pump. Perfusion pressure was recorded via a side arm of the arterial cannula using a Statham P 23 dB transducer. Flow rate was adjusted to 3 ml/min which gave a baseline pressure of 20 - 30 mmHg. NA (1 μg dissolved in 0.05 ml Krebs bicarbonate buffer) or KCl (10 mg in 0.05 ml buffer) were infused into another side arm of the arterial cannula within 15 sec at 4 min intervals. Each injection produced a transient rise in pressure which returned to baseline pressure within 1 - 2 min. Piretanide was added to the perfusate in increasing concentrations (0.34; 0.69; 1.38 or 2.76; 5.52; 11.04 mmol/l). At each concentration, agonist perfusion was performed four times at 4 min intervals followed by a piretanide-free contraction period.

The left descending bovine coronary artery and several of its primary branches were cut into spiral strips (2 - 3 cm long and 2 - 3 mm wide) and immersed in 4° C oxygenated Krebs solution. The strips were later superfused with oxygenated Krebs solution at 37° C at a rate of 5 - 6 ml/min. The solution contained a mixture of antagonists to inhibit the activity of endogenous acetylcholine, catecholamines, 5-hydroxytryptamine or histamine according to Gilmore et al. [12]. Changes in lengths were isotonically recorded with an initial tension of 2 g. Strips were superfused up to 3 hours before the effect of any substance was studied. Reactivity of the artery strips was tested with PGE_2 (100 ng/ml) and PGI_2 (100 ng/ml). The effect of piretanide was tested in concentrations of 0.28, 1.38 and 2.76 mmol/l in a solution of 10 ml oxygenated Krebs buffer.

Spontaneously hypertensive (SH) rats and normotensive Sprague Dawley rats were anaesthetized with ether and bilaterally nephrectomized. Twenty-four hours later, the animals were again anaesthetized and the trachea was cannulated. Rats were pithed through the right orbit with a steel rod and immediately respirated with room air (1 ml/100 g). Blood pressure was recorded from a carotid artery using a Statham P 23 dB transducer and a Hellige amplifier-recorder system. Heart rate was obtained from the pressure signal. Intravenous bolus injections were given into a tail vein. Duration of the experiment was 60 min which consisted of a control period of 30 min commencing after administration of 1 ml/kg i.v. saline (not shown) and a drug period of 30 min beginning after piretanide which was dissolved in 1 ml saline/kg i.v. Diastolic blood pressure was evaluated from the end of the control period and at 5, 10, 20 and 30 min after administration of piretanide.

Experiments in the ganglion-blocked ANG II-supported rat were carried out modifying the method described by Brown and Worcel [13]. Male Sprague Dawley rats were anaesthetized with pentobarbital sodium (Nembutal[R], Abbott, Belgium). Blood pressure was measured in a cannulated carotid artery using a Statham P 23 dB transducer. The left jugular vein and the penile vein were cannulated for drug administration. The trachea was cannulated for artificial respiration. Pentolinium was administered in a dose of 10 mg/kg i.v., phenoxybenzamine was given in a dose of 5 mg/kg i.v. Blood pressure was allowed to stabilize for 30 min. Subsequently the rats were infused with ANG II (1.5 /ug x kg^{-1} x min^{-1}; 0.02 ml/min) via a Unita BII (Braun Melsungen, FRG) perfusor. Following a second 30 min stabilization period, piretanide was administered in a dose of 10 mg/kg i.v. (10 mg/ml). Mean arterial blood pressure was evaluated at 0, 10, 20, 30, and 40 min after administration of piretanide.

The coronary flow was measured using the hearts of female heparinized guinea pigs. The ascending aorta was cannulated and connected to a non-recirculating perfusion system (hydrostatic pressure 75 cm H_2O). A perfusion period of 20 - 30 min against a load of 2 g was allowed for equilibration. Krebs-Henseleit bicarbonate solution was equilibrated with carbogen (pH 7.4, 38° C). Osmolality of the buffer was kept constant by adjusting the amount of NaCl. The coronary flow was measured by means of a drop counter. Piretanide dissolved in Krebs-Henseleit solution was given by infusion (1 mg x ml^{-1} x min^{-1}) above the aortic cannula into the inflow.

RESULTS

The effect of piretanide on thoracic aorta strips is shown in figures 1 - 3. In rat thoracic aorta strips, piretanide dose-dependently attenuated NA- and KCl-induced contractions (Fig. 1). The contractions induced by NA (10^{-7} mol/l) and KCl (32.7 mmol/l) were inhibited with an IC_{50} of 1.68 mmol/l and 1.65 mmol/l respectively.

The concentration-response curves of piretanide in ANG II-contracted guinea pig aorta strips are shown in Fig. 2. The contractions were inhibited with an IC_{50} of 1.38 mmol/l piretanide at an ANG II concentration of 1.9 x 10^{-8} mol/l.

In rabbit aorta strips (Fig. 3), the contractions induced by NA (10^{-6} mol/l) were inhibited with an IC_{50} of 1.9 mmol/l piretanide. With KCl, dose-response curves could not be established.

In the rat mesenteric vascular bed, piretanide inhibited the NA- and KCl-induced pressure increase as illustrated in Fig. 4. The vasoconstrictor response to NA and KCl is inhibited by piretanide in a dose-related manner when added to the perfusate. After NA- and K^+-induced vascoconstriction, an IC_{50} for piretanide of 0.5 mmol/l and 4.9 mmol/l was calculated respectively.

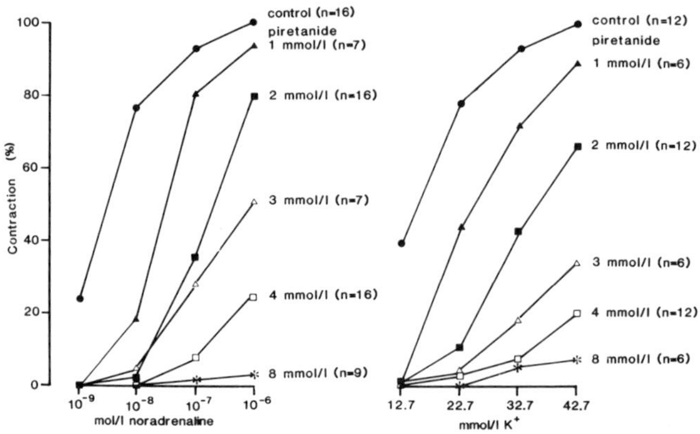

Fig. 1. Effect of piretanide on rat thoracic aorta strips stimulated either with NA or with KCl.

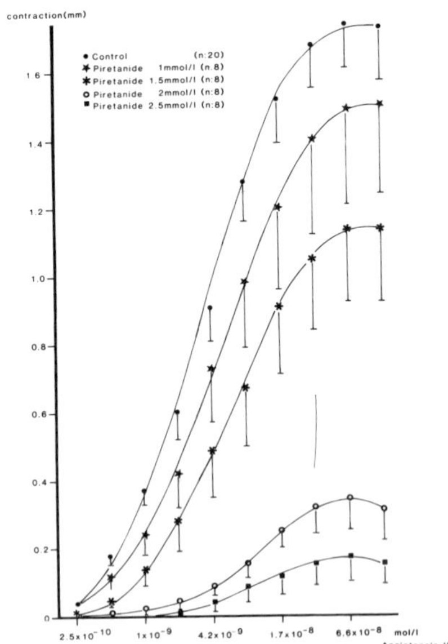

Fig. 2. Effect of piretanide on guinea pig thoracic aorta strips stimulated with ANG II. Values are mean ± SEM.

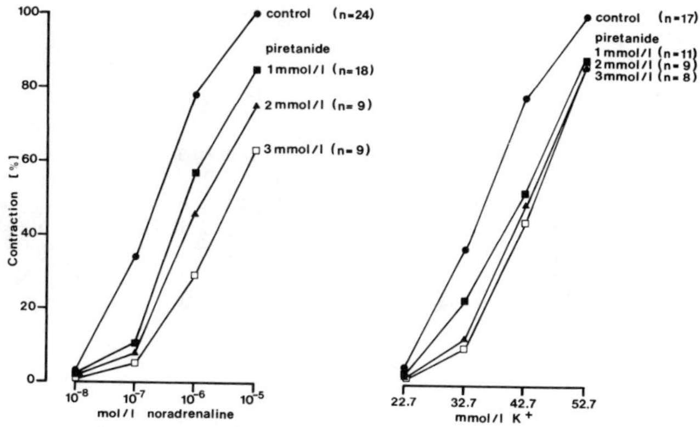

Fig. 3. Effect of piretanide on rabbit thoracic aorta strips stimulated either with NA or with KCl.

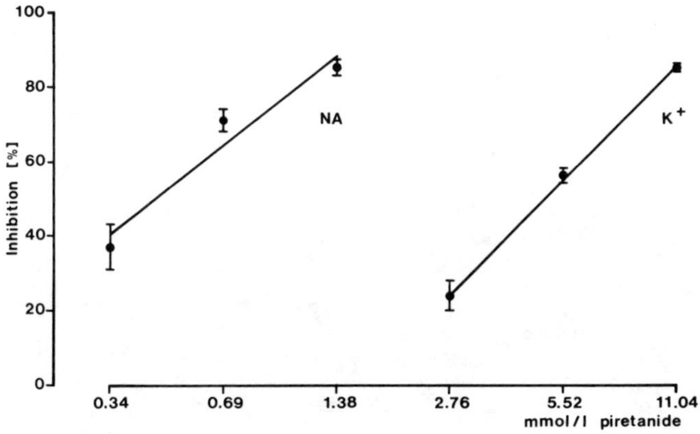

Fig. 4. Effect of piretanide perfusion of the rat mesenteric vascular bed. The preparations are stimulated either with NA (1 μg) or with KCl (10 mg). Results are mean $\pm$ SEM (n = 6).

The relaxation of bovine coronary artery strips by superfused piretanide is demonstrated in Tab. 1. Piretanide in concentrations of 0.28, 1.38 and 2.76 mmol/l caused a marked concentration-dependent decrease in tension with an IC_{50} of 0.94 mmol/l.

Table I. Effect of piretanide on bovine coronary artery strips. Values (mean ± SEM, n = 10) are per cent of initial response to 100 ng/ml PGI_2.

Piretanide concentration (mmol/l)	Relaxation (%)
0.28	11 ± 2
1.38	52 ± 7
2.76	95 ± 10

The effects of piretanide on blood pressure in bilaterally nephrectomized pithed rats are shown in figures 5 and 6. In Sprague-Dawley rats (Fig. 5), the lowest dose of 3 mg/kg i.v. caused a significant reduction in diastolic blood pressure. A further decrease was observed after 10 and 30 mg/kg piretanide. Heart rate was not affected. SH rats were less susceptible to the effect of piretanide. Only doses of 10 and 30 mg/kg piretanide i.v. significantly decreased the diastolic blood pressure (Fig. 6).

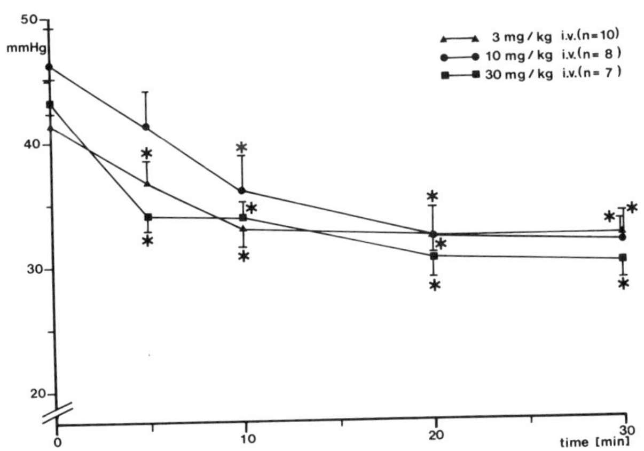

Fig. 5. Effect of piretanide on the diastolic blood pressure of bilaterally nephrectomized pithed normotensive rats. Results are mean ± SEM. An asterisk denotes $p < 0.05$ (t-test).

In the ganglion-blocked ANG II-supported rat, mean arterial pressure (MAP) was 128 ± 7 mmHg at the end of the stabilization period after ANG II. Piretanide (10 mg/kg i.v.) reduced the MAP significantly (Fig. 7). The pressure difference was - 18 ± 5 mmHg within 40 min.

In isolated guinea pig hearts, the initial coronary flow was 5.59 ± 0.21 ml x g^{-1} x min^{-1} (Fig. 8). Infusion of piretanide (1 mg x ml^{-1} x min^{-1}) produced an increased flow up to 8.53 ± 0.23 ml x g^{-1} x min^{-1} (+ 53 %, $p < 0.01$). At the end of the infusion, the coronary flow reached control values again. The vehicle in the volume used did not affect the flow registered.

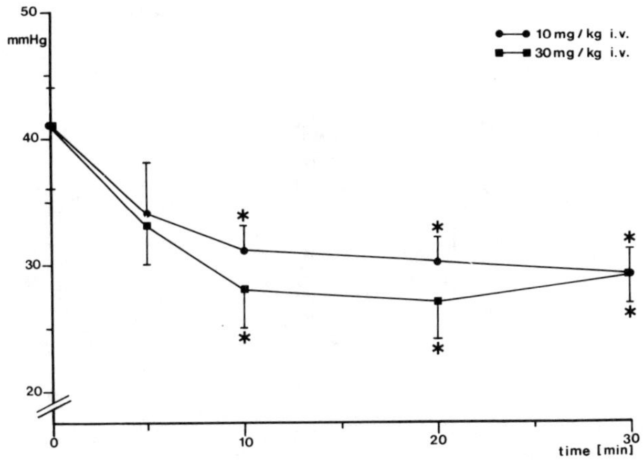

Fig. 6. Effect of piretanide on the diastolic blood pressure of bilaterally nephrectomized pithed SH rats. Values are mean ± SEM, n = 9). An asterisk denotes $p < 0.05$ (t-test).

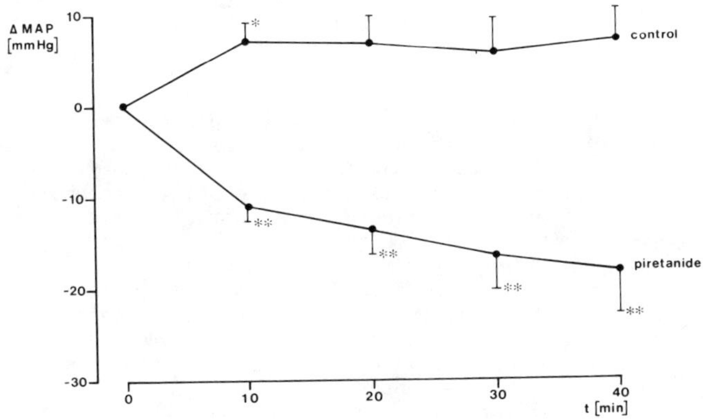

Fig. 7. Effect of piretanide on mean arterial pressure of ganglion-blocked ANG II-supported rats. Values are mean ± SEM, n = 6. An asterisk denotes $p < 0.05$, two asterisks $p < 0.01$ (t-test).

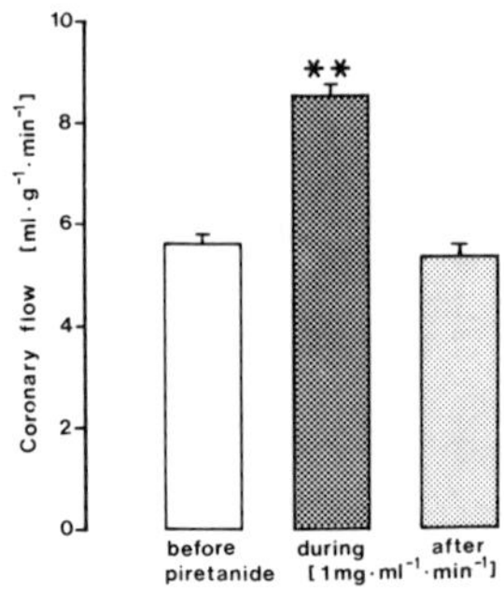

Fig. 8. Effect of piretanide on the coronary flow in 10 isolated guinea pig hearts. Mean ± SEM ($p < 0.01$, t-test) are indicated.

DISCUSSION

Clinical data suggest that piretanide is a valuable antihypertensive agent for long-term treatment of mild to moderate hypertension [5 - 7]. In double-blind controlled studies, piretanide significantly reduced systolic and diastolic blood pressure. Although the therapeutic value of diuretics in essential hypertension has been established, the antihypertensive effect of a diuretic is not necessarily related to its salidiuretic potency. Thus, an extrarenal site of action has to be considered. Evidence for such an extrarenal vascular effect on the venous system and its capacitance vessels has been evaluated in a plethysmographic study in healthy volunteers [14] and in patients recovering from myocardial infarction [4, 5]. Direct effects of piretanide on vessels has been shown in experiments with isolated rat aorta and portal vein [15].

In addition to these findings resulting mostly from studies on the venous system, the present studies reveal a distinct arterial action of piretanide in numerous isolated vascular tissue preparations. These include large vessels like rat, guinea pig, and rabbit thoracic aorta and bovine coronary artery but also smaller vessels like the rat mesenteric artery bed.

The results demonstrate an in vitro relaxant effect of piretanide on vascular smooth muscle. In all experimental models piretanide dose-dependently attenuated the vascular reactivity to vasoconstrictor agents like noradrenaline, angiotensin II and PGE_2. There is a discrepancy as far as the Ca^{++} influx is concerned between rabbit thoracic aorta strips and the rat mesenteric vascular bed on the one hand and rat thoracic aorta strips on the other hand. Piretanide seems to reduce the Ca^{++}-influx in rat aorta but had little effect in the two other experiments mentioned above.

A direct relaxant effect of piretanide on vascular smooth muscle is also shown in vivo using bilaterally nephrectomized pithed rats in which a renal site of action is excluded. These findings are supported by the experiments in ganglion-blocked rats in which a direct blood pressure-lowering effect of piretanide could be also observed.

From these experimental results one may conclude that the antihypertensive effect of piretanide [6, 7] is not only due to its volume and salt depletion but also due to its direct action on resistance and capacitance vessels.

REFERENCES

1. E. Klaus, H.G. Alpermann, G. Caspritz, W. Linz, and B. Schölkens, Arzneim.-Forsch./Drug Res. 33, 1273-1276 (1983).
2. P. Lund-Johansen, Acta med. scand. 187, 509-518 (1970).
3. W. Merkel, D. Bormann, D. Mania, R. Muschaweck, and M. Hropot, Eur. J. med. Chem. 11, 399-406 (1976).
4. W. Nechwatal, A. Stange, H. Sigel, P. Kress, A. Resch, and M. Stauch, Herz Kreislauf 14, 91-96 (1982).
5. H. Valette, J.-L. Hebert, B. Raffestin, A. Lockhart, and E. Apoil, J. cardiovasc. Pharmacol. 2, 103-111 (1980).
6. P.S. Gupta and M.L. Dave, Curr. ther. Res. 30, 468-476 (1981).
7. W. Dols, J. Freude, M. Verho, and B. Rangoonwala, Curr. Med. Res. Opin. 8, 649-658 (1983).
8. B. Biamino and P. Kruckenberg, Amer. J. Physiol. 217, 376-382 (1969).
9. R. Towart, J. cardiovasc. Pharmacol. 4, 895-902 (1982).
10. D.D. McGregor, J. Physiol. (Lond.) 177, 21-30 (1965).
11. M.S. Manku and D.F. Horrobin, Prostaglandins 12, 369-376 (1976).
12. N. Gilmore, J.R. Vane, and J.H. Wyllie, Nature 218, 1135-1140 (1968).
13. N.L. Brown and M. Worcel, European J. Pharmacol. 92, 285-289 (1983).
14. H. Valette, P. Duhaze, and E. Apoil, Brit. J. clin. Pharmacol. 7, 219 (1979).
15. G. Biamino and H. Huckauf, in: Diuretika, J. Rosenthal and H. Knauf, eds. (edition medizin, Weinheim - Deerfield Beach/Florida - Basel 1980) pp. 51-58.

ANTIHYPERTENSIVE ACTION OF CHRONIC TREATMENT WITH PIRETANIDE IN SPONTANEOUSLY HYPERTENSIVE RATS

Thomas Unger, Thomas Fleck, Detlev Ganten, Rudolf E. Lang
German Institute for High Blood Pressure Research and Department of Pharmacology, University of Heidelberg, Im Neuenheimer Feld 366, D-6900 Heidelberg, F.R.G.

ABSTRACT

Chronic oral treatment with piretanide (50 mg/kg/day p.o.) lowered blood pressure in adult stroke prone spontaneously hypertensive rats (SHRSP) and, to a lesser degree, in normotensive Wistar Kyoto rats (WKY). After 4 weeks of treatment tachyphylaxis to the antihypertensive action occurred and the dose had to be doubled to be effective. In young (6 week old) SHRSP the development of hypertension was prevented during a 4 week treatment period with piretanide (50 mg/kg/day).

In all groups the effects on blood pressure were accompanied by diuresis. However,this effect was much greater in the WKY than in the SHRSP. Natriuresis was moderate if at all present and a kaliuresis was not observed. Piretanide produced a marked stimulation of the plasma renin angiotensin system (RAS) throughout treatment in all groups. This could be an explanation for the tachyphylaxis observed in the adult rats.

Our results demonstrating the antihypertensive efficacy of piretanide in SHRSP are consistent with the hypothesis that the mechanisms may include factors other than volume reduction induced by natriuresis.

INTRODUCTION

Piretanide (Arelix[R]) is a recently developed diuretic with the main site of action in the ascending limb of the loop of Henle (1,2). Evidence is accumulating that this compound has antihypertensive properties in patients with essential hypertension (3,4) and that the blood pressure lowering action is accompanied by a relatively mild diuresis.

In this study we have investigated the antihypertensive action of chronic oral piretanide treatment in the spontaneously hypertensive rat, the experimental model of hypertension most closely resembling human essential hypertension. Particular attention has been paid to the question whether the effects on blood pressure could be directly related to the diuretic or natriuretic actions of the drug.

MATERIALS AND METHODS

Experiments were carried out in spontaneously hypertensive rats of the stroke prone Okamoto-Aoki strain (SHRSP) and their normotensive Wistar Kyoto controls (WKY) bred in Heidelberg since 1975. Rats were housed singly throughout the experiments and were kept under controlled temperature, humidity and light

Diuretics, Jules B. Puschett, Editor

period. Food (Altromin^R) containing 120 meq sodium/kg and 220 meq potassium/kg was offered ad libitum.

Piretanide was dissolved in distilled water adjusted to pH 7.5 with 2N NaOH and added to the drinking fluid (demineralized water). The drug solution volumes were adjusted to the individual water intake of the animals to ensure correct dosage. The drug was made up freshly every three days. Control SHRSP and WKY received demineralized water instead of the drug solution but were otherwise kept under identical conditions as the experimental animals.

Experiment 1: Effect of chronic oral treatment with piretanide on blood pressure, urinary parameters and the plasma renin angiotensin system (RAS) in adult SHRSP and WKY

Six month old SHRSP and WKY (n:8 per group) were treated orally with piretanide for three months. The dose was 50 mg/kg/day for the first seven weeks, and was increased to 100 mg/kg/day for the rest of the treatment period. Rats were kept in metabolic cages starting one week before treatment (adaptation period) for the first 4 weeks of treatment, then for one week at the end of each of the following two months of treatment. Urine was collected before treatment, and after 1,3,7 days and 2,4,8 and 12 weeks of treatment for determination of urinary volume and sodium and potassium excretion. Blood was taken from the retroorbital venous plexus under light ether anaesthesia before treatment and after 3 days, 1,4,8 and 12 weeks of treatment for measurement of plasma renin concentration (PRC) and plasma angiotensin II (ANGII). Systolic blood pressure was measured by tail plethymography under light ether anaesthesia before treatment and at weekly intervals during treatment.

Experiment 2: Effect of chronic oral treatment with piretanide on blood pressure, urinary parameters and plasma RAS in young SHRSP

Six week old SHRSP (n:9) were treated with piretanide (50 mg/kg/day) for 4 weeks. Rats were kept in metabolic cages throughout treatment. Urine was sampled twice weekly, and blood pressure was measured before and after 3 days, 1,2,3, and 4 weeks of treatment.

Urinary electrolytes and the Na^+ and K^+ content of the food were measured by flame photometry. Plasma PRC and ANGII were determined by radioimmunoassay as described elsewhere (5). Results are reported as means $\pm$ SEM. Students t-test for unpaired observation was used for comparison of treated and untreated groups, and differences were accepted at the $2P<0.05$ level.

RESULTS

Experiment 1:

In adult SHRSP, piretanide lowered systolic blood pressure markedly in the initial phase of treatment (FIG.1). However, after 4 weeks blood pressure returned to hypertensive levels. When the dose was doubled, blood pressure fell again and remained significantly reduced until the end of the treatment period. A similar picture, though less pronounced, was seen in the WKY (FIG.1).

In both strains the temporal pattern of blood pressure changes was paralled by increases in water intake and urinary volume which were more marked in the WKY than in the SHRSP (FIG.2).

In the treated SHRSP the urinary sodium excretion was elevated only after one week ($p<0.01$) but otherwise similar as in the controls (FIG.3), while in the treated WKY a decreased urinary sodium excretion was observed initially, and again from the 4th to the 12th week of treatment (FIG.3). A similar pattern was observed in both strains with respect to urinary potassium excretion.

The plasma RAS was markedly and consistantly stimulated in the SHRSP (FIG.4) and WKY throughout treatment.

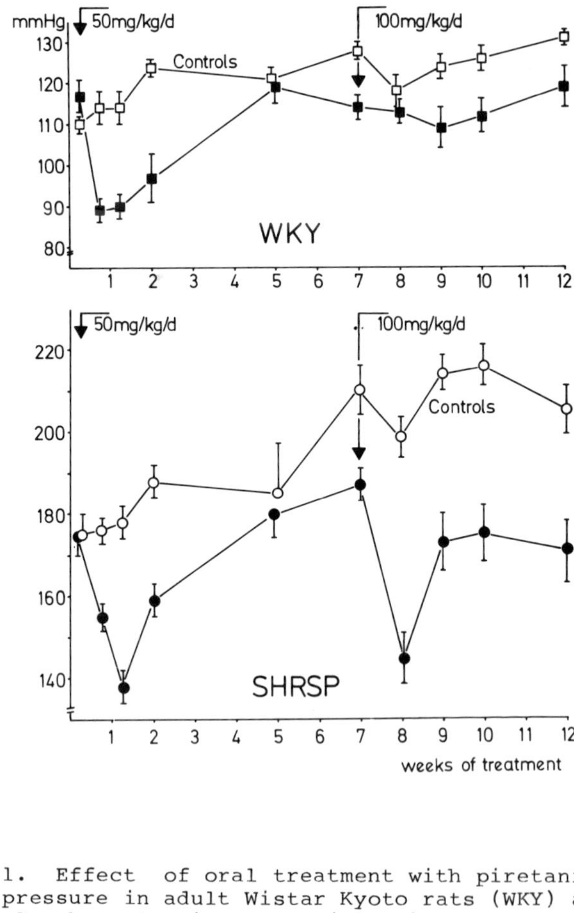

FIG. 1. Effect of oral treatment with piretanide on systolic blood pressure in adult Wistar Kyoto rats (WKY) and spontaneously hypertensive rats (SHRSP). Note the escape from the antihypertensive action after 4 weeks of treatment.

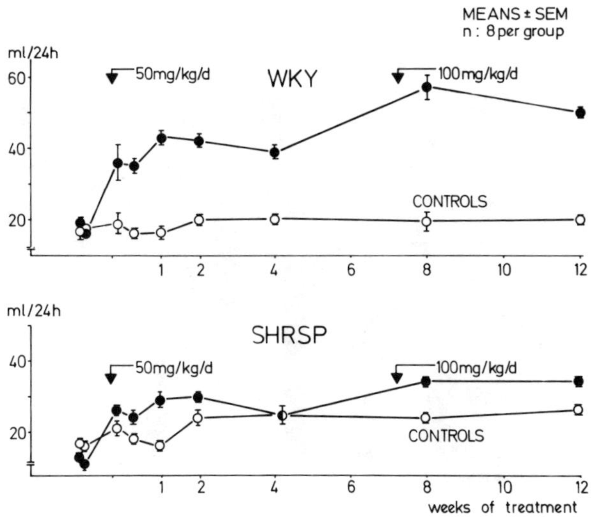

FIG. 2. Urinary volume during chronic oral treatment with piretanide in adult WKY (upper panel) and SHRSP (lower panel)

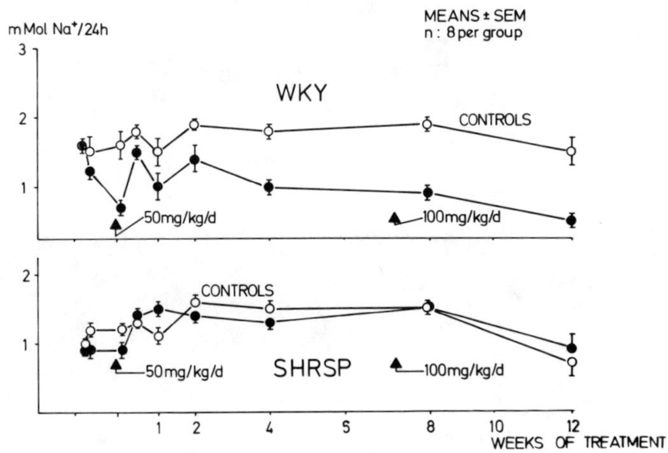

FIG. 3. Urinary sodium excretion during chronic oral treatment with piretanide in adult WKY (upper panel) and SHRSP (lower panel)

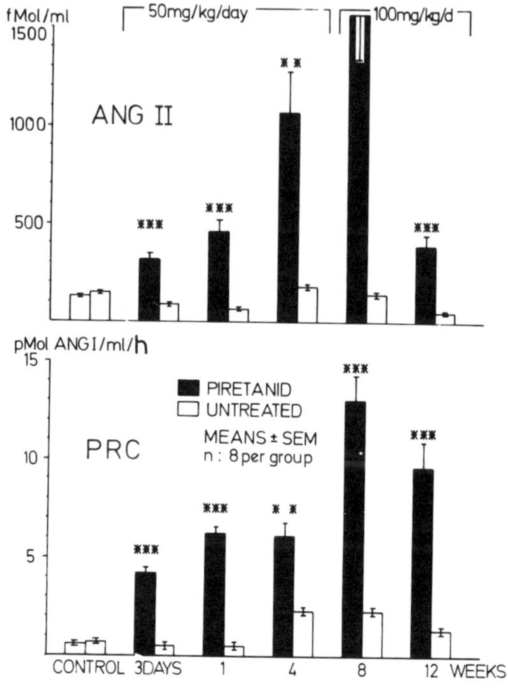

FIG. 4. Plasma renin concentration (PRC) and plasma angiotensin II (ANGII) during chronic oral treatment with piretanide in adult SHRSP

Experiment 2:

In young SHRSP, piretanide prevented the further development of hypertension, which was seen in the untreated group, and produced a marked increase in urinary volume (FIG.5). The urinary sodium excretion was increased initially but unchanged later. However, the balance between sodium intake and urinary excretion was lower in the treated than in the untreated SHRSP throughout treatment (FIG.6). In contrast, urinary potassium excretion and potassium balance in the treated SHRSP were not consistently different from those in the untreated controls (FIG.7).

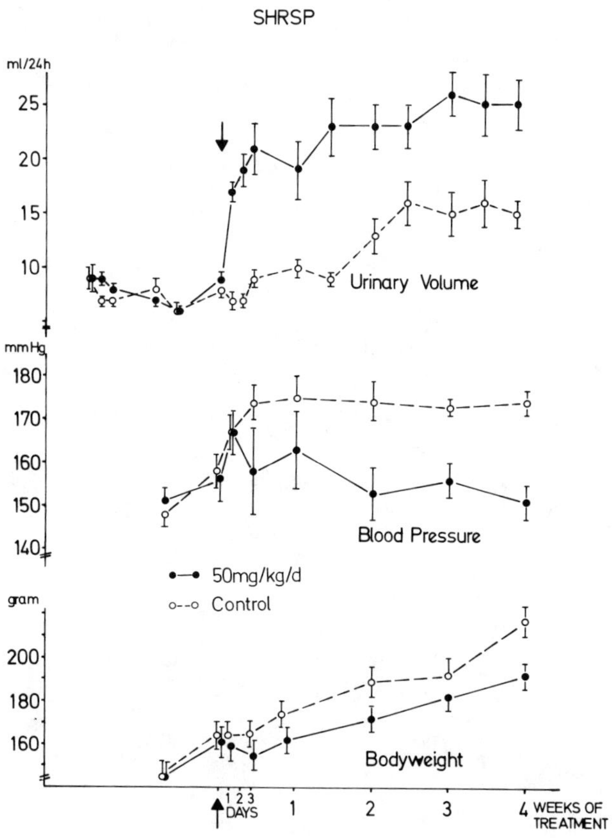

FIG. 5. Urinary volume, blood pressure and bodyweight during chronic oral treatment with piretanide in young SHRSP

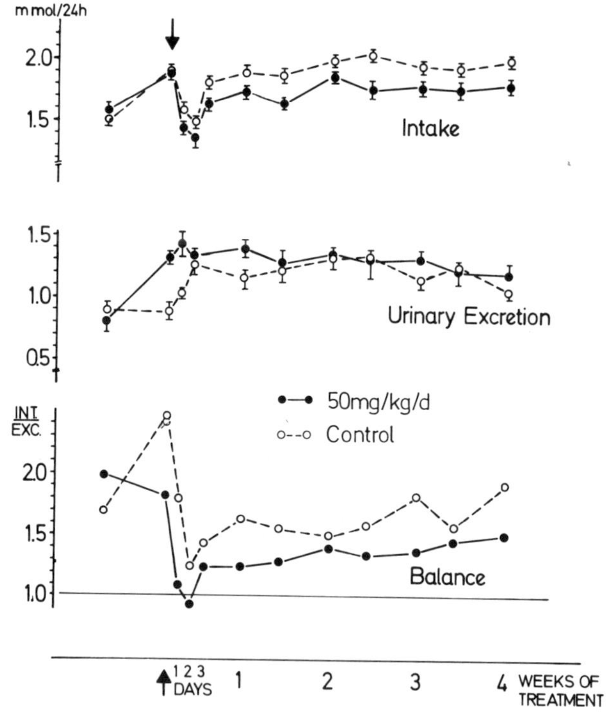

FIG. 6. Sodium intake, urinary sodium excretion, and balance between sodium intake and excretion during chronic oral treatment with piretanide in young SHRSP

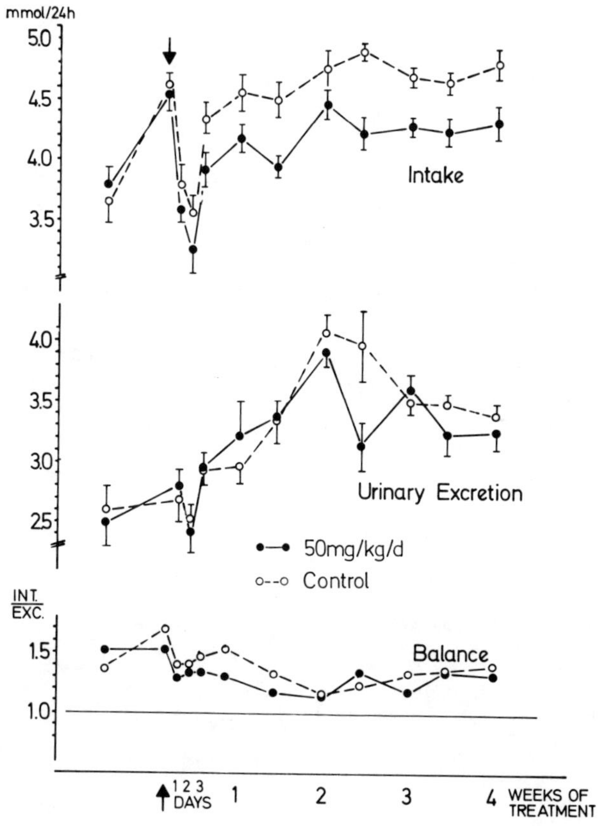

FIG. 7. Potassium intake, urinary sodium excretion, and balance between potassium intake and excretion during chronic oral treatment with piretanide in young SHRSP

DISCUSSION

Piretanide proved to be an effective antihypertensive agent in SHRSP, and also lowered blood pressure in normotensive WKY. Its effects on blood pressure were invariably associated with a marked diuresis, but the natriuresis, if at all present, was less than one might have expected. A loss of potassium was not observed in this study, except for one time point (one week of treatment) in the adult SHRSP. The antihypertensive action appeared to be better in young SHRSP during the development of high blood pressure than in adult SHRSP with established hypertension. In the latter, the dose of the drug had to be increased after 4 weeks of treatment because of marked tachyphylaxis for both the antihypertensive and diuretic actions. Since tachyphylaxis to the blood pressure effects also occurred in the WKY, it cannot be ascribed to factors such as progressive kidney damage in the hypertensive animals. However, this phenomenon could be explained by the stimulation of compensatory mechanisms such as the plasma RAS. Indeed, the plasma concentrations of ANGII measured in the treated animals were sufficient to produce marked pressor and antinatriuretic effects alone.

The increase in water intake and diuresis during treatment was exaggerated in the WKY when compared with the SHRSP, which, on the other hand, showed the greater antihypertensive responses. This is yet another observation pointing to the fact that the chronic blood pressure lowering action of diuretics cannot be explained solely on the basis of a reduced plasma volume, but may be due to mechanisms unrelated to diuresis. These include direct vasodilatation, reduction of vascular reactivity, loss of sodium from the vascular wall or release of vasodilating agents such as prostaglandins or bradykinin, as has recently been reviewed by Struyker-Boudier et al. (6).

In line with this hypothesis is the demonstration of direct vascular effects of piretanide in several in vitro models (7), although the functional significance of this observation remains to be established in vivo.

REFERENCES

1. M. Omoso, K. Fujimoto, T. Sakaguchi, K. Yamamoto, H. Iwao, Y. Abe, Arzneim.-Forsch./Drug Res. 33(9), 1277-1280 (1983).

2. B. Odling, B. Beermann, G. Selen, A.E.G. Persson, J. Pharm. Exp. Therap. 225(3), 742-746 (1982).

3. W. Dols, J. Freude, M. Verho, B. Rangoonwala, Curr. Med. Res. Opinion 8 , 649-658 (1983).

4. P.S. Gupta, M.L. Dave, Curr. Ther. Res. 30, 468 (1981).

5. J.F.E. Mann, A.K. Johnson, D. Ganten, Am. J. Physiol. 238, R372-R377 (1983).

6. H.A.J. Struyker-Boudier, J.F.M. Smits, J.C.S. Kleinjans, H. van Essen H, Clin. Exp. Hyper. A5(2), 209-223 (1983).

7. E. Klaus, G. Alpermann, G. Caspritz, W. Linz, B. Schölkens, Arzneim.-Forsch./Drug. Res. 33(II)9, 1273-1276 (1983).

EFFECT OF DIURETIC TREATMENT ON THE PRESSURE RESPONSE TO ACUTE PROPRANOLOL AND LABETALOL INFUSION IN ESSENTIAL HYPERTENSION.

R.FOGARI and L.CORRADI
Department of Internal Medicine, University of Pavia, Pavia, Italy

INTRODUCTION

The relationship between sympathetic activity and sodium balance is still a complex matter and remains to be defined. Many causes have been implicated in the pathogenesis of essential hypertension and both the state of sodium homeostasis and adrenergic activity are important factors. (1-4)
The purpose of this study is to investigate the connection between the state of sodium balance and the adrenoreceptor responsiveness. To study this problem the effect of chronic diuretic treatment on the blood pressure response either to acute alpha and beta blockade or to acute beta blockade alone was evaluated.

METHODS

13 essential hypertensive subjects (all male, WHO I - II, mean age 45,8, range 33-54) were studied.
Diagnosis of essential hypertension was established by excluding known causes of hypertension. None of the subjects exibited cardiac failure, cardiac arrhytmias, diabetes or disorders of the respiratory system.
All of them were given a costant diet containing 100 mEq Sodium and 60 mEq Potassium daily.
Labetalol 1 mg/Kg and Propranolol 0,2 mg/Kg were intravenously administrated, in two differet days, to all patients before and after 4 weeks Chlorthalidone treatment (50 mg/daily).
Every time each perfusion was performed in 10 minutes and blood pressure and heart rate were monitored.

RESULTS

Fig.1 and 2 outline the effect of chronic Chlorthalidone treatment on blood pressure response to propranolol and Labetalol.
Before diuretic treatment Labetalol acute infusion reduced blood pressure (-28,5/16,3 mmHg) without modifying heart rate; in contrast Propranolol significantly alowed heart rate without reducing blood pressure. After 4 weeks Chlorthalidone treatment Labetalol induced an ever greater blood pressure decrease (-47,5/35,2 mmHg) and it was such a drop that in some cases it needed to stop the infusion before ending; heart rate never changed.
In the same conditions Propranolol decreased blood pressure significantly much less (-13,4/5,1 mmHg) and slowed heart rate again.

Diuretics, Jules B. Puschett, Editor

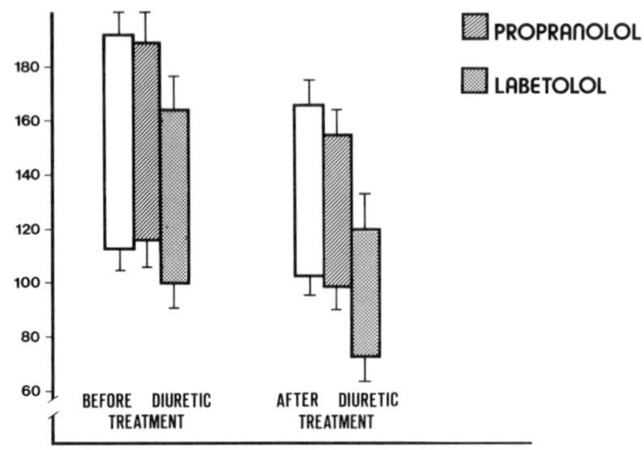

FIG. 1. Effects of acute Propranolol and Labetalol infusions on systemic blood pressure before and after Chlorthalidone treatment.

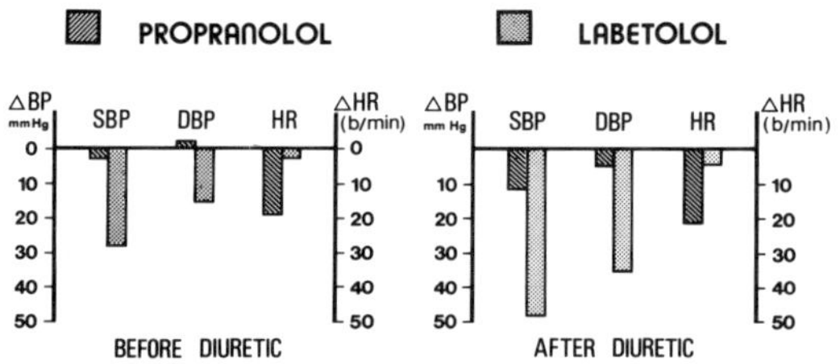

FIG. 2. Effect of chronic Chlorthalidone treatment on the blood pressure and heart rate response to acute Propranolol and Labetalol infusion.

DISCUSSION

Chlorthalidone chronic treatment of essential hypertensives gave rise to a remarkable and significant increase of the hypotensive (either systolic or diastolic) response to Labetalol acute infusion. On the contrary the same diuretic treatment induced only a very slight, and mostly systolic, hypotensive response to propranolol acute infusion.

These results suggest that diuretic treatment mainly enhances the vascular alpha adrenoceptor sensitivity to acute adrenergic blockade.

It is known that sodium may condition vascular reactivity to humoral vasoactive substances; on the other hand there is a considerable evidence that sodium depletion leads to an higher norepinephrine release from the nerve endings: it could be responsible for modifying the number and the affinity of the adrenergic receptors in the cell membranes. If the alpha-receptors were reduced in the periferal vasculature either in number or in responsiveness, it could explain why the activity of the adrenoreceptor blocking drugs is much more dramatic. (5-9)

REFERENCES

1. T.Kawasaki, C.S.Delea, F.C.Bartter, and H.Smith, Am.J.Med. 64,193,1978.
2. M.C. Khosla, I.Page, and F.M.Bumpus, Biochem.Pharm. 28,2867,1979.
3. L.K. Dahl, Am.J.Clin.Nutr. 25,231,1972.
4. J. De Champlain, J.Clin.Endocrinol.Metab. 6,633,1977.
5. F.C.Luft, L.I.Rankin, D.P.Henry, R.Bloch, and C.E.Grim, Hypertension 1, 261,1979.
6. S. Shah, I.Khatri, and E.D.Freis, Am.Heart J. 95,611,1978.
7. J. De Champlain, L.Krakoff, and J.Axelrod, Circ.Res. 24-25, suppl.1,75, 1969.
8. M.S.Romoff, G.Keusch, V.M.Campese, M.S.Wang, R.M.Friedler, P.Weidmann, and S.G.Massry, J.Clin.Endocr.Metab.48,26,1979.
9. M.G.Nicholls, W.Kiowski, A.Zweifler, S.Julius, M.A.Schork, and J.Greenhouse, Hypertension 2,29,1980.

COMPARISON OF THE EFFECTS OF HYDROCHLOROTHIAZIDE-AMILORIDE (MODURET) AND HYDROCHLOROTHIAZIDE ALONE ON BLOOD PRESSURE AND SERUM POTASSIUM IN MILD TO MODERATE ESSENTIAL HYPERTENSION

ALEXANDER G. LOGAN, MD, FRCP(C), *AND PIERRE LAROCHELLE, MD, PhD, FRCP(C)**
*Department of Medicine, Mount Sinai Hospital, Toronto, Ont., Canada M5G 1X5 (416-596-4301); **Institut de Recherches Cliniques de Montréal, 110 avenue des Pins ouest, Montréal, Qué., Canada H2W 1R7

INTRODUCTION

The most common and most serious electrolyte disturbance associated with thiazide therapy is a fall in serum and whole body potassium. The incidence of hypokalemia has been reported to be close to 50% with chronic administration (1). Many patients complain of weakness, fatigue, lassitude, muscle cramps and/or paresthesia which fortunately are usually reversible with potassium repletion. Of greater concern, however, is the possibility that diuretic-induced hypokalemia increases the risk of sudden death (2-4).

To minimize hypokalemia with chronic diuretic therapy, antikaliuretic agents such as amiloride have been combined with a thiazide. The present study was undertaken to compare the blood pressure lowering effect, the frequency of hypokalemia and the tolerability of a combination tablet of hydrochlorothiazide-amiloride (Moduret) with hydrochlorothiazide alone in adult patients with essential hypertension.

METHODS AND RESULTS

The study was limited to ambulatory patients of either sex between the ages of 18 and 70 years with essential hypertension whose supine diastolic blood pressure (Korotkoff Phase V), untreated for at least two weeks, lay in the range of 95 to 109 mmHg and whose serum potassium was 3.5 mmol/L or higher. Patients were drawn from 42 centres across Canada and gave their informed consent at entry. After a single-blind, placebo-controlled, prerandomization period of 2 to 4 weeks duration, patients were randomly assigned to receive, double-blind, either hydrochlorothiazide 50 mg - amiloride 5 mg combination tablet or hydrochlorothiazide 50 mg once daily. If diastolic blood pressure was > 90 mmHg after 2 weeks, the drug dosage was doubled. All patients were treated for 8 weeks.

There were 338 patients who were entered into the double-blind phase of trial. Of these, 27 were later excluded because they failed to meet the entry criteria with the most frequent reason being a diastolic blood pressure outside the acceptable range (18 patients). Other protocol violations included failure to keep scheduled appointments (12 patients), serum potassium below 3.5 mmol/L (8 patients), non-compliance with medication (7 patients) and use of other medication concomitantly (9 patients). Of the remainder, 15 patients had severe adverse effects from the medication, 2 had poorly controlled hypertension and 266 completed all phases of the study (133 in each group).

The mean age (52.2±10.6 vs 53.8±11.2 years), proportion of men (64 vs 55%) and mean weight (78.8±15.0 vs 76.2±14.5 kg) of the patients on hydrochlorothiazide - amiloride and hydrochlorothiazide respectively were not statistically significantly different. The effect of treatment

Diuretics, Jules B. Puschett, Editor

on blood pressure and pulse are described in Table I; the changes in the values of serum potassium, in Table II, III and IV; and the adverse experiences associated with each of the treatments, in Table V.

TABLE I. Change in blood pressure and pulse in supine and upright positions.

	Hydrochlorothiazide-Amiloride Blood Pressure			Hydrochlorothiazide Blood Pressure		
	Systolic (mmHg)	Diastolic (mmHg)	Pulse (bpm)	Systolic (mmHg)	Diastolic (mmHg)	Pulse (bpm)
Supine						
Entry	156±15	99±4	75±10	157±17	99±6	75±12
Week 8	138±16*	88±9*	77±12*	138±15*	87±8*	76±11
Change	-18±16	-11±9	2±10	-19±16	-12±8	1±11
Upright						
Entry	155±14	101±5	79±10	156±16	101±5	79±13
Week 8	136±15*	90±8*	82±11*	136±14*	90±8*	80±13
Change	-19±17	-11±9	3±11	-20±17	-11±9	2±11

* Significantly different from week 1 value ($p < 0.01$)

TABLE II. Change in serum potassium values (mmol/L)

	Hydrochlorothiazide - Amiloride	Hydrochlorothiazide
Entry	4.23±0.43	4.16±0.41
Week 8	3.91±0.46*+	3.69±0.48+
Change	-0.31±0.47*	-0.47±0.52

* Significantly different from corresponding value for hydrochlorothiazide - treated group ($p < 0.02$)
\+ Significantly different from entry value ($p < 0.02$)

TABLE III. Categorical change by number and percentage in serum potassium values.

Group	Time Period	Potassium (mmol/L) Range < 3.5	3.5 - 4.5	> 4.5
Hydrochlorothiazide - Amiloride	Entry	-	102 (76.7%)	31 (23.3%)
	Week 8*	18 (13.5%)	109 (81.9%)	6 (4.5%)
Hydrochlorothiazide	Entry	-	110 (82.7%)	23 (17.3%)
	Week 8	37 (28.7%)	87 (67.4%)	5 (3.9%)

* Significant difference between drugs ($p < 0.05$)

TABLE IV. Number and percent of patients who had reduction or increase in serum potassium of more than 0.6 mmol/L at week 8

	Hydrochlorothiazide - Amiloride* n(%)	Hydrochlorothiazide n(%)
Reduction of 0.6 mmol/L	24 (18.1%)	46 (35.7%)
No change outside limits	104 (78.2%)	79 (61.2%)
Increase of 0.6 mmol/L	5 (3.8%)	4 (3.1%)

* Significant difference between drugs ($p < 0.01$)

TABLE V. Adverse reactions during the trial

Event	Hydrochlorothiazide - Amiloride (n)	Hydrochlorothiazide (n)
Serum potassium < 3.0 mmol/L	1	3
Intolerable side effects*	4	4
Acute myocardial infarction	1	0
Poorly controlled hypertension	2	0
Symptomatic hypotension	1	1

* Include severe cramps, headaches, vertigo, dizziness and gastrointestinal disturbances

DISCUSSION AND CONCLUSION

The drug of first choice in the treatment of mild and moderate essential hypertension is the subject of considerable debate. Diuretics are the recommended first-step drug in North America, but thiazide-induced hypokalemia is of concern because of the possible link between this biochemical abnormality and sudden death (2-4). In the present study, both hydrochlorothiazide - amiloride and hydrochlorothiazide reduced blood pressure to a similar degree and were equally well tolerated. On the other hand, significantly more patients on hydrochlorothiazide had a serum potassium of less than 3.5 mmol/L and a reduction in potassium concentration of more than 0.6 mmol/L. In light of growing concern about the cardiovascular sequalae of hypokalemia, a potassium-sparing diuretic like hydrochlorothiazide-amiloride (Moduret) is preferrable to hydrochlorothiazide alone in the drug treatment of hypertension.

REFERENCES

1. F.G. McMahon, Management of Essential Hypertension (Futura, Mount Kisco, NY 1978).
2. Multiple Risk Factor Intervention Trial Research Group, JAMA 248, 1465-1477 (1982).
3. A. Helgeland, Amer. J. Med. 69, 725-732 (1980).
4. T.O. Morgan, J.B. Myers, and W. Adam in: Frontiers in Hypertension Research, J.H. Laragh, F.R. Buhler, and D.W. Seldin, eds. (Springer-Verlag, New York 1981) pp. 62-64.

COMPARISON OF THE EFFECTS OF MUZOLIMINE AND A FIXED COMBINATION OF HYDROCHLOROTHIAZIDE AND AMILORIDE IN MILDLY TO MODERATELY HYPERTENSIVE PATIENTS.

P. WICKER, M.D., and J. CLEMENTY, M.D.
Hôpital Cardiologique du Haut-Lévêque, 33604 Bordeaux-Pessac, France.

INTRODUCTION

Diuretics, together with beta-adrenergic blocking agents, are currently the most widely prescribed antihypertensive drugs. The Joint National Committee on Detection, Evaluation and Treatment of High Blood Pressure has recommanded diuretics as first-line therapy in most forms of hypertension (1), since they provide effective and adequate control in most hypertensive patients, and are usually well tolerated (2, 3).

In this article, a comparison of the efficacy and tolerance of muzolimine, a new loop diuteric, and a fixed combination of hydrochlorothiazide and amiloride in mild to moderate hypertensive patients is reported.

METHODS.

Patients were considered as eligible for entry into this double-blind, double-dummy study if they had mild to moderate hypertension (a supine diastolic blood pressure (DBP) of between 90 and 115 mm Hg). At their first visit, patients who met the above-mentionned inclusion criteria were enrolled into a placebo lead-in period. They were given placebo tablets for 3 to 4 weeks. At the end of this lead-in period, patients whose supine DBP was still over 90 mm Hg and below 115 mm Hg were randomly allocated to treatment with either 20 mg of muzolimine per day and a placebo matching hydrochlorothiazide and amiloride, or to a combination of hydrochlorothiazide (50 mg/day) and amiloride (5 mg/day) and a placebo matching muzolimine. Patients were subsequently seen at monthly intervals, for five months. Dosages of each active medicament were fixed throughout the study, and patients who did not respond to either regimen at these dosages were excluded.

All data reported are expressed as mean $\pm$ SD. The statistical significance of differences in results between the two groups was evaluated via a Student's t-test. Within each treatment group, values on entry and at each subsequent follow-up visit were subjected to an analysis of variance.

Response to treatment was also analysed by categorizing the results as follows :

- normalization : DBP below 9P mm Hg,
- improvment : DBP not normalized but decreased by more than 10 % ,
- failure : DBP not normalized and decreased by 10 % or less.

RESULTS.

Seventy-one patients were entered into the placebo lead-in period. Ten patients responded to placebo and were excluded. Sixty-one patients therefore were allocated to active treatment. Five of these were excluded from the final analysis because of poor cooperation. Fifty-six patients therefore from the basis of this report. Twenty-seven received muzolimine and 29 hydrochlorothiazide plus amiloride. Both groups were similar with regard to all prerandomization characteristics and duration of follow-up (4.7 months in both groups).

Blood pressure.

Both muzolimine and hydrochlorothiazide plus amiloride induced highly significant decreases in mean supine SBP and DBP (Table I). All values on follow-up over five months were significantly different from prerandomiza-

Diuretics, Jules B. Puschett, Editor

tion values ($p < 0,001$). The magnitude of changes in SBP and DBP was not statistically different between both groups.

TABLE I. Effects of five months of therapy with muzolimine or hydrochlorothiazide + amiloride on supine blood pressure in mildly to moderately hypertensive patients (mean ± SD).

	INITIAL VALUES	DURATION OF TREATMENT (months)				
		1	2	3	4	5
Number of patients						
- Muzolimine	27	27	26	26	25	22
- Combination	29	29	29	28	26	25
S B P (mm Hg)						
- Muzolimine	178±17	160±15	155±14	153±16	153±15	150±13
- Combination	172±15	157±13	150±13	150±13	147±14	147±12
D B P (mm Hg)						
- Muzolimine	103±6	91±8	86±8	87±10	85±9	84±10
- Combination	101±8	91±7	86±10	86±10	83±10	81±9

Categorization of the results as outlined above revealed that similar percentages (approximately 80 %) of patients in both groups experienced either normalization or improvment in DBP.

Heart rate and body weight.

Neither treatment induced any noticeable changes in supine or standing heart rate. A reduction in body weight occurred in both groups (muzolimine 3.4 Kg, combination 1.33 Kg), but the decreases were not statistically significant.

Serum potassium levels and other laboratory findings.

In both groups, serum potassium levels decreased. However, the changes were small (muzolimine 0.14 mmol/l, combination 0.18 mmol/l) and not significant. In addition, there were no significant differences between the groups as regards the magnitude of decrease in serum potassium.

As expected, blood uric acid levels increased slightly but not significantly. Fasting blood sugar and serum creatinine levels remained remarkably constant. None of the other laboratory tests (haemogram and the usual blood chemistry investigations) gave abnormal results.

Side effects.

During the trial, similar percentages of patients in the two groups (muzolimine 44 %, hydrochlorothiazide plus amiloride 55 %) complained of side effects. In most cases, side effects were mild. None was so severe that treatment had to be interrupted.

DISCUSSION.

Muzolimine is a new, nonsulfonamide diuretic belonging to the pyrazolinone group. Studies in man and animals have demonstrated that the site of action of muzolimine is located in the ascending limb of the loop of Henle (4). However, unlike other high-ceiling diuretics, muzolimine has a prolonged duration of action (4) which makes it suitable for long term treatment of hypertension.

Our results demonstrate that muzolimine is an effective antihypertensive agent. Supine and standing SBPs and DBPs were significantly reduced, by 15 to 20 %, by both muzolimine and the combination. These results are similar to those reported in previous studies with thiazide diuretics alone, as reviewed by Mc Mahon (3), and in more recent papers (5, 6).

As expected, muzolimine induced a slight but not significant decrease in serum potassium. The magnitude of this reduction (0.14 mmol/l) was similar to that previously reported in hypertensive patients when given other high-ceiling diuretics, such as furosemide (3). When thiazide diuretics are given alone, the decrease in serum potassium is usually more marked, ranging from 0.4 to 0.8 mmol/l (3). It was noteworthy that the reduction in potassium in both treatment groups was identical, and that no patient developed hypokalaemia.

The incidence of side effects in the two groups was somewhat higher than reported in previous studies on the combination of hydrochlorothiazide and amiloride (3, 6). This findings may be attributable to the fact that our patients were specifically and precisely questionned regarding possible side effects. The possibility therefore exists that various side effects in fact unrelated to treatment were listed.

CONCLUSION.

This study demonstrates the utility of muzolimine in mild to moderate hypertension. The drug was as effective as hydrochlorothiazide and amiloride. No serious adverse reactions to muzolimine were noted in this five - month trial.

REFERENCES.

1 . The Joint National Committee on Detection, Evaluation, and Treatment of High Blood Pressure : the 1980 report of the Joint National Committee on Detection, evaluation, and treatment of high blood pressure. Arch. Intern. Med. 140, 1280,(1980).

2 . Berglund, G. and Andersson, O. : Beta-blockers or diuretics in hypertension ? A six year follow-up of blood pressure and metabolic side effects. Lancet. 1 , 744, (1981).

3 . Mc Mahon, F.G. Management of Essential Hypertension. (Futura Publishing Company, Mount Kisco, 1978).

4 . Mussche, M. and Lameire, N. The mechanism of action of Bay g 2821 : a new diuretic. Curr. Med. Res. Opin. 4, 462, (1977).

5 . Veterans Administration Cooperative Study Group on Antihypertensive Agents : Comparative effects of ticrynafen and hydrochlorothiazide in the treatment of hypertension. N. Engl. J. Med. 30, 293 (1979).

6 . Multicenter Diuretic Cooperative Study Group : Multiclinic comparison of amiloride, hydrochlorothiazide, and hydrochlorothiazide plus amiloride in essential hypertension. Arch. Intern. Med., 141, 482 (1981).

ARE DIURETICS EFFECTIVE IN SALT-INDUCED HYPERTENSION IN DAHL-S-RATS?

BERNWARD GARTHOFF, WOLFGANG EBSEN, STANISLAV KAZDA, AND GEORG LUCKHAUS
Institutes of Pharmacology and Toxicology, Bayer AG, P.O.Box 101709,
D 5600 Wuppertal 1, Fed. Rep. Germany

INTRODUCTION

It was suggested that salt-induced hypertension in Dahl-S-rats (DS) is caused by the inability of the DS-kidneys to eliminate sodium chloride. Diuretics by facilitating sodium excretion, should prevent hypertension in DS rats whose blood pressure would otherwise increase to accomplish pressure natriuresis (1).

However, reports on the preventive effects of thiazides in DS are contradictory. In 6 week-old DS rats, a thiazide diuretic was not at all effective in preventing the initial marked rise of blood pressure when treatment was started concomitantly with feeding 8% NaCl diet (2).

To further clarify the effectiveness of diuretics in salt-induced hypertension, we treated DS rats by adding the more potent loop diuretics furosemide and muzolimine to a high salt diet.

METHODS

Groups of nine to ten female rats (Brookhaven colony) were treated with the following diets at the prehypertensive age of 6 weeks:
Group I: 8% NaCl diet
Group II: 8% NaCl diet plus muzolimine (800 ppm)
Group III: 8% NaCl diet plus furosemide (800 ppm)
Group IV: low NaCl diet (= 0.4% NaCl)
Blood pressure was measured at weekly intervals with the "tail cuff" method in conscious animals. At the end of the experiments (8 weeks), surviving animals were sacrificed by decapitation and blood samples were used for analysis. Heart wet weight was determined; relative values (organ weight per 100 g body weight) were used for evaluation. Histopathological investigations were performed in all tissues of the animals. Tissue samples were stained by standard procedures, and scored in a "blind" manner.

RESULTS

DS control rats (n=10) developed high blood pressure within 8 weeks, starting with a systolic blood pressure of 100 ± 4 mm Hg and reaching 229 ± 14 mm Hg (see Tab. 1). Three out of ten rats died as the results of malignant hypertension. Those rats receiving furosemide with the high salt diet also developed hypertension (211 ± 9 mm Hg after eight weeks), but increase in blood pressure was delayed, and none of the ten rats died. Muzolimine given with the high salt diet prevented hypertension, blood pressure remaining nearly as normal as that of normotensive DS control rats on low salt diet (148 ± 3 mm Hg versus 131 ± 3 mm Hg).

Hypertension induced cardiac hypertrophy (relative heart weight 482 ± 40 mg/100 g b.w. in the high salt DS) was significantly reduced in the muzolimine group only ($p < 0.01$), with the heart weight being approximately the same as that of normotensive DS controls on low salt diet (357 ± 9 mg/100 g versus 323 ± 7 mg/100 g). Heart weight in the furosemide treated group was 410 ± 12 mg/100 g (n.s.).

Diuretics, Jules B. Puschett, Editor

TABLE I. Blood pressure in salt-loaded rats (DS)

Group	Systolic blood pressure (mm Hg) [a)] 0	3	8 weeks
I	100±4 (10)[b)]	156±2 (10)	229±14 (7)
II	101±3 (9)	139±3 (9)[c)]	148± 3 (9)[c)]
III	100±3 (10)	148±4 (10)	211± 9 (10)
IV	100±4 (9)	124±2 (9)[c)]	131± 3 (9)[c)]

[a)] mean ± SEM   [b)] surviving animals   [c)] $p < 0.05$ vs. controls I

Histopathological (see Tab. 2) and clinicochemical results (data not shown) paralleled these findings. Malignant hypertensive arteriopathy, especially pronounced in the kidneys of DS rats on 8% NaCl, were characterized by periarteritis, medial hypertrophy and fibrinoid degeneration of the intima. The degree of this was less severe under furosemide treatment, but only with muzolimine a marked prevention of arteriopathy was achieved. There was slight dilation of the distal tubule and enlargement of the tubular epithelial cells as an index of diuretic activity in the treated DS rats.

TABLE II. Degree of hypertensive arteriopathy

	surviving animals	alterations severe	moderate	slight	none
I	7/10	2/10	3/10	2/10	2/10
II	9/ 9	0/ 9	0/ 9	1/ 9	8/ 9
III	10/10	1/10	1/10	3/10	5/10
IV	9/ 9	0/ 9	0/ 9	0/ 9	9/ 9

SUMMARY

Results obtained in hypertension prevention studies with loop diuretics in salt-loaded DS rats, demonstrate that there is a preventive effect of diuretic treatment on mortality with both muzolimine and furosemide, but only muzolimine exerts a sustained effect in preventing high blood pressure and its sequelae.

In contrast to what has been speculated, i.e. that the preventive effect depends on the age of DS rats at which diuretics and salt are started (3), our results suggest that the beneficial effect of diuretic treatment in salt-induced hypertension is merely dependent on the efficacy of the employed diuretic.

REFERENCES

1. L.Tobian, J.Lange, J.Iwai, K.Hiller, M.A.Johnson, and P.Goossens, Hypertension 1, 316-323 (1979).
2. J.Iwai, E.V.Ohanian, and L.K.Dahl, Circ. Res. 40, I 131-I 134 (1977).
3. J.P.Rapp, Hypertension 4, 753 (1982).

HEMODYNAMIC EFFECTS OF TRIPAMIDE, A NEW HYPOTENSIVE DIURETIC IN THE TREATMENT OF ESSENTIAL HYPERTENSION

TERUO TSUYUSAKI, MASAAKI MURAYAMA, SOTARO HAYASHI AND RYUICHI KIKAWADA
Department of Internal Medicine, Kitasato University School of Medicine, 1-15-1 Kitasato, Sagamihara, Kanagawa 228, Japan

ABSTRACT

Many diuretics, when used in patients with essential hypertension (EH), usually decrease cardiac output (CO) and increase total peripheral resistance (TPR) in early stage of treatment (acute phase), and within 4 weeks CO recovers to normal and TPR begins to decrease (retard reaction). Therefore we compared the hemodynamic effects of tripamide with those of usual diuretics.

Fifteen to 30 mg/day of tripamide was administered orally in 25 patients with EH. Systolic time intervals (STI) were analyzed with Blumberger-Holldack's method [1, 2] and cardiac pump performance with Wezler's method [3]. According to hemodynamic pattern the patients were divided into high TPR type, high CO type, and normal (N) type. Significant reductions in systolic pressure (Ps)(-12.3%, $p<0.001$) and diastolic pressure (Pd)(-10.5%, $p<0.001$) were observed. In high TPR type (N:12), during acute phase (1–2 weeks) of tripamide treatment, TPR decreased (2724→2514 dyne·sec·cm^{-5}, -7.7%) with little changes in CO (3.66→3.86 l/min, +5.5%), isovolumic contraction time (ICT)(-3.5%), preejection period (PEP)(+2.6%) and ejection time (ET)(+2.3%). In the following periods (2–4 weeks, 1–3 months, 3–6 months, 6–12 months) the decrease in TPR persisted. In N type (N:9) similar tendency was observed. These results suggest that tripamide caused significant decrease in Ps and Pd, and that, in high TPR type and N type, tripamide induced the same hemodynamics as retard reaction from early stage of treatment in contrast to other diuretics.

INTRODUCTION

Tripamide is a newly synthesized antihypertensive diuretic that has both hypotensive action and a mild but long-lasting diuretic action [4, 5] (Fig. 1). As for its hypotensive effect, it is reported that tripamide reduces blood pressure in the studies with DOCA-salt hypertensive rats and old spontaneously hypertensive rats [5]. Clinically its hypotensive effect is being estimated, however, its effect on hemodynamics in hypertension is not sufficiently elucidated. The purpose of the present study is to clarify the influences of tripamide upon hemodynamics in essential hypertension and to compare the hemodynamic effects of tripamide with those of other diuretics.

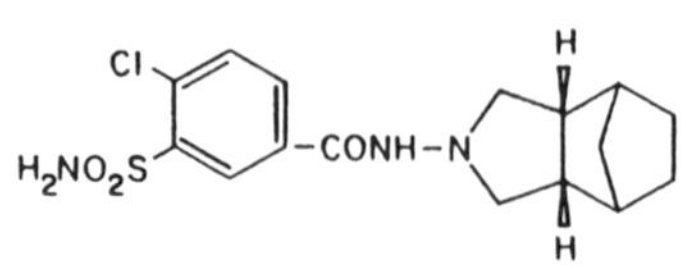

FIG. 1. Chemical structure of tripamide.

Diuretics, Jules B. Puschett, Editor

METHODS

Fifteen to 30 mg/day of tripamide was administered orally in 25 patients with EH between 34 and 79 years old (13 males and 12 females, mean age 58.9± 11.8 years). Blood pressure (BP) was measured with a cuff type sphygmomanometer. Systolic time intervals were analyzed with Blumberger-Holldack's method [1, 2] and cardiac pump performance with Wezler's method [3]. For this purpose carotid and femoral artery pulse waves, phonocardiogram and electrocardiogram were recorded simultaneously using the Mangograph 81 (Elma-Schönander CO). About these methods more explanations are described in other papers [6, 7]. According to hemodynamic pattern before treatment the patients were divided into high TPR type (TPR>2300 dyne•sec•cm^{-5}), high CO type (CO>6.3 l/min), and normal (N) type. As hemodynamic effects of antihypertensive drugs differ according to the duration of treatment, the effects of tripamide were estimated in the following periods: 1 week–2 weeks, 2 weeks–1 month, 1–3 months, 3–6 months, 6 months–1 year and more than 1 year.

RESULTS

1) Antihypertensive effect

At first the mean values of Ps and Pd before and during the treatment with tripamide were compared in 25 hypertensive patients. On an average, there were significant decreases in Ps (175→154 mmHg, -12.3%, p<0.001) and Pd (100→89 mmHg, -10.5%, p<0.001). Comparing each patient's response respectively, a significant decrease (p<0.05) in Ps was observed in 72.0% of the patients and that in Pd was in 60.0%.

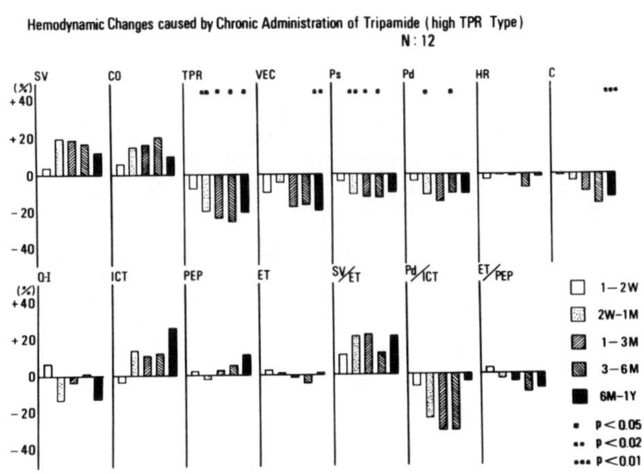

FIG. 2. In high TPR type, from early stage of the treatment with tripamide, significant decreases in TPR, Ps and Pd were observed.

2) Effects on hemodynamics

In high TPR type, during early phase (1 week–2 weeks) of treatment with tripamide, there appeared the decreases in Ps (-4.0%), Pd (-4.0%), heart rate (HR) (-3.3%), volume elasticity coefficient (VEC) (-9.7%) and TPR (-7.7%), accompanied by increases in stroke volume (SV) (+3.8%) and CO (+5.5%). There were little changes in Q-I (+7.0%), ICT (-3.5%), ET (+2.3%), ET/PEP (+2.5%) and SV/ET (+11.1%). However, in the period of 2–4 weeks of tripamide treatment, significant reductions in Ps (-10.7%, $p<0.02$), Pd (-11.5%, $p<0.05$), and TPR (-20.3%, $p<0.02$) were observed. At the same time, the values of SV (+19.8%) and CO (+14.9%) increased. In the periods of 1–3 months, 3–6 months, 6–12 months, and more than 1 year, almost the same tendency persisted (Fig. 2). Through all the periods treated with tripamide, there were remarkable decreases in Ps, Pd and TPR, and increasing tendencies in SV, CO and SV/ET. There were no significant changes in the value of ET/PEP.

In N type, the decreasing tendencies in Ps and Pd were observed, however, there were no significant changes in TPR, HR and STI.

In M type (though only 3 cases), the reductions in Ps (-6.1%), SV (-4.0%), and CO (-4.8%) were shown in acute phase (1–2 weeks), however, almost no changes in TPR (-0.6%), HR (-0.8%), and VEC (-2.1%) were observed. In the period of 3–4 weeks, the decreasing tendency in blood pressure persisted with little change in TPR.

DISCUSSION

Tripamide is a new antihypertensive drug that is reported to have an interesting feature of dissociation of antihypertensive and diuretic effects [5]. In small doses, it lowers the blood pressure chiefly through arteriolar vasodilating effects, and at larger doses, it can exert both vasodilating and diuretic effects . According to Igarashi [5], oral use of 1–100 mg/kg of tripamide did not influence on the BP in normotensive rat, however, in DOCA-salt hypertensive rats 1–10 mg/kg of tripamide induced significant decrease in BP over 3–9 hours, and also in spontaneously hypertensive rats, hypotensive effects of tripamide was observed by repeated administration more than 1 week. In the present study, antihypertensive effect of tripamide began to appear in the period of 1–2 weeks of the treatment and it became statistically significant in the period of 2–4 weeks. As to hemodynamic changes in these periods, a decrease in TPR was distinct especially in high TPR type and no decreases in SV and CO were observed. Many diuretics, when used in patients with EH, especially in high TPR type, usually decrease CO and increase TPR in early stage of treatment (acute phase) and within 4 weeks CO recovers to normal and TPR begins to decrease (retard reaction). In high CO type, however, even after several weeks the decrease in SV and CO lasts and the decrease in TPR is not manifest. In the treatment of EH, in which the elevation of TPR is supposed to be playing an important role , the appearance of retard reaction is very important. In this respect, in the present study, tripamide induced the same hemodynamics as retard reaction from early stage of treatment in high TPR type, and in N type no increase in TPR was seen from early stage of treatment. These results suggest that tripamide might influence on hemodynamics in EH more adequately than other diuretics.

REFERENCES

1. K. Blumberger, Arch. Kreisl. forsch. 6, 203-292 (1940).
2. K. Holldack, Dtsch. Arch. Klin. Med. 198, 71-91 (1951).
3. K. Wezler, Verh. dtsch. Ges. Kreisl. forsch. 15(Anhang), 18-19 (1949).
4. M. Kobayashi, et al. Shinryo to Shinyaku 16, 1001-1010 (1979).
5. T. Igarashi, et al. Shinryo to Shinyaku 16, 1253-1261 (1979).
6. R. Kikawada, et al. Jpn. Circul. J. 39, 755-764 (1975).
7. T. Tsuyusaki, et al. Asean J. of Clinical Sciences 2, 439-446 (1981).

EFFECTS OF TRIPAMIDE ON CARDIAC OUTPUT AND VASCULAR RESISTANCE IN SPONTANEOUSLY HYPERTENSIVE RATS.

T. IGARASHI, Y. NAKAJIMA AND T. SAEKI
Department of Pharmacology,Tsukuba Research Laboratories, Eisai Co., Ltd., Toyosatomachi, Ibaraki, Japan

INTRODUCTION

Tripamide is a new antihypertensive drug with a mild but long-acting sodium uretic action [1,2]. In a previous paper [2], we reported that tripamide reduced blood pressure even after a single dosing in acute studies with DOCA-salt hypertensive rats and spontaneously hypertensive rats (SHR), and that the antihypertensive action was more remarkably manifested by repeated administration. These findings were obtained using an indirect determination of blood pressure with a tail-cuff method. The present study aimed to investigate the antihypertensive effect of single and repeated dosing with tripamide by a direct determination of blood pressure on the one hand and to clarify effects of tripamide on cardiac output and vascular resistance in connection with the mechanism of action on the other. Propranolol, an adrenergic beta-blocker was chosen as a reference drug, since it reduces cardiac output and increases vascular resistance in acute studies but reduces vascular resistance by repeated administration resulting in blood pressure reduction.

This paper includes a brief description of a new methodology with which we tried to determine cardiac output in unrestrained conscious rats.

MATERIALS AND METHODS

Experiments were carried out with male SHR (40-55 weeks old, 400-450 g). The amimals were housed under conditions of 23 ± 2 C temperature, 55 ± 5% humidity and 12 hour lighting (7:00-19:00). They were fed a pellet diet and had free access to tap water.

For the determination of blood pressure and cardiac output, two polyethylene catheters were implanted in the body under ether anesthesia on the day before the experiment. One (PE-10, Clay Adams) was used for rapid injection of ice-cold saline into the vena cava superior in the vicinity of the opening to the right atrium. The other (PE-50, Clay Adams) was used to determine blood pressure in the aortic arch. A thermoelement (TW-300, Tokai Irika) was placed in the aortic arch through the aortic catheter to measure blood temperature. Both catheters were passed subcutaneously to the back of the neck and exteriorized through a small stab wound.

During the experiment, the animals were housed in individual cages, 16 x 24 x 13 cm^3. The aortic catheter was connected to a transducer (MPU-0.5A, Nihon Kohden) in order to record phasic and mean blood pressure. Heart rate was counted by a tachometer (AT-600G, Nihon Kohden) triggered by the blood pressure pulse. Cardiac output was estimated from the thermo-dilution curve after an injection of 0.1 ml of ice-cold saline into the vena cava superior. The thermoelement was connected to an electronic thermometer (Shincorder TTA-100, Shinei). Blood pressure and heart rate were recorded on a polygraph (RM-600, Nihon Kohden) and aortic blood temperature on a pen-writing recorder.

Tripamide (Eisai) and propranolol hydrochloride (ICI) were prepared in gum arabic solution and given by stomach tube. Control animals received the vehicle alone.

The thermodilution method based on the Fick principle for the determination of cardiac output has some problems when it is applied to the hemodynamic analysis in small animals such as rats. The limited amount of the indicator, e.g., 0.1 ml of 0°C saline, makes the relative amount of the indicator lost in the implanted catheter not negligible. The amount of thermodiffusion into the

Diuretics, Jules B. Puschett, Editor

tissue during lung circulation should be also taken into account. Therefore, it seems impossible to determine exactly the absolute value of cardiac output by the thermodilution method in conscious rats. However, if the amount of thermo-loss remains nearly constant in individual animals, the declining gradient of the thermodilution curve would reflect the relative change in cardiac output, as indicated by the Fick principle. The thermodilution method has the advantages that no withdrawal of blood is necessaray and that the determination can be easily repeated at short time-intervals. In fact, we could detect transient changes in cardiac output which was caused by an intravenous injection of isoproterenol with this method.

RESULTS

At the beginning of the experiment, blood pressure of test animals was in a range of 180-220 mmHg in systole, 130-160 mmHg in diastole and heart rate was 300-380. Changes in heart rate, mean blood pressure, cardiac output and vascular resistance during three days of the experiment are shown in Fig. 1.

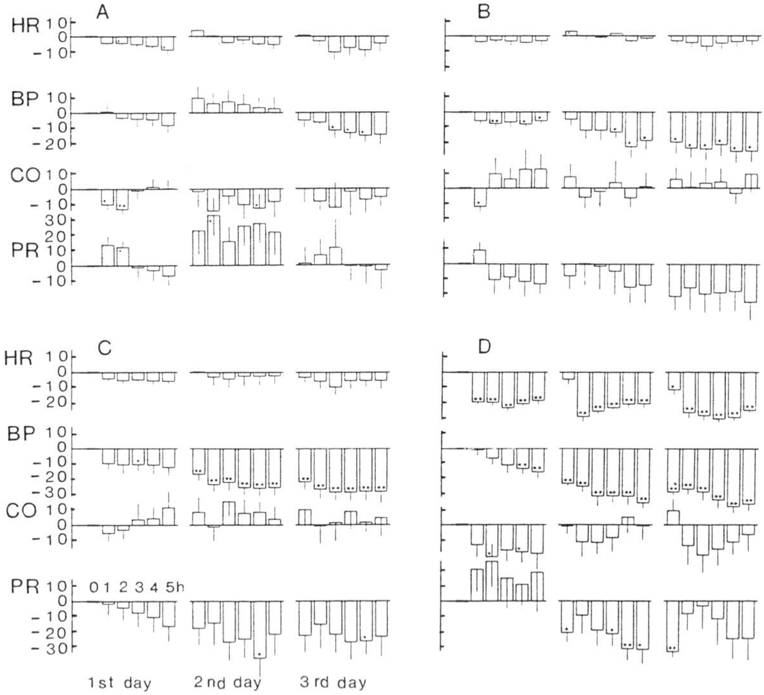

Fig. 1. Changes in heart rate (HR), mean blood pressure (BP), cardiac output (CO) and vascular resistance (PR) in SHR during three days of experiment. Ordinate: Percent change compared to the pre-value of the first dosing day (mean ± S.E.). Statistical significance of differences from the pre-value (paired t-test) is shown by * (0.01 < P < 0.05) or ** (P < 0.01). Abscissa: Time course (hours) after drug-administration. Drugs were given by stomach tube once a day for three consecutive days. A: Control group treated with the vehicle (gum arabic solution), n=8. B: 4 mg/kg of tripamide, n=7. C: 40 mg/kg of tripamide, n=7. D: 40 mg/kg of propranolol, n=7.

In the control group, in which the animals were given the vehicle alone once a day for three consecutive days, blood pressure tended to increase on the second experimental day and fell significantly on the third day. Fluctuations in heart rate were less than 10%, while those in cardiac output were around 15%. Heart rate and cardiac output tended to decrease. The reduction in cardiac output was statistically significant at several time points. The vascular resistance estimated from the ratio of blood pressure to cardiac output varied in a range from -10% to +33% of the pre-value of the first experiment day.

Reduction in blood pressure after the first dosing of 4 mg/kg of tripamide was less than 10%, but statistically significant. With the repeated administration of tripamide on the second and third days, the antihypertensive effect became more remarkable. Heart rate and cardiac output fluctuated, but remained within the range of the controls. In the group given 40 mg/kg of tripamide, blood pressure was reduced by 10% on the first day, and 20-30% on the second and third days, while heart rate and cardiac output remained unchanged. Therefore, the antihypertensive action of tripamide could be accounted for by a reduction in vascular resistance.

In the group treated with 40 mg/kg of propranolol, heart rate and cardiac output decreased after each dosing and returned to the pre-value within 24 hours, while blood pressure gradually fell after the first dosing and remained lowered on the second and third days. Vascular resistance tended to increase for several hours after the dosing not only on the first day but also on the second and third days.

DISCUSSION

The above-mentioned hemodynamic effects of propranolol may suggest the propriety of the method used for cardiac output determination in the present study. Similar to clinical observations, propranolol reduced blood pressure in two ways, i.e., by decreasing cardiac output on the first dosing day and by decreasing vascular resistance on the second and third days.

The findings of the present study on the antihypertensive effect of tripamide well support the results of our previous paper [2]. Both systolic and diastolic blood pressures were reduced by a single dosing of 4 or 40 mg/kg of tripamide and the effect manifested more remarkably by repeated administration. The reduction in blood pressure could be accounted for by the decrease in vascular resistance since cardiac output remained unchanged throughout the three-day treatment with tripamide. However, it still remains unknown whether the reduction in vascular resistance by tripamide is caused by its renal effect [1,3] or through a direct effect on the vascular smooth muscles [4].

REFERENCES

1. M. Kobayashi, N. Mori, T. Tomiuga and T. Igarashi, Shinryo to Shinyaku 16, 1001-1010 (1979) (in Japanese).
2. T. Igarashi, Y. Nakajima and M. Kobayashi, Shinryo to Shinyaku 16, 1253-1261 (1979) (in Japanese).
3. D. C. Brater and S. Anderson, Clin. Pharmacol. Ther. 34, 79-85 (1983).
4. H. Asada, T. Itoh, H. Suzuki, Y. Ito and H. Kuriyama, Gen. Pharmac. 13, 215-223 (1982).

A CLASSIFICATION OF ESSENTIAL HYPERTENSIVE PATIENTS ACCORDING TO THE ERYTHROCYTE Na TRANSPORT ABNORMALITIES: A NEW STRATEGY FOR MONITORING THE MANAGEMENT OF HIGH BLOOD PRESSURE.

RICARDO GARAY*, CORINNE NAZARET*, EVELYNE DESCHAMPS DE PAILLETTE, GERARD JUIN, AND PIERRE BRAQUET.
* INSERM U7/CNRS LA 318. Hôpital Necker. Paris 75015 and I.H.B. 17, av. Descartes, Le Plessis Robinson, France.

ABSTRACT

A detailed kinetic study of the interaction of internal Na with different erythrocyte Na transport systems has recently permitted the distinction of different subgroups of essential hypertensive patients (Pump ⊖, Co ⊖, Counter ⊕ and Leak ⊕). On the other hand, <u>in vitro</u> experiments have shown that cicletanide, a new diuretic and antihypertensive agent, stimulates K fluxes in human erythrocytes.

Herein, we provide results on the <u>in vivo</u> effect of cycletanide in 45 essential hypertensive patients previously characterized according to the above classification. Blood samples were drawn before and after 1, 4 and 8 months of treatment. Results indicate that the antihypertensive efficiency of the compound depends on the magnitude of the K-flux stimulation and on the subgroup to which the hypertensive belongs. Thus measurement of ion fluxes in human erythrocytes may be used as a test for monitoring the management of hypertension.

INTRODUCTION

Na movements across human red cell membranes are mediated by several transport systems: i) a Na,K pump which exchanges internal Na for external K using the energy supplied by the hydrolysis of ATP, ii) a Na,K cotransport system which catalyzes coupled movements of Na and K across the cell membrane and iii) a one:to:one Na:Na (or Na:Li) countertransport system. The inhibition of these transport systems unmasks a residual Na flux with kinetic properties consistent with the ground membrane Na-leak.

A detailed kinetic analysis of Na fluxes in erythrocytes from essential hypertensive patients has recently shown the existence of at least 4 subgroups of hypertensives: <u>Pump ⊖ hypertensives</u>: showing low pump affinity for internal Na and high maximal pump rate, ii) <u>Co ⊖ hypertensives</u>: characterized by low cotransport affinity for internal Na and low or normal maximal cotransport rate, iii) <u>Counter ⊕ hypertensives</u>: characterized by low countertransport affinity for internal Na and high maximal countertransport rate and iv) <u>Leak ⊕ hypertensives</u>: showing increased Na-leak (1,2). A study of the apparent affinity of the Na,K cotransport system for external K has permitted to divide the Co ⊖ hypertensives in three subgroups (symmetric, asymmetric and antisymmetric) according to the presence of low, normal or high K affinity (3)

We have previously observed that natriuretic furopyridines such as cicletanide are able to stimulate K movements across human red cell membranes <u>in vitro</u> (4). The study of structural analogues showed that the intensity of this effect is strongly correlated with the natriuretic activity. On the other hand, the mechanism of action of cicletanide appears to involve a K-dependant, prostacyclin generation in the vascular wall (5).

The above results led us to investigate here the <u>in vivo</u> effects of cicletanide on blood pressure and erythrocyte K fluxes in 45 essential hypertensive patients previously characterized according to the above classification.

Diuretics, Jules B. Puschett, Editor

PATIENTS

45 essential hypertensive patients (25 males,20 females) aged from 30 to 70 years old,were included in this study. All the hypertensive patients were on free Na diet and none was treated with antihypertensive drugs for at least one month before the study. Initial mean blood pressure ranged from 132 to 155 mmHg.

Starting from time 0, all hypertensives received 150 mg of cicletanide per day (see Figure 1).

METHODS

Venous blood was drawn into heparinized tubes at various monthly intervales (see Figure 1). Erythrocyte Na and K fluxes, Na and K contents and cell volume were measured by methods used and detailed in previous studies (1,3,4)

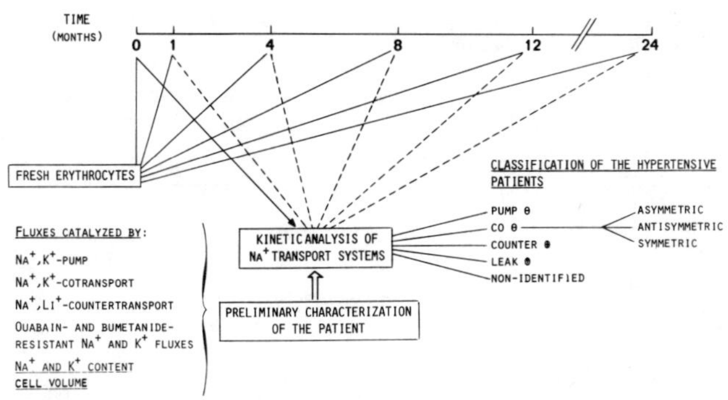

FIG 1. Protocol for the study of Na and K transport in erythrocytes from 45 essential hypertensive patients treated with 150 mg of cicletanide per day.

RESULTS

This study will be continued for 2 years. Here we present preliminary results obtained during the first 4 months of treatment.

Antihypertensive treatment with cicletanide has no significant effect on erythrocyte Na and K contents, cell volume and fluxes catalyzed by the Na,K pump, Na,K cotransport and Na,Li countertransport systems and Na leak. Conversely, we observed a significant increase in ouabain and bumetanide-resistant K fluxes (see Figure 2). This effect is correlated with the decrease in blood pressure (Fig.2).

31 out of the 45 hypertensives included in this study have been already characterized according to a previous classification (1,2,3). Table 1 shows values of mean blood pressure after 4 months of treatment. It appears from this Table that cicletanide treatment is more effective in Asymmetric Co ⊖ hypertensives than in Counter ⊕ or Pump ⊖ hypertensives.

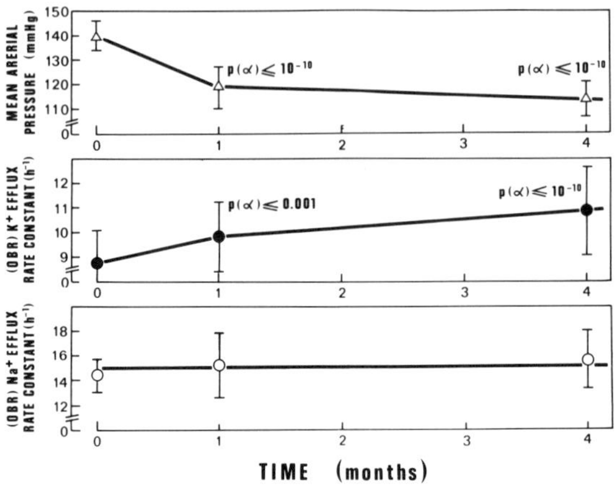

FIG. 2. Stimulation of erythrocyte K fluxes by antihypertensive treatment with cicletanide. Values are given as mean$\pm$SD.

TABLE I. Mean blood pressure (mmHg) in different subgroups of essential hypertensive patients treated for 4 months with 150mg per day of cicletanide.

Subgroup	Mean blood pressure(mmHg)
Pump ⊖	119.8 $\pm$ 2.1 (4)
Antisymmetric Co ⊖	115.0 $\pm$ 6.2 (3)
Asymmetric Co ⊖	109.0 $\pm$ 2.9 (5)
Symmetric Co ⊖	117.0 $\pm$ 6.8 (4)
Counter ⊕	119.1 $\pm$ 9.5 (9)
Leak ⊕	113.8 $\pm$ 7.5 (6)

Values in this Table are given as mean$\pm$SD

DISCUSSION

The population of essential hypertensive patients is heterogeneous regarding erythrocyte Na transport abnormalities (1,2,3). On the other hand, antihypertensive drugs may act, directly or indirectly, on transmembrane ion transport. Preliminary results obtained here with cicletanide indicate that the antihypertensive efficiency of the compound depends on the magnitude of the K-flux stimulation and on the subgroup to which the hypertensive belongs.

REFERENCES

1. R.P.Garay, C.Nazaret, P.Hannaert and M.Price.Eur.J.Clin.Invest. 13, 311, 1983.
2. R.P.Garay et.al. Phys.Chem.Transm.Ion.Mot. (Elsevier) 645, 1983.
3. M.Price, P.Hannaert, G.Dagher and R.Garay. Hypertension (in press).
4. R.P.Garay et.al. Bioch.Pharm. (in press).
5. P.Braquet,C.Deby,R.Garay et.al. The Lancet i,1218, 1983.

SECTION III

DIURETICS AND BETA BLOCKERS IN HYPERTENSION

BETA-ADRENERGIC ANTAGONISTS AND ANGIOTENSIN CONVERTING ENZYME INHIBITORS: COMPARISON AND INTERACTION WITH DIURETICS. A SUMMARY OF VETERANS ADMINISTRATION COOPERATIVE STUDIES.

BARRY J. MATERSON, M.D.
Miami Veterans Administration Medical Center, Medical and Research Services, and the Department of Medicine, University of Miami, Miami, FL 33125 USA.

INTRODUCTION

In 1960, George Perera, a distinguished investigator based at Columbia University College of Physicians and Surgeons, published a paper on the drug treatment of hypertension in which he concluded that, over a seven-year period, there was no beneficial effect of treatment on survival [1]. These patients had a maximum pre-treatment blood pressure that averaged 224/132 mmHg and they were treated with drugs such as hexamethonium, pentolinium, mecamylamine, rauwolfia and hydralazine. Over seven years, 16 of the 29 patients in each group (55%) died, the most common causes being congestive heart failure, stroke and myocardial infarction. Dr. Perera was cautious in his conclusions, but suggested that "the burden of proof, that drugs which lower the arterial pressure will prolong the lives of patients with primary hypertension who do not have the accelerated form of disease, must rest with those who make such claims".

Four months later, Dupler et al [2] reviewed "in simple, practical form the present status of the management of essential hypertension" based on their experience with private patients at the University of Pennsylvania. Their initial therapy was reserpine. When 39/49 patients failed to respond, they added the new drug, hydrochlorothiazide, and achieved control in all but 10 patients. When hydralazine was added, 8 of these last 10 had an excellent or good response. Curiously, non-diuretic initial therapy now seems to have come full circle.

In 1967, Dr. Edward D. Freis and the Veterans Administration Cooperative Study Group on Antihypertensive Agents published the landmark paper demonstrating the efficacy of antihypertensive therapy in reducing morbidity and mortality in the treatment group when compared to a placebo treated control group [3]. What accounted for this striking difference? The simple answer is diuretics. The first study was performed before the availability of orally active diuretic agents. The available drugs were associated with extremely noxious adverse effects including orthostatic hypotension, constipation, difficulty in initiating urination, sexual dysfunction and depression. Reserpine and hydralazine had been available since the early 1950's, but high doses were required for therapeutic effect and this effect was soon lost owing to extracellular fluid volume expansion. In addition, they were associated with severe adverse effects of their own including depression and a systemic lupus erythematosis-like syndrome. When diuretics became available, it became possible to use lower doses of reserpine and hydralazine in combination so that a highly effective triple therapeutic regimen could be devised that was associated with relatively few adverse effects.

As each subsequent class of antihypertensive drugs has evolved, it has become evident that their efficacy is enhanced by combination with a diuretic drug. This paper will focus mostly on beta-adrenergic

Diuretics, Jules B. Puschett, Editor

antagonists and the enhancement of their effect by diuretics. Although numerous examples exist in the literature, discussion will be limited to the several Veterans Administration Cooperative Studies Group papers in which the enhancing effect of diuretics was demonstrated.

THE FIRST VETERANS ADMINISTRATION PROPRANOLOL STUDY

Partial results of the first Veterans Administration Cooperative study dealing with propranolol [4] are displayed in Table I. It is interesting that in this study of mild to moderately hypertensive patients, the combination of reserpine and hydrochlorothiazide was just as effective as the triple regimen of propranolol, hydralazine and hydrochlorothiazide. Propranolol used alone was associated with the approximate decrement in blood pressure and success rate that has been demonstrated with hydrochlorothiazide alone. In the parallel group of patients that was treated with propranolol plus hydrochlorothiazide, an additive effect on blood pressure was evident as was an increase in the percent of patients controlled from 52 to 81%. This same general relationship also obtained for the group of patients treated with propranolol plus hydralazine. The group that received hydrochlorothiazide in combination with propranolol and hydralazine had a substantially greater reduction in blood pressure as well as an increase in the percent of patients controlled from 72 to 92%. Overall, this study demonstrated that reserpine combined with hydrochlorothiazide remained a highly effective regimen although it was associated with a high percentage of nasal stuffiness. Propranolol was clearly demonstrated to be useful as single-drug therapy. The addition of diuretic markedly enhanced the efficacy of propranolol and a combination of propranolol plus hydralazine. Other than nasal stuffiness, there were no significant differences in clinical side effects between the regimens. The regimens that included diuretic had hypokalemia and hyperuricemia more frequently.

Table I. Results of the first Veterans Administration trial on propranolol [4].[a)]

Regimen	R + T	P	P + T	P + H	P + H + T
N	75	81	77	75	75
BP Reduction	26.6/16.7	11.6/9.0	24.7/14.5	14.9/12.7	27.5/18.3
% Controlled[b)]	88	52	81	72	92
% Controlled at Level 1	67	26	56	43	73
% Requiring Level 4	8	40	8	28	9
% K <3.2 mEq/L	9.3	2.4	10.3	1.3	9.3
% Uric Acid >8.9 mg/dL	37.3	3.7	28.5	5.3	28.0

a) R = reserpine; T = hydrochlorothiazide; P = propranolol; H = hydralazine; N = number in group; BP = blood pressure in mmHg.
b) Controlled means a diastolic BP <90 mmHg and ≥ 5mmHg decline from baseline. Level 1 = reserpine 0.3mg plus hydrochlorothiazide 105mg; propranolol 120mg; propranolol 120mg plus hydrochlorothiazide 105mg; propranolol 120mg plus hydralazine 105mg; or propranolol 120mg plus hydrochlorothiazide 105mg plus hydralazine 105mg. These total doses were given divided three times daily. Level 4 was the same as Level 1 for reserpine, hydrochlorothiazide and hydralazine, but was 480mg for propranolol.

THE SECOND VETERANS ADMINISTRATION PROPRANOLOL STUDY

The results of the above study suggested that propranolol given alone was approximately as effective as hydrochlorothiazide given alone. The second study was designed to address the question whether one drug was superior to the other in terms of efficacy and/or adverse effects and to test the validity of the algorithm calling for diuretic as the initial drug treatment of hypertension [5].

We recruited 906 ambulatory men in seven VA Medical Centers for this prospective, randomized double-blind trial. Of these, 683 met the blood pressure (diastolic BP 95-114 mmHg) and compliance criteria for randomization after a four-week single-blind placebo period.

Patients received either 40mg of propranolol twice daily or 25mg of hydrochlorothiazide twice daily. After two weeks, if goal BP (diastolic BP <90 mmHg) had not been achieved, the drug was increased to the next blinded level. Possible total daily doses of propranolol were 80, 160, 240, 320, 480 and 640mg; those for hydrochlorothiazide were 50, 100 and 200mg. Because there were twice as many propranolol dose levels as for hydrochlorothiazide, every other hydrochlorothiazide blinded "increase" was actually not a change in dose. When patients were at goal BP on two consecutive visits, they became eligible for entry into the long-term phase of the trial. Patients who reached the maximum drug dose, but not goal BP, could still be entered into the long-term trial if they were compliant and if their BP was <100 mmHg and ≥ 6 mmHg below their BP at randomization.

Results

Propranolol (N = 340) lowered BP from 146.0 ± 14.4 (mean $\pm$ SD)/101.6 ± 4.6 to $134.8 \pm 16.3/90.5 \pm 7.6$ compared to hydrochlorothiazide which lowered BP from $146.5 \pm 15.8/101.3 \pm 4.5$ to $128.8 \pm 12.2/89.4 \pm 6.5$. The reduction of systolic BP by hydrochlorothiazide was greater than that by propranolol ($P<.001$) as was diastolic BP ($P=.03$). The heart rate decreased from 77 to 61 bpm with propranolol and increased from 77 to 79 with hydrochlorothiazide.

If analysis had ceased at this point, it would have been possible to conclude that hydrochlorothiazide was superior to propranolol for initial therapy of hypertension. The study population, however, was 56.8% black compared with 11.8% blacks in the general population of the United States. When the data were analyzed by race (Table II), a racial effect on therapeutic efficacy was evident.

Removal of patients from the protocol for medical reasons occurred in 3.8% of the patients taking propranolol and 1.7% of those receiving hydrochlorothiazide, but this was not a statistically significant difference.

This study suggested that white patients were likely to have equal benefit from the two drugs, but that black patients responded less to propranolol and far better to hydrochlorothiazide. The choice of an initial antihypertensive drug for white patients could therefore be made on the basis of facts other than efficacy alone; e.g., relative contraindications, co-indications such as migraine, angina pectoris or essential tremor, convenience of titration, patient acceptance and cost.

Of interest is the fact that some patients responded to "dummy" increases in the dose of hydrochlorothiazide. Of the total patients who achieved goal BP while taking hydrochlorothiazide, 18.5% did so after two additional weeks on 50mg, 10.0% on two additional weeks on 100mg and 9.5% after one additional week on 200mg. This was probably due to additional time for the drug to exert its effect and is a lesson to the clinician to be patient as blood pressure approaches goal. It may take as long as six months for the full effect of a thiazide diuretic on hypertension to be reached [6].

Table II. Racial differences in the effect of propranolol and hydrochlorothiazide on blood pressure.[a)]

	Propranolol		Hydrochlorothiazide	
	White	Black	White	Black
Reduction of Systolic Blood Pressure	13.2±13.1	8.2±12.2*	15.3±12.0	20.3±14.3*
Reduction of Diastolic Blood Pressure	12.6± 6.6*	9.5±7.0*	10.9± 5.7*	13.0± 7.0*
% Reaching Goal	61.7	53.3*	55.3	71.3*
% ≤ 140mmHg Systolic	68.0*†	64.1*†	81.6*†	87.7*†
% ≥ 160mmHg Systolic	9.4*	7.1	1.4*	1.8
% ≥ 100mmHg Diastolic	8.6†	17.6†	10.6	7.6
% Increase Systolic	14.1*†	24.1*†	7.1*	7.0*
% Increase Diastolic	3.1†	10.0†	5.7	4.7

a) Blood pressure recorded as mean ± SD in mmHg. * indicates a statistically significant (P<.05) difference between the effect of the two drugs in the same race. † indicates a statistically significant (P<.05) difference between the two races taking the same drug.

The Chronic Treatment Phase

Of the original 683 randomized patients, 394 entered the long-term treatment phase and 302 completed the 12-month study [7]. There was a tendency for blood pressure to increase over the year for patients of both races taking either drug. White patients taking propranolol had a blood pressure increase of 6.6/5.3 mmHg compared with 2.2/0.5 for those taking hydrochlorothiazide (P<.001). Black patients taking propranolol had a blood pressure increase of 7.7/3.2 mmHg compared with 1.6/1.5 mmHg for those taking hydrochlorothiazide (P<.001). At one year, white patients taking propranolol had blood pressure reduced 10.6/11.5 mmHg from baseline; the hydrochlorothiazide group was 14.7/12.0 mmHg from baseline. Black patients taking propranolol had blood pressure reduced 5.6/11.3 mmHg from baseline; for hydrochlorothiazide the reduction was 19.9/14.0 mmHg. Therefore, the tendency for loss of control was greater for propranolol than hydrochlorothiazide irrespective of race. The diuretic continued to be more effective in blacks and propranolol about the same as hydrochlorothiazide in whites.

More terminations for medical reasons occurred in the propranolol treated group than the hydrochlorothiazide group (35 vs 11; P<.001). Most of these (25 propranolol, 3 hydrochlorothiazide) were due to loss of control of blood pressure to diastolic >104 mmHg or greater than the baseline blood pressure in two successive visits or any single visit >119 mmHg. Seven propranolol patients were terminated from the study because of drug side effects (wheezing, syncope, impotence, depression, hallucinations) while only one patient was dropped because of hydrochlorothiazide associated muscle cramps. Complaints that were reported in more than 1% of patient visits for propranolol were insomnia (2.6%), swelling of the hands (2.6%), vivid dreams (1.9%), diarrhea (1.5%) and impotence (2.0%). For hydrochlorothiazide, the complaints were insomnia (1.0%), swelling of hands (1.0%), diarrhea (9.7%), impotence (2.9%), constipation (1.6%) and numbness (1.5%).

In summary, this complex study showed that propranolol and hydrochlorothiazide were equally effective in white patients, but there was a tendency toward loss of control with time. In black patients in particular, but also in the general study population, hydrochlorothiazide appeared to be effective, at least as safe, less expensive, and associated with fewer premature terminations than propranolol.

Evaluation of the Renin-Angiotensin system

Additional questions posed in this trial related to the ability to predict drug response by means of renin profiling and renin response to intravenous furosemide. We determined plasma renin activity (PRA) and responsiveness at baseline and after treatment with either propranolol or hydrochlorothiazide [8]. Special care was taken to use assay methods previously approved by the Laragh-Sealey group (see [8] and its references for details).

Low renin profiles were found in 56%, normal in 33% and high in 11% of our patients. This is a greater preponderance of low renin profiles than in the general population [9]. Black patients and older patients of both races had lower initial PRA and renin responsiveness. Although the high renin patients tended to respond better to propranolol and the low renin patients to hydrochlorothiazide, this was by no means absolute. Treatment failures and loss of control occurred randomly across renin profile groups.

Our data were generally consistent with the volume-vasoconstrictor analysis of essential hypertension. They do not support the concept, however, that response can be predicted based on pre-treatment renin profiling. The slight clinical differences in response to treatment with hydrochlorothiazide vs. propranolol do not appear to warrant the cost or effort involved in renin profiling.

Racial Differences in Electrolyte Excretion

It is not known why blacks tend to have a greater prevalence of hypertension and also low renin profile. We performed urinary electrolyte excretion studies on the patients in this trial [10] and found that there was no racial difference in urine sodium excretion (184 ± 108 mEq/24 hours for whites, 176 ± 117 for blacks), but that blacks excreted significantly ($P < .001$) less urine potassium (45 ± 39 mEq/24 hours for blacks, 73 ± 41 for whites). The urinary Na/K excretion ratio correlated significantly with systolic blood pressure. One hypothesis is that blacks comsume less dietary potassium and thereby initiate the events leading to higher blood pressure, volume expansion, low renin and low aldosterone.

THE VETERANS ADMINISTRATION STUDY ON NADOLOL AND BENDROFLUMETHIAZIDE

That the lessons learned from the prior studies on propranolol and hydrochlorothiazide were not limited to these drugs was demonstrated by a study of patients receiving nadolol or bendroflumethiazide alone or the combination [11].

We randomized 365 men with diastolic blood pressure of 95-114 to once-daily treatment with nadolol (80-240mg), bendroflumethiazide (5-10mg) or the combination. Non-responders were treated single-blind by the addition of hydralazine (50-200mg).

Goal blood pressure was attained by 46% of the patients taking diuretic, 49% of those receiving beta-blocker and 85% of patients on the combination. The addition of hydralazine controlled 60% of those previously not at goal. Blood pressure changes are displayed in Table III.

Table III. Blood pressure reduction after 12 weeks of therapy.[a)]

	Bendro (68)	Nadolol (104)	Combination (136)
Systolic Blood Pressure			
Whites (130)	13.3±2.0	17.2±2.3	22.9±1.7
Blacks (178)	19.9±2.4	5.8±2.1	27.3±2.1
Diastolic Blood Pressure			
Whites	10.2±1.7	15.6±1.2	17.7±0.8
Blacks	12.4±1.5	9.6±0.9	18.1±1.0

a) Blood pressure displayed as mean ± SE in mmHg. Numbers in parentheses are numbers in each group. Refer to [11] for statistical analysis.

This study tended to confirm the racial differences found in the second propranolol trial, but the diuretic racial effect was less and the beta-blocker racial effect was much greater. The combination of diuretic with beta-blocker abolished the racial differences. The findings are also of interest when compared to the first VA propranolol trial. Propranolol alone controlled 52% of patients compared with 49% for nadolol. Propranolol plus hydrochlorothiazide controlled 81% compared with 85% for nadolol plus bendroflumethiazide. Propranolol plus hydralazine controlled 72% of patients; nadolol plus hydralazine controlled 75%. Propranolol/hydrochlorothiazide/hydrazaline controlled 88%; nadolol/bendroflumethiazide/hydralazine controlled 93%. As before, adverse effects were few and medical terminations very low.

THE OXPRENOLOL VS PROPRANOLOL TRIAL

This study was designed to compare oxprenolol vs propranolol as "Step-2" therapy in patients who had not achieved goal blood pressure with hydrochlorothiazide alone [12]. When hydrochlorothiazide 25mg thrice daily was administered to 313 patients who were anticipated to be non-responders, 39 (12.5%) achieved goal blood pressure and had to be excluded. Propranolol (120 to 360mg per day) added to the diuretic controlled only 50% of the patients (goal was <90mmHg and ≥5mmHg reduction from baseline) and oxprenolol plus diuretic controlled 27%. The reason for this poor response compared with the prior studies is not clear. Compliance was a more difficult problem in this patient population and the reporting of adverse effects was strikingly higher. Twenty-four percent of the patients taking propranolol plus diuretic complained of impotence as a new side effect.

It is interesting that a clinical trial designed and performed by experienced personnel in a similar population can be at variance with previous studies by the same group. The patient population may have been different in that the clinic personnel recruited many patients that were known non-responders to diuretic in order to be assured enough patients for randomization to the study drugs.

THE VETERANS ADMINISTRATION CAPTOPRIL TRIAL

Obviously, beta-adrenergic antagonists are not the only antihypertensive medications whose efficacy is enhanced by diuretics. The Veterans Administration Cooperative Study Group on Antihypertensive Agents has also performed trials on hydrochlorothiazide plus prazosin or hydralazine [13], hydrochlorothiazide plus bethanidine or guanethidine [14] and chlorthalidone plus small doses of reserpine [15].

Our most recent study is of the angiotensin converting enzyme inhibitor, captopril [16-19]. In summary, we found that captopril lowered blood pressure effectively in doses much lower than had been used previously, that the addition of hydrochlorothiazide to the captopril had an additive effect on blood pressure reduction, and the addition of diuretic abolished the racial difference between response of blacks and whites to captopril alone. Captopril, like propranolol, was less effective alone in our black population.

CONCLUSIONS

A series of large clinical trials conducted by the Veterans Administration have clearly established the importance of diuretic drugs either as primary or adjustive therapy for the treatment of hypertension. As new drugs with novel mechanisms of action become available, their role as initial therapy will become defined, but it is nearly certain that the efficacy of any such drug will be enhanced by a diuretic.

Finally, it is important to keep in mind that the results of trials such as those cited here pertain to large groups of patients and do not necessarily obtain for a given individual. Therapeutic decisions must continue to rest on specific indications and co-indications, contraindications, simplicity of titration and dosing schedule, patient acceptance, potential undesirable effects, and cost.

ACKNOWLEDGEMENTS

The Veterans Administration studies cited above were from the Cooperative Studies Program of the Veterans Administration Medical Research Service. Ms. Clydie Mae Denson prepared the manuscript.

REFERENCES

1. Perera GA: Antihypertensive drug versus symptomatic treatment in primary hypertension. Effect on survival. J. Amer. Med. Assoc. 173, 11-13 (1960).
2. Dupler DA, Greenwood RJ, Connell JT: Present status of the treatment of hypertension. J. Amer. Med. Assoc. 174, 123-126 (1960).
3. Veterans Administration Cooperative Study Group on Antihypertensive Agents: Effects of treatment on morbidity in hypertension. Results in patients with diastolic blood pressures averaging 115 through 129 mm Hg. J. Amer. Med. Assoc. 202, 116-122 (1967).
4. Veterans Administration Cooperative Study Group on Antihypertensive Agents: Propranolol in the treatment of essential hypertension. J. Amer. Med. Assoc. 237, 2303-2310 (1977).
5. Veterans Administration Cooperative Study Group on Antihypertensive Agents: Comparision of propranolol and hydrochlorothiazide for the initial treatment of hypertension. I. Results of short-term titration with emphasis on racial differences in response. J. Amer. Med. Assoc. 248, 1996-2003 (1982).
6. Soghikian K, Bartenbach DE: Influence of dosage and duration of therapy on the rate of response to methychlothiazide in essential hypertension. South Med. J. 70, 1397-1404 (1977).
7. Veterans Administration Cooperative Study Group on Antihypertensive Agents: Comparison of propranolol and hydrochlorothiazide for the initial treatment of hypertension. II. Results of long-term therapy. J. Amer. Med. Assoc. 248, 2004-2011 (1982).
8. Freis ED, Materson BJ, Flamenbaum W: Comparison of propranolol or hydrochlorothiazide alone for treatment of hypertension. III. Evaluation of the renin-angiotensin system. Am. J. Med. 74, 1029-1041 (1979).
9. Ganguly A, Weinberger MH: Low renin hypertension: a current review of definitions and controversies. Am. Heart J. 98, 642-652 (1979).
10. Veterans Administration Cooperative Study Group on Antihypertensive Agents: Urinary Na^+/K^+ ratio is much higher in blacks and correlates with diastolic blood pressure in hypertensive patients. Cardiovascular Disease Epidemiology Newsletter (Abstract), 31-37 (1982).
11. Veterans Administration Cooperative Study Group on Antihypertensive Agents: Efficacy of nadolol alone and combined with bendroflumethiazide and hydralazine for systemic hypertension. Amer. J. Cardiol. 52, 1230-1237 (1983).
12. Veterans Administration Cooperative Study Group on Antihypertensive Agents: Oxprenolol vs propranolol: a randomized, double-blind, multiclinic trial in hypertensive patients taking hydrochlorothiazide. Hypertension 3, 250-256 (1981).
13. Veterans Administration Cooperative Study Group on Antihypertensive Agents: Comparison of prazosin with hydrazaline in patients receiving hydrochlorothiazide. A randomized double-blind clinical trial. Circulation 64, 772-779 (1981).
14. Veterans Administration Cooperative Study Group on Antihypertensive Agents: Multi-clinic controlled trial of bethanidine and guanethidine in severe hypertension. Circulation 55, 519-525 (1977).
15. Participating Veterans Administration Medical Centers: Low doses v standard dose of reserpine. A randomized, double-blind, multiclinic trial in patients taking chlorthalidone. J. Amer. Med. Assoc. 248, 2471-2477 (1982).

16. Veterans Administration Cooperative Study Group on Antihypertensive Agents: Captopril: Evaluation of low doses, twice daily doses, and the addition of diuretic for the treatment of mild to moderate hypertension. Clinical Science 63, 443s-445s (1982).
17. Veterans Administration Cooperative Study Group on Antihypertensive Agents: Racial differences in response to low-dose captopril are abolished by the addition of hydrochlorothiazide. Brit. J. Clin. Pharmacol. 14, 97s-101s (1982).
18. Veterans Administration Cooperative Study Group on Antihypertensive Agents: Low-dose captopril for the treatment of mild to moderate hypertension. II. Long-term results. Hypertension 5(Supp III), III-139 - III-144 (1983).
19. Veterans Administration Cooperative Study Group on Antihypertensive Agents: Low-dose captopril for the treatment to mild to moderate hypertension. I. Results of a fourteen week trial. (Accepted for publication in the Archives of Internal Medicine, 1984).

BETA-BLOCKERS AS FIRST-STEP THERAPY OF HYPERTENSION

JOSE CARLOS PENA, M.D. and MARGARITA FERNANDEZ, M.D.
Department of Nephrology and Mineral Metabolism, Instituto Nacional De LA Nutricion Salvador Zubiran. Calle Unsco De Quiroga No. 15, Del Tlalpan. 14000 Mexico O.F. Mexico

Beta-adrenoreceptors blocking drugs are known to reduce elevated blood pressure since 1964, when three reports demonstrating this effect were published (1,2,3).
Interest in these compounds increase over the years and today we are discussing beta-blockers as first choice antihypertensive therapy; there are several reasons for this approach: good antihypertensive effect, a possible action against fatal ischemic heart disease, and relatively few and mild side effects (4,5). Furthermore some kind of central action that helps to decrease arterial pressure has also been postulated(6).

MECHANISM OF ACTION OF BETA-BLOCKERS

Sympathetic stimulation produce nor-adrenaline release and accelerates the heart rate. Noradrenaline receptors sites can be divided into three groups: alpha sites stimulated only by the natural neurotransmitter noradrenaline and beta 1 and beta 2 sites estimulated both by noradrenaline and the synthetic catecholamine, isoprenaline (isoproterenol). Beta-1 receptors increase the force and rate of contraction of heart muscle, beta 2 receptors dilate arterioles and bronchioles. The beta-blocking drugs supress these effects by occupying receptor sites with molecules similar in structure to natural neurotransmitters (4).

The effect of beta-blockade in arterial pressure was unexpected, and is still very imperfectly understood.

Reduction of cardiac output.- Beta adrenoreceptors antagonists, especially propranolol reduce cardiac output (7). This effect is seen especially when patients are studied under conditions associated with high sympathetic drive to the heart. Thus, the reduction in cardiac output is invariably pronounced when the patient is studied during physical excercise whereas the decrease in cardiac output may not be found, or it may be very slight, especially when sympathetic tone is low. Consequently, the fall in blood pressure that can be induced by beta blockade in the supine resting patient is not very marked. In a relatively large serie of patients, it has been found that sytolic pressure diminishes by 15 to 20% and diastolic pressure by 10 to 15%. These values show little change in the upright position. This absence of postural hypotension gives the beta blockers one of their major advantages over other antihypertensive drugs, such as post-ganglionic sympathetic inhibitors.
The situation changes when the rise in pressure provoked by physical excercise is considered. This increase, that is more pronounced in hypertensive than in normotensive individuals affects systolic pressure and is strongly inhibited by beta-blockers, The explanation is relatively simple: during strenuous physical excercise, sympàthetic tone is greatly enhanced and the effects of this enhancement on the heart are inhibited by beta-blockade. The increase in cardiac output and in systolic blood pressure during excercise is less marked following beta blockade.

Diuretics, Jules B. Puschett, Editor

Unfortunately this reduces substantially the capacity for heavy physical excercise in normal young volunteers (12). The reduction in CO is not enough to explain the decrease in BP. For example propranolol lowers CO long before blood pressure. Tarazi et al (8) assume that this delay is the result of adaptive changes in vascular flow resistance secondary to the persistent fall in CO.

Modulation of central blood pressure regulation.- One strong argument against a direct influence of beta adrenoreceptor antagonist on the central nervous system (CNS), is the lack of correlation between the ability of these drugs to penetrate the blood-brain barrier and their antihypertensive effect (6). For instance the antihypertensive effects of lipophilic beta-blocking drugs, such as propranolol, wich pass readely into the brain are in man not significantly different from those caused by compounds with a low lipophilicity such as: sotalol, practolol and timolol, wich permeate only to a limited extent the blood-brain barrier (9,10).

Inhibition of renin release.- The regulation of the renin-angiotensin system is a highly complex process. In the present context, however, were are interested solely in the influence exerted on these regulatory mechanism by the sympathetic system (11). Stimulation of the sympathetic system produces an increase release of renin. This effect and consequently the rise in the blood levels of Angiotensin I and Angiotensin II, can be inhibited by beta-adrenoreceptor antagonists.

Angiotensin II, in addition to its other well know effects on smooth muscle and on aldosterone production influences sympathetic activity at various sites levels. Via the area postrema, increased blood angiotensin levels can enhance the activity of sympathetic nervous centers, promote ganglionic transmission and the biosynthesis or release of nor-epinephrine (12). Thus the sympathetic system both stimulate and is stimulated by the renin-angiotensin system. If other mechanism were not to exert a breaking effect on this mutual activation, a vicious cycle would result. Conversely, it is understandable that inhibition of renin release by a β-adrenoreceptor antagonist should reduce the activity of both systems.

Buhler et al divided their series of patient with essential hypertension into those with high, normal and low renin levels (13). They found that blood pressure was lowered more markedly in the high-renin groups than in the normal and specially the low-renin groups (14). There are many reports indicating that reduction of renin is not of primary importance in the antihypertensive action of beta-blockers. In several studies, for instance no correlation was seen between the renin values and the reduction in blood pressure. There was also no relationship between the decrease in blood pressure and the plasma renin values in patients previously receiving diuretics and then given propranolol. Following the substitution of pindolol for propranolol, the low renin values quickly returned to normal, but the reduction in blood pressure persisted. Similar results were observed when propranolol was replaced by atenolol (15).

Resetting of the Baroreceptors.- Prichard and Gillam (2) suggested that the anti-hypertensive action of beta-adrenoreceptor antagonists might be secondary to resetting of the baroreceptors. Propranolol, for example, reduce the carotid-sinus reflex in the cat and the dog. This effect occurres only after chronic treatment. In hypertensive patients findings were contradictory (16,17). The role of baroreceptor in the hypotensive action of beta blockers thus remain uncertain.

Restoration of vascular relaxation sensitivity and structural changes in the vessel well.- The prolonged blockade of vascular beta adrenergic receptors may protect the relaxation mechanism involving cyclic AMP synthesis from being desensitized. Beta agonists (isoproteronol) decrease the number of beta receptors and desensitization to beta stimuli. Chronic beta-blockade increase the number of beta receptors (18). Vascular beta-receptors are linked as a subunit to receptors for other vasoactive substances and coupled also to the catalytic subunit of adenylate-cyclase; cathecolamines would reduce the sensitivity of the receptor cyclase complex through interaction with beta-adrenergic subunits (19). Beta blockade allows the restoration to other various endogenous vasodilators that normally are obliterated.

Effects on plasma volume.- It seems unlikely that a decrease in plasma volume plays any part in the antihypertensive action of beta blockers as was originally proposed by Tarazi et al (20).

In hypertensive patients blood pressure becomes adjusted to a higher level whenever this level is reduced by acting on one of the determinant variables. Reflex-induced mechanisms modify the other variables in such a way that the original blood pressure level remains constant. When the blood pressure is lowered by decreasing CO, the activation of the sympathetic and renin-angiotensin system will occur in acute experiments. Norepinephrine and angiotensin II release counter balance the decrease in CO by an increase in peripheral vascular resistances. In long term reductions aldosterone production would result in an increased blood volume and blood pressure. This type of adjustements would be expected after decreasing CO and probably even produce a slight antihypertensive effect.

On the basis of this observations it must be concluded that beta blockers must have different sites of action; the effect on the heart reduces CO and some other action must counteract or block peripheral vasoconstriction. From their effects on peripheral vascular resistance, it is apparent that beta receptors antagonists do in fact, possess such properties: peripheral resistance decreases after a period of latency or reverts to normal values despite the persistent reduction of CO. These effects my be secondary to the following mechanisms:

a) reduction of sympathetic tone mediated by an effect on central peripheral structures or both, b) improvement in the sensitivity of vascular smooth muscle mediators of vasodilatation, c) inhibition of renin secretion. In addition to the reduction in CO, any or all the factors mentioned may participate in the antihypertensive action of beta blockers.

PHARMACODYNAMIC PROPERTIES OF BETA BLOCKERS

All of the beta-blocking drugs are specific antagonists. Thus, stimulation of beta-adrenoreceptors in the heart, irrespective of the manner they evoke the response, can be blocked by the beta-adrenergic antagonists. However, the response to agents that stimulate contractility of the heart by other pathways, such as calcium or digitalis is unaffected (4).

Potency of beta blockers.- Beta blocking potency is judged by the inhibition of tachycardia produced by isoproterenol (21). Pindolol and timolol are the must potent, and acetobutolol and sotalol are the least potent. All drugs are compared against propranolol.

Membrane stabilizing potency.- This effect is also expressed as "quinidine like" or "local anesthetic" effect. But is not related to the antiarrhytmic action of beta blockers or anti-hypertensive effect.

Intrinsic sympathomimetic activity (ISA).- Some of the beta-blockers have a partial agonist activity on the heart (Table 1). The maximum response obtained is lower than the one obtained with isoproterenol or norepinephrine.

TABLE I. Pharmacodynamic and pharmacokinetics of beta-blockers

Beta-blocker	ISA	Cardio-selectivity	Half Life Hours	Route of Excretion	Effect on GFR	Lipid Solubility
Propranolol	—	No	3.5-6	Liver		+
Metoprolol	—	Yes	3-4	Liver	?	+
Nadolol	—	No	20	Kidney	—	—
Atenolol	—	Yes	7	Kidney	?	—
Pindolol	+	No	3-4	Kidney and liver	—	+
Timolol		No	4	Kidney and liver	?	—
Oxprenolol	+	No	2-3	Liver	?	+
Labetalol		No	8	Liver	—	—

GFR = Glomerular filtration rate
ISA = Intrinsic sympathomimetic activity

On theoretical grounds if may be postulated that beta-blockers displaying ISA are less likely to induce cardiac insufficiency than beta-blockers devoid of such activity. Therapeutic studies have yet to demonstrate this supossition.

There is no good evidence that beta blocking drugs with ISA are inherently safer in patients at risk from beta-blockade (asthmatics) than those without ISA. However pindolol, a drug with high ISA, has been shown to be broncho-protective in many patients intolerant to propranolol because of bronchospasm (22).

Cardioselectivity.- Beta blockers may be classified as selective and non-selective (Table I). When employed in low doses, cardioselective blockers inhibit the cardiac beta receptors (beta 1) but exert little influence in the bronchial and vascular beta-receptors (beta-2). These agents will be safer to use in patients with bronchial asthma. In practice, cardioselectivity is diminished at the doses required for the treatment of hypertension. Cardioselectivity is dose dependent and decreases or disappears when larger doses are used (23).

The half life, route of excretion and lipid solubility are depicted in Table I and also its effect on glomerular filtration rate (GFR).

BETA BLOCKERS IN THE TREATMENT OF HYPERTENSION

In the past two decades was clearly established that treatment of arterial hypertension prevents cardiovascular disease. Although not so long ago hypertension was considered the result and not the cause of vascular disease.

From a total of 7,000 hypertensive patients reported in six prospective studies (24,25,26,27,28,29), 3,367 (48%) were untreated and 3,652 (52%) were treated; cerebrovascular disease especially stroke clearly decrease with treatment. In contrast the effect of anti-hypertensive therapy on coronary heart disease (CHD) is inconsistent and not clearly beneficial. Furthermore, there is variation among studies in the incidence of complications caused by CHD in untreated patients. For purpose of analysis CHD includes: sudden death and fatal and non-fatal infarction.

In two of the six studies active therapy actually increased morbidity associated with CHD. In the Goteborg study the 40 percent reduction in CHD is attributed to the high number of patients on beta-blocking drugs. Finally the analysis of all treated groups showed no effect on the incidence of CHD complications.

One of the reasons to explain these findings, may be that CHD is multifactorial. Hence, blood pressure control alone may have limited values in a disease where other non-hypertensive risk factors might be worsened or unchanged.

Evenwhen drug treatment of hypertension did not reduce CHD, beta-blocking agents are invariably effective in decreasing death rate and number of recurrent myocardial infarctions in secondary prevention trials (30). The results obtained with the secondary prevention trials suggests that inhibition of sympathetic function via beta-receptor blockade may be useful to prevent the CHD complications in a hypertensive population.

Beta blockers are now confirmed as effective antihypertensive agents and have been recomended for initial treatment, providing the contraindications to their use are observed. This acceptance stems from two major factors. The side-effects of beta blockers compared to other drugs have been well documented. They cause little or no postural hypotension; the sexual disturbances are minimal or non-existent. Headaches and palpitations as seen with vasodilators, or depression which can follow the use of reserpine or methyldopa, are infrequently seen. The treatment of hypertension in the young patient with these drugs permit a free way of life and good compliance. This is due to a lack of side effects and that the drug can be taken once a day (4,6,30).

The reduction in blood pressure by beta blockers shows a marked variation among individual subjects; but an average fall of 15 to 20% in systolic and 10 to 15% in diastolic blood pressure can be expected. These falls are similar to the ones observed with thiazide diuretics, an occur at rest an during excercise. When given as a first step drug, a clinically satisfactory response is seen in 20 to 50% of cases. Use in combination with a diuretic the number of patients controlled increases to 70 to 88%. The possible advantages of this combination are that beta blockers will reduce the effect of the diuretic-induced increase in catecholamines and the estimulation of the renin-angiotensin system. There is also some evidence that beta blockers increase the plasma levels of potassium (31) and it has been suggested that this is due to a decrease in plasma renin activity. The combination of a diuretic with a beta blocker may protect the patient from the effects of hypokalemia while increasing the antihypertensive response.

Beta-blockers monotherapy reduces blood viscosity and platelet aggregation (32). So far beta blockers have not been found to induce clinically relevant long-term changes in glucose tolerance or serum lipids, although the problem needs further clarification (33). Most importantly, by effect of their pharmacological action, beta blockers attenuate the response to sympathetic cardiac stimulation and the effects of stress-induced increases in free fatty acids, thereby preventing dangerous dysrhytmias and reducing the threat of sudden death. If one contrast the favourable rheological, electrophysiological and metabolic effects of beta-blockers with the unfavourable effects of diuretics, one is bound to acknowledge the cardioprotective potential of antihypertensive therapy based on beta-blockers.

CONTRAINDICATIONS AND SIDE EFFECTS

When beta blockers are prescribed patients with cardiac failure, left ventricular insufficiency and bronchial asthma, must be excluded. Heart-block beyond first degree, also constitutes a formal contraindication to the use of these compounds (4,6,7). Beta adrenoreceptor blockade reduce cardiac rate, thus patients with bradycardia should be treated with caution. In our group of patients pulse rate below 55 was seen in 17/77 patients and below 50 in only 5/66. In these five patients beta blockers were discontinued.

Diabetes mellitus is frequently associated with ischemic heart disease and hypertension and beta blockers play an important role in the treatment if these patients (4). In 14 type II diabetics treated with beta blockers of 73 hypertensive patients, no evidence of hypoglycemia was detected. Hypoglycemia occurred with the use of propranolol in insulin dependent diabetics. There is evidence of a delayed recovery from insulin induced hypoglycemia with propranolol. Atenolol and metoprolol have little or no effect on the recovery of insulin induced hypoglycemia; although further work is necessary. It would seem reasonable to suggest that cardioselective agents can be used without greatly disturbing the control of diabetic patients. Other side effects seen with beta-blockers include central effects such as: sleep disturbances and dizziness, gastrointestinal effects such as nausea and abdominal discomfort and general effects such as tiredness and fatigue. In rare ocassion dermatological and ophtalmological manifestations have been seen. Practolol has been the only beta blocker to be discontinued, because of the multiple and severe complications and side effects. Occulo-mucocutaneous syndrome was described following the long term use only of this drug (34,35).

All patients must be warned about stopping suddenly the treatment with beta blockers. The withdrawal syndrome may occur especially in patients with ischemic heart disease or severe angina. The use of beta blockers can be continued prior to surgery only if appropriate anesthetic agents are used such as those that affect the circulation as little as possible, an with minimal or no activation of the sympathetic system (6).

The treatment of hypertension associated with pregnancy with beta adrenergic antagonists has been questioned; mainly because of the effects on the fetus or newborn and the possibility that these effects may interfere with the course of labor and delivery. Recent reports of the use of oxaprenolol, metoprolol and propranolol in high risk pregnant patients with hypertension described satisfactory control of the blood pressure and succesful outcome of delivery, fetal growth, and perinatal morbidity and mortality (36,37,38).

CONCLUSIONS

The experience of different group to advocate beta blockers as first line drugs in the treatment of hypertension, strongly points to the following findings:

a) They reduce the incidence of myocardial infarction and sudden death.
b) They improve lipid levels and do not alter the glucose tolerance test.
c) The side effects are minimal and can be overcome.
d) The serum potassium is maintained within normal limits.
e) Used as a single drug they can control blood pressure in more than 40 percent of hypertensive patients.
f) When used in association with a second drug (diuretic, alfa adrenergic-blocker or vasodilator) the percentage of good control increase to 80 percent of the hypertensive population.

REFERENCES

1. BNC Prichard, Br. Med. J. 1: 1227-1228 (1964)
2. BNC Prichard, and PRS Gillam, Br. Med. J. 21: 725-727, (1964)
3. G. Schroder, G. and L. Werko, Clin. Pharmacol. Ther. 5: 159-164 (1964)
4. W.H. Frishman, Clinical Pharmacology of the beta-adrenoreceptor blocking drugs (Appleton-Century Crofts/

New York, 1980)
5. J.H. Laragh. Am. J. Med. 55: 261-274 (1973)
6. M. Meier et al, Pharmacology of Antihypertensive drugs. A. Scriabine, ed. (Raven Press, New York 1980) pp. 179-194
7. J.D. Fitzgerald, Pharmacology of Antihypertensive Drugs. A. Scriabine, ed. (Raven Press, New York, 1980) pp. 195-208
8. R.C. Tarazi and H.P. Dustan, Am. J. Cardiol. 29: 633-740, (1972)
9. M.G. Myers, et al, J. Pharmacol. Exp. Ther. 192: 327-335, (1975)
10. Zweiten et al, J. Cardiovasc. Pharmacol. 1: 85-96 (1979)
11. S. Oparil and E. Haber, N. Engl. J. Med. 291: 387-401, 446-457, (1974)
12. R.H. Roth, Fed. Proc. 31: 1358-1364, (1972)
13. F.R. Buhler, N. Engl. J. Med. 287: 1209-1214, (1972)
14. F.R. Buhler, J.H. Laragh, et al, Am. J. Cardiol. 32: 511-522 (1973)
15. A. Amery, et al, Postgrad. Med. J. (Suppl 4) 52: 102-108, (1976)
16. Hanson, L. et al, Acta Med. Scand. 196: 27-34 (1974)
17. G. Simon, W. Koiwski, and St. Julius, Clin. Pharmacol. Ther. 22: 293-298, (1977)
18. G. Glaubiger and R.J. Lefkowitz, Biochem. Biophys. Res. Commun. 78: 720-725, (1977)
19. M.S. Amer. Science 179: 807-809, (1973)
20. R.C. Tarazi, H.P. Dustan, and E. Bravo, Postrag. Med. J. (Suppl 4) 52: 92-106 (1976)
21. H.J. Waal-Mannings, Drugs 12: 412-441, (1976)
22. W. Frishman, R. Dans, J. Stron, et al. Am. Heart, J. 98: 393, (1979)
23. JTL, Lertora, et al, J. Clin. Invest. 56: 719-724, (1975)
24. Veterans Administration Cooperative Study, JAMA 213: 1143-1152, (1970)
25. W. Smith-Mc Fate, Circ. Res. 40 (Suppl. 1): 98-105, (1977)
26. R. Reader, G.E. Baner, A.E. Doyle, et al. Lancet 11: 1261-1267, (1980)
27. A. Helgeland, Am. J. Med. 69: 725-732, (1980)
28. G. Berglund, et al, Lancet 7: 1-5, (1978)
29. A.M. Perry, Jr. et al. Ann. NY Acad, Sci. 304: 254-266, (1978)
30. L. Krakoff: Cardiovascular Rev and Reports 4: 319-324, (1983)
31. R.M. Pearson, et al, Br. Med. J. 1: 933-936, (1976)
32. H.W. Bucher and P. Stucki, Experientia 25: 280-284, (1965)
33. S.P. Allison, M.I. Chamberlain and J.E. Miller, Diabetologia 5: 339-342, (1969)
34. P. Wright, Br. Med. J. 1: 395-398, (1975)
35. H.J. Waal-Mainning, Drugs 10: 336-341, (1975)
36. P.H. Tcherdakoff et al, Br. Med. J. 2: 670, (1978)
37. B. Sandstrom. Obstet. Gynecol. 6: 385, (1978)
38. E.D. Gallery et al, Abstracts. 5th Meeting Int. Soc. Hypert. Paris (1978) pp. 92

A NOVEL APPROACH IN THE TREATMENT OF HYPERTENSION: NON-DIURETIC DIURETICS.

GERARD E. PLANTE,* and CLAUDE ROBILLARD,**
Department of Physiology-Pharmacology* and Family Medicine,**
University of Sherbrooke, Sherbrooke, Quebec, Canada, J1H 5N4

INTRODUCTION

It has been well demonstrated that mild or moderate untreated arterial hypertension is associated with higher incidence of morbidity and mortality (1). The chronic use of traditional diuretics is associated with a significant number of side effects related to intermediary or ionic metabolic disturbances:sodium and potassium depletion, metabolic alkalosis, hyperuricemia, glucose intolerance, hypercalcemia, hyperlipidemia (2). The more recent introduction of beta blockers as first step therapy in hypertension is not devoid either of significant clinical and biological side effects: bradycardia, heart failure, inadaptation to hypoglycemia, impaired peripheral microcirculation, bronchospasm (3). The chemical structure of indapamide is closely related to that of most diuretic agents, with the exception of the thiazide nucleus which characterizes most traditional diuretics (4). The mechanisms of action of indapamide on blood pressure are not well established. A number of studies have shown that indapamide reduces peripheral resistance in hypertensive patients (5). It is possible that this action results from the local production of vasodilatory prostaglandins (6), from a modification of ionic metabolism in the vascular smooth muscles, or finally, from an eventual effect on the cellular metabolism of divalent anions (G.E. Plante et al., unpublished observations).

METHODS

The present study was designed to compare the clinical response and the biological tolerance to hydrochlorothiazide (HTC:50mg per day) and to indapamide (IND:2.5mg per day) a non-thiazide diuretic. Twenty-four patients suffering from benign essential hypertension (recumbent diastolic pressure at rest ranging between 95 and 110 mm of Hg) were included in this double blind study. All patients were submitted to a placebo period ranging between 4 to 6 weeks. The patients were given HCT and IND in a double blind manner for a period of 12 consecutive weeks. They were examined at weekly intervals during the first month, and at monthly intervals thereafter. Eleven patients received HTC, 8 females and 3 males, whereas IND was given to 13 patients, 7 females and 6 males. Mean age, as well as body weight, were comparable in the two groups.

RESULTS

Systolic and diastolic pressure values in supine and upright positions are shown in Table I. The slight reduction in systolic and diastolic supine values during HCT treatment was not statistically significant. In contrast, supine values for patients treated with IND decreased significantly from placebo to active treatment periods. Pressure values measured in the upright position are also shown: in HCT-treated patients, the slight fall in systolic pressure was not statistically significant. In contrast, the drop in systolic pressure for IND-treated patients was significant: $p<0.05$. The reduction in diastolic pressure was significant: $p<0.05$ and <0.01 in HCT and IND-treated patients, respectively. The degree of reduction in systolic and diastolic pressure from placebo to active treatment is best shown in Fig. 1 for IND and HCT-treated patients: in the upper portion of this figure, both systolic and diastolic pressure decreased significantly. In contrast, HCT-treated patients only had an 8mm Hg fall in diastolic pressure in the upright

Published 1984 by Elsevier Science Publishing Co., Inc.
Diuretics, Jules B. Puschett, Editor

position.

TABLE I. Systolic and diastolic pressure, kaliemia and uricemia during prior therapy, placebo and active treatment periods. (mean ± 1SE).

		Prior therapy	Placebo period	Active treatment
Systolic supine	HCT	137 ± 4	147 ± 3	139 ± 3
	IND	142 ± 3	138 ± 3	126 ± 4[a]
Diastolic supine	HCT	92 ± 2	93 ± 3	89 ± 2
	IND	94 ± 2	93 ± 2	83 ± 2[b]
Systolic upright	HCT	144 ± 3	150 ± 3	139 ± 4
	IND	142 ± 6	139 ± 2	127 ± 5[a]
Diastolic upright	HCT	96 ± 2	98 ± 3	90 ± 3[a]
	IND	96 ± 2	98 ± 2	84 ± 2[b]
Kaliemia (mEq/l)	HCT	3.6 ± 0.1	4.2 ± 0.2	3.4 ± 0.1[b]
	IND	3.5 ± 0.2	3.9 ± 0.1	3.6 ± 0.1[a]
Uricemia (mg/dl)	HCT	6.0 ± 0.7	5.2 ± 0.4	7.3 ± 0.6[b]
	INC	6.5 ± 0.4	6.2 ± 0.4	6.7 ± 0.3

[a)] $p<0.05$ [b)] $p<0.01$ for sifnificance between placebo and active treatment.

Total serum proteins, calcemia, blood urea nitrogen, serum sodium and chloride values as well as serum creatinine were measured during each experimental period. No significant change obtained for these parameters in both HCT and IND-treated patients (data not shown). In contrast, the pattern of serum potassium and uricemia during each experimental period was different in HCT and IND patients, as shown in Table I. Serum potassium fell during HCT, and a smaller decrement obtained in IND-treated patients. Thiazide-treated patients developed hyperuricemia during active treatment. In contrast, IND failed to influence this parameter.

DISCUSSION

The main objective of chronic diuretic therapy in essential hypertension is the reduction in arteriolar smooth muscle reactivity, which determines peripheral resistance. Recent studies suggest that smooth muscle ionic metabolism is impaired in essential hypertension (7). It would appear that the reduction of intracellular sodium in these muscle cells, as well as the concomitant variations in intracellular calcium represent the basis for the pharmalogical action of diuretics when administered chronically. However, the diuretic effect of thiazides is accompanied by a series of biological consequences, responsible for most of the side effects reported with this category of drugs. As shown in Fig. 2, inhibition of the tubular transport of sodium results in increased natriuresis which lead progressively to extracellular volume contraction: this phenomenon is responsible for elevation of serum uric acid, and occasionally proteins and calcium. Urinary sodium losses under certain circumstances may lead to hyponatremia: this side effect has recently been reported to be deleterious in ageing patients (8). Almost all diuretics are associated with increased urinary potassium excretion and negative potassium balance. This abnormality may be associated with metabolic alkalosis and would appear to be responsible for carbohydrate intolerance seen in most patients treated with traditional diuretics. Fig. 2 clearly depicts the imbalance between the main objective of diuretic therapy, shown on the left hand side, and the numerous metabolic side effects resulting from the diuretic action of most traditional preparations used in hypertensive patients.

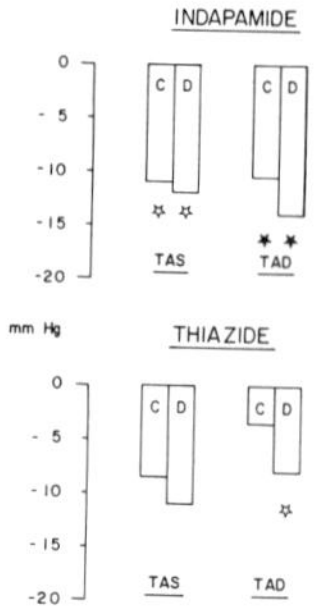

Fig. 1. Fall in systolic (TAS) and diastolic (TAD) pressure in supine (C) and upright (D) positions during IND or HCT. White and black stars for P values less than 0.05 and 0.01 respectively.

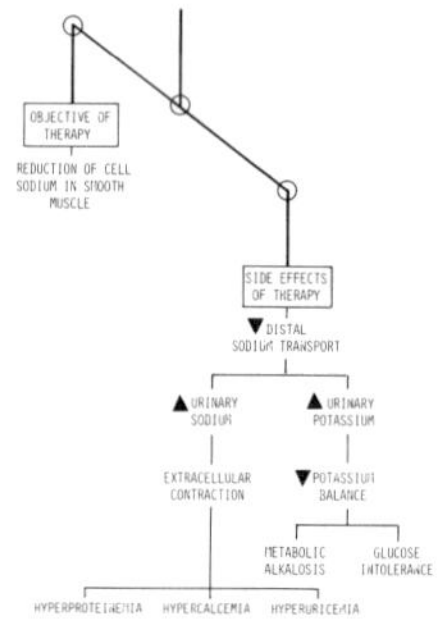

Fig. 2. Objective of traditional diuretic therapy and expected side effects reported in hypertensive patients.

CONCLUSIONS

The results obtained in the present study indicate that IND, as compared to HCT, has several advantages. The hypotensive action of this substance is well-documented. Several other clinical studies (9, 10) as well as the present series of patients, indicate that urinary potassium losses and hypokalemia are minimal in IND-treated patients. In addition this drug does not produce hyperglycemia nor hyperlipidemia as recently demonstrated by Weidmann and co-workers (11). Finally, hyperuricemia is seldom observed in patients treated with IND, in contrast to HCT-treated patients. The introduction of IND in clinical medicine represents a major step in the therapy of arterial hypertension.

REFERENCES

1. V.A. Cooperative Study Group, JAMA 213, 1143-1152 (1970).
2. G.E. Plante and C. Robillard, Curr. Med. Res. Opin. 8, Suppl. 3, 205-212 (1983).
3. W. Frishman, R. Silverman, R. Strom, J. Elkayam, and E. Sonnenblick, Amer. Heart J. 98, 256-262 (1979).
4. D.B. Campbell, A.R. Taylor, Y.W. Hopkins, and J.R.B. Williams. Curr. Med. Res. Opin. 5, Suppl. 1, 13-24 (1977).
5. R.I. Ogilvie, Curr. Med. Res. Opin. 8, Suppl. 3, 199-204 (1983).
6. M. Lebel, J.H. Grose, L.J. Belleau and S. Langlois, Curr. Med. Res. Opin. 8, Suppl. 3, 228-234 (1983).
7. R.P. Garay, J.L. Elghore, G. Dagher, and P. Mayer, N. Eng. J. Med. 302, 769-771 (1980).
8. N. Ashraf, R. Locksley, and A.I. Arieff, Am. J. Med. 70, 1163-1168 (1981).
9. R.A. Vukovich, M. Zisblatt, F. Caroso, M. Losi, J. Barton, W.E. Schotz, E. Webb, J. Eff, R. Bronstein, and E.S. Neiss, Curr. Med. Res. Opin. 8, Suppl. 3, 257-271 (1983).
10. A. Mimran, J.J. Zambrowski, and T. Coppolani, Curr. Med. Res. Opin. 8, Suppl. 3, 253-256 (1983).
11. P. Weidmann, M.G. Bianchetti, and R. Mordasini, Curr. Med. Res. Opin. 8, Suppl. 3, 272-284 (1983).

ANTIHYPERTENSIVE THERAPY IN PATIENTS ABOVE 60 YEARS.A MULTICENTRE TRIAL OF THE EUROPEAN WORKING PARTY ON HIGH BLOOD PRESSURE IN THE ELDERLY(EWPHE).

P.W.de Leeuw (on behalf of all collaborators on the EWPHE).
Dept of Med, Zuiderziekenhuis, Groene Hilledijk 315, 3075 EA Rotterdam, The Netherlands.

SUMMARY

Over 800 hypertensive patients above the age of 60 years have now been entered into the double-blind multicentre trial of the European Working Party on High Blood Pressure in the Elderly (EWPHE). Half were treated with one capsule daily containing 25 mg hydrochlorothiazide and 50 mg triamterene and half were given matching placebo. If blood pressure control was insufficient a second capsule was given and, if necessary, up to 2 g of methyldopa daily.

Prior to randomisation no significant differences were present between the two groups. A significant blood pressure difference between the groups was obtained during the initial phase of the trial and maintained during 5 years of follow-up. No major disturbances in serum sodium or serum potassium were observed. However, serum creatinine and serum uric acid rose in the active - treatment group, while it did not so in the placebo-group.

INTRODUCTION

Hypertension is one of the major risk factors for stroke and coronary heart disease in both middle aged and elderly subjects [1,2] , but controlled trials of antihypertensive agents in these age groups have shown either no difference or some possible but not necessarily statistically significant benefit [3-9].

Because of the uncertainties regarding treatment in aged people, the European Working Party on High Blood Pressure in the Elderly (EWPHE) initiated a study to assess the effects of antihypertensive drug therapy in patients above the age of 60 years. Therefore, a double-blind, multicentre trial was designed, which started in 1973.

Patients and methods

Study protocol

Elderly patients with high blood pressure are admitted to the study if they fulfil certain criteria. The positive (selection) criteria are as follows: 1) age of 60 years or more; 2) sitting blood pressure (average of readings on three separate visits) on placebo between 160 and 239 mm Hg for systolic and between 90 and 119 mm Hg for diastolic pressure; 3)patient's willingness to co-operate and to be followed-up regularly (informed consent).

Negative (exclusion) criteria are: 1) curable causes of blood pressure elevation; 2) certain complications, i.e. retinopathy grade III or IV, congestive heart failure, enlarging aortic aneurysm, severe renal failure, past history of cerebral or subarachnoid haemorrhage; 3)co-existing diseases such as hepatitis or cirrhosis, gout, malignancy etc.

Patients are stratified for each collaborating centre according to age, sex, and the presence or absence of cardiovascular complications; subsequently they are randomly allocated to an active-treatment or placebo-treatment group for the duration of the study.

At first, all patients receive 1 capsule containing either 25 mg hydrochlorothiazide and 50 mg triamterene, or a matching placebo.The dosage may be increased, after not less than 2 weeks, to 2 capsules per day.

Diuretics, Jules B. Puschett, Editor

If the blood pressure remains high after 1 month, alpha-methyldopa in the treated group or matching placebo in the other group can be added.

Patients may end the study for one of the following reasons: 1) by completion of 7 years observation; 2) by being lost to follow-up; 3) by interruption of all study treatment during more than 3 months; 4) by meeting one of the specific study terminating events, including death, cerebral or subarachnoid haemorrhage, development of hypertensive retinopathy grade III or IV, enlarging or dissecting aneurysm, congestive heart failure not controllable without diuretics or antihypertensive drugs, hypertensive encephalopathy, increase in left ventricular hypertrophy and a rise in blood pressure exceeding the defined limits.

Results

On June 1, 1983, a total number of 843 patients had been admitted into the trial. In general no significant differences between the two groups were found on admission.

The average age was 71.9 years; mean body weight was 67.0 kg for an average height of 1.59 m.

The intake of the diuretic was relatively constant over the total trial period; only a few patients were taking methyldopa after 3 months, while from one year on the methyldopa intake averaged around 317 mg daily.

In the placebo group, both systolic and diastolic blood pressure fell significantly ($p < 0.001$) after 3 months of treatment; subsequent changes in pressure were small and not significant. In the actively treated group a greater fall in blood pressure was noted; this was mainly due to the administration of the diuretic. After 3 months the systolic and diastolic blood pressures continued to decrease in the actively-treated group probably as a consequence of the administration of methyldopa. At 5 years the average sitting blood pressure was 20/9 mm Hg higher in the placebo treated group than in the actively-treated group.

At no time during the first five years was there a significant difference in body weight between the two groups.

The serum creatinine levels were similar in both groups on admission. In the placebo group serum creatinine did not change but during the trial serum creatinine was significantly higher in the actively treated group than in the placebo group ($p < 0.001$). In this active treatment group, the change in sitting systolic blood pressure over the first three months was inversely correlated with the change in serum creatinine.

The serum uric acid level was not significantly different between both groups on admission. In the placebo group no significant change was observed but in the active treatment group serum uric acid increased by 0.07 mmol/l during the first year and remained high during the subsequent years $p < 0.001$).

The combination of thiazide diuretic and a potassium sparing agent provoked only small changes in serum potassium; but the small differences in serum potassium level between active and placebo treatment group reached statistical significance ($p < 0.001$).

The serum sodium concentrations were similar in both groups on admission and subsequent changes were small and statistically insignificant. The fasting blood glucose level did not change significantly in the placebo treated group during the first three years, but rose significantly in the actively treated group ($p < 0.05$).The serum cholesterol level was similar in both groups during the run-in period. Over time a slight decrease was noted in the two groups, but so far no significant difference has emerged between the placebo and the active-treatment group.

Discussion

The ultimate goal of antihypertensive therapy is to reduce mortality and morbidity while maintaining the quality of life. The purpose of the present multicentre trial is to evaluate whether this aim can be achieved in elderly subjects.

So far, a significant blood pressure difference between the groups seems to have been achieved already at three months of therapy and this difference is well maintained during the 5 years of observation. Therefore, the present trial might be expected to detect a difference in stroke incidence, although it is not clearly established for how long such a difference in blood pressure has to be maintained or whether a reduction in pressure from a previously high level has the same beneficial effect as that calculated from observed casual blood pressure differences in epidemiological studies not involving intervention[1].

Furthermore, one has to realise that any potential benefit resulting from the fall in blood pressure may be offset by unwanted side effects of treatment. Serum creatinine and uric acid , indeed, rose during the first three months of active treatment and remained elevated as compared with the placebo group during follow-up observation.

The reduction in pressure was maintained without major disturbances in the serum potassium level; this may be the result of using triamterene as a potassium-sparing compound in the diuretic. Serum sodium also was not adversely affected.

Glucose intolerance also is a major risk factor for coronary artery disease and in this study a significant increase in fasting blood glucose was observed in the active-treatment group without such changes in the control group. On the other hand, no major differences were found with respect to cholesterol, suggesting that the spontaneous decrease in this variable which seems to occur at high age [10] is not altered by the thiazide-methyldopa treatment.

In conclusion, the results of the present study indicate that effective lowering of blood pressure with combination of diuretics and alpha-methyldopa is associated with a rise in serum creatinine and uric acid, while glucose tolerance is impaired. Therefore, the balance between the potential benefit associated with blood pressure reduction and the possible harm related to enhancement of other risk factors remains to be determined.

REFERENCES

1. W.B. Kannel, T.R. Dawber, P. Sorlie, and P.A. Wolfe, Stroke 7, 327-331 (1976).
2. A. Amery, H. Wasir, C. Bulpitt, et al., Acta Cardiol 33, 443-467(1978).
3. A.B. Carter, Lancet i, 485-489 (1970).
4. Hypertension-Stroke Co-operative Study Group, JAMA 229, 409-418 (1974).
5. M.E. Sprackling, J.R.A. Mitchell, A.H. Short, G. Watt, Br Med J 283, 1151-1153 (1981).
6. Report by the Management Committee, Med J Aust 2, 398-402 (1981).
7. Veterans Administration Co-operative Study on Antihypertensive Agents, JAMA 202, 1028-1034 (1967).
8. Veterans Administration Co-operative Study on Antihypertensive Agents, JAMA 213, 1143-1152 (1970).
9. Veterans Administration Co-operative Study on Antihypertensive Agents, Circulation 45, 991-1004 (1972).
10. A. Amery, W. Birkenhäger, C. Bulpitt et al., Acta Cardiol 37,235-244 (1982).

HEMODYNAMIC CHANGES FOLLOWING WITHDRAWAL OF LONG-TERM THIAZIDE TREATMENT IN ESSENTIAL HYPERTENSION

P. VAN BRUMMELEN,
Department of Nephrology, University Hospital,
2333 AA LEIDEN, The Netherlands

ABSTRACT

In 13 patients with essential hypertension blood pressure, cardiac output, plasma volume and renin were measured before treatment, during long-term hydrochlorothiazide and at weekly intervals during 4 weeks placebo following withdrawal of the drug. The fall in blood pressure during hydrochlorothiazide was accompanied by non-significant changes in cardiac output and plasma volume and a rise in renin. Withdrawal of the drug was followed by a gradual rise in blood pressure and rapid increases in plasma volume and body weight. Cardiac output rose transiently and renin was suppressed. Different hemodynamic patterns were found for responders and non-responders to diuretic treatment. The results question the importance of body fluid volume depletion for the long-term antihypertensive effect of thiazide diuretics and indicate that slow-acting processes, by far outlasting the halflife of these drugs, are involved.

INTRODUCTION

The mechanism underlying the antihypertensive effect of thiazide diuretics has not been fully clarified. According to most authors blood pressure (BP) is lowered by a fall in peripheral resistance (TPR) [1,2] but a decrease in cardiac output (CO) was found during chlorthalidon [2]. Data on changes in plasma volume (PV) and renin are also controversial [1,3]. Discontinuation of thiazides is followed by rapid expansion of body fluid volumes and suppression of renin [4], whereas BP rises slowly. These findings were taken as evidence that continuous hypovolemia is a key factor for the antihypertensive action of thiazides. In the present study, BP, CO, PV and renin (PRC) were measured in patients with essential hypertension, before, during and at weekly intervals, after withdrawal of long-term treatment with hydrochlorothiazide (HCT). A comparison was made between patients with and without a good BP response to HCT.

PATIENTS AND METHODS

Thirteen patients (mean age 40.8 years) with uncomplicated essential hypertension participated. All had a diastolic BP above 100 mmHg when untreated. After stopping all antihypertensive medication placebo was given for 4 weeks (placebo I). Subsequently patients received HCT 50 mg b.i.d. as the only drug for 3 to 12 months (mean 8 months). Then HCT was discontinued and placebo given for 4 weeks (placebo II). At the end of placebo I, after long-term HCT and 1,2,3 and 4 weeks after discontinuation of HCT, BP, body weight, CO, PV and PRC were determined. CO was measured by radiocardiography and PV by determining the distribution volume of 99mTC-albumin. PRC was measured by radioimmunoassay. Student's t-test for paired and unpaired observations was used to determine the statistical significance of differences.

Diuretics, Jules B. Puschett, Editor

RESULTS (table I and figure 1)

BP was lowered by HCT ($p<0.001$). In 8 patients the fall in mean BP was more than 10% (responders). After discontinuation of HCT BP rose gradually. At the end of placebo II it was higher when compared with values during HCT ($p<0.01$) but still below the levels during placebo I ($p<0.01$). A rise in BP during placebo II was only seen in responders. Long-term HCT treatment was accompanied by a reduction in body weight ($p<0.01$). In the first week after stopping HCT it increased ($p<0.001$) followed by a gradual decline. At the end of placebo II it was still above the level during HCT ($p<0.05$). Changes in body weight were similar in responders and non-responders. During HCT CO and total peripheral resistance (TPR) were not significantly different from values at the end of placebo I. In responders TPR was lowered ($p<0.01$). In non-responders CO was lowered ($p<0.05$) and TPR increased ($p<0.05$). Discontinuation of HCT was followed by a transient increase in CO and reduction in TPR. Values for these variables were not different at the end of both placebo periods. In non-responders, stopping HCT was followed by an increase in CO and a decrease in TPR, which were maximal after 1 week. In responders a gradual increase in TPR was found with relatively small changes in CO. After long-term HCT, PV was not different from values during placebo I. Withdrawal of HCT was followed by an increase in PV which was maximal after 1 week ($p<0.001$). It decreased hereafter but was still significantly elevated at the end of the 4th week. Similar changes were found in responders and non-responders. PRC increased during HCT ($p<0.001$). Within 1 week after discontinuation of HCT PRC was suppressed to values below the original levels ($p<0.001$).

TABLE 1. Mean values (± SEM) for mean BP, body weight and PRC at the end of placebo period I, after long-term HCT and 1 and 4 weeks after withdrawal (placebo period II) (Reproduced with permission from P. van Brummelen [6]).

	PLACEBO PERIOD I	HYDROCHLORO THIAZIDE	PLACEBO PERIOD II	
			1 week	4 weeks
Mean BP (mmHg)	117.9 ± 4.2	103.3 ± 3.0	107.3 ± 2.9	111.2 ± 3.5
Body Weight (kg)	80.8 ± 2.3	79.5 ± 2.4	80.7 ± 2.4	80.1 ± 2.6
PRC (μU/ml)	74.2 ± 5.8	168.7 ± 19.3	58.4 ± 7.8	56.6 ± 4.7

DISCUSSION

For the whole group of patients BP was lowered by HCT without significant changes in CO, TPR of PV, but with a significant fall in body weight. In responders, however, BP was lowered by way of a fall in TPR, which is in agreement with several other studies [1,2]. The small fall in BP of the non-responders was due to a decrease in CO partly compensated for by an increase in TPR. In this group a tendency to a greater degree of PV depletion was found, which, together with the higher PRC levels, could explain the observed hemodynamic pattern [5]. Discontinuation of HCT was followed by a transient expansion of PV and body weight and a gradual rise in BP, which is in accordance with a previous study [4]. The suppression of renin in this situation has also been reported. The findings that BP after withdrawal of HCT did not parallel the changes in PV and body weight and that volume changes were similar whether or not a rise in BP was observed question the importance of PV reduction for the BP lowering of long-term thiazide treatment. The slow rise in BP after withdrawal of HCT was accompanied by a transient rise in CO and a subsequent increase in TPR. These findings could be interpreted as evidence for whole body auto-regulation of tissue perfusion to be reponsible for the rise in BP. However, the differences between responders and non-responders suggest that the initial increase in CO is not decisive for the subsequent rise in TPR. Four weeks after discontinuation of thiazide therapy BP, PV and PRC had not yet returned to pretreatment values. Also, it takes several months to achieve a maximal reduction in BP during thiazide therapy [5]. These findings suggest that slow acting processes, by far outlasting the half-life of these drugs, are involved in their antihypertensive effect. The nature of these processes remains to be established.

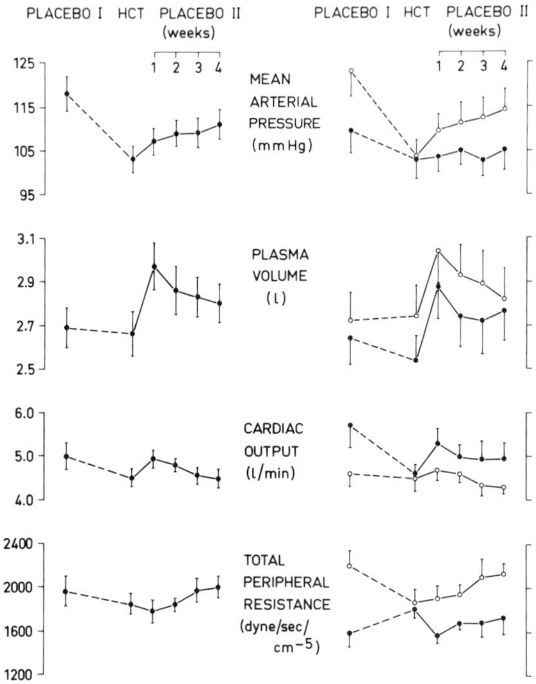

Figure 1. Mean values (±SEM) for mean arterial pressure, PV, CO and TPR, in both placebo periods and during long-term HCT treatment. Values are given for all patients (left panel) and for responders (open circles) and non-responders (closed circles) to long-term thiazide therapy separately (right panel) (Reproduced with permission from P. van Brummelen)[6]

REFERENCES

1. J. Conway in: Antihypertensive Agents, Handbook of Experimental Pharmacology 39, F. Gross ed. (Springer Verlag, Berlin 1977) pp 477-494.
2. P. Lund-Johansen, Acta Med. Scand. 187, 509-518 (1970).
3. P. van Brummelen, and M.A.D.H. Schalekamp, Acta Med. Scand. 207, 259-264 (1980).
4. R.C. Tarazi, H.P. Dustan, and E.D. Frohlich, Circulation 41, 709-717 (1970).
5. P. van Brummelen, A.J. Man in 't Veld, and M.A.D.H. Schalekamp, Clin. Pharmacol. Ther. 27, 328-336 (1980).
6. P. van Brummelen, and M.A.D.H. Schalekamp, Drugs Exptl. Clin. Res. 6, 695-701 (1980).

DIRECT VASCULAR EFFECTS OF SOME DIURETICS IN ANIMAL MODELS; EFFECTS IN THE RAT MESENTERIC ARTERY

MICHIKO HANDA,* KAZUOKI KONDO**, YU IGARASHI,* AND TAKAO SARUTA*
*Department of Internal Medicine, School of Medicine, Keio University, 35, Shinanomachi, Shinjuku-ku, Tokyo, Japan; **Department of Clinical Pharmacology, Jichi Medical School, Kawachi-gun, Tochigi, Japan

ABSTRACT

The effects of four different diuretics, tripamide, indapamide, furosemide and hydroflumethiazide on the vascular responses to norepinephrine and potassium chloride were studied in the perfused rat mesenteric vascular bed. Tripamide inhibited the potassium-induced vasoconstriction in a dose related manner, while on the norepinephrine-induced response, its inhibitory effect was slight. In contrast to tripamide, indapamide induced only slight changes in the vascular responses to norepinephrine and potassium chloride. Furosemide inhibited norepinephrine-induced vasoconstriction but showed no inhibitory effect on potassium-induced vasoconstriction. Hydroflumethiazide affected neither norepinephrine- nor potassium-induced vasocnstriction. None of the diuretics changed the basal pressure.

These results suggest that tripamide and furosemide have direct vascular actions independent from their renal actions, which may contribute to their antihypertensive effects.

It is also suggested that the vascular action of tripamide may be, different from that of furosemide, due to the inhibition of the transmembrane calcium movement.

INTRODUCTION

Diuretics are well known for their effectiveness in the treatment of hypertension. It is generally believed that diuretics lower blood pressure by reducing intravenous sodium and water volume. However, mechanisms other than the actions on the kidney, such as a vascular action, may play a role in the antihypertensive effect of diuretics. Previous studies reported that some diuretics attenuated the pressor response to vasoconstriction substances in vivo [1][2][3][4]. However, it still remains controversial as to whether the change in vascular responsiveness induced by diuretics is due to plasma volume reduction or to direct effects of these agents on the vascular bed. Recently, tripamide and indapamide, newly developed non thiazide diuretics, are suggested to have both renal and vascular actions.

In the present study, using isolated rat mesenteric vascular bed, we examined the effects of four different diuretics, hydroflumethiazide, furosemide, tripamide and indapamide, on the vascular contraction induced by norepinephrine and potassium chloride, and attempted to determine whether these diuretics had a direct vascular action or not.

METHODS

Male rats of Wistar strain, weighing about 300 g, were used. The isolated superior mesenteric vascular bed was prepared as described by McGregor [5]. The superior mesenteric artery was cannulated under ether anesthesia. The vascular bed was dissected out, and perfused by a peristaltic

Diuretics, Jules B. Puschett, Editor

flow inducer (Master flex pump, Cole-Parmer) with Krebs bicarbonate buffer (150 mM sodium, 4.3 mM potassium, 1 mM magnesium, 2.5 mM calcium, 1.7 mM phosphate, 25 mM bicarbonate, remaining anion chloride and 11.1 mM glucose) at 37°C bubbled with 5% carbon dioxide in oxygen. The pH of the solution was 7.4. The perfusion pressure was recorded via a side arm of the arterial cannula using a Nihon Koden MPU-0.5 transducer, the flow rate being adjusted to give a steady perfusion pressure of 25-35 mmHg. The actual flow rate was around 4 ml/min, which is not greatly divergent from the expected superior mesenteric artery flow rate in an adult rat. The flow rate was constant during each experiment. We confirmed in a previous study [6] that, under the conditions described here, the preparation remained remarkably stable with no significant changes in baseline pressure for at least 2 hrs.

When injected into the arterial cannula, norepinephrine (L-arterenol bitartrate, Sigma) or potassium chloride produced dose-related rises in pressure. The maximum pressure rise which could be achieved with these substances was usually in the region of 80-100 mmHg. For each substance, we determined a dose which gave an approximately 50% maximal response and employed this in all subsequent experiments. The doses actually used were 20 mg of norepinephrine and 2 mg of potassium chloride. Each substance was dissolved in 0.05 ml of buffer and injected at 5 min intervals into the cannula. Each injection produced a transient rise in pressure, which returned to the base line within about 1 min. The vasoconstrictor responses to norepinephrine or to potassium ions remained constant (±10%) for at least 2 hrs. At the beginning of each experiment, three responses to norepinephrine or to potassium chloride were obtained. The mean value of these three amplitudes was taken to represent 100%, and all subsequent responses were expressed as a percentage of this mean initial response.

The tested drugs were hydroflumethiazide (Rontyl®; Sankyo Co., Ltd.), furosemide (Lasix®; Hoechst Japan Ltd.), tripamide (Normonal®; Eisai Co., Ltd.) and indapamide (Natrix®; Selvier Lav.). Progressively increasing concentration of hydroflumethiazide ($3x10^{-7}$-$3x10^{-5}$ M), furosemide ($3x10^{-7}$-$3x10^{-5}$ M), tripamide (10^{-8}-10^{-5} M) and indapamide (10^{-8}-10^{-5} M) were added to the perfusate. For each concentration, perfusion was continued for 15 min, and at the end of this time, the amplitude of the pressor response to norepinephrine or potassium chloride was determined. Norepinephrine and potassium were tested on different preparations.

Six experiments were performed in each study. The results were expressed as means ± SD. Comparisons were made by student's t test.

RESULTS

Hydroflumethiazide

Hydroflumethiazide, added to the perfusate at concentrations of ($3x10^{-7}$-$3x10^{-5}$ M), did not change the basal pressure. Neither did it induce any change in the vascular response to norepinephrine or to potassium chloride.

Furosemide

Furosemide, when added to the perfusate, did not alter the basal pressure but inhibited the vascular response to norepinephrine in a dose related manner. The vascular contraction induced by potassium chloride was not affected by furosemide.

Tripamide (Fig. 1)

Tripamide, when added to the perfusate at concentrations of 10^{-8}-10^{-5} M, did not change the basal pressure. It significantly attenuated the potassium induced vasoconstriction but only slightly attenuated the vasoconstriction induced by norepinephrine. In the presence of 10^{-5} M of tripamide, potassium-induced contraction was 49±8% of the control response, while norepinephrine-induced vasoconstriction was 92±6%.

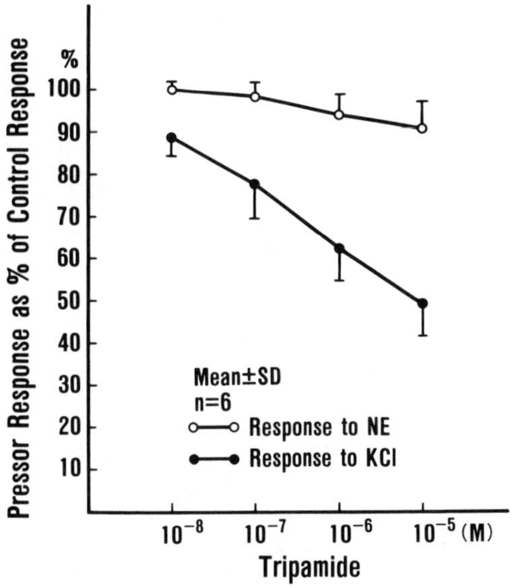

FIG. 1. The effect of tripamide on the vascular responses to norepinephrine (open circles) or to potassium chloride (closed circles). The pressor responses to norepinephrine or to potassium chloride are expressed as a percentage of the mean amplitude of three control responses obtained prior to adding the drug in the perfusate. The vertical bars indicate S.D.

Indapamide (Fig. 2)

Indapamide, when added to the perfusate at concentrations of 10^{-8}-10^{-5} M, did not change the basal pressure. It induced only a slight change in the responses to norepinephrine and potassium chloride. In the presence of 10^{-5} M of indapamide, potassium-induced contraction was 90±8% of the control response, and norepinephrine-induced contraction was 94±5%.

DISCUSSION

In the present study, it was found that furosemide attenuated the vascular response to norepinephrine and tripamide attenuated the vascular contraction induced by potassium chloride. Hydroflumethiazide and indapamide, however, did not induce significant changes on vascular contractions. These results suggest that tripamide and furosemide act directly on the vascular bed, and affected the vasoconstrictor response to potassium chloride or to norepinephrine.

There are several reports [1][2] suggesting that thiazide diuretics may attenuate pressor response to norepinephrine or angiotensin II *in vivo* in various experimental animals. On the other hand, there are reports that this effect of thiazide is dependent on the diuretic effects, since

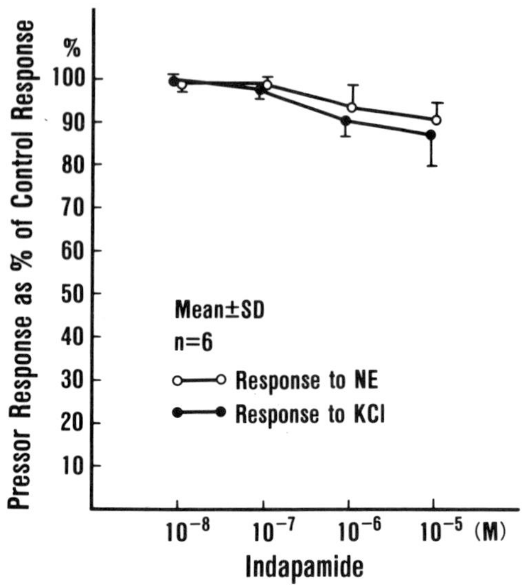

FIG. 2. The effect of indapamide on the vascular responses to norepinephrine (open circles) or to potassium chloride (closed circles). The pressor responses to norepinephrine or to potassium chloride are expressed as a percentage of the mean amplitude of three control responses obtained prior to adding the drug in the perfusate. The vertical bars indicate S.D.

replenishment of sodium and water abolished this attenuating effect [3][4]. And in our present study, we found that hydroflumethiazide did not affect the vascular response induced by norepinephrine or potassium chloride. Therefore, it is suggested that thiazide may not have a direct vascular action on the peripheral vascular bed.

There are also reports [7][8] about furosemide, that furosemide may have a direct vasodilatory effect because if administered to patients with heart failure, there is a reduction in preload with a resulting improvement in hemodynamics before the obvious diuretic effects set in. We found that furosemide attenuated the vascular resopnse to norepinephrine in the rat mesenteric artery.

In contrast to furosemide, tripamide significantly attenuated the potassium induced vasoconstriction but only slightly attenuated the vasoconstriction induced by norepinephrine. In the perfused rat mesenteric artery we used in this experiment, the potassium induced vasoconstriction is immediately abolished in a calcium-free medium, whereas in such a medium, norepinephrine still produces contractions which are 70-80% maximal [9]. This suggests that potassium acts primarily to promote entry of calcium from extracellular fluid, whereas norepinephrine primarily releases calcium from intracellular stores. In fact, in this vascular bed, nifedipine and diltiazem, both are calcium antagonists, also significantly attenuated the potassium induced vasoconstriction with a slight change in the norepinephrine response [10]. Therefore, it is suggested that the vascular action of tripamide is similar to that of calcium antagonists, such as nifedipine and diltiazem, which interfere directly with the transmembrane calcium supply. The report by Asada et al. [11] is in good accordance with our results. They observed that, in guinea pig mesenteric artery, tripamide, in a concentration below 10^{-7} g/ml (2.7×10^{-7} M) suppressed the spike evoked by outward current pulses in the presence of 3-5 mM TEA (tetraethylammonium-Cl) without modifying the membrane potential and resistance. This implies that this agent may suppress the calcium influx through calcium channel since the spike evoked in the guinea pig mesenteric artery was enhanced in NaCl-free solution, suppressed in $MnCl_2$ containing solution and blocked by calcium-antagonists.

It also should be noted that this effect of tripamide is apparent within the physiological concentrations. As the mesenteric vascular bed is known to be uniformly constricted in hypertensive animals and is thought to be important in the regulation of blood pressure, tripamide may be an important agent clinically with its action on the peripheral vascular bed in a similar manner as calcium-antagonists, which may contributes to its hypotensive effect.

On the other hand, indapamide, though its chemical structure is similar to tripamide (Fig. 3), induced only slight changes in the vascular response to norepinephrine and potassium chloride. This finding does not necessarily indicate that the vascular action of indapamide is quite different from tripamide, since it might exert some vasoactive effects at higher concentrations. Actually there is a report [12] suggesting that indapamide showed calcium-channel blocking action in the rabbit portal vein at high concentrations. Nevertheless, at concentrations below 10^{-5} M, vascular action of indapamide was not as evident as tripamide.

In summary, our study revealed that tripamide and furosemide have direct vascular actions independent from their renal actions, which may contribute to their antihypertensive effects. It is also suggested that the vascular action of tripamide may be similar to that of calcium antagonists, such as nifedipine and diltiazem, which suppress the calcium inward current during the activation of the membrane.

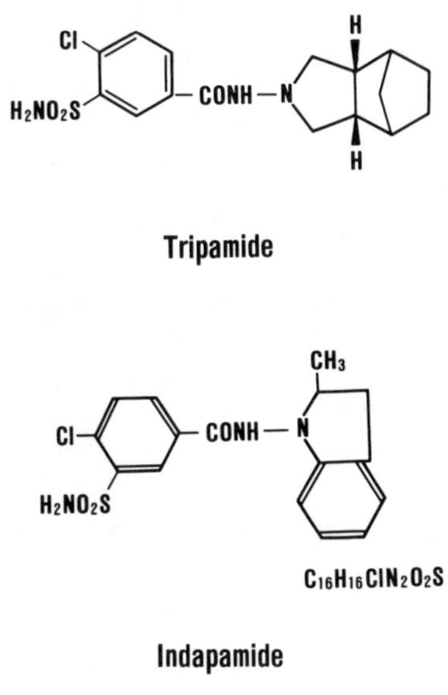

FIG. 3. The chemical structures of tripamide and indapamide.

REFERENCES

1. Beavers, W.K. and Blackmore, W., Effect of chlorothiazide on vascular reactivity. Proc. Soc. Exp. Biol. Med. 98, 133-135 (1958).
2. Fröhlich, E.D., Thurman, A.E., Pfeffer, M.A., Brobmann, G.F. and Jacobson, E.D., Altered vascular responsiveness: Initial hypotensive mechanism of thiazide diuretics. Proc. Soc. Exp. Biol. Med. 140, 1190-1196 (1972).
3. Freis, E.D., Wanko, A., Schnaper, H.W. and Fröhlich, E.D., Mechanism of the altered blood pressure responsiveness produced by chlorothiazide. J. Clin. Invest. 39, 1277-1281 (1960).
4. Weinberger, M.H., Ramsdell, J.W., Rosner, D.R. and Geddes, J.J.L., Effect of chlorothiazide and sodium on vascular responsiveness to angiotensin II. Am. J. Physiol. 223, 1049-1051 (1972).
5. McGregor, D.D., The effect of sympathetic nerve stimulation on vasoconstrictor responsiveness in perfused mesenteric blood vessels in the rat. J. Physio. (Lond) 177, 21-31 (1965).
6. Kondo, K., Okuno, T., Konishi, K., Saruta, T. and Kato, E., Effect of potassium and ouabain on the vascular reactivity to norepinephrine in the rat mesenteric artery. J. Canad. Physiol. Pharm. 57, 908-912 (1979).
7. Dikshit, K., Vyden, J., Forrester, J.S., Chatterjee, K., Prakash, R., and Swan, H.J.C., Renal and extrarenal effects of furosemide in congestive heart failure after acute myocardial infarction. N. Engl. J. Mde. 288, 1087-1090 (1973).
8. Mtabaj, J.P., Manku, M.S. and Horrobin, D.F., Vascular action of furosemide and bumetanide on the rat superior mesenteric vascular bed; interactions with prolactin and prostaglandins. Can. J. Physiol. Pharmacol. 54, 357-364 (1976).
9. Kondo, K., Manku, M.S., Horrobin, D.F., Boucher, R. and Genest, J., Potentiation of pressor effects of noradrenarine and potassium ions in the rat mesenteric arteries by physiological concentration of angiotensin I; Effects of prostaglandin E_2 and cortisol. Clin. Sci. Mol. Med. 53, 233-239 (1977).
10. Kondo, K., Suzuki, H., Okuno, T., Suda, M. and Saruta, T., Effects of nifedipine, diltiazem and verapamil on the vasoconstrictor resonses to norepinephrine and potassium ions in the rat mesenteric artery. Arch. int. Pharmacodyn. 245, 211-217 (1980).
11. Asada, H., Itoh, T., Suzuki, H., Ito, Y. and Kuriyama, H., Effects of N-(4-azo-endo-tricyclo[5.2.1.0.$^{2.6}$]-decan-4-YL)-4-chloro-3-sulfamoylbenzamide(E614;tripamide) on vascular smooth muscles. Gen. Pharmac. 13, 215-223 (1982).
12. Gargouil, Y.M. and Mironeau, J., Effects of indapamide on excitation-contraction coupling in smooth muscle of the mammalian portal vein. Curr. med. Res. Opin. (Supp. 1) 5, 55-59 (1977).

PATIENT SELECTION AND ASSESSMENT OF BLOOD PRESSURE IN CLINICAL TRIALS

RITA A. CAREY, Ph.D., ROY Z. EBY, M.S., MIRZA A. BEG, M.D., CHARLES F. McNALLY, M.D., MICHAEL J. FOX, M.D.
Smith Kline & French Laboratories, 1500 Spring Garden Street, Philadelphia, PA 19101

ABSTRACT

A new method for selecting patients with mild-to-moderate hypertension (M-HBP) who are appropriate for clinical trials and a technique for assessing statistically significant decreases in diastolic blood pressure (D-BP) resulting from drug therapy are described. This procedure defines M-HBP, eliminates subjects whose D-BP decreases while on placebo, and eliminates subjects with highly variable D-BP. Subjects are then selected for the study if the following criteria are met: 1) the average weekly D-BP for a 4-week placebo period is not <95 nor >115 mmHg, .2) the average weekly D-BP does not decrease, 3) the range of 12 DPB values recorded over a 4-week placebo period is not greater than 28 mmHg. To assess small but significant changes in D-BP in clinical trials, the technique of recording 3-DBP at not <30 min. intervals was used. In a study of 63 patients, an assessment was made of D-BP following therapy compared to placebo. A decrease of 4 mmHg was statistically significant ($P <.01$).

INTRODUCTION

The conduct of clinical trials on antihypertensive agents requires that patients be selected who have stable pre-therapy blood pressure values and that modest but statistically significant changes in blood pressure consequent to therapy can be identified.

The severity of hypertension must be accurately measured pre-therapy and those patients whose blood pressure falls within a range recognized by clinicians as either mild, moderate or severe hypertension should be selected for study. Patients who respond positively to placebo therapy or those whose baseline blood pressure is highly variable should not be admitted into a clinical trial. To date, no procedure for selecting patients or for measuring small but statistically significant changes in diastolic blood pressure of mildly hypertensive patients is totally satisfactory. This methodology was developed, therefore, to identify a sample population of mildly hypertensive patients for clinical trials and to evaluate the therapeutic effect of new antihypertensive medications on diastolic blood pressure.

Diuretics, Jules B. Puschett, Editor

METHOD

Patient Selection

Following a complete history and physical, the prospective subject is placed on placebo therapy for four weeks. Each week three measurements of supine blood pressure are recorded. The subject is supine for five minutes prior to the first measurement and the time between each subsequent measurement is a minimum of 30 minutes. Thus, twelve independent measurements of supine blood pressure are obtained during the placebo period. The average of the twelve diastolic blood pressure measurements, the average of the three diastolic blood pressures recorded on each single day and the range (high minus low) of the twelve diastolic blood pressure measurements are calculated. Subjects who meet all the following criteria are selected for study: 1) the overall average diastolic blood pressure for the four-week period is not less than 95 nor more than 115 mmHg, 2) the average weekly diastolic blood pressure does not decrease from week-to-week, 3) the range of diastolic blood pressure is not greater than 28 mmHg. A range of 28 from twelve observations is equivalent to a standard deviation of 8.5.

Assessment of Drug Effect

To assess the effect of the experimental antihypertensive medication, supine and standing diastolic blood pressure was measured at weekly intervals for four weeks. On each day, three supine and standing diastolic blood pressure values were recorded at intervals of not less than 30 minutes.

RESULTS

The usefulness of this methodology for selecting patients and for evaluating the therapeutic effect of an experimental antihypertensive agent has been demonstrated in a multicenter clinical trial. Sixty-three patients satisfied the entry criteria described above and entered into a double-blinded clinical trial designed to compare the antihypertensive effects of drug A and drug B. The mean changes in diastolic blood pressure at weeks 1, 2, 3 and 4 of drug therapy compared to placebo values are shown in figure one. Small changes from placebo of less than 4 mmHg achieved statistical significance ($P < .01$).

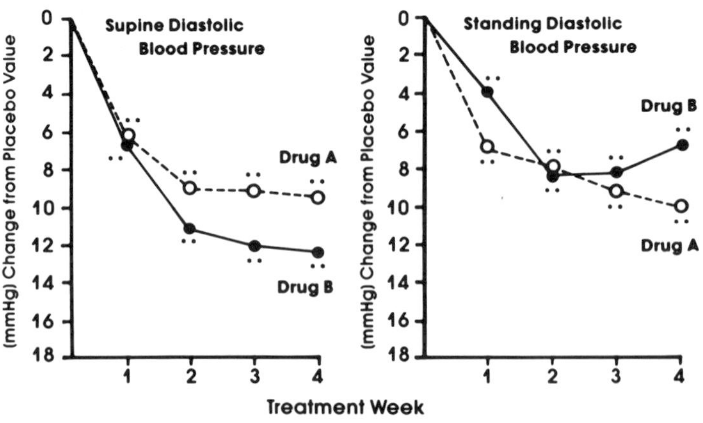

FIG. 1. Mean changes in supine and standing diastolic blood pressure for a four-week treatment period. Both drug A and drug B were associated with significant ($p < .01$) decreases in blood pressure.

DISCUSSION

This report describes a new method of selecting mildly hypertensive patients for clinical trials and for assessing the efficacy of antihypertensive medications in this population. The success of these procedures is also demonstrated.

Clinical investigators have recognized numerous potential sources of error in determining blood pressure by sphygmomanometry. These include inaccurate measurements attributed to equipment, such as improper cuff size[2], poor calibration of aneroid manometers[8] and malfunctioning exhaust valves[1]. Technique may vary between examiners, or the same examiner may allow slight changes in procedure which affect blood pressure. Procedural variability includes recording blood pressure when the patient's back is supported versus sitting on a table[9], or with the arm supported versus in isometric contraction[7]. A cuff applied at the improper level[5] or not centered over the artery[3] will also introduce technical error. Changing physiological or psychological state of a patient introduces variability in blood pressure. Diurnal changes in blood pressure may occur[4] The physical stress of exercise from which a patient is not fully recovered and psychological stress, including the presence of the examiner[6] are associated with variability in blood pressure.

A successful clinical trial requires that the equipment, technical and patient sources of variability are eliminated or reduced to a minimum. Further, it is necessary to take additional precautions for proper patient selection and accurate blood pressure measurements throughout the experimental period. With careful consideration of patient enrollment and precise blood pressure recordings, data can be collected which will yield statistically significant results from small, but clinically important changes in blood pressure.

REFERENCES

1. Conceicao S, Ward MK, Kerr DNS: Defects in sphygmonanometers: An important source of error in blood pressure reading. Brit Med J 1:886-889.
2. Geddes LA, Whisler SJ: The error in indirect blood pressure measurement with the incorrect size of cuff. Am Heart J 96:4-8, 1978.
3. Karvonen MJ, Telivgo LJ, Jarvinen EJK: Sphygmamanometric cuff size and accuracy of indirect measurement of blood pressure. Am J Cardiol 13:688-693, 1964.
4. Littler WA, Honour AJ, Carter RD et al: Sleep and blood pressure. Brit Med J 3:346-348, 1975.
5 Mitchell PL, Parlin, RW, Blackburn H: Effect of vertical displacement of the arm on indirect blood pressure measurement. N Engl J Med 271:72-74, 1964.
6. Richardson DW, Honour AJ, Fenton GW et al: Variation in arterial pressure throughout the day and night. Clin Sci 26:445-460, 1964.
7. Silverberg DS, Shemesh E, Iaina A: The unsupported arm. Brit Med J 2:1331, 1977.
8. Thulin T, Andersson G, Schersten B: Measure of blood pressure - a routine test in need of standardization. Postgrad Med J 51:390-395, 1975.
9. Viol GW, Goebel M, Lorenz GL et al: Seating as a variable in clinical blood pressure measurement. Am Heart J 98:813-814, 1979.

DIVISION OF ANTIHYPERTENSIVE DIURETICS INTO TWO CATEGORIES

W. P. LEARY,* A. J. REYES,** AND K. VAN DER BYL*
*Department of Clinical Pharmacology, University of Natal, Durban, South Africa; **Universidad de la República and Fundación Procardias, Montevideo, Uruguay

ABSTRACT

Diuretics are first choice antihypertensives. As monotherapy, thiazide-type diuretics control blood pressure in at least 65% of unstratified cases of essential hypertension. Pressure responses to antihypertensives follow linear or power functions of time. Power diuretics (e.g. indapamide) decrease pressure significantly in the first week; thereafter pressure follows a decreasing power function stabilising in 10-15 weeks. Linear diuretics (e.g. hydrochlorothiazide) reduce arterial pressure insignificantly during the first week; thereafter pressure follows a decreasing linear function, stabilising in 12-16 weeks. Power antihypertensives should be prescribed first in most patients and linear agents reserved for cases with impaired peripheral blood flow.

INTRODUCTION

Not all diuretics are effective monotherapy for essential hypertension. Antihypertensive diuretics are identified by their ability to control blood pressure as monotherapy, in at least 65% of patients in representative unstratified samples of the total population of essential hypertensives treated for 16 weeks [1]. Loop diuretics do not fall within this definition and should be reserved for hypertensive crises, resistant hypertension or hypertension accompanied by chronic renal failure. Early distal tubule diuretics, including thiazides, indapamide and xipamide, are effective antihypertensives but reduce pressure at different rates during the first 3-4 months of treatment.

The objective of the present study was to describe the time course of the blood pressure falls during the first 3 months of monotherapy with various diuretics.

PATIENTS AND METHODS

The experiments involved 155 patients with mild to severe uncomplicated essential hypertension who received monotherapy with a diuretic or a combination of diuretics or a diuretic and reserpine. Pressure was measured weekly at the same time of day using the standard indirect technique and average values analysed.

RESULTS AND DISCUSSION

Daily doses of indapamide 2,5 mg, xipamide 5, 10, 20 (FIG. 1) and 40 mg, hydrochlorothiazide 100 mg plus amiloride 10 mg and hydrochlorothiazide 50 mg + reserpine 0.5 mg caused a significant fall in blood pressure, P, during the first week of

Diuretics, Jules B. Puschett, Editor

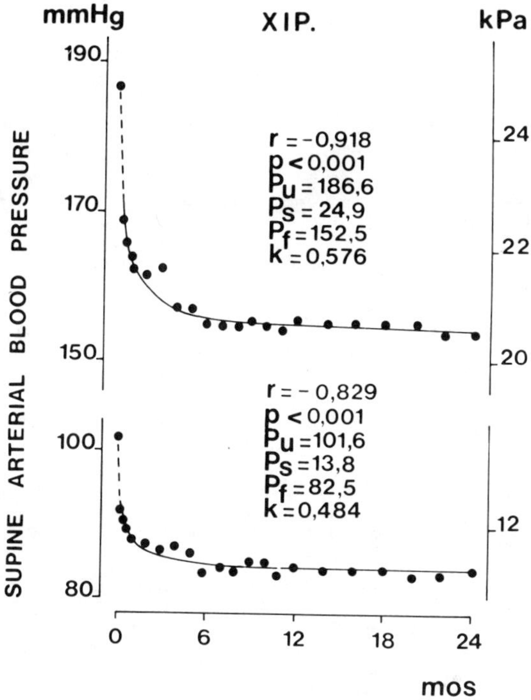

FIG. 1. Time course of responses of mean supine systolic and diastolic pressures, P, of 25 patients, to monotherapy with xipamide for 24 months. All cases received 20 mg.day^{-1} for 4 weeks; thereafter 20 (n=16), 30 (n=4), 40 (n=3) or 10 (n=2) mg was maintained. mos = months. From Castro and Reyes [2], by courtesy of Sístole.

treatment and rapid reduction thereafter, fitted by a decreasing power function of time, t

$$P = P_f + (P_u - P_f - P_s) \exp(-k \cdot \ln t), \quad (1)$$

where P_u is the pre-treatment pressure value, P_s is the difference between P_u and theoretical P after one week, P_f is a theoretical limit value to which P tends upon indefinite prolongation of treatment and k is a constant governing the rate of pressure fall.

Daily doses of cyclothiazide 10, hydrochlorothiazide 25-50 (FIG. 2) and tizolemide 100 mg.day^{-1} reduced pressure negligibly in the first week, pressure falling gradually thereafter, fitted by a linear function of time.

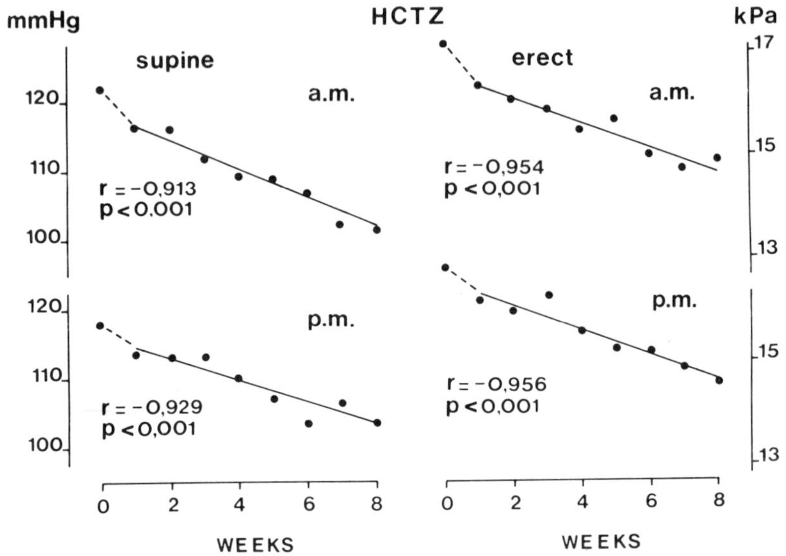

FIG. 2. Time course of responses of mean supine and erect, morning and afternoon blood pressures (mmHg, kPa) of 15 patients to monotherapy with hydrochlorothiazide. All received 25 $mg.day^{-1}$ for 4 weeks; thereafter a dose of 25 (n=8) or 50 (n=7) $mg.day^{-1}$ was maintained. From Leary and Reyes [3], by courtesy of Current Therapeutic Research.

where P_d is the difference between P_u and theoretical P for t = 0 and b is the slope of the function.

The models consistently fitted blood pressures. The exclusion of non-responders to treatment did not change the response pattern. Linear diuretics showed similar parametric features irrespective of dose. However, power antihypertensive xipamide exhibited a higher velocity of response at higher doses.

Since the incidence of complications in hypertensives correlates linearly with the pressure values at any time, power diuretics should be prescribed first in most cases. Linear diuretics should be reserved for cases with impaired regional flow.

REFERENCES

1. A.J. Reyes, and W.P. Leary, S. Afr. J. Contin. Med. Educ. in press (1984).
2. M. Castro, and A.J. Reyes, Sístole 31, 57-62 (1981).
3. W.P. Leary, A.J. Reyes, and R. Espinas, Curr. Ther. Res. 31, 201-208 (1982).

UP 788-42, A NEW DIURETIC β-BLOCKING AGENT

A. CLOAREC, M. CAZES, D. PROVOST, C. DELCHAMBRE, AND R. DEGHENGHI
Laboratoires UPSA, B.P. 325, 92506 Rueil Malmaison Cedex, France

ABSTRACT

UP 788-42, 1-[2-carbethoxy-4(2'-thienylcarboxamido)-phenoxy]-3-terbutylamino-2-propanol, HCl is a new drug combining in the same molecule diuretic and β-blocking properties. Both activities are demonstrated in normotensive conscious rats after oral dosing. UP 788-42 like hydrochlorothiazide shows a moderate diuretic profile totally different from that of propranolol.

INTRODUCTION

A common therapeutic approach for hypertensive diseases is the combination treatment of a diuretic and a β-blocking drug. Although propranolol does not possess appreciable diuretic properties in man, the fact that it has weak diuretic activity in rats was considered encouraging. We reasoned that we needed a β-blocking drug with more potent diuretic activity in animals to evidence a measurable effect in man. We report the diuretic and β-blocking properties of a novel compound designed to possess both properties.

MATERIALS AND METHODS

Diuretic activity in rats and monkeys : Fasted Sprague Dawley rats with free access to water were used. The rats received a water load of 2.5 ml/kg of body weight and then were given per os the vehicle or test substances. The rats were housed in groups of two in metabolism cages. Urine was collected for the 0-6 hours period and was analysed for electrolytes in total volume by standard methods. In monkeys, protocol used was closely related to that described above. Four drug naive Cynomolgus monkeys were used and dosed by oral gavage a dose volume of 25 ml/kg with either vehicle or test compound.

β-blocking activity in conscious rats : Chronic implanted Sprague Dawley rats were used. Before and 1.50, 3.50, 5.50 and 24 hours after oral administration of test compounds, β blockade was assessed by serial construction of dose-response curves for IV isoprenaline-induced tachycardia or hypotension. From these curves ED_{50} were determined by linear regression. ED_{50} is the dose of isoprenaline eliciting 50 % of the maximal effect observed (+174±6 beats/min or -42±1 mmHg). ED_{50} were taken as a measure of β-blocking effects.

RESULTS

Diuretic activity of UP 788-42 is shown in table 1 and in figure 1.

TABLE 1. Urinary output and electrolyte excretion in Cynomolgus monkeys.

UP 788-42 per os	Diuresis (ml) mean ± SEM	Na^+ (mEq) mean ± SEM	K^+ (mEq) mean ± SEM	Cl^- (mEq) mean ± SEM
0	44.7 ± 4.08	5.42 ± .52	5.06 ± .45	1.81 ± .16
3 mg/kg	26.1 ± 3.84	4.22 ± .54	3.21 ± .47	1.47 ± .32
10 mg/kg	106.8 ± 13.80*	14.43 ± 2.02*	12.80 ± 1.40*	3.41 ± .40*
30 mg/kg	89.0 ± 15.61	11.70 ± 1.51*	10.60 ± 2.01	1.85 ± .19

n=4, * $p<.05$. Study performed in HRC by JE Davies, DR Algate and DJ Beard.

FIG. 1. Urinary output and electrolyte excretion in rats.

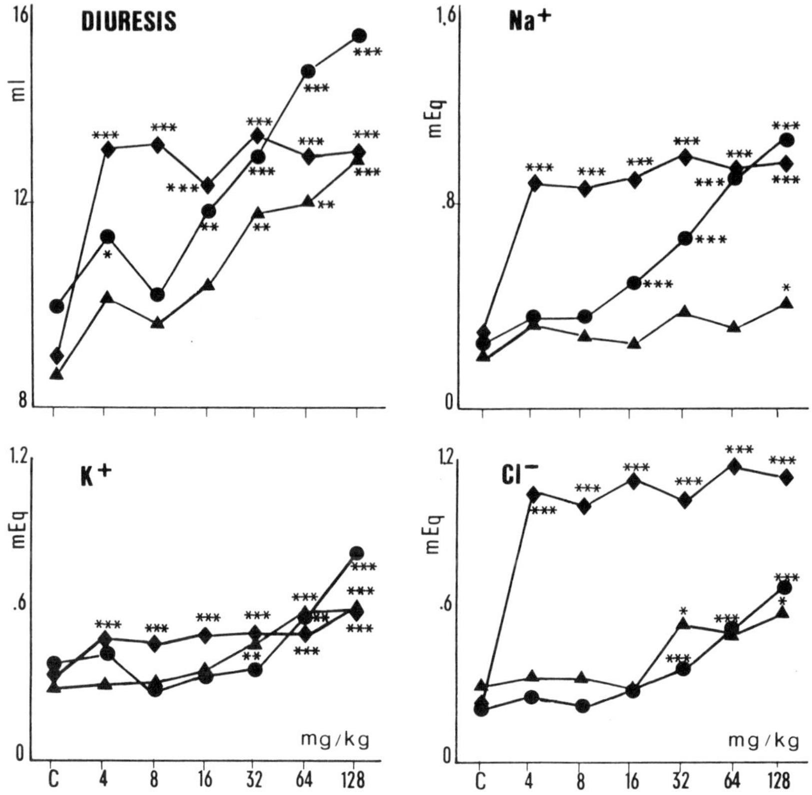

n=6; ● UP 788-42, ▲ propranolol, ◆ hydrochlorothiazide administered per os. Significance of the difference to controls (C) : * p<.05, ** p<.01, *** p<.001.

In rats and monkeys, UP 788-42 administered per os, induces a significant salidiuretic effect. In monkeys the dose of 10 mg/kg causes a strong diuretic effect with increase in the excretion of sodium, chloride and potassium ions. At the dose of 30 mg/kg, the increase of diuresis and output of sodium and chloride ions is somewhat less marked than that produced by the dose of 10 mg/kg. At the highest dose there is however virtually no increase in potassium excretion. In rats UP 788-42 causes a significant dose related increase of diuresis. As expected hydrochlorothiazide induces a diuretic effect which is maximal from the dose of 4 mg/kg. Propranolol only exerts a moderate activity on urinary output at high dosages. UP 788-42 and hydrochlorothiazide provoke a strong urinary sodium excretion which is concurrent with their diuretic activity. In contrast propranolol is unable to modify natriuresis. In our experimental conditions hydrochlorothiazide is more chloruretic than UP 788-42. Propranolol and UP 788-42 only have a weak effect on the excretion of chloride ions. Up to 32 mg/kg, UP 788-42 induces a potassium excretion similar to that of control group. At higher dosages its kaliuretic properties are comparable to those observed with hydrochlorothiazide. Propranolol increases potassium excretion from the dose of 32 mg/kg.

Figure 2 shows cardiac (β_1) and vascular (β_2) β-adrenoceptor blocking activities of UP 788-42 and propranolol, administered p.o. in conscious rats.

FIG. 2. Cardiac and vascular β-blocking activities in the conscious rat.

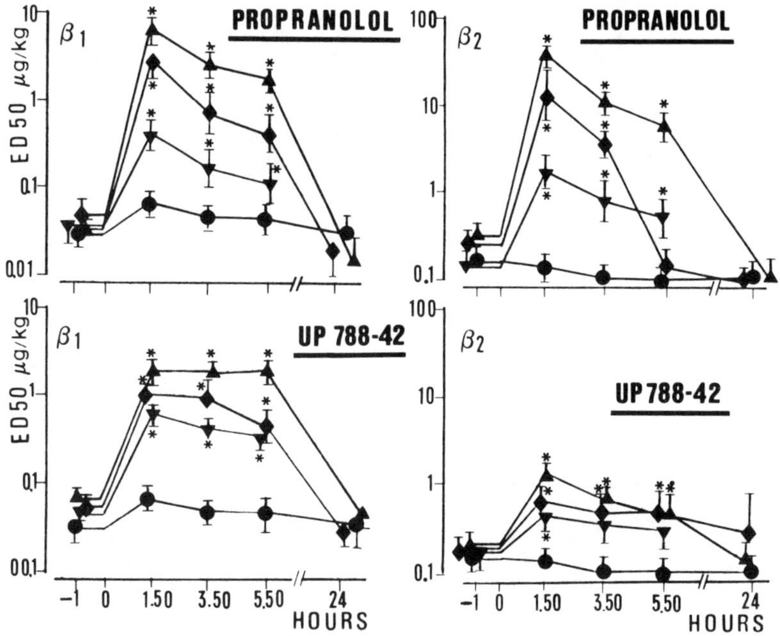

n=5-9 rats; ● placebo group, ▼ 8 mg/kg, ◆ 16 mg/kg, ▲ 32 mg/kg administered p.o. Each point represents ED_{50} and its 95 % confidence limits, * $p<.05$ significance to control values (1 hour before oral administration).

Vehicle in placebo group has virtually no effect on isoprenaline-induced tachycardia (β_1) or hypotension (β_2). UP 788-42 and propranolol induce a reduction of sensitivity for isoprenaline with a maximal effect at 1.50 hour. The degree of reduction depends both on time after administration and on doses of drugs. Maximal β_1 blocking effects of UP 788-42 are of a lesser degree than those of propranolol. In case of UP 788-42, β_1 blocking effect keeps almost constant until 5.50 hours whereas β-blocking effect of propranolol gradually decreases. UP 788-42 induces quite a weak β_2 blockade in comparison with that of propranolol and its effect on β_1 adrenoceptors.

CONCLUSION

β_1 blocking action of UP 788-42 is slightly weaker than that of propranolol, but unlike it, it shows cardioselective properties. UP 788-42 like hydrochlorothiazide has the profile of a moderate diuretic drug with good excretion of sodium, it seems to induce a lesser excretion of potassium and chloride. UP 788-42 presents a totally different diuretic profile from that of propranolol which only acts on dilution of urine. This work provides evidence that, at least in rats and monkeys, UP 788-42 possesses diuretic and β-blocking properties of obvious interest for the treatment of hypertension.

SECTION IV

DIURETICS, CALCIUM AND MAGNESIUM METABOLISM

EFFECTS OF DIURETICS ON THE DISTAL CONVOLUTED TUBULAR TRANSPORT OF CALCIUM

LINDA S. COSTANZO
Department of Physiology and Biophysics, Medical College of Virginia, Richmond, Virginia, USA.

In order to preserve homeostasis, the kidney normally reabsorbs more than 99% of the Ca filtered by the glomeruli. The proximal tubule reabsorbs 65% of the filtered load, the loop of Henle 25% and the distal convoluted tubule 9% (1). The magnitude of Ca reabsorption in each of these segments can be influenced by a variety of experimental manipulations. In general, maneuvers which alter proximal tubule Na and water absorption cause proportional changes in Ca absorption, such that volume contraction increases Ca reabsorption and volume expansion, parathyroid hormone or Diamox administration decrease Ca reabsorption (2). The thick ascending limb of Henle has both passive and active Ca transport (3,4). Furosemide diminishes Ca transport in proportion to NaCl transport by inhibiting the lumen positive potential difference in this segment (5). This action forms the basis for furosemide-induced calciuresis. The thick ascending limb also contains PTH-sensitive adenylate cyclase (6) and responds to high doses of PTH with increased Ca transport rates (7). In contrast to the more proximal segments, Ca transport in the distal tubule is characterized by its dissociation from Na transport (2). The distal convoluted tubule and connecting tubule are the major sites of the Ca-retaining action of PTH (5,8). Thiazide diuretics (9) and amiloride (10) enhance distal Ca reabsorption while simultaneously diminishing Na reabsorption. Alkalosis and phosphate loading also increase Ca transport rates; conversely, acidosis and phosphate depletion inhibit Ca transport (2). Thus, the distal nephron is a site for Na-independent regulation of Ca reabsorption; it is also a site where an inverse relationship between Na and Ca transport can occur.

The best studied example of the dissociable nature of distal Na and Ca transport is that occurring during treatment with thiazide diuretics. Data from Yendt and collaborators are typical of those obtained in hypercalciuric patients treated with hydrochlorothiazide (11). On the first day of drug treatment, urinary Na excretion increases while Ca excretion is unchanged; thus, Ca and Na excretion are dissociated. On subsequent days of thiazide therapy, the dissociation continues as Na excretion returns to pre-drug values and Ca excretion falls below control.

One possible explanation for this pattern of results is that diminished Ca excretion is contingent upon the volume contraction which chlorothiazide produces. We therefore evaluated the direct renal effects of chlorothiazide in volume expanded dogs (13). Chlorothiazide was infused into the left renal artery of 5 normal dogs at 1mg/min. A comparison was made between the renal function of the left kidney before and during drug infusion as well as comparison of the left and right kidneys. Neither glomerular filtration rate nor ultrafilterable Ca concentrations changed over the course of the experiments. Drug infusion produced a mainly unilateral natriuresis; the mean clearance ratio for Na increased by 80% on the infused side, from 0.085 to 0.153, $p < 0.05$. In contrast, the clearance ratio for Ca actually fell by 25% from 0.064 to 0.048 on the infused side, $p < 0.01$. Consequently, the ratio between Ca and Na clearances, fell on the experimental side form 0.81 to 0.39, $p < 0.001$. Only small changes in these parameters could be demonstrated on the contralateral side. These experiments demonstrated that the hypocalciuric

Diuretics, Jules B. Puschett, Editor

action of thiazides is exerted directly on the kidney; the effect is independent of alterations in extracellular fluid volume, since volume contraction should have affected both kidneys to the same extent. Similar experiments were performed in 5 thyro-parathyroidectomized dogs and the results were comparable to those from intact dogs. We therefore also concluded that thiazide induced Ca retention is not mediated by changes in circulating parathyroid hormone levels.

Kunau and collaborators demonstrated that thiazides inhibit NaCl transport in the distal convoluted tubule (13). As originally suggested by Walser (14), we proposed that the drugs' hypocalciuric action also occurs in the distal tubule. To test this hypothesis, we performed free flow micropuncture in rats to characterize distal Ca reabsorption and examine the effects of chlorothiazide (9). The results showed that the tubular fluid entering the distal convoluted tubule has a Ca concentration lower than that in plasma ultrafiltrate. The luminal concentration continues to dicline along the length of the distal tubule and fractional Ca reabsorption amounts to 8% of the filtered load. Taken together with the well known lumen negative potential difference (15), these data demonstrate active Ca transport by the distal convoluted tubule.

In order to examine the components of net Ca reabsorption, the efflux from lumen to blood, and the backflux from blood to lumen, we performed stationary microperfusion experiments (9). Selected distal tubular segments were punctured with micropipettes containing droplets of ion-free isosmotic raffinose sealed between columns of mineral oil. A column of oil was injected into the tubule and at zero time the raffinose droplet was injected into the lumen to split the oil columns. The aqueous droplet was allowed to sit in the lumen for varying periods of time and was then re-aspirated and analyzed for its Ca concentration. Ca backflux, determined in this manner, was negligible and we concluded that the Ca permeability of the distal convoluted tubule is extremely low. When we examined Ca efflux from isosmotic raffinose droplets, initially containing either 9mM Ca or 2.5mM Ca, we found that the luminal Ca concentration declined as a function of contact time. We concluded from these efflux data that the reabsorptive flux of Ca is dependent upon the luminal Ca concentration and suggested that this concentration dependence might result in load dependency of distal Ca transport.

In order to test the load dependency of distal Ca transport directly, we developed the technique of *in vivo* microperfusion of rat distal convoluted tubules (9). Distal tubules were perfused with an artificial solution simulating early distal fluid containing 14-C inulin to measure water reabsorption. The collected fluid was analyzed for its Ca, Na and inulin concentrations and the values were compared to those measured in the perfused fluid. Reabsorptive rates for Ca, Na and water were then calculated. The length of perfused segments was measured after experiments by injecting Microfil into the tubules and determining the length of the rubber cast. 21 distal convoluted tubules were microperfused in this fashion with either a control solution or one containing 5×10^{-4}M chlorothiazide. The delivered load of Ca and Na was varied by changing the rate of the microperfusion pump. Na and Ca reabsorptive rates were measured in each perfused segment as a function of the delivered load. In control tubules, Na reabsorption varied as a linear function of the load up to Na delivery rates which were 3 times the physiological rate, wihtout evidence of saturation; fractional reabsorption was constant at 85%. In the presence of chlorothiazide, Na reabsorption was significantly diminished for any given load, such that fractional reabsorption was reduced to 48%. Chlorothiazide inhibited Na transport whether it was present in the lumen alone or on both sides of the epithelium, consistent with a luminal site of drug action. Contrasting results were obtained for Ca. Under control conditions, Ca reabsorption, like Na reabsorption, increased in proportion to the Ca load, with fractional reabsorption being 68%. When chlorothiazide was present, Ca transport in the distal segments was actually increased for any level of delivered load, increasing Ca reabsorption to virtually 100%. Drug- enhancement of Ca transport also occurred from the luminal aspect of the distal cells. Thus, evidence was obtained for an inverse relationship between Na and Ca transport by the distal convoluted tubule; the inhibition of Na transport and enhancement of Ca transport can explain the well-known natriuretic and hypocalciuric actions of thiazide diuretics.

Kriz and Kaissling and their collaborators have recently documented the morphologic heterogeneity of the distal convolution (16,17). In the rat, there are no less than 4 distinct cell types intermingled, whose functional characteristics have yet to be described. In light of this heterogeneity, we were interested in determining the site of action of thiazides within the distal tubule more precisely. We therefore modified our technique so that we could separately perfuse early and late distal convoluted tubules (10). Early tubules were described as those in which the post macula densa segment appears on the kidney surface; late tubules are described as those in which the juction with another distal tubule is on the kidney surface. The position of the perfused segments was determined by a latex cast. After microperfusion, Microfil was injected to fill the entire distal convoluted tubule from the macula densa to the junction to the junction with another distal tubule. After microdissection, the entire distal tubular length was measured and thereafter referred to as 100%. The perfused segment's length was also measured as well as it's distance from the macula densa and expressed as percent of the total length. Any tubule falling predominantly within the first 50% of the distal tubule was referred to as "early"; any tubule falling predominantly within the last 50% was referred to as "late".

Perfused distal tubules, characterized according to localization, were evaluated for their transport properties. Fluid transport, Na transport and Ca transport were measured in 15 early and 14 late tubules. Only fluid reabsorption differed between the two groups, early tubules giving a mean value of 0.36±0.05 nl/min-mm and late tubules giving a value of 1.13±0.09 nl/min-mm, $p < 0.001$. The observation of higher osmotic water flow in the late rat distal convolution is consistent with the appearance of ADH-sensitive adenylate cyclase in the late portion of the rat distal tubule as described by Morel (6) and the osmotic equilibration of late distal tubular fluid with peritubular blood, described by Gottschalk and co-workers (18).

Having obtained these baseline transport rates for early and late tubules, the effects of chlorothiazide in early as compared to late tubules was assessed. Eight early tubules and seven late tubules were perfused with both a control and chlorothiazide-containing solution. Thus, each tubule served as it's own control. Chlorothiazide inhibited Na transport in each of the early distal tubules, the mean value decreasing from 131±12 pmole/min-mm to 89±10 pmole/min-mm, $p < 0.001$. In contrast, only two of the late tubules responded with a modest decrease in Na transport. The location of thiazide-enhancement of Ca transport was similar. Each early distal convoluted tubule responded to chlorothiazide with an increased rate of Ca transport, the mean value increasing from 3.24±0.29 pmole/min-mm to 4.00±0.18 pmole/min-mm, $p < 0.01$. On the other hand, late distal convoluted tubules were not, on the average, affected by the drug. We concluded that chlorothiazide is natriuretic and hypocalciuric because it specifically interacts with a cell present predominantly in the early distal convoluted tubule.

Our experiments with thiazides prompted us to question whether other distal diuretics might also enhance Ca transport in association with inhibition of Na transport. Early experiments showed that amiloride is hypocalciuric in dogs (19). We confirmed these results in rats receiving an infusion of 5% mannitol (10). Amiloride infusion did not alter GFR or ultrafilterable Ca concentrations. However, fractional Ca excretion declined significantly from 12% to 7.4%, $p < 0.05$. The ratio of Ca to Na clearance also decreased, from 0.69±0.13 to 0.46±0.01, $p < 0.01$.

To further investigate the site of action of amiloride, early and late tubules were perfused with control solutions and 10^{-5} M amiloride-containing solutions at constant delivered load (10). A localization opposite to that for chlorothiazide obtained. Amiloride inhibited Na transport from 143±12 to 87±9 pmole/min-mm in late distal convoluted tubules, $p < 0.01$. Only two of the seven early tubules responded to amiloride, and on the average, amiloride did not inhibit early distal tubular Na reabsorption. Amiloride enhanced Ca transport in the late distal tubule from 3.60±0.49 to 4.73±0.69 pmole/min-mm, $p < 0.005$. Ca transport in early tubules was affected to only a small extent or not at all. Thus amiloride inhibited Na transport and enhanced Ca transport in the same portion of the rat distal convoluted tubule. It seemed reasonable to suggest that the two effects on ion transport might be related. We therefore examined the change in Ca reabsorption as a function of the change in Na reabsorption for every tubule perfused. In general, the larger the decrease in Na reabsorption, the larger the increase in Ca reabsorption, suggesting a relationship between the two different effects.

It is conceivable that enhanced transepithelial Ca transport is secondary to amiloride-induced inhibition of Na transport. One possible mechanism for these inverse effects of amiloride is as follows. Na and Ca may passively enter the late distal tubular cell from the lumen down their respective electrochemical gradients. Na is extruded from the cell against an electrochemical gradient by the Na-K pump in the peritubular membrane. Ca may be actively extruded via a Ca pump utilizing ATP (20) or via a Ca-Na exchange process (21). The latter derives the energy for Ca extrusion from the inward Na gradient. Alterations in the Na gradient across the peritubular membrane should result in changes in the extrusion rate of Ca.

It is known that amiloride blocks apical Na channels in responsive epithelia (22). The resulting decrease in Na conductance of the luminal membrane should result in decreased intracellular Na ion activity and decreased net transepithelial Na movement. A second consequence could be an increase in the rate of Ca extrusion-coupled Na entry across the peritubular membrane due to the more favorable Na gradient; secondarily, Ca transport would be increased. This model remains to be tested with measurements of intracellular Na and Ca ion activities.

There is one additional feature to the story of distal hypocalciuric diuretics. The early studies of amiloride in dogs also described the additive hypocalciuric effects of thiazides and amiloride (19). Amiloride when added to a maximally effective dose of thiazide produced additional enhancement of renal Ca reabsorption. At the time, we suggested that the additivity was the result of different sites or different mechanisms of diuretic action. To examine this question, we recently microperfused 2 long distal convoluted tubules containing both early late segments with three solutions: (1) control, (2) containing a maximal dose of chlorothiazide (5×10^{-4}M) and (3) containing the same thiazide dose plus amiloride (10^{-5} M). In both tubules, chlorothiazide alone inhibited Na transport and enhanced Ca transport. Addition of amiloride further increased Ca transport with a small additional inhibition of Na transport.

This additivity may have therapeutic implications for the treatment of hypercalciuria. We studied 7 children who were hypercalciuric from treatment with pharmacologic doses of vitamin D for underlying disorders. All were receiving hydrochlorothiazide to lower urine calcium excretion. When we added amiloride to the thiazide regimen, there was significant additional lowering of urinary calcium excretion (23). Addition of amiloride also prevented thiazide-induced hypokalemic alkalosis as a result of it's K-sparing effect. Leppla and co-workers reached similar conclusions from studies in hypercalciuric adults (24).

In summary, chlorothiazide and amiloride have similar effects on distal Na and Ca reabsorption. Both diuretics inhibit Na and enhance Ca transport. The two diuretics apparently interact with different cell types in the distal convoluted tubule as thiazide's actions were confined to the early distal tubule and amiloride's to the late distal tubule. We conclude that separate sites of action are at least in part responsible for drugs' additive hypocalciuric actions.

ACKNOWLEDGEMENTS

The author's work was supported by a grant from N.I.H. (AM-28358). L. Costanzo is an Established Investigator of the American Heart Association.

REFERENCES

1. W.E. Lassiter, C.W. Gottschalk, and M. Mylle. Am.J. Physiol. 204: 771-775 (1963).
2. R.A. L. Sutton and J. H. Dirks. In the The Kidney , 2nd Edition, B.M. Brenner and F.C. Rector, eds. (Saunders), pp. 551-618 (1981).
3. J.E. Bourdeau and M.B. Burg. Am.J. Physiol. 236: F357-F364 (1979).
4. W.N. Suki, D. Rouse, R.C. Ng and J.P. Kokko. J. Clin . Invest. 66: 1004-1009 (1980).
5. G.R. Shareghi and L. C. Stoner. Am. J. Physiol. 235: F367-F375 (1978).
6. F. Morel. Am. J. Physiol. 240:F159-F164 (1980).
7. J.E. Bourdeau and M. Burg. Am. J. Physiol. 239: F121-F126 (1980).
8. L. S. Costanzo and E. E. Windhager. Am. J. Physiol. 239: F478-F485 (1980)
9. L. S. Costanzo and E. E. Windhager. Am. J. Physiol. 235: F492-F506 (1978)
10. L. S. Costanzo. Am . J. Physiol. In press (1984).
11. E. R. Yendt, R. J. A. Gagne and M. Cohanim. Am. J. Med. Sci. 251: 107-118 (1966).
12. L. S. Costanzo and I. M. Weiner. J. Clin.Invest. 54: 628-637 (1974).
13. R. T. Kunau, D. R. Weller and H. L. Webb. J. Clin. Invest. 56:401-407 (1975).
14. M. Walser. In Renal Pharmacology . (Appleton-Century-Crofts). pps:21-41 (1971).
15. F.S. Wright. Am. J. Physiol. 220: 624-638 (1971).
16. W. Kriz, B. Kaissling and M. Pszolla. In New Aspects of Renal Function H. G. Vogel and K. J. Ullrich, eds. (Excerpta Medica), pps. 67-79 (1978).
17. B. Kaissling. Am. J. Physiol. 243: F221-F226 (1982).
18. C. W. Gottschalk and M. Mylle. Am. J. Physiol. 196:927-936 (1959).
19. L. S. Costanzo and I. M. Weiner. Am. J. Physiol. 239: 67-73 (1976).
20. A. Doucet and A.I. Katz. Am. J. Physiol. 242: F346-F352 (1982).
21. P.A. Friedman, J.F. Figueiredo, T. Maack and E. E. Windhager. Am. J. Physiol. 240: F558-F568 (1981).
22. T. U. L. Biber. J. Gen. Physiol. 58: 131-144 (1971).
23. U. Alon, L.S. Costanzo and J. C. M. Chan. Min. Elec. Metab., in press (1984).

EFFECTS OF DIURETICS ON MAGNESIUM METABOLISM

Ezequiel Bellorín-Font, José Weisinger, Virgilio Paz Martínez
Centro Nacional de Diálisis y Trasplante (M.S.A.S.) and
Division of Nephrology. Hospital Universitario de Caracas.
P.O.Box 47365. Los Chaguaramos. Caracas. Venezuela.

ABSTRACT

Diuretic therapy is associated to urinary magnesium losses. This cation, the second most abundant in intracellular fluids,is involved in several metabolic processes. Its metabolism is regulated by glomerular filtration and tubular reabsorption.The loop of Henle reabsorbs the bulk of the filtered load, with little reabsorption occurring in the proximal and distal tubule. Loop diuretics induce profound urinary losses of magnesium by inhibition of chloride transport in the loop of Henle. Thiazide induce mild magnesuria in vivo by mechanisms not clearly defined,whereas potassium-sparing diuretics may produce magnesium retention.Magnesuria induced by diuretics may result in magnesium deficiency.This alteration could lead to altered potassium and calcium metabolism by mechanism probably mediated by deppresion of enzyme and biochemical functions of the cell.

INTRODUCTION

One of the aspects somewhat overlooked during diuretic therapy is the impact of these agents on magnesium metabolism. However, magnesium depletion associated to the use of diuretics was initially reported in 1952 in patients with congestive heart failure treated with ammonium chloride and mercurial diuretics (1). Subsequently, it has been shown that thiazide and loop diuretics can induce substancial urinary losses of magnesium (2-7). On the other hand potassium-sparing diuretics do not have this effect, and indeed may produce magnesium retention (8-9).

In a series of 5.100 consecutive patients seen at a general diagnostic clinic, diuretic therapy was the second most commom cause of hypomagnèsemia after diabetic acidosis (10). It should be pointed out, however, that in a great number of cases, the deficiency of this element may not be of suficient degree to induce clear clinical situations. Furthermore, changes in plasma levels of magnesium do not always reflect the status of body magnesium. But, regardless of this, alterations of magnesium metabolism are of prime importance since this cation has profound regulatory functions in several biochemical processes.

Magnesium is the second most abundant cation in intracellular fluids and the fourth in extracellular fluids, and plays a key role in many metabolic processes, which include among others: oxidative phosphorilation, activation of Na-K-ATPase, generation of cyclic nucleotides, metabolism of deoxyribonucleic and ribonucleic acids, protein synthesis and many other reactions involving hydrolisis of adenosine triphosphate (ATP). Therefore , alterations in magnesium metabolism have tha potential for impairing many biochemical functions of the cell and to result in serious clinical consequences.

MAGNESIUM METABOLISM

On average, subjects on a normal diet ingest between 25 and 30 mEq of magnesium per day (11,12). Of this amount, 25 to 60 percent are absorbed in the ileum (13,14), and close to 30 percent are excreted in the urine. Under normal conditions endogenous fecal secretion of magnesium is minimal (15).

Diuretics, Jules B. Puschett, Editor

But there is no convincing evidence of physiological control of magnesium in the intestine. Therefore, the kidney becomes the major site of body magnesium regulation.

Within the plasma, the ultrafilterable fraction of magnesium accounts for aproximately 80 percent of the total. The remaining 20 percent of total magnesium is bound to albumin.Direct sampling by mycropuncture of glomerulus in the Munich-Wistar rat has shown a ratio of glomerular fluid to plasma magnesium of 0.8 (16). In the proximal tubule, however, magnesium concentration rises with respect to ultrafilterable magnesium, reaching a ratio of tubular fluid to ultrafiltrate magnesium concentration (TF/UFMg) of 1.5 ; indicating that in this segment only 15 to 30 percent of the filtered load is reabsorbed (17). Micropuncture studies of the proximal tubule in experiments in which the luminal membrane was exposed to variable concentrations of magnesium have shown an increase in the collected to perfusate concentration ratio of magnesiun with water reabsorption along the tubule. This rise is independent of intraluminal magnesium concentration over the range of 0 to 20 mEq/l (19). It was also shown in these studies that magnesium reabsorption in this segment was altered by factors that affected sodium reabsorption such as volume expansion. Therefore, volume contraction induced by diuretics may also affect magnesium reabsorption.

The bulk of magnesium reabsorption occurs in the thick ascending limb of the loop of Henle. This portion of the nephron reabsorbs about 60 percent of the filtered load of magnesium (17-19). Studies by Quamme and coworkers (19) recently showed that in the presence of normal plasma magnesium , the fractional reabsorption of this ion remained constant at approximately 70 percent of the delivery load as luminal magnesium was increased from 0 to 10 mEq/l. At higher concentrations, magnesium reabsorption declined. This demonstrates a great capacity of the loop of Henle to increase absolute magnesium reabsorption. In contrast, during hypermagnesemia, fractional reabsorption of magnesium decreased markedly to around 20 percent of the delivery load. Calcium reabsorption was also decreased by hypermagnesemia. Furthermore, hypercalcemia retards magnesium reabsorption (19), suggesting that a calcium-magnesium interaction may occur probably on the contraluminal membrane of the ascending limb cell.

The mechanism of magnesium reabsorption in the ascending limb is still unclear, but it seems to be voltage-dependent. Thus, active chloride transport would be the major driving force for magnesium reabsorption. Loop diuretics like furosemide, ethacrynic acid and others could, then, increase magnesium excretion by inhibiting chloride transport in this segment.

Unlike the loop of Henle, the distal tubule has a small capacity for magnesium reabsorption, accounting for only 2 to 5 percent of the filtered load (19). This transport occurs against an electrochemical gradient, pressumably by an active mechanism.

In summary, magnesium is reabsorbed in the proximal tubule following changes in salt and water reabsorption. The loop of Henle reabsorbs close to 60 percent of filtered magnesium by voltage-dependent mechanisms and, the distal tubule plays only a minor role in overall magnesium handling.

EFFECTS OF DIURETICS ON MAGNESIUM HANDLING IN THE KIDNEY

According to the above physiological review of magnesium handling in the kidney, diuretics could conceivably affect magnesium reabsorption in a variety of ways: 1., by inducing volume contraction; 2., by inducing changes in electrical potentials accross the cell membrane; 3., by direct inhibition of possible active mechanism controlling magnesium reabsorption; and, 4., by altering enzymes involved in solute reabsorption.

Diuretics acting at the proximal tubule, like carbonic anhidrase inhibitors do not significantly alter magnesium excretion. These agents induce a small decrease in proximal reabsorption, but the loop of Henle probably reabsorbs most of the increased delivery of magnesium. The increased excretion of magnesium showed in previous studies could also be explained by inhibition of distal hydrogen secretion by carbonic anhidrase inhibitors (3,20). However, the overall effect of these drugs on magnesium excretion is minimal.

Diuretics acting at the loop of Henle, like furosemide and ethacrynic acid, are well known to alter magnesium metabolism by inducing magnesuria (2,3,20-22). However, cumulative losses leading to severe magnesium depletion wil occur only when the doses are high, the interval of administration is short, or when other causes of hypomagnesemia are also present. For instance, magnesium depletion associated to loop diuretics has been shown with increasing frequency in areas were the magnesium content in water and food is low (24).

The action of furosemide appears to be in the ascending loop of Henle, probably through inhibition of chloride transport. Quamme showed that during microperfusion experiments in the rat, furosemide decreased fractional magnesium reabsorption from nearly 80 per cent to 30 percent, whereas sodium reabsorption was decreased to only 50 per cent (23). This profound effect of furosemide on magnesium reabsorption has important implications in the chronic use of this diuretic such as in the treatment of symptomatic hypercalcemia. In fact, as mentioned previously, hypercalcemia per se causes magnesuria and may induce some degree of hypomagnesemia. Administration of furosemide in these cases may agravate magnesium losses and result in symptomatic hypomagnesemia.

Another factor that may contribute to the magnesium handling in the kidney is parathyroid hormone (PTH). Its role in magnesium excretion is less well defined as compared to that in calcium and phosphorus excretion. The data on the effect of PTH on magnesium handling in the kidney has been controversial and,an increase in magnesium excretion as well as increased magnesium reabsorption have been reported in response to PTH (20). However, the former is most probably due to the hypercalcemia induced by PTH, which may induce magnesuria itself and overcome the effect of PTH. Indeed, in most recent studies in humans and experimental animals, injections of PTH decreased fractional excretion of magnesium (20,24,25). Micropuncture studies in the hamster demonstrate that magnesium transport is increased by PTH (20). Furthermore, cyclic AMP may mimic this effect, suggesting that the action of PTH on magnesium reabsorption is mediated by the generation of cyclic AMP at the contraluminal membrane of the tubular cell (24,25). Thus, it is possible that inhibition of PTH-sensitive adenylate cyclase by diuretics could result in increased urinary losses of magnesium.

Recently, we have analyzed this possible mechanism by examining the effect of furosemide on basal and PTH-dependent adenylate cyclase activity in basolateral membrane preparations of normal dogs. In these experiments , the magnesium concentration in the incubation medium was varied from 0 to 40 mM, furosemide (1mM) produced a significant decrease in PTH-dependent adenylate cyclase activity, at all Mg concentrations in the medium. Basal enzyme activity was not affected by furosemide, suggesting that the effect of the diuretic was specific for the PTH-dependent enzyme activity. The afinity of the enzyme for magnesium was not altered (26). At present, however, the significance of this effect in the final action of furosemide on magnesium metabolism in vivo remains to be studied.

Thiazide diuretics are known to exert their natriuretic effect primaryly in the distal tubule. Early studies in vivo by Parfitt have shown that chlorothiazide induces a modest increase in magnesium excretion (21). These observations have been confirmed by others (3,9,27). However, the nature of the effect of thiazide diuretics on magnesium reabsorption is not well known. Micropuncture experiments by Wong et al in the hamster demonstrated little or no effect of thiazides on magnesium reabsorption (28). One possibility, then, is that these diuretics may increase magnesium excretion by inhibiting carbonic anhidrase activity in the proximal tubule. The resulting increased delivery of magnesium may escape reabsorption in the ascending limb of Henle, thus accounting for the variable magnesiuric effect reported in some clinical studies.

Finally, as opposed to most diuretic agents, potassium-sparing diuretics acting at the distal tubule may increase magnesium reabsorpeion. Previous studies have demonstrated reduced levels of muscle magnesium in patients with congestive heart failure (8,9), particulary in those receiving the combination of diuretics and digitalis. More recently it has been shown that in patients with congestive heart failure treated with furosemide, the addition of amiloride results in a decrease in the urinary output of magnesium. This was reflected in an increase in both plasma and lymphocite magnesium (8). Other studies have also shown an increment in muscle magnesium after addition of amiloride or spironolactone to patients treated with chlorothiazide (9). Spironolactone decreases urinary losses of magnesium in patients with aldosteronism. The mechanism of this magnesium conserving effect of potassium-sparing diuretics is not clearly stablished. It has been postulated that this effect could be due to enhaced magnesium reabsorption in the proximal tubule in response to the volume contraction induced by this agents. In addition, amiloride could enhance distal tubule reabsorption of magnesium as a result of inhibition of sodium reabsorption. This magnesium-retaining effect of these diuretics may be of help to avoid magnesium losses during long-term therapy with loop diuretics or thiazides. In fact, preliminary observations by Ryan et al, suggest that long-term treatment with amiloride is succesful at maintaining lymphocite magnesium levels in patients with congestive heart failure (9).

INTERACTION OF MAGNESIUM DEFICIENCY WITH POTASSIUM AND CALCIUM METABOLISM.

It has been recognized for long time that magnesium and potassium metabolism are closely interdependent. Thus, changes in the serum levels of one ion cause alterations of the other in the same direction (29). Recent reports have stressed this point by the observation of potassium deficiency and increased urinary losses of potassium associated to hypomagnesemia (6, 30-33). In these cases, attempts to restore potassium balance are difficult, unless magnesium is previously replaced. Moreover, magnesium supplementation alone can restore potassium balance towards normality (31).

The failure of the cell to take potassium under these conditions suggest that the lack of magnesium prevents the cell from stablishing a normal transcellular gradient for potassium. As previously mentioned, magnesium is required for the activation of the Na-K-ATPase, the enzyme system responsable for maintaining the gradient of sodium and potassium across the cell membrane (29). Ethacrynic acid and furosemide enhibit renal ATPase in kidney membrane preparations of different animal species (34). But there is no clear evidence that the effect of these agents on sodium and magnesium reabsorption in the kidney is a direct consequence of this inhibition. However, magnesium losses induced by diuretics or other conditions may deppress the function of the Na-K-ATPase at different levels. This would lead to impaired pumping of sodium out and potassium into the cell and, as a consequence, the excess of potassium in the extracellular fluid will be lost in the urine. Upon magnesium replacement, the Na-K-ATPase would acquire its normal activity, thus restoring the balance of potassium.

The interaction of magnesium deficiency with calcium metabolism is also of particular interest. Hypocalcemia has been observed in conjuction with severe magnesium depletion (12,34-36). Moreover in these patients and experimental animals, low or inapropriately low levels of PTH are almost constant features of the syndrome (12,34-36). This association of hypocalcemia, "functional hypoparathyroidism" and hypomagnesemia is most frequently observed in patients with decreased gastrointestinal absorption of magnesium or in animals subjected to a low magnesium diet for variable periods of time. However, it is conceivably that the syndrome could also occour due to increased urinary losses of magnesium such as that induced by potent diuretics.

Clinical and experimental studies indicate that the origen of hypocalcemia in states of magnesium depletion is multifactorial and, that end -

organ ressistance to the action of PTH as well as impaired secretion of this hormone are probably the principal mechanisms (12,20,34-36). Most of the actions of PTH in target cells are mediated through the generation of cyclic AMP by the enzyme adenylate cyclase (37-40). At the same time, this enzyme, which in the parathyroid gland is partly responsable for PTH secretion , depends on magnesium for activation (40-42). Therefore, one possibility is that hypomagnesemia may impair the function of adenylate cyclase in bones and parathyroid glands. Recent studies by Freitag et al (43) using the isolated perfused bone system have demonstrated that in dogs rendered magnesium depleted by dietary manipulations the generation of cyclic AMP by the isolated perfused bone in response to PTH infusion is blunted as compared to that in the normal dog bones. Suggesting that the end-organ ressistance to the action of PTH in hypomagnesemia ia at least in part, a consequence of altered adenylate cyclase activation in bone.

There is no confirmed evidence that a similar mechanism operates within the parathyroid gland. However, it has been demonstrated that the stored (pre-formed) PTH is controled by the adenylate cyclase system in response to calcium and other stimuli, whereas the secretion of newly synthesind hormone depends primarily from the levels of ionized calcium, but with no influence of the adenylate cyclase (44). Moreover, in hypomagnesemia with low levels of plasma PTH, the intravenous injection of magnesium restores PTH secretion within minutes (36). Suggesting that alterations in the secretion of the preformed PTH rather that an impaitment in de novo synthesis of the hormone is the principal defect. Bellorín-Font et al (41), have demonstrated that the adenylate cyclase in hyperplastic parathyroid glands and parathyadenomas have an increased sensitivity to the activating effect of magnesium compared to that in the normal gland tissue. Since the inhibitory action of calcium in this enzyme activity is competitive with respect to magnesium, the increased sensitivity to this cation results in a decrease in the inhibitory effect of calcium, so that the concentration of calcium required to inhibit adenylate cyclase activity in the hyperfunctioning glands is considerable higher than that in the normal parathyroid tissue (41). Therefore, it migth be possible that in hypomagnesemia a reverse alteration could occur, rendering the adenylate cyclase inhibited at very low calcium concentrations. This would deppress the portion of parathyroid hormone secretion controled by this enzyme system.

CONCLUSIONS

In conclusion, diuretic therapy is a frequent cause of alteration of magnesium metabolism. The abnormalities that these agents induce in the homeostasis of this important cation, particulary magnesium depletion, may result in derrangements of several biochemical and metabolic functions of the cell, with potentially seriuos consequences for the patient. Therefore a word of caution should be rised with regard to the need of monitoring magnesium levels in patients on long-term diuretic therapy, and to the convenience of megnesium supplementation, particulary in the high risk patients.

AKNOLEDGMENTS

This work was supported in part by Grant s1-1309 of the Consejo Nacional de Investigaciones Científicas y Tecnológicas (CONICIT). The authors wish to thank Miss Jeannette Humpierres for her technical assistance and , Miss Inés Mayorca for her secretarial work.

REFERENCES

1. H.E.Martin, J. Mehl, M. Wertman, Clinical Studies of Magnesium Metabolism Med. Clin. N. Amer 36, 1157-1164 (1952).
2. C.G. Duarte Effects of ethacrynic acid and furosemide on urinary calcium phosphate and magnesium. Metabolism 17, 867-876, 1968.
3. G. Eknoyan, W.N. Suki, and M. Martinez-Maldonado.Effect of diuretics on urinary calcium, and magnesium in thyroparathyroidectomized dogs. J. Lab Clin. Med. 76, 257-266 (1970).
4. P.Limb, E. Jacob. Magnesium deficiency in patients on long-term diuretic therapy for heart failure. Br. Med. J.3, 620-622, 1972.
5. W.E.C. Wacker, A.F.Parisi. Magnsesium metabolism. N. Engl. J. Med. 278, 658-663, 712-717, 771-776, (1968).
6. P.O. Wester, T. Dyckner. Diuretic treatment and magnesium losses. Acta. Med. Scand. Suppl 647, 145-152. (1981)
7. Reyes, A. J., Leary, W.P. The magnesiuric effect of a single dose of furosemide in healthy adults.Curr.Ther.Res 32, 406-416 (1982).
8. M. Ryan, M.F. Ryan, T.B. Counihan. The effect of diuretics on lymphocite magnesium and potassium. Acta. Med. Scand; Suppl 647, 153-161 (1981).
9. L. Widman, T. Dyckner and P.O. Wester. Effect of moduretic and aldactone on electrlytes in skeletal muscle in patients on long-term diuretic therapy. Acta. Med. Scand (suppl) 661, 33-35 (1982).
10. C.E. Jackson, D.W.Meier. Routine Serum magnesium analysis. Correlation with clinical state in 5,100 patients. Ann. Int. Med. 69,743-748 (1968).
11. M.S. Seeling. Requirements of magnesium by normal adult: Summary and analysis of published data. Am.J. Clin. Nutr. 14.246-252 (1964).
12. E. Slatopolsky, R. Rosenbaum, P.Mennes, and S. Klahr. The hypocalcemia of magnesium depletion. S. Massry, E. Ritz, A. Rapado. (Editors). Homeostasis of phosphate and other minerals. Plenum Publishing Corporation , 263-271 (1978).
13. R.G. King and S.W. Stanbury. Magnesium metabolism in primary hyperparathyroidism. Clin. Sci, 39, 218-232 (1970).
14. P.G. Branan, P.Vergne-Marini, C.Y.C.Pack, A.R. Hull, and Fordtran, J.S. Magnesium absorption in the human small intestine. Results in normal subjects, patients with chronic renal disease, and patients with absortive hypercalciuria. J. Clin. Invest 57, 1412-1418 (1976).
15. L.V. Avioli, J. Berman. Magnesium 28 Kinetics in man. J. Appl. Physiol. 21, 1688-1964 (1966).
16. C.Le Grimellec, P. Poujeul, and C. Rouffignac. 3-H-Inulin and electrolyte concentrations in Bowmans capsule in rat kidney. Comparision with artificial ultrafiltration. Pflugers Arch. 354: 17-28 (1975).
17. G.A. Quamme, N.L. Wong, J.H. Dirks,N. Roinel, C. de Rouffignac and F Morel, Magnesium handling in the dog kidney: A micropuncture study. Pflugers Arch.377, 95-99 (1978).
18. M. Brunnette, N.Vigneault,and S Carriere. Micropuncture Study of Magnesium transport along the nephron in the young rat. AM. J. Physiol, 227, 891-896 (1974).
19. G.A. Quamme, and J.H. Dirks. Intraluminal and contraluminal magnesiun on magnesium and calcium transfer in the rat nephron. AM. J.Physiol 238, (Renal fliud Electrolyte Physiol.7), F187-F198 (1980).
20. R.Sutton and J.H.Dirks. Renal Handling of calcium, phosphate and magnesium. In The kidney. B. Brenner and F. Rector (Editors) W.B. Saunders, Phyladelphia. London,Toronto.P.P. 551-618 (1981).
21. A.M. Parfitt. The acute effects of mersalyl, chlorothiazide and manitol on the renal excretion of calcium and other ions in man. Clin. Sci. 36, 267-282 (1969).
22. Leary,W.P.,Reyes, A.J. Piretanide in the treatment of hypertension. Effects on arterial blood pressure and several blood variables. S.Afr. Med.J.60, 925-928 (1981).
23. G.A. Quamme. Effect of intraluminal furosemide on calcium and magnesium transport in the loop of Henle and the role of PTH. Kidney Int 14:642,

(1978).
24. M.A. Burnatowska, C.A. Harris, R.A. Sutton and J.H. Dirks. Effects of PTH and cAMP on renal handling of calcium, magnesium amd phosphate in the hamster.AM. J. Physiol. 233: F 514-518 (1977).
25. C.A. Harris, M.A. Burnatowska, J.F.Seely, R.A. Sutton, G.A. Quamme and J.H.Dirks. Effects of parathyroid hormone on electrolyte transport in the hamster nephron. AM. J. Physiol 236: F 342-348 (1979).
26. E.Bellorín-Font, J.R.Weisinger, V. Paz Martínez. Unpublished Observa - tions.
27. E.R. Yendt and M, Cohamin. Prevention of calcium stone with thiazides. Kidney Int. 13, 397-409 (1978).
28. N.L.M. Wong, G.A. Quamme, J.H. Dirks. Effect of chlorothiazide on renal calcium and magnesium handling in the hamster. Can.J. Physiol. Pharmacol 60, 1160-1165 (1981).
29. R.E. Cronin, J.P. Knochel. Magnesium deficiency. Advances in Internal Medicine G.H.Stollerman (Editor). Year Book Medical Publishers Inc. p.p. 509-533 (1983).
30. T. Dyckner and Per Ola Wester.Relateion between potassium, magnesium and cardiac arrhitmias. Acta Med. Scand. Suppl 647, 163-169 (1981).
31. M.E. Shils. Experimental human magnesium defficiency. Medicine 48,61-85 (1969).
32. E.B. Flink. Magnesium deficiency. Etiology and Clinical spectrum. Acta. Med. Scand. Suppl 647, 125-137 (1981).
33. W.P. Leary, and A.J. Reyes. Diuretics, magnesium, potassium and sodium. S.A. Medical J. 61, 279-280 (1982).
34. J. Levy, S.G. Massry, J.W. Coburn et al. Hypocalcemia in magnesium depleted dogs. Evidence for reduced responsiveness to parathyroid hormone, and relative failure of parathyroid gland function. Metabolism 23, 323-335 (1974).
35. L.R. Chase, Slatopolsky,E. Secretion and metabolic efficacy of para - thyroid hormone in patients with severe hypomagnesemia. J.Clin.Endo - crinol. Metab. 38, 363-371 (1974).
36. C.A. Anast, J.L. Winnocker, L.R. Forte, et al. Impaired release of parathyroid hormone in magnesium deficiency. J.Clin.Endocrinol Metab. 42, 707-717 (1976).
37. L.R.Chase, and G.D. aurbach. Renal adenyl cyclase. Anatomically separate sites for parathyroid hormone and vasopressin. Science 159, 545-547 , (1968).
38. R.A. Nissenson, and C.D. Arnaud. Properties of the parathyroid hormone - receptor-adenylate cyclase system in chicken renal plasma membranes. J. Biol. Chem. 254, 1469-1475 (1979).
39. G.V. Segre, M.Rosenblatt, B.L.Reinier, J.E. Mahaffey, and J.T. potts Jr. Characterization of parathyroid hormone receptors in canine renal cortical plasma membranes using a radioidinated sulfur-free hormone a - nalog.J. Biol. Chem. 254, 6980-6986 (1979).
40. E.Bellorín-Font, and K.J. Martin. Regulation of the PTH-receptor-cyclase system of canine kidney: effects of calcium, magnesium and guanine nucleotides. AM. J. Physiol.241 (Renal Fluid Electrolyte Physiol.10), F364-F373 (1981).
41. Ezequiel Bellorín-Font, K.J. Martin, J.J. freitag, C.B. Anderson, G. Sicard,E. Slatopolsky, and S. Klahr. Altered adenylate cyclase kinetics in hyperfunctioning human parathyroid glands. J. Clin.Endocrinal. Metab. 52, 499-507 (1981).
42. E.Bellorín-Font, J.Tamayo, K.J. Martin. Regulation of PTH-receptor-adenylate cyclase system of canine kidney: influence of Mn^{2+} on effects of Ca^{2+}, PTH, and GTP. AM. J. Physiol.242 (Renal Fluid Electrilyte Physiol. 11), F 457-F462 (1982).
43. Freitag,J.F., Martin,K.J., Conrades,M.B., Bellorín-Font,E., Teitelbaum, S., Klahr,S., and Slatopolsky,E. Evidence for skeletal resistance to parathyroid hormone in magnesium deficiency.Studies in isolated perfused bone. J. Clin Invest 64:1238-1244,1979.

44. Morrisey, J.J., Cohn, D.V. Regulation of secretion of parathormone and ecretory protein I from separate intracellular pool by calcium dibuty - ryl cyclic AMP and isoproterenol. J.Cell.Biol. 82: 93 - 99,1979.

EFFECT OF THIAZIDE DIURETICS ON CALCIUM METABOLISM

SHAUL G. MASSRY
Division of Nephrology and Department of Medicine, University of Southern California School of Medicine, Los Angeles, California.

Several aspects of calcium metabolism are affected by the use of thiazide diuretics. These include urinary calcium, serum calcium, bone, and intestinal absorption of calcium.

The acute administration of thiazide diuretics usually produces calciuria, but the increment in calcium clearance is smaller than that of sodium clearance (1-4). This dissociation between urinary sodium and calcium excretion during the acute administration of thiazides is due to events that take place in the distal tubule (5) where these agents enhance calcium reabsorption (6).

The chronic administration of thiazidesis associated with hypocalciuria (7-10). The mechanisms responsible for this phenomenon are complex and multiple; they may include extracelluler volume depletion, presence of parathyroid hormone (PTH) and a direct action of the diuretic on the distal tubular transport of calcium. Two detailed studies in man showed that both extracellular volume depletion and intact parathyroid glans are required for the thiazide-induced hypocalciuria (9, 10). Indeed, Brickman et al (9) demonstrated that a) hypocalciuria fails to occur if the sodium losses produced by the thiazides are quantitatively replaced, and b) patients with hypoparathyroidism do not exhibit hypocalciuria despite volume depletion. These observations were confirmed by Parfitt (10). These data have led to the suggestion that thiazides may potentiate the action of PTH on the distal reabsorption of calcium.

Other data in patients with hypoparathyroidism and parathyroidectomized animals deemphasize the role of PTH in the genesis of the thiazide-induced hypocalciuria. Porter et al (11) found that patients with hypoparathyroidism receiving sodium-restricted diet display a moderate decrease in urinary calcium during chronic treatment with thiazides. Jorgensen (12) reported that thiazide diuretics caused a fall in urinary calcium in parathyroidectomized rats. Furthermore, the dissociation between the clearances of sodium and calcium during thiazide administration to dogs is not affected by parathyroidectomy (13). Finally, Costanzo and Windhager (6), utilizing free flow micropuncture and in situ microperfusion techniques, have shown that thiazides enhance calcium reabsorption in the distal convoluted tubules.

The short or long term administration of thiazide diuretics may be associated with an increase in the total concentration of serum calcium in normal subjects (14,15) and in patients with a variety of clinical conditions (16-21). This phenomenon has been reported in patients with juvenile osteoporosis (16), those with primary hyperparathyroidism (9,16-18), patients undergoing chronic hemodialysis (19), patients with hypoparathyroidism receiving vitamin D (9, 10, 20) and those with malignant diseases (21). In many of these patients overt hypercalcemia developed.

Several factors may be responsible for the increase in levels of serum calcium. First, hemoconcentration of serum proteins probably account in part for the augmented serum calcium concentration. However, in many studies the administration of thiazides also caused a rise in the diffusible or the ionized (11, 15, 22) moieties of serum calcium indicating that a true elevation in serum calcium has occurred. Second, the thiazide-induced hypocalciuria may contribute to the rise in serum levels of calcium. However, the demonstration that hypercalcemia occurs in patients with no renal function (19) and in those with hypoparathyroidism without a significant change in urinary calcium (9, 10, 20) indicates that the renal effects of thiazides are not essential for the thiazide-induced rise in serum calcium. Third, because of the above considerations, it has been suggested that thiazides may potentiate the action of PTH on bone and/or have a direct action on bone resulting in enhanced release of calcium from the skeleton

Diuretics, Jules B. Puschett, Editor

into the extracellular space (9). The studies of Popovtzer et al (22) strongly support the hypothesis that thiazide diuretics potentiate the action of PTH on bone. They found that within two hours after the administration of chlorothiazides to normal subjects, the serum concentration of both total and ionized calcium rose transiently. Similar treatment with thiazides produced a sustained elevation in serum calcium levels in patients with primary hyperparathyroidism but had no effect on those with hypoparathyroidism. The simultaneous infusion of PTH to the latter patients restored the calcemic response to thiazide therapy. In addition to these observations, the data of Porter, et al (11) lend support for the notion that thiazides may have a direct action on bone. They showed that chronic administration of chlorothalidone to patients with hypoparathyroidism was associated with normalization of the serum concentration of ionized calcium.

Malluche et al (23) provided the evidence that thiazides act directly on bone. They demonstrated that chronic administration of hydrochlorothiazide to parathyroidectomized dogs maintained serum calcium levels within normal values and produced an increase in osteocytic index and urinary hydroxyproline excretion. Their findings indicate that thiazides stimulate osteocytic osteolysis. If the direct effect of thiazides on bone is potentiated by PTH or is additive to the action of PTH, one would expect that treatment with this drug should produce or aggravate hypercalcemia in patients with primary or secondary hyperparathyroidism. Indeed, several investigators have reported that hypercalcemia develops or worsensin such patients (9, 10, 19, 22)

The available data on the effects of thiazide diuretics on intestinal calcium absorption are contradictory. An increase (24, 25), a decrease (26, 27) or no change (26) has been reported. Since the chronic administration of thiazides is associated with renal calcium retention, the patients should increase body content of calcium tremendously unless other adaptive adjustments are made. One would expect that either intestinal absorption of calcium is decreased or endogenous calcium secretion is enhanced to offset renal calcium retention. Definite answers to these questions are not available as yet.

The interaction between thiazide diuretics and calcium homeostasis may have important clinical implications. Indeed, the hypocalciuric effect of these agents has been utilized successfully in the treatment of renal calcium stones (24). The effects of thiazides on serum calcium level led to their therapeutic use for the treatement of the hypocalcemia of hypoparathyroidism (11) and as provocative agents for the detection of occult hyperparathyroidism (18, 21). Thiazide diuretics are being used for the treatment of hypertension, and it is possible that their effects on renal calcium retention plays a role in their antihypertensive action. This is being postulated in view of recent observations suggesting that high calcium intake reduces blood pressure (28).

REFERENCES

1. C.G. Durate. Metab. 17, 420-429 (1968).
2. A.M. Parfitt. Clin. Sci. 36, 267-282 (1969).
3. I. Sotornik, O. Schuck and J. Strilerna. Experientia 25, 591-592 (1969)
4. G. Eknoyan, W.N. Suki and M. Martinez-Maldonado. J. Lab. Clin. Med. 76, 257-266 (1970).
5. B.R. Edwards, P.G. Baer, R.A.L. Sutton and J.H. Dirks. J. Clin. Invest. 52, 2418-2427 (1973).
6. L. S. Costanzo and E.E. Windhager. Am. J. Physiol. 235, F492-F506 (1978).
7. B.A. Lamberg and B. Kuhlback. Scand. J. Clin. Lab. Invest. 11, 351-357

(1959).
8. B.A. Higgins, J.R. Nassim, J. Collins and A. Hilb. Clin. Sci. 27, 457-462 (1964).
9. A.S. Brickman, S.G. Massry and J.W. Coburn. J. Clin. Invest. 51, 945-954 (1972).
10. A.M. Parfitt. J. Clin. Invest. 51, 1879-1888 (1972).
11. R.H. Porter, B.G. Cox, D. Heaney, T.H. Hostetter, P.J. Stienbaugh and W.N. Suki. N. Engl. J. Med. 298, 577-581(1978).
12. F. S. Jorgensen. Acta Pharmacol. Toxicol. 30, 296-307 (1971).
13. G.A. Quamme, N.L.M. Wong, R.A.L. Sutton and J.H. Dirks. Am. J. Physiol. 229, 200-205 (1975).
14. H. Seitz and Z.F. Jaworksi. Can. Med. Assoc. J. 90, 414-420 (1969).
15. R.M. Stote, L.H. Smith, D.M. Wilson, W.J. Dube, R.S. Goldsmith and C.D. Arnaud. Ann. Intern. Med. 77, 587-591 (1972).
16. A.M. Parfitt. N. Engl. J. Med. 281, 55-59 (1969).
17. E. Paloyan, M. Forland and J.R. Picklman. J. Am. Med. Assoc. 210, 1243-1245 (1969).
18. P. Adams, T.M. Chalmers, L.F. Hill and B. McN. Truscott. Br. Med. J. 4, 582-585 (1970).
19. M.H. Koppel, S.G. Massry, J.H. Shinaberger, D.L. Hartenbower and J.W. Coburn. Ann. Inter. Med. 72, 895-901 (1970).
20. A.M. Parfitt. Ann. Inter. Med. 77, 557-563 (1972).
21. J. Sode, J.J. Sabol, C.R. Meloni and J.J. Canary. Clin. Res. 17, 550 (1969).
22. M.M. Popovtzer, V.L. Subryan, A.C. Alfrey, E.B. Reeve and R.W. Schrier. J. Clin. Invest. 55:1295-1302 (1975).
23. H.H. Malluche, W. Meyer-Sabellek, F.R. Singer and S.G. Massry. Miner. Elect. Metab. 4, 89-96 (1980).
24. E.R. Yendt, R.J.A. Gagne and M. Cohanin. Am. J. Med. Sci. 251, 449-460 (1966).
25. F.S. Jorgensen and I. Transbol. Acta. Med. Scand. 195, 33-36 (1974).
26. V. Ehrig, J.E. Harrison and D.R. Wilson. Metabolism 23, 139-145 (1974).
27. E.R. Yendt and M. Cohanim. Kidney Intl. 13, 397-409 (1978).
28. D.A. McCarron, C.D. Morris and C. Cole. Science 217, 267-269 (1982).

THERAPY OF HYPERCALCEMIA WITH DIURETIC AGENTS

JESUS H. DOMINGUEZ, University of Pittsburgh School of Medicine, Renal-Electrolyte Division, Pittsburgh, PA 15261, U.S.A.

Hypercalcemia is a medical complication frequently observed in unselected hospitalized patients [1]. In the vast majority of these individuals the underlying disorder produces an abnormal increase in bone resorption, table 1. The form of presentation of hypercalcemia varies widely, from the most common, the asymptomatic patient, to the second most common, that presenting as hypercalcemic crisis [1]. In the first case, usually there is time for a complete diagnostic evaluation preceding any therapeutic intervention. In the second case, when the development of hypercalcemia is associated with a severe compromise of neurological, renal or cardiac function, the hypercalcemia should be viewed as a medical emergency and therapy must be initiated as early as possible. The initial therapy of this condition should be directed to the correction of hypovolemia and related electrolyte abnormalities. If bone resorption is the cellular mechanism responsible for the hypercalcemia, the use of rapid inhibitors of bone resorption, such as calcitonin and glucocorticoids [2] is recommended. Once euvolemia and correction of blood electrolyte abnormalities have been achieved, the administration of loop diuretics contributes to the overall effort to attenuate the hypercalcemia during the acute treatment period (first 24 hours).

TABLE I. A classification of Hypercalcemia

INCREASED BONE RESORPTION

1. Primary hyperparathyroidism
2. Malignancy
3. Thyrotoxicosis
4. Chronic granulomatous diseases
5. Immobilization
6. Vitamin D and A intoxication

INCREASED INTESTINAL ABSORPTION OF CALCIUM

1. Vitamin D intoxication
2. Sarcoidosis
3. Milk - alkali syndrome

INCREASED RENAL TUBULAR REABSORPTION OF CALCIUM

1. Thiazide therapy
2. Familiar hypocalciuric hypercalcemia

ACUTE AND CHRONIC RENAL FAILURE

1. Following severe hyperphosphatemia
2. Failure of the skeleton to mineralize
3. Hyperparathyroidism
4. Unknown

The successful use of loop diuretics in the acute treatment of hypercalcemia was first described by Suki in 1970 [3]. The rationale for the use of loop diuretics in hypercalcemia derived from the discovery that these

Diuretics, Jules B. Puschett, Editor

drugs promote large urinary losses of calcium in humans [4] and animals [5, 6]. The effectiveness of these drugs in the removal of systemic calcium was later supported by studies in the hypercalcemic dog [7]. In this animal model it was found that the acute administration of furosemide decreased the elevated serum calcium concentration in proportion to the calciuric response evoked by the diuretic. Furthermore, these dual responses to the administration of the loop diuretic appear to be present over a wide range of glomerular filtration rates [3, 7]. In contrast, in hypoparathyroid humans, while furosemide also produced a uniformed decrease in the concentration of ionized calcium, the excretion of urinary calcium was not always enhanced by the drug [8].

Over the past decade, the site of action of loop diuretics, as well as their mode of action have been extensively investigated. Burg and associates demonstrated that these drugs act on the thick ascending limb of Henle [9-11]. In this nephron segment the diuretics decrease the lumen positive transtubular potential difference [9-11]. Evidence obtained from several laboratories has demonstrated that this lumen positive potential difference is actually the main driving force for calcium reabsorption in this cortical segment [11-14]. However, other investigators have provided evidence for an active calcium reabsorptive process as well [15-17]. Furthermore, in the cortical thick ascending limb, calcium reabsorption is also stimulated by parathyroid hormone [14, 17-19]. This effect of the hormone occurs independently of changes in the transtubular potential difference and is also reproduced by cyclic AMP analogs [14, 18, 19]. These findings demonstrate that in addition to the electrical forces prevalent in the lumen, humoral stimulation of cell transport, mediated by the activation of adenylate cyclase, also participates in the reabsorption of calcium in the cortical thick ascending limb. The effect of furosemide on calcium reabsorption has been examined in the thick ascending limb. It has been possible to show that when the diuretic is present in the lumen, it inhibits the absorption of calcium in the absence [16] and also in the presence of parathyroid hormone [20]. Since furosemide attenuates the activation of renal adenylate cyclase [21, 22], one wonders whether or not the antagonism of the diuretic to the action of the hormone is in part the result of inhibition of the enzyme produced by furosemide in the thick ascending limb.

In contrast, conclusive evidence for extrarenal effects of furosemide that might contribute to its hypocalcemic action has been lacking. In an in vitro bone resorption system that measures the % release of labeled bone calcium from live fetal rat bones kept in culture for 5 days [23], furosemide at concentrations of 10^{-4} and 10^{-3}M progressively attenuated the activation of bone resorption produced by near maximal concentrations of parathyroid hormone. This inhibitory effect of furosemide on bone resorption in vitro, was also shared by acetazolamide at the same molar concentrations, table 2. These data suggest that these diuretic agents directly antagonize the activation of bone resorption at high concentrations perhaps by acting on bone carbonic anhydrase. Although this cannot be the only explanation for these results since the inhibitory concentrations used in this work were much higher than those expected for only an effect on bone carbonic anhydrase [24]. It is also possible that the inhibitory action on bone carbonic anhydrase plays only a part in their pharmacological effect and that other cellular functions that participate in bone resorption are affected by the diuretic agent.

In summary, the clinical use of loop diuretics in hypercalcemia has proven to be an effective acute therapeutic option (first 24 hours). In this situation, their use should be initiated only after correction of the fluid and electrolyte disturbances associated with severe hypercalcemia. Their use demands of a careful accounting and prompt replacement of fluid and electrolyte losses. If the underlying pathological process is a disorder of bone resorption, as most commonly occurs, the diuretic agent should be used in association with the rapid inhibitors of bone resorption available at this time [2].

The experimental evidence supports the notion that loop diuretics have a hypocalcemic action and that this action is the result of their calciuric effect. Any other extrarenal effect that could participate in the lowering of serum calcium remains yet to be proven. In this communication it was reported that preliminary work appears to suggest that furosemide also antagonizes the activation of bone resorption in vitro. These observations have to be confirmed using lower doses of the diuretic agents, or their analogs, as well as a much more detailed study of the earlier time courses of drug action.

TABLE II. Effect of furosemide and acetazolamide on bone resorption in vitro, n = 4

	$\%^{45}$Ca released		
Additions	Basal	PTH*	PTH/Basal ratio
None	26 ± 2	76 ± 4	2.9
Furosemide 10^{-4}M	31 ± 4	60 ± 7	1.9
Furosemide 10^{-3}M	21 ± 1	25 ± 1	1.2
Acetazolamide 10^{-4}M	30 ± 3	54 ± 4	1.8
Acetazolamide 10^{-3}M	22 ± 1	32 ± 2	1.4
Dead Bone	16 ± 1	---	---

*1-34 bPTH 4 x 10^{-8}M
Values are Means ± S.E.

REFERENCES

1. G.R. Mundy, D.H. Cove, and R. Fisken, Lancet. 1:1317-1320 (1980).
2. M.L. Binstock and G.R. Mundy, Ann. Intern. Med. 93:1269-1272 (1980).
3. W.N. Suki, J.J. Yium, M.V. Mindeu, C. Saller-Herbert, G. Eknoyane, and M. Martinez-Maldonado, New Engl. J. Med. 283:836-840 (1970).
4. F.E. Demartini, A.M. Briscoe, and C. Ragan, Proc. Soc. Exp. Biol. Med. 124:320-324 (1967).
5. C.G. Duarte, Metabolism. 17:867-876 (1968).
6. G. Eknoyan, W.N. Suki, and M. Martinez-Maldonado, J. Lab. Clin. Med. 76:257-266 (1970).
7. S.C. Ong, R.J. Shalhoub, P. Gallagher, L.D. Antoniov, and J.M. Brian O'Connell, Proc. Soc. Exp. Biol. Med. 145:227-233 (1974).
8. P.A. Gabow, T.J. Hanson, M.M. Popovtzer, and R.W. Schrier, Ann. Intern. Med. 86:579-581 (1977).
9. M. Burg, L. Stoner, J. Cardinal, and N. Green, Am. J. Physiol. 225:119-124 (1973).
10. M. Burg and N. Green, Kidney Int. 4:301-308 (1973).
11. M. Burg, Kidney Int. 22:454-464 (1982).
12. G.R. Shareghi and L.C. Stoner, Am. J. Physiol. 235:F367-F375 (1978).
13. J.E. Bourdeau and M.B. Burg, Am. J. Physiol. 236:F357-F364 (1979).

14. G.R. Shareghi and Z.S. Agus, J. Clin. Invest. 69:759-769 (1982).
15. A.S. Rocha, J.B. Magaldi, and J.P. Kokko, J. Clin. Invest. 49:974-983 (1977).
16. M. Imai, Pflügers Arch. 374:255-263 (1978).
17. W.N. Suki, D. Rouse, R.C.K. Ng, and J.P. Kokko, J. Clin. Invest. 66: 1004-1009(1980).
18. M. Imai, Pflügers Arch. 390:145-151 (1981).
19. J.E. Bourdeau and M.B. Burg, Am. J. Physiol. 239:F121-F126 (1980).
20. J.E. Bourdeau, S.L. Buss, and G.G. Vurek, J. Pharmacol. Exp. Ther. 221:815-819 (1982).
21. H. Ebel, Naunyn-Schmeideberg's, Arch. Pharmacol. 281:301-314 (1974).
22. J. Thode, Acta Pharmacol. et Toxicol. 49:285-289 (1981).
23. L.G. Raisz and I. Niemann, Endocrinology, 85:446-452 (1969).
24. J.B. Puschett and M. Goldberg, J. Lab. and Clin. Med. 71:666-677 (1968).

THE ROLE OF DIURETICS IN THE THERAPY OF RENAL STONE DISEASE

Zalman S. Agus, M.D.

Renal Electrolyte Section, Dept. of Medicine, Hospital of Univ. of Pennsylvania, 860 Gates Pavilion, 3400 Spruce Street Philadelphia, PA 19104

INTRODUCTION

Thiazide diuretics assumed prominence in the treatment of nephrolithiasis approximately 15 years ago with the publication of Yendt describing his experience [1]. The rationale for their use related to the observation that chronic administration was associated with a sustained reduction in urinary calcium excretion as described by Dr. Costanzo and the assumption that urinary calcium excretion was a risk factor for kidney stone formation. Since that time, a large experience has developed confirming their effectiveness[2]. It has been suggested that diuretics would be most effective in those patients with stones and increased urinary calcium excretion ("idiopathic hypercalciuria") and more recently, it has been suggested that their use be restricted to a particular subgroup of these patients--i.e., those with the so-called "renal leak" type of idiopathic hypercalciuria [3-5]. It is now our belief, and the belief of others as well [6-8], that rigid separation of patients into various subgroups is no longer useful and that reduction of urinary calcium excretion is beneficial to most if not all patients with calcium stones. Oral administration of phosphate is also an effective way to reduce calcium excretion but the experience is not as extensive as with thiazides. At the moment, the choice between these two modalities depends predominantly upon the ease of administration and the choice of side effects. I shall review briefly nephrolithiasis, the association with hypercalciuria, the issue of pathogenesis and classification of idiopathic hypercalciuria, and the usefulness of thiazides in this disorder.

URINE CALCIUM AS A RISK FACTOR

Nephrolithiasis is a relatively common disorder affecting 1-10% of the population in various estimates. The types of stones formed include uric acid, ammonium phosphate (triple-phosphate) cystine and calcium oxalate or calcium phosphate. Calcium stones are the most common, accounting for 70-80% in most series. Calcium tends to precipitate as oxalate in acid urines and phosphate in alkaline urines. As urine is usually acid, calcium oxalate stones are the most common variety. Exceptions to this statement include patients with primary hyperparathyroidism, renal tubular acidosis, and urinary tract infection, situations wherein the urine pH may be relatively alkaline (pH >5.5-6.0).

The pathogenesis of calcium stone disease remains unclear, but a number of risk factors have been suggested. These include reduced urine volume and/or increased urinary calcium in the urine. Increased oxalate and decreased citrate excretion would decrease the ability of urine to chelate calcium and prevent precipitation. Magnesium has also been promoted as a factor which increases the solubility of calcium oxalate and decreased magnesium excretion has been suggested as a risk factor. Finally, recent studies have shown that increasing concentrations of uric acid decrease the solubility and enhance the crystallization of calcium oxalate. Thus, it has been suggested that increased uric acid excretion

Diuretics, Jules B. Puschett, Editor

(hyperuricosuria) may adversely affect the patient with calcium nephrolithiasis [9,10].

Several studies have attempted to assess the frequency with which these various factors occur in patients with stone disease. We have recently conducted a survey of our patients referred for evaluation of stone disease compared to an age and sex-matched control population. In our studies, approximately 50% of patients had 24-hour urinary calcium excretion values which exceeded 280 mg, a value exceeded by only 15% of the control population. In contrast, the prevalence of hyperuricosuria, increased oxalate excretion or decreased urine volume was not different in the affected and control populations. We did not evaluate citrate excretion, but earlier studies suggested the occurence of hypocitraturia in stone formers and more recent studies have shown a prevalence of 30-50% of low values in both normocalciuric and hypercalciuric stone-forming patients [11,12]. Most investigators agree that increased calcium excretion is a very important risk factor and hence the focus on therapeutic agents which lower urinary calcium excretion. It should be pointed out that hypercalciuria alone does not account for calcium nephrolithiasis. Thus, 50% of patients have 24-hour excretion rates of less than 280 mg. Studies to date have not been able to define precisely the value below which calcium excretion ceases to be important. Based upon studies comparing values in relapsing patients to non-relapsers [13], it has been suggested that a value of 150-200 mg is a reasonable target goal. It seems likely that the lower the rate of urinary calcium excretion, the less likely calcium stones are to form.

IDIOPATHIC HYPERCALCIURIA

The association of recurrent nephrolithiasis and hypercalciuria (greater than 280 to 300 mg per 24 hours) in the absence of hypercalcemia was described many years ago by Albright [14] and is referred to as the syndrome of idiopathic hypercalciuria. For many years, two alternative hypotheses were considered to explain the pathogenesis of this disorder. The first suggests that the primary defect resides in the GI tract, producing increased absorption of calcium. This tends to elevate serum calcium and suppress PTH secretion. As PTH is an important stimulator of tubular calcium transport, suppression of secretion results in decreased reabsorption and increased excretion. Alternatively, a primary defect in renal tubular calcium transport could lead to increased calcium excretion. These two mechanisms have different implications for total body calcium balance, PTH levels, and, ultimately, therapy as follows:

	RENAL HYPERCALCIURIA	ABSORPTIVE HYPERCALCIURIA
PTH level	Increased	Suppressed
Calcium balance	Negative	Positive
Effect of dietary calcium restriction	Little	Reduced calcium excretion
Appropriate therapy	Increase renal reabsorption (thiazides)	Decrease gut absorption (cellulose phosphate dietary restriction)

Various investigators have presented evidence for the existence of both types of hypercalciuria. Thus patients were described with elevated levels of PTH and increased calcium excretion, despite dietary restriction, consistent with a renal etiology [3,4]. Other patients, however, exhibit dietary dependence without elevated levels of PTH, consistent with an absorptive defect [3,4]. Proponents of these subtypes point out that therapy should theoretically be different. Thus, in a patient with a primary hyperabsorption of calcium, it would seem inappropriate to enhance tubular reabsorption of calcium with thiazides and more reasonable to attempt reduction of intestinal calcium absorption with a drug such as cellulose phosphate. Conversely, reducing calcium absorption in a patient with a primary renal leak would theoretically aggravate negative calcium balance. Thiazide therapy would be the drug of choice in this group. There is now compelling evidence, however, to suggest that patients do not easily fall into these various subgroups. Thus, many recent studies have been unable to document elevated levels of PTH in patients with fasting hypercalciuria. Similarly, positive calcium balance cannot be documented in the majority of patients with so-called absorptive hypercalciuria when calcium intake is reduced and, in fact, many go into negative calcium balance [8]. For these reasons, many investigators currently believe that idiopathic hypercalciuria should be regarded as a single entity [6-8]. The therapeutic approach consists of increasing urine volume, reducing urinary calcium excretion, and avoiding negative calcium balance.

EFFECTS OF THIAZIDE DIURETICS IN NEPHROLITHIASIS

It is well documented that thiazide diuretics, in contrast to other diuretics discussed elsewhere, reduce calcium excretion by increasing tubular reabsorption. Several recent, but limited, studies suggest that amiloride may also lower urinary calcium excretion in hypercalciuric patients [15-17] but this drug has not yet been evaluated as a single agent. Its potential use in combination with thiazides is discussed below. The use of thiazides to treat calcium stone disease is based upon this hypocalciuric effect and the clinical impression from uncontrolled studies that stone formation rate is reduced.

It is useful to point out that there are few, if any, controlled studies which definitely document the efficacy of thiazides in the prevention of nephrolithiasis. There are numerous studies which demonstrate a reduction in stone formation rate as compared to pre-treatment [1,2]. This effect has been demonstrated in both hypercalciuric and normocalciuric stone formers. Placebo studies have shown, however, that exposure to a stone clinic, with increased fluid ingestion and urine volume, is also associated with a marked reduction in stone formation rate which persists for several years [18,19]. In one randomized study, thiazides could not be shown to be better than placebo after one year of therapy [20].

Thiazides have other effects upon urinary composition which may affect the propensity for stone formation. Urine volume increases. Urine pyrophosphate excretion also increases.This compound may retard formation, growth and aggregation of crystal nuclei. Urine magnesium excretion tends to increase in some studies [21] but not all [20]. As mentioned above, there is no evidence for altered magnesium excretion as a risk factor in patients with nephrolithiasis, but increased magnesium excretion may increase the solubility of calcium oxalate in urine.

Finally, thiazide administration is associated with a reduction in urine citrate excretion [17,21]. Hypocitraturia may be observed in 30-50% of calcium stone formers and may be an important contributing risk factor. Two important regulators of urinary citrate excretion include the serum potassium and the serum pH. Thus, increasing serum potassium and metabolic alkalosis both increase citrate excretion. Thiazides induce both hypokalemia and metabolic alkalosis. In the few studies available in calcium stone formers, the effects on potassium seem to predominate as urine citrate excretion usually falls after institution of therapy. As amiloride tends to reduce calcium excretion and decreases potassium secretion, it might be reasonable to combine these two drugs and produce better results. Very few studies are currently available comparing the combination to either drug alone. In a recent study, no beneficial effect of the combination on urinary citrate could be demonstrated although there was a further slight lowering of urine calcium excretion with addition of amiloride [17]. In these patients, however, relatively small doses of drugs were used and the addition of amiloride did not prevent hypokalemia, so that the issue of citrate excretion remains to be more definitively evaluated. It should be pointed out that triamterene should not be used in this situation because of recent reports of triamterene stone formation [22,23].

Other than hypokalemia and asthenia, the usual side effects associated with thiazide administration, the only other complication associated with the use of thiazides for calcium nephrolithiasis is refractoriness to the hypocalciuric effect. In most reported series, thiazides effectively reduce urinary calcium excretion in 90-95% of patients. In those patients appearing to be refractory to the drug, superimposition of sodium restriction is almost always effective [24], suggesting that mild contraction of the extracellular fluid volume is a necessary component of the chronic sustained hypocalciuric effect. Alternatively, it may be possible to superimpose amiloride, but the data are not yet available from studies using this regimen in thiazide resistant patients.

SUMMARY

Calcium stones represent approximately 75% of nephrolithiasis. The risk factor most commonly observed in these patients, when compared to non-stone forming patients, is increased urine calcium excretion. At present, there is no compelling evidence for the existence of various subgroups of idiopathic hypercalciuria and the necessity of applying different therapeutic approaches. Thiazide diuretics effectively reduce urine calcium excretion by 50-60% in the vast majority of individuals and have been shown to be associated with a reduction in stone formation rates although carefully controlled studies have not been done. Other potential benefits of thiazide therapy in these patients include an increase in urine volume and an increase in magnesium excretion. Citrate excretion tends to fall and this may be a reflection of the hypokalemia induced by these drugs. As amiloride also reduces calcium excretion and raises potassium, it might be expected that the combination of these agents will further reduce calcium excretion and additionally increase citrate excretion, or at least prevent the thiazide induced decrease. Experience with this regimen is at the momemt too limited to state whether or not these expectations will be borne out.

REFERENCES

1. E.R. Yendt, Canad. Med. Ass. J. 102, 479 (1970).
2. F.L. Coe, Ann. Int. Med. 87, 404 (1977).
3. C.Y.C. Pak, M. Ohata, E.C. Lawrence, and W. Snyder, J. Clin. Invest. 54, 387 (1974).
4. C.Y.C. Pak, P. Peters, M. Hurt, M. Kadesky, M. Fine, D. Reisman, F. Splann, C. Carmela, and A. Freeman, Am. J. Med. 71, 615 (1981).
5. C.Y.C. Pak, M. Nicar, and C. Northcutt, Contrib. Nephrol. 33, 136 (1982).

6. A. Wasserstein, and Z.S. Agus, In: Controversies in Nephrology, R. Narins, ed. (Churchill Livingstone, Inc., N.Y., 1984) In Press.
7. M. Peacock, Contrib. Nephrol. 33, 152 (1982).
8. F.L. Coe, M.J. Favus, T. Crockett, A.L. Strauss, J.H. Parks, A. Porat, C.L. Gantt, and L.M. Sherwood, Amer. J. Med. 72, 25 (1982).
9. C.Y.C. Pak, O. Water, L. Arnold, K. Holt, C. Cox, and D. Barilla, J. Clin. Invest. 59, 426 (1977).
10. F.L. Coe, Kidney Int. 13, 418 (1978).
11. M.J. Nicar, C. Skurla, K. Sakhaee, and C.Y.C. Pak, Urology 21, 8 (1983).
12. D. Rudman, M.H. Kutner, S.C. Redd, W.C. Waters, G.G. Gerron, and J. Bleier, J. Clin. Endo. and Metabolism 55, 1052 (1982).
13. A.L. Strauss, F.L. Coe, L. Deutsch, and J.H. Parks, Amer. J. Med. 72, 17 (1982).
14. F. Albright, P. Henneman, P.H. Benedict, and A.P. Forbes, Proc. Royal Soc. Med. 46, 1077 (1953).
15. G.N. Maschio, N. Tessitore, A. D'Angelo, A. Fabris, F. Pagano, A. Tasca, G. Graziani, A. Arnoldi, M. Surian, G. Colussi, A. Mandressi, A. Trinchieri, F. Rocco, C. Ponticello, and L. Minetti, Am. J. Med. 71, 623 (1981).
16. U. Alon, L.S. Costanzo, and J.C.M. Chan, Abst. Am. Soc. Nephrol. 16, 1A (1983).
17. D. Leppla, R. Browne, K. Hill, and C.Y.C. Pak, J. Clin. Endo. and Metabolism 57, 920 (1983).
18. B. Ettinger, Amer. J. Med. 61, 200 (1976).
19. D.H. Hosking, S.B. Erickson, C.J. Van Den Berg, D.M. Wilson, and L.H. Smith, J. Urol. 130, 1115 (1983).
20. D. Scholz, P.O. Schwille, and A. Sigel, J. Urol. 128, 903 (1982)
21. E.R. Yendt and M. Cohanim, Kidney Int. 13, 397 (1978).
22. B. Ettinger, N.O. Oldroyd, and F. Sorgel, JAMA, 244, 2443 (1980).
23. K.M. Patel, J. Urol. 126, 230 (1981).
24. E. Cunningham, F.H. Oliveros, and L. Nascimento, Clin. Pharmacol. Therap. 32, 642 (1982).

USE OF DIURETICS IN THE INVESTIGATION OF CLINICAL DISORDERS OF DIVALENT CATION METABOLISM

ROGER A. L. SUTTON, DM. FRCP, FRCP(C)
Department of Medicine
University of British Columbia
Vancouver, B.C. Canada.

INTRODUCTION

The application of techniques of micropuncture and renal tubule microperfusion in experimental animals has greatly increased our knowledge of the normal renal handling of calcium and magnesium during the past decade[1]. Furthermore the renal tubular sites and mechanisms of action of diuretic drugs upon calcium and magnesium transport have been examined in several studies. Each of the major classes of diuretic drugs has characteristic effects on the reabsorption of these ions. Carbonic anhydrase inhibitors such as acetazolamide inhibit the proximal tubular reabsorption of calcium[2] (together with sodium) but have little effect on urinary calcium excretion. The loop diuretics including furosemide can virtually abolish the normal ability to lower tubule fluid sodium, calcium and magnesium concentrations at the end of the loop to levels substantially below those in plasma ultrafiltrate[3]. This inhibition of calcium and magnesium reabsorption in the thick ascending limb of Henle's loop probably results from abolition of the lumen positive transepithelial potential difference in this segment[4], and is associated with a striking and approximately parallel acute increase in the urinary excretion of these cations[3]. This increased calcium and magnesium excretion during furosemide therapy may[5] or may not[6] be sustained, depending perhaps on the extent to which urinary sodium losses are replaced. If volume contraction occurs, this may blunt the rise in calcium and magnesium excretion by enhancing their absorption in the proximal (and perhaps in the distal) tubule. The thiazide diuretics, including chlorthalidone[7] and metolazone[8] have a unique dissociating effect on sodium and calcium reabsorption, which is now known to result from a direct stimulation of calcium reabsorption, associated with inhibition of sodium reabsorption, in the distal convoluted tubule[9]. Magnesium reabsorption is affected very little, either acutely or chronically, by thiazide diuretics, perhaps because the distal convoluted tubule is a less important site for the reabsorption of this cation[10]. The effects of the distal potassium-sparing diuretics (including spironolactone, triamterene, and amiloride) upon divalent cation reabsorption have been less studied: each tends to decrease the urinary calcium to sodium ratio[11], but to a less striking degree than the thiazides. Recently amiloride has been shown to have a thiazide-like effect in the distal convoluted tubule[12] in addition to its familiar effect in the collecting duct where the lumen negative transepithelial potential difference is inhibited, and consequently the tubular secretion of divalent cations such as calcium may be decreased[13]. If such a component of tubular calcium secretion exists under normal conditions, it is probably very small.

Diuretic agents are therefore available for administration to humans which selectively alter calcium and magnesium transport at several different tubule sites. We have examined the effects of these agents in several clinical disorders that are associated with abnormal calcium or magnesium excretion, including idiopathic hypercalciuria, familial hypocalciuric

Published 1984 by Elsevier Science Publishing Co., Inc.
Diuretics, Jules B. Puschett, Editor

hypercalcaemia, and various renal magnesium wasting syndromes. A major problem in such studies is the selection of control subjects with whom the patients may be appropriately compared.

IDIOPATHIC HYPERCALCIURIA

The commonest underlying metabolic anomaly to be identified in patients with calcium containing renal calculi is so-called idiopathic hypercalciuria, in which the urinary calcium excretion is increased despite a normal plasma calcium level. The underlying cause of this disorder has been the subject of controversy for many years; in particular it is unclear whether the abnormality usually results from the primary intestinal hyperabsorption of calcium, from a primary defect in the renal tubular reabsorption of calcium, or even from excessive resorption of skeletal calcium, which must presumably be intermittent since the disorder is not usually associated with osteopenia. Several investigators have noted that patients with idiopathic hypercalciuria frequently have fasting hypophosphatemia which does not appear to be attributable to increased PTH levels: since the plasma phosphate level is determined primarily by proximal renal tubular phosphate reabsorption, this observation would be consistent with the presence of an abnormality of proximal tubular function in idiopathic hypercalciuria. To examine this possibility further we determined the responses of 36 idiopathic calcium stone patients and 20 matched normal control subjects to single oral doses of hydrochlorothiazide (100 mgms.) or acetazolamide (500 mgms.) which were administered following an overnight fast[14]. During a two hour period preceding diuretic administration, urinary excretion (expressed as the ion/creatinine ratio) of sodium and magnesium was not different between normals and stone patients, whereas mean (fasting) calcium excretion was almost two-fold higher in the patients. (fig. 1) Twenty of the thirty six stone patients had fasting urinary calcium excretions significantly above the upper limit defined for local normal subjects.

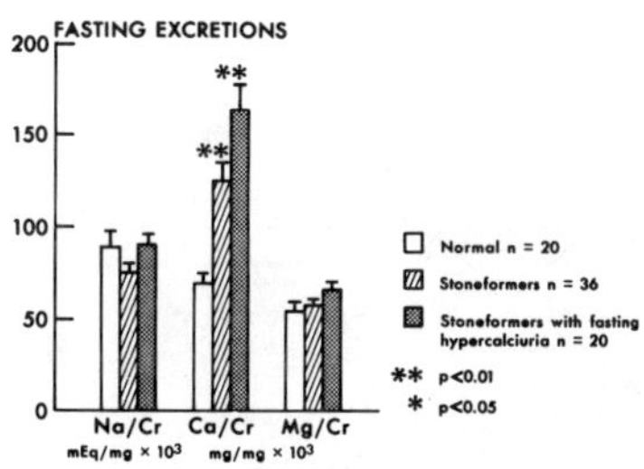

FIG. 1. Excretions of Na, Ca and Mg in 2-hour urine collection following overnight fast, expressed as ion/creatinine ratios, in normal subjects (n=20), all calcium stoneformers (n=36), and calcium stoneformers with fasting hypercalciuria (n=20) (mean $\pm$ S.E.). Data from reference [14].

In response to hydrochlorothiazide the stone patients showed a significantly greater increment in sodium, calcium and magnesium excretion than the normal subjects and these responses were greatest in the patients with fasting hypercalciuria. (fig. 2)

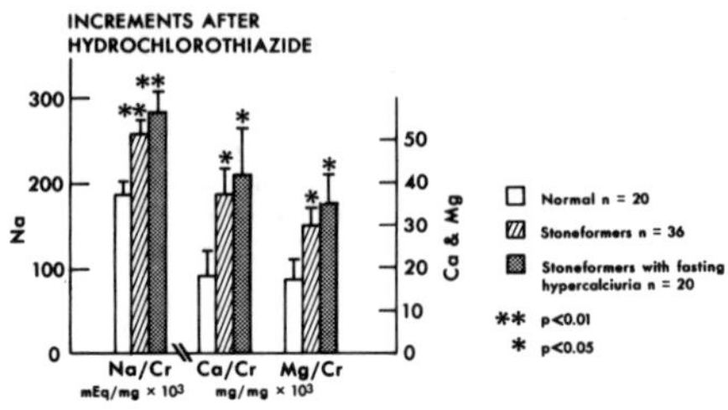

FIG. 2. Differences in Na, Ca and Mg excretion, expressed as ion/creatinine ratio, in 4-hour period following 100 mg hydrochlorothiazide p.o compared with a control day on which no drug was given. Subjects as in fig. 1 Data from reference [14].

By contrast, in response to acetazolamide the increment in sodium excretion was lower in stone patients than in controls, whereas the increments in calcium and magnesium excretion were not different. (fig. 3)

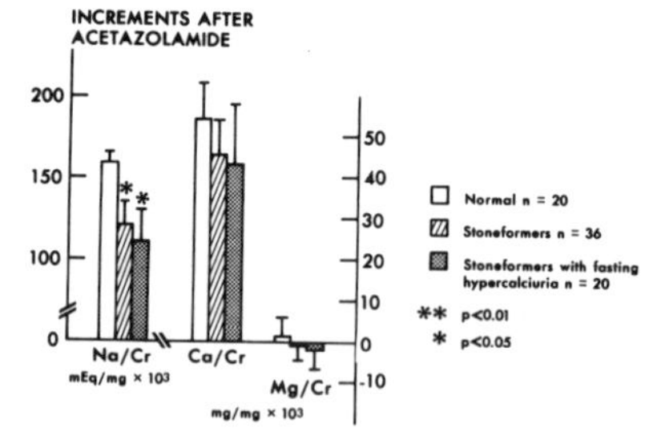

FIG. 3. Differences in Na, Ca and Mg excretion, expressed as ion/creatinine ratio, in 4-hour period following 500 mg acetazolamide p.o. compared with a control day on which no drug was given. Normal subjects (n=10), all calcium stoneformers (n=13), stoneformers with fasting hypercalciuria (n=6). Data from reference [14].

We interpreted these data as suggesting a defect in proximal tubular reabsorption (presumably involving sodium, calcium, magnesium and phosphate) in calcium stoneformers, particularly in those with fasting hypercalciuria. Such a defect would increase fluid delivery to more distal nephron segments, resulting in an exaggerated response to thiazide, while an already decreased proximal reabsorption would result in a blunted response to an agent acting within the proximal tubule such as acetazolamide. The existence of a defect in proximal reabsorption has also been suggested by studies of free water clearance in patients with idiopathic hypercalciuria, which also demonstrated that the abnormality was not corrected during acute or chronic phosphate administration, and presumably therefore was not a consequence of phosphate depletion[15]. Micropuncture studies in the spontaneously hypercalciuric rat[16] suggest that reabsorption of calcium (but not sodium) is impaired in the proximal tubule. The relevance of such a putative proximal defect to the pathophysiology of hypercalciuria is far from clear. Since sodium wasting is not apparent in idiopathic hypercalciuria during fasting, presumably the more distal nephron segments are able to reabsorb the increased delivered sodium load.

Furthermore, in the hypercalciuric rat, although delivery of calcium to the late superficial proximal tubule was increased, delivery to the early and late superficial distal tubules was not different from that of normal rats. Thus in both human idiopathic hypercalciuria, and in the rat model, hypercalciuria may be the result of an additional abnormality of calcium transport in the later nephron segments. In any event there is persuasive evidence suggesting the presence of a proximal tubular lesion in idiopathic hypercalciuria. Coe has suggested that a lesion at this site could also account for the abnormal (increased) calcitriol levels that are frequently observed in idiopathic hypercalciuria. This increased calcitriol production could in turn be responsible both for enhanced intestinal calcium absorption and increased skeletal calcium resorption. The observation by Coe et al[17] that, while ingesting very low calcium intakes, stone patients show persistent urinary calcium wasting as well as significantly higher plasma calcium levels than normal subjects is consistent with the presence of increased skeletal calcium resorption.

FAMILIAL HYPOCALCIURIC HYPERCALCAEMIA (FHH)

This disorder[18], inherited as an autosomal dominant, resembles primary hyperparathyroidism (PHP) in that it is associated with chronic stable hypercalcaemia and normal or elevated plasma parathyroid hormone (PTH) and urinary cyclic AMP levels. However it differs with respect to the family history, the early age of onset, the usually benign course, the tendency towards an increase (rather than a decrease as in PHP) in the plasma magnesium level, and the strikingly low urinary calcium excretion rate, which averages about 1/3 of that in PHP. The parathyroid glands may show mild hyperplasia in FHH and subtotal parathyroidectomy usually does not result in correction of hypercalcaemia. The pathophysiology of this disorder is not understood: in particular, the reason for the striking hypocalciuria is unclear. Two studies have recently been published in which responses to diuretic agents have been examined in an attempt to clarify the nature of the abnormality of renal calcium handling in FHH. We [19 - 21] compared the responses of parathyroid intact FHH and PHP patients who showed similar degrees of hypercalcaemia and similar PTH levels, to chlorothiazide, bicarbonate or furosemide. Chlorothiazide or sodium bicarbonate caused a similar fall in the urinary Ca/Na ratio in both groups, whereas furosemide increased the calcium excretion much more in FHH than in PHP, abolishing the pre-existing differences in the Ca/Na ratio (fig. 4).

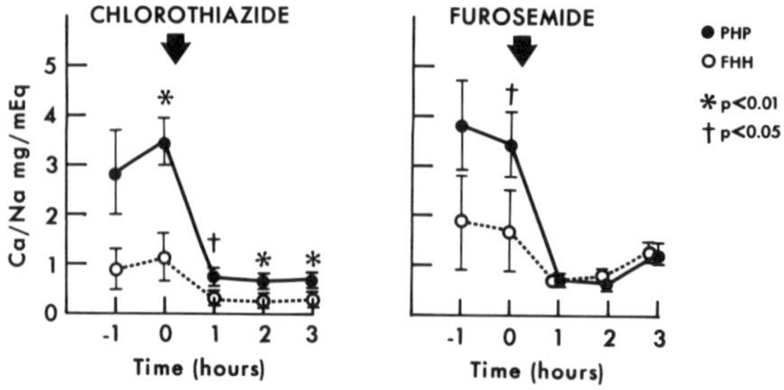

FIG. 4. Acute effect of chlorothiazide (500 mg i-v), or furosemide (40 mg i-v) on urinary Ca/Na ratio in patients with primary hyperparathyroidism (PHP, n=4) and familial hypocalciuric hypercalcemia (FHH, n=3). Values are mean $\pm$ S.E. Data from reference [21].

Attie and colleagues[22] compared totally parathyroidectomized FHH patients with parathyroidectomized normal controls. The hypocalciuria clearly persisted despite the absence of PTH in the FHH patients, and is therefore not a result of hypersensitivity to the hypocalciuric effect of PTH. The administration of acetazolamide did not influence the hypocalciuria in FHH, while ethacrynic acid produced a greater increment in calcium excretion in FHH than in controls and tended to abolish the characteristic hypocalciuria. Both of these studies suggest that tubular calcium hyperabsorption in FHH is probably occurring in the thick ascending limb of Henle's loop, the site of action of both furosemide and ethacrynic acid. An inhibitory effect of hypercalcaemia on calcium and magnesium reabsorption has been demonstrated in Henle's loop[23]. It is possible that, in FHH, both the normal effect of hypercalcaemia at this site, as well as its effect on the parathyroid glands are blunted, leading to enhanced tubular calcium and magnesium transport as well as a failure of PTH suppression by the hypercalcaemia.

SYNDROMES OF RENAL MAGNESIUM WASTING

Hypomagnesaemia associated with renal magnesium wasting occurs in several clinical circumstances. These include diuretic therapy (particularly furosemide), post-obstructive diuresis, osmotic diuresis (as in diabetic ketoacidosis) as well as both congenital and acquired disorders of the renal tubule. The congenital disorders include a rare syndrome of selective renal magnesium wasting with or without potassium wasting[24, 25] as well as some cases of Bartter's Syndrome. An acquired defect of renal magnesium conservation occurs rarely with aminoglycoside toxicity [26] and frequently following cis-platinum nephrotoxicity[27]. The site and nature of the renal tubular defect which leads to magnesium wasting is not known in any of these disorders. However, since the thick ascending limb of Henle's loop is the major site of magnesium reabsorption[10], it seems likely that the defect in these disorders may involve this segment of the renal tubule. We have recently had the opportunity to study four patients with persistent renal magnesium wasting following cis-platinum therapy for testicular tumors, as well as two affected members of a sib-ship of 5, of whom 3 have renal magnesium wasting, hypokalaemia, metabolic alkalosis, hyperreninaemia and hyperaldosteronism. These latter individuals probably have a variant of Bartter's Syndrome. All of these 6 individuals that we have studied have renal magnesium wasting, hypomagnesaemia, normocalcemia, normal PTH levels, and striking hypocalciuria. Thus in both disorders renal magnesium wasting is associated with a PTH-independent enhancement of tubular calcium reabsorption. In preliminary studies we have examined the responses of these subjects to oral or intravenous furosemide. In response to oral furosemide, the cis-platinum patients[28] had similar increments in sodium excretion to those of normal controls, but significantly greater increments in calcium excretion. These preliminary data suggest that the enhanced calcium reabsorption that causes the hypocalciuria in this disorder may be occurring in the thick ascending limb, where furosemide inhibits absorption. The hypocalciuria persists during magnesium infusion and therefore does not appear to be caused by the hypomagnesemia. It is possible that magnesium absorption may be impaired and calcium absorption enhanced in the thick ascending limb of Henle's loop. Such a defect might result if the permeability of this segment to magnesium were decreased while permeability to calcium were increased, so that the driving force would result in the reabsorption of more calcium and less magnesium than usual. In the two siblings with familial magnesium wasting, the responses to furosemide appear to be similar to those of the cis-platinum patients. For other reasons the site of the tubular defect in Bartter's Syndrome has been thought to be the thick ascending limb of Henle's loop[29], and it is therefore tempting to speculate that this may also be the site of abnormal divalent cation reabsorption in Bartter's Syndrome and its variants.

Acknowledgement. The contributions of the following collaborators to the studies reported above are gratefully acknowledged: Dr. V. Walker, Dr. H. Watanabe, Dr. V. Mavichak, Dr. C. Coppin, Dr. J.H. Dirks, and Dr. N.L.M. Wong. The studies were supported by M.R.C. (Canada) grant MT-5279.

REFERENCES

1. R.A.L. Sutton, and J.H. Dirks in: The Kidney, B.M. Brenner and F.C. Rector, eds. (W.B. Saunders & Company, Philadelphia 1981) pp. 551-618.
2. L.H. Beck, and M. Goldberg, Am J Physiol 224: 1136-1142 (973).
3. B.R. Edwards, P.G. Baer, R.A.L. Sutton, J.H. Dirks, J. Clin. Invest. 52, 2418-2427 (1973).
4. J.E. Bourdeau, S.L. Buss, and G.G. Vurek, J. Pharm. Exp. Therapeutics 22, 815-819 (1982).
5. B.L. Warshaw, S.K. Annand, A. Kerian, and E. Liberman, Pediatric Research 14, 1118-1121 (1980).
6. H. Toft and J. Roin, Brit. Med. Journal 1, 437-438 (1971).
7. E. Gursel, New York State J. Med, 399-405 (1970).
8. E. Cunningham, F.H. Oliveros, and L. Nascimento, Clin. Pharmacol Ther. 32, 642-645 (1982).
9. L.S. Costanzo, and E.E. Windhager, Am. J. Physiol. 235, F492-F506 (1978).
10. G.A. Quamme, and J.H. Dirks, Am. Journal of Physiol. 238, F187-F198 (1980).
11. L.S. Costanzo, and I.M. Weiner, Am. J. Physiol. 230, 67-73 (1976).
12. L.S. Costanzo, M.P. Conrad, and L.S. Beahm, Abstracts of the 15th Annual Meeting of the American Society of Nephrology, pp 4A (1982).

13. J.E. Bourdeau and R.J. Hellstrom-Stein, Am. J. Physiol. 242: F285-F292, (1982).
14. R.A.L. Sutton and V. Walker, New Eng. J. Med. 302. 709-713 (1980).
15. Y. K. Lau, A. Wasserstein, G. R. Westby, P. Bosanac, M. Grabie, P. Mitnick, E. Slatopolsky, S. Goldfarb, Z.S. Agus, Min. Electrolyte Metab. 7, 237-249 (1982).
16. K. Lau and B.K. Eby, J. Clin. Invest. 70, 835-844, (1982).
17. F.L. Coe, M.J. Favus, T. Crockett, A.M. Strauss, J.H. Parks, A. Porat C.L. Gantt, L.M. Sherwood, Am. J. Med. 72, (1982).
18. S.J. Marx, New Eng. J. Med. 303, 810-811 (1980).
19. H. Watanabe and R.A.L. Sutton, Clin. Res. 29: 74A, (1981).
20. H. Watanabe and R.A.L. Sutton, Clin. Res. 29, 426A, (1981).
21. H. Watanabe, and R.A.L. Sutton, Kidney International 24, 353-357 (1983).
22. M.F. Attie, J.R. Gill, Jr., J.L. Stock, A.M. Spiegel, R.W. Downs, Jr., M.A. Levine, and S.J. Marx, J. Clin. Invest. 72. 667-676 (1983).
23. G.A. Quamme, Can. J. Physiol. Pharmacol. 60, 1275-1280 (1982).
24. H.J. Gitelman, J.B. Graham and L.G. Welt, Trans. Ass. Amer. Phys. 79, 221-235 (1966).
25. R.A. Evans, J.N. Carter, C.R.P. George, R.W. Walls, R.C. Newland, G.D. McDonnell, and J.R. Lawrence, Quarterly J. Med. New Series L., 197, 39-52 (1981).
26. R.S. Bar, H.E. Wilson, and E.H. Mazzaferri, Ann. Int. Med. 82, 646-650 (1975).
27. R.L. Schilsky, and J. Anderson, Ann. Int. Med. 90, 929-933 (1979).
28. R.A.L. Sutton, V. Mavichak, V.R. Walker, N.L.M. Wong, J.H. Dirks, and C.M.L. Coppin, Abstracts of VIIIth International Conference on Calcium Regulating Hormones, Kobe, Japan, p-160 (1983).
29. J.R. Gill, and F.E. Bartter, Am. J. Med. 65, 766-772 (1978).

SECTION V

DIURETIC MECHANISMS AND SITES OF ACTION

EVIDENCE FOR A ROLE OF THE TAMM-HORSFALL PROTEIN IN THE TUBULAR ACTION OF FUROSEMIDE-LIKE LOOP DIURETICS

J. Greven, B. Kölling, B. v. Bronewski-Schwarzer, M. Junker, B. Neffgen, R. M. Nilius

Abt.Pharmakologie der RWTH Aachen, Schneebergweg, D-5100 Aachen, FRG

ABSTRACT

The present study describes the dependence on Na^+, K^+ and Cl^- of ^{14}C-furosemide binding to the Tamm-Horsfall (TH) protein, a renal epithelial glycoprotein localized in the cell membranes of the thick ascending limb of Henle's loop. The TH protein was isolated from human urine and purity was checked by SDS gel electrophoresis which showed one single band corresponding to a molecular weight of 100 000.
The TH protein was found to bind ^{14}C-furosemide in a saturable manner. A Scatchard type analysis of the binding isotherm revealed a bell-shaped plot suggesting the presence of positive cooperativity. This was also indicated by a Hill coefficient of 1.53. Specific furosemide binding required the presence of Na^+. Binding could be further increased by K^+ and Cl^-. The concentrations of Na^+, K^+ and Cl^- at which half-maximal furosemide binding was reached amounted to 1.5-3.3 mmol/l for Na^+, 14 mmol/l for K^+ and 78 mmol/l for Cl^-. At Cl^- concentrations > 100 mmol/l, furosemide binding to the TH protein decreased.
Furosemide congeners which were diuretically active also displaced labeled furosemide from its binding site on the Tamm-Horsfall protein. Diuretically inactive furosemide derivatives and loop diuretics chemically not related to furosemide did not affect furosemide binding. The apparent affinities of the diuretically active furosemide congeners to the TH protein corresponded well with their apparent affinity to the Na^+-K^+-$2Cl^-$ transport system in the thick ascending limb of Henle's loop as determined by Schlatter et al. (1983).
It is concluded that the TH protein has binding sites for Na^+,K^+ and Cl^-. Furosemide, its diuretically active congeners and Cl^- are thought to share the same binding sites on the TH protein. These data would be compatible with the assumption that the TH protein fulfills a transport function for Na^+,K^+ and Cl^- in the cell membranes in the thick ascending limb of Henle's loop. The inhibitory effect of furosemide and its diuretically active analogs on active transport might then be due to competitive displacement of Cl^- from the TH protein.

Diuretics, Jules B. Puschett, Editor

INTRODUCTION

Recent studies employing immunofluorescence microscopy suggested the presence of the Tamm-Horsfall (TH) protein, a renal epithelial glycoprotein, along the surface membranes of the cells of the thick ascending limb of Henle's loop (TAL) (1). This protein was first isolated by Tamm and Horsfall (2, 2a) from human urine by repeated precipitation in 0.58 M NaCl solution. It was originally utilized for inhibition of viral hemagglutination.

The renal origin of the TH protein, its localization in the distal part of the nephron, its presence in all mammalian kidneys so far studied (3, 4, 5, 6, 7), the relation of its presence to the oncogenetic development of the loop of Henle (3)and its appearance in amniotic fluid in relation to the occurrence of a functional thick ascending limb of Henle's loop in the fetus (8) suggested an important role of this protein for the function of the loop of Henle. However, its true function remained obscure up to now. Sikri et al. (9) and Hoyer et al. (10) speculated that the TH protein may entrap water and might therefore be responsible for the low water permeability of the distal segments of the nephron. However, the TH protein contains nearly 30% carbohydrate components (11, 12) which might interact with electrolytes, a possibility which is presumably of greater physiological significance.

The present study reports on the binding of the loop diuretic furosemide to the TH protein derived from human urine, and the dependence of binding on the presence of Na^+, K^+ and Cl^-. Furosemide, the classical loop diuretic, was thought to constitute a valuable tool for the evaluation of a possible role of this protein in electrolyte transport.

METHODS

The TH protein was isolated from human urine by the method originally described by Tamm and Horsfall (2a). Purity of the TH protein was checked by SDS gel electrophoresis which showed one single band corresponding to a molecular weight of 100 000 (Fig. 1). Binding of ^{14}C-furosemide (specific activity 8 mCi/mmol) was determined utilizing an Amicon ultrafiltration system at 0^oC. The incubation medium always contained 4 mmol/l Tris buffer and ions, as indicated in the legends to the figures. The pH was adjusted to 8.0.

Binding of ^{14}C-furosemide was observed over a broad range of pH, declining sharply at pH < 5.5 and > 10. The centrifugation technique used did not allow the determination of the time course of association in short time intervals. The minimum centrifugation time required to obtain sufficient filtrate for accurate measurements was 2 min. Furosemide binding had already reached its maximum within this time.

RESULTS

1. Na^+ - and K^+-dependent binding of furosemide to the TH protein.

Fig. 2 shows that the binding of ^{14}C-furosemide (8 x 10^{-5} mol/l) to the TH protein depends on the presence of Na^+ in the incubation medium. There was no binding at all at zero NaCl. The binding increased with rising NaCl concentration and reached saturation at NaCl concentrations above 5 mmol/l. The increase in binding with rising NaCl concentration was entirely due the increase in Na^+ and not in Cl^- concentration as indicated by the fact that 10 mmol/l choline-Cl^- did not affect furosemide binding at all.

Linear transformation of the binding isotherm revealed that half-maximal binding was reached at a Na^+ concentration of 1.5 x 10^{-3} mol/l. In a previously published experiment (13, 14), furosemide binding was determined at Na^+ concentrations ranging from 0 to 100 mmol/l. In these experiments, Cl^- concentration was kept constant by replacing choline-Cl^- isotonically with NaCl. Under these conditions, a similar Na^+ concentration of 3.3 x 10^{-3} mol/l at half-maximal binding could be determined.

As can be seen from Fig. 3, furosemide binding in the presence of 10 mmol/l Na^+ may be further stimulated by adding K^+ to the incubation medium. In these experiments, nitrate was used as an anion. Nitrate (utilized as $NaNO_3$) was found not to affect binding within the concentration range used for KNO_3. Furosemide binding was saturable at concentrations above 40 mmol/l. A K^+ concentration at halfmaximum saturation of about 14 mmol/l was estimated although the scatter of the values at the low K^+ concentrations prevented exact determination by linear transformation of the binding isotherm. In contrast to the Na^+-dependent furosemide binding, the K^+-dependent furosemide binding could not be abolished by a large excess of unlabeled furosemide (10^{-2} mol/l).

2. Equilibrium binding of ^{14}C-furosemide to TH protein

Since Na^+ stimulated specific furosemide binding, the binding isotherms at different ^{14}C-furosemide concentrations were determined at the Na^+ concentration where maximal binding was attained (10 mmol/l). Nitrate was used as an anion because Cl^- was suspected to interfere with the furosemide binding, especially when the concentration ratio Cl^- to furosemide would have become higher at low furosemide concentrations. Fig. 4 shows binding of ^{14}C-furosemide to TH protein at increasing ^{14}C-furosemide concentrations with and without Na^+. In the absence of Na^+, a linear increase of binding was observed which was entirely due to the unspecific binding of ^{14}C-furosemide to the membranes. In the presence of Na^+, ^{14}C-furosemide binding reached saturation. By adding a large excess of unlabeled furosemide (10^{-2} mol/l), ^{14}C-furosemide binding was depressed to the values observed in the absence of Na^+. The apparent affinity of furosemide to the TH protein was estimated to be 1.6 · 10^{-5} mol/l.

Scatchard and Hill analyses of the specific furosemide binding are depicted in Fig. 5. The Scatchard plot is bell-shaped with a maximum near the center of the plot. The maximum number of binding sites amounted to 1.7 nmol/mg protein.A Hill coefficient of 1.53 was deduced from the Hill plot.

3. Displacement of ^{14}C-furosemide from TH protein by Cl^- and loop diuretics

Fig. 6 depicts the dependence of furosemide-binding on the Cl^- concentration in the incubation medium. The NaCl concentration amounted to 10 mmol/l and the Cl^- concentration was increased by utilizing choline as cation. Furosemide binding increased up to a Cl^- concentration of 100 mmol/l and decreased subsequently with increasing Cl^- concentrations. To exclude the possibility that the shape of the binding curve was attributable to changes in osmolality, sufficient amounts of mannitol were added to the incubation medium to keep osmolality at all Cl^- concentrations in an identical range. From the ascending part of the curve, which was further analyzed in a separate set of experiments, an apparent Cl^- affinity of 78 mmol/l to the TH protein and a Hill coefficient of 3.7 was deduced (The Hill coefficients for the Na^+- and K^+-dependent furosemide binding were not significantly different from 1).

Displacement studies with unlabeled diuretics suggest that drugs which are chemically related to furosemide displace furosemide from its binding side on the TH protein. The affinity of the diuretically active furosemide congeners to the TH protein corresponded fairly well with their affinity to the transport system in the thick ascending limb, as described by Schlatter et al. (15).

DISCUSSION

The results of this study suggest that the TH protein derived from human urine specifically binds ^{14}C-furosemide. Scatchard and Hill analyses of the binding isotherm revealed the presence of positive cooperativity. The binding of furosemide depended on the presence of Na^+ and could be further increased by K^+. This may indicate that the TH protein has binding sites for these ions and furosemide may be considered as an indicator for ion binding. The Na^+ and K^+ concentrations at half-maximum furosemide binding may then be assumed to reflect the apparent affinity of these ions to the TH protein. Since K^+ further stimulated furosemide binding when the Na^+-binding sites had been saturated it seems reasonable to conclude that two independent binding sites for these ions exist on the TH protein. Due to the low apparent affinities, direct measurements of ion binding to the TH protein were not possible with the technique used.

Cl^- concentrations of more than 100 mmol/l decreased furosemide binding whereas at lower concentrationsfurosemide binding was enhanced. It is noteworthy that at chloride concentrations > 50 mmol/l the viscosity of the TH solution increased and the change in ^{14}C-furosemide binding might be due to the formation of high mulecular weight aggregates induced by increasing chloride concentration. Alternatively, the shape of the ^{14}C-furosemide binding curve observed might be explained by the presence of positive cooperativity, assuming an increase of the association rate constant with increasing protein occupancy. A mathematical treatment and a computer simulation for such a binding system has been published (16) and the properties of this model of cooperativity fit best with the present experimental data, assuming that Cl^- and furosemide share the same binding sites on the TH protein. The model predicts bell-shaped Scatchard plots and a hook in the low dose region of the displacement curves. Following this model, the unusual increase of furosemide binding at low Cl^- concentrations may be explained in the following way. Preincubation of a low concentration of Cl^- will enhance the association rate constant. If labeled furosemide is subsequently added, the increase in the association rate constant due to the presence of Cl^- will counterbalance the reduction in free binding sites induced by the unlabeled species and more labeled furosemide may be bound than in the absence of Cl^-. If the concentration of Cl^- is further increased, the transient increase in furosemide-binding will be followed by a progressive decrease of binding, since now Cl^- displaces labeled furosemide from its binding sites. The high Cl^- concentrations needed for displacement seem reasonable if one takes into account the apparent affinity of Cl to the TH proteins of 78 mmol/l.

Interestingly, similar conclusions were recently drawn by Kinne and coworkers, who investigated the binding of N-methylfurosemide (NMF) to plasma membrane vesicles isolated from the rectal glands of the dogfish Squalus acanthias (17). These membranes contain a Na^+, K^+, Cl^- cotransport system with characteristics similar to that of the thick ascending limb of Henle's loop. The ionic dependence of NMF binding to the membranes was very similar to that observed in this study with human TH protein. A halfmaximal stimulation of NMF was observed at a Na^+ concentration of about 0.5 mmol/l. Binding could also be further increased by K^+, and a similar affinity of K^+ (about 12 mmol/l) to the membranes as in our study to TH protein can be deduced from the binding isotherm. Furthermore, NMF binding to the membranes could be depressed by increasing Cl^- concentration to 600 mmol/l. Cooperativity of binding, however, could not detected in this system.

In addition to membranes from shark rectal gland Forbush and Palfrey (18) isolated membranes from dog kidney (19)and established the necessity of the presence of Na^+, K^+ and Cl^- for binding of the furosemide derivatives bumetanide and benzmetamide. Cl^- again inhibited bumetamide binding at higher concentrations.

It seems useful to compare also the binding data of this study with the characterics of the Na^+, K^+, $2Cl^-$ cotransport system of the thick ascending limb of Henle's loop, which has been recently evaluated ingenuously by Greger and coworkers (20-25). Greger suggested a halfmaximal stimulation of active transport at a Na^+ concentration of 3.6 mmol/l (20). This value may indicate the Na^+ affinity to the transport carrier and agrees with the affinity of Na^+ to the TH protein. Furthermore, the curve for the Cl^- dependence of active transport revealed a sigmoidal shape which was assumed to indicate the presence of two Cl^- transport sites on the carrier molecule. The halfmaximal stimulation of transport was observed at an apparent Cl^- concentration of 49 mmol/l (23). This value again may indicate the affinity of Cl- to the transport system and is compatible with the conclusions of the present study concerning the Cl^- binding to the TH protein. With respect to K^+, the affinity of this ion to the transport carrier has been observed by Greger to lie in the range of 0.5 to 1 mmol/l and therefore seems to be somewhat smaller than the K^+ affinity as derived from furosemide binding to TH protein and to rectal gland plasma membranes.

Taken together, there is a striking similarity between the data concerning the binding of N-methylfurosemide to rectal gland plasma membrane vesicles and the binding of furosemide to the TH glycoprotein. Furthermore, the stoichiometry of the cotransport of Na^+,K^+ and $2Cl^-$ and the affinity of Cl^- and Na^+ to the transport carrier as derived from electrophysiological studies on isolated thick ascending limb of Henle's loop of rabbits by Greger and coworkers are mirrored by the suggested binding of these ions to the TH protein. In addition, the affinities of the diuretically active furosemide congeners to the TH protein and to the transport system in the thick ascending limb are compatible. The fact that loop diuretics not related chemically to furosemide were unable to displace furosemide from its binding sides on the TH protein, would agree with the conclusion of Schlatter et al. (15) that these diuretics may have a mode of tubular action different from that of furosemide and its derivatives.

The Na^+, K^+ and $2Cl^-$ transport carrier may, therefore, be assumed to be closely related to or even identical with the TH protein, although the mechanism connecting binding with subsequent transport remains speculative. The inhibitoryaction of furosemide and its chemically related congeners on transport might then be explained by a competitive displacement of Cl- from the TH protein.

This assumption would require as further evidence a tissue distribution of the TH protein corresponding to the localization of the cotransport system. Indeed, according to Hoyer and Seiler (1), the tubular distribution of the TH protein precisely corresponds to revised morphologic limits of the thick ascending limb, where the cotransport system is primarily localized in the kidney. The TH protein is absent in the glomeruli, proximal tubules, the descending limb of the loop of Henle and the collecting ducts. Interestingly, it is also not present in the macula densa cells (9, 10, 26). This finding may be of major physiological relevance, since the macula densa cells contain also no or only little Na^+,K^+-ATPase on the basolateral cell side (27).

There is some controversy with respect to the presence of the TH protein in the cell membranes of the distal convoluted tubule. Hoyer and Seiler suggested that the presence of TH protein on the luminal surface of the tubular cells distal to the thick ascending limb reflects absorption related to urinary excretion of TH protein (1). On the other hand, Sikri et al. asserted synthesis of TH protein also in the cells of the distal convoluted tubule (9,26). The latter suggestion might be related to the findings of a recent study in rats which indicated that the distal convoluted tubule may also contain a furosemide-sensitive NaCl cotransport system in the luminal cell membrane (28-30). The immunofluorescence studies published regularly demonstrate a strong positive staining reaction along the luminal cell membrane suggesting localization of the TH protein mainly in the luminal border of the cells. Positive staining reactions of the tubular cytoplasma in the Golgi region may provide evidence for synthesis of the protein in this region. Adult humans excrete TH protein in urine in an amount of some 50 mg/day (31, 32), suggesting that it may be dissolved out from the luminal membrane during passage of urine. The half life has been determined in rabbits to be only 9 hrs (33), emphasizing the high rate of synthesis of this glycoprotein.

Some findings, however, are not readily explained in terms of a suggested carrier function of the TH protein. Positive staining reactions for TH protein were also found on the basal cell borders and the lateral intercellular membranes of the thick ascending limb and distal convoluted tubules (9, 10, 26).A role of TH protein in several tubular interstitial diseases has been postulated (1). However, basal deposits - in contrast to the most massive and consistent luminal staining - were some times capricious (26).

The Na^+, K^+, $2Cl^-$ cotransport system is not restricted to the kidney and has been identified in several extrarenal tissues such as erythrocytes,colon, trachea, cornea, Ehrlich's ascites tumor cells and the rectal gland of the dogfish. The transport molecule may be assumed to be very similar in all these tissues. Evidence is accumulating that the origin of TH-like glycoproteins is not exclusively renal and its presence in erythrocyte membranes has been reported recently (34). Further studies are needed to prove the presence of the TH or a similar protein in the other tissues where the Na^+, K^+, $2Cl^-$ transport has been identified. The similarity between binding of furosemide to the TH protein and to the membranes of the rectal gland, however, is striking.

Acknowledgements:

The secretarial work of E. Abrahams is gratefully acknowledged. ^{14}C-furosemide and its unlabeled congeners were generously supplied by Dr. Hropot, Dr. Bremer and Dr. Lang from Hoechst AG, Frankfurt/M.
We thank Dr. Oemar and Dr. Ehrich, Kinderklinik der Medizinischen Hochschule Hannover, for performing the molecular weight determination of the TH protein.

1

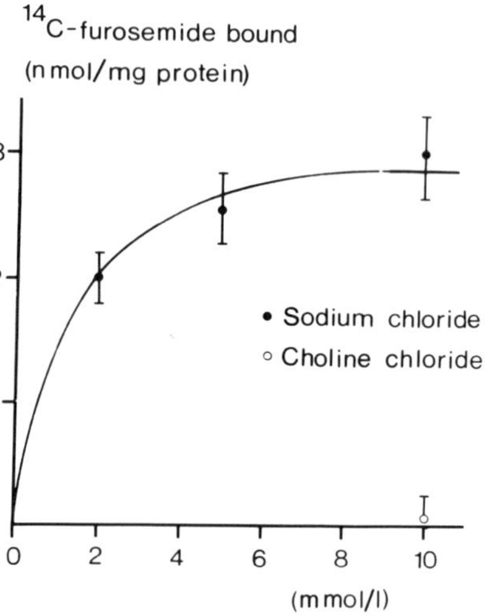

14C-furosemide bound
(nmol/mg protein)
Sodium chloride
Choline chloride
(mmol/l)

2

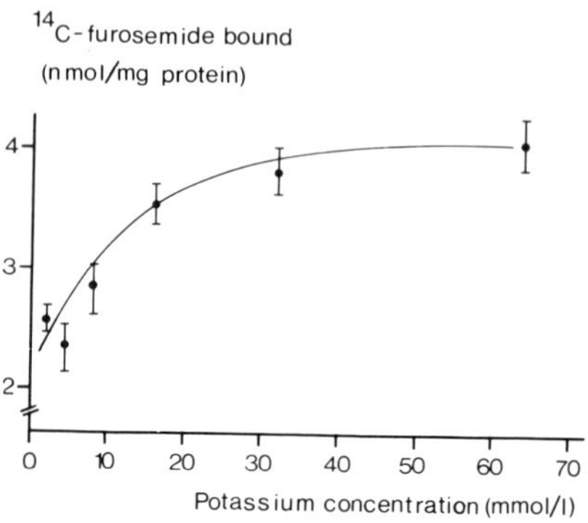

14C-furosemide bound
(nmol/mg protein)
Potassium concentration (mmol/l)

3

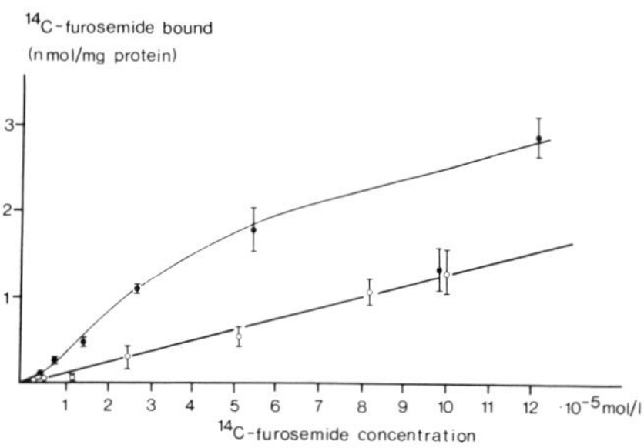

14C-furosemide bound
(nmol/mg protein)
10-5mol/l
14C-furosemide concentration

4

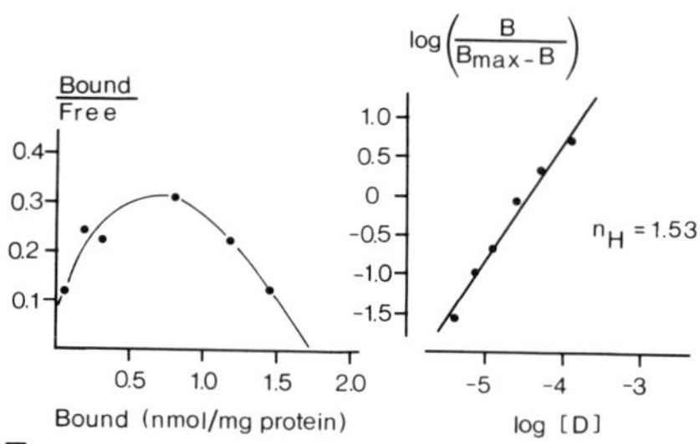

Bound
Free
Bound (nmol/mg protein)
log (B / Bmax - B)
nH = 1.53
log [D]

5

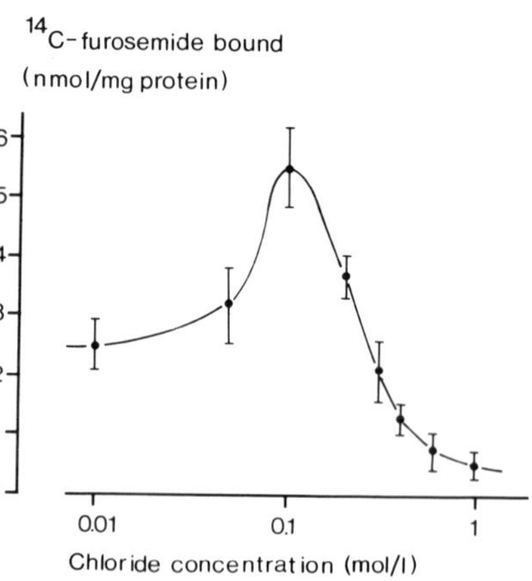

14C-furosemide bound
(nmol/mg protein)
Chloride concentration (mol/l)

6

Legends

Fig. 1: SDS gel electrophoresis of TH protein.

Fig. 2: Na^+-dependent binding of ^{14}C-furosemide to TH protein. Binding was determined at 0^oC after 30 min incubation of 8 x 10^{-5} mol/l ^{14}C-furosemide in a medium consisting of 2.5 mg/ml TH protein, 4 mmol/l Tris (pH 8.0) and increasing concentrations of NaCl. The effect of 10 mmol/l choline Cl^- on furosemide binding is shown too. Each value is the mean ±SEM of 8 experiments.

Fig. 3: K^+-dependent binding of ^{14}C-furosemide to TH protein in the presence of Na^+. Binding was determined at 0^oC after 30 min incubation of 8 x10^{-5} mol/l ^{14}C-furosemide in a medium consisting of 2.5 mg/ml TH protein, 4 mmol/l Tris (pH 8.0), 10 mmol/l $NaNO_3$ and increasing concentrations of KNO_3.
Each value is the mean ±SEM of 4-8 experiments.

Fig. 4: Equilibrium binding of ^{14}C-furosemide to TH protein. The binding isotherms were determined at 0^oC after 30 min incubation of increasing ^{14}C-furosemide concentrations in a medium consisting of 2.5 mg/ml TH protein, 4 mmol/l Tris (pH 8.0) in the presence (upper curve) or absence (lower line) of 10 mmol/l $NaNO_3$. The unspecific binding of ^{14}C-furosemide to the filtration membranes in the absence of TH protein is shown too (squared point). Each value is the mean ± SEM of 4 experiments.

Fig. 5: Scatchard and Hill analyses of the binding site of ^{14}C-furosemide on the TH protein. The Scatchard plot is non linear and concave down. The Hill plot reveals a Hill coefficient of 1.53 for the furosemide binding site.

Fig. 6: Displacement of labeled furosemide by Cl^-. The binding was determined at 0^oC after 30 min incubation of 8 x 10^{-5} ^{14}C-furosemide in a medium consisting of 2.5 mg/ml TH protein, 4 mmol/l Tris buffer (pH 8.0), 10 mmol NaCl and increasing concentrations of choline Cl^-. Sufficient mannitol was added to the incubation medium to keep the osmolality constant at all concentrations. In a separate set of experiments, mannitol was found not to affect furosemide binding.
Each value is the mean ±SEM of 4 experiments.

REFERENCES

1. Hoyer, J. R., Seiler, M. W. 1979. Pathophysiology of Tamm-Horsfall protein. In: "Proteinuria", Guest Edts.: J. W. Boylan & B.. van Liew, Kidney Int., Vol. 16 (No.3), pp. 279-289

2. Tamm, I., Horsfall, F. L., Jr. 1950. Characterization and separation of an inhibitor of viral hemagglutination present in urine. Proc. Soc. Exp. Biol. Med. 74: 108-114

2a. Tamm, I., Horsfall, F. L., Jr. 1952. A mucoprotein derived from human urine which reacts with influenza, mumps, and Newcastle disease viruses. J. Exp. Med. 95: 71-97

3. Hoyer, J. R., Resnick, J. S., Michael, A. F., Vernier, R. L. 1974. Ontogeny of Tamm-Horsfall urinary glycoprotein. Lab. Invest. 30: 757-761

4. Cornelius, C. E., Mia, A. S., Rosenfeld, S. 1965. Ruminant urolithiasis VII. Studies on the origin of Tamm-Horsfall urinary mucoprotein and its presence in ovine calculous matrix. Invest. Urol. 2: 453-457

5. Marr, A. M. S., Neuberger, A., Ratcliffe, W. A. 1971. Rabbit Tamm-Horsfall urinary glycoprotein: Chemical composition and subunit structure. Biochem. J. 122: 623-631

6. Dunstan, D. R., Grant, A. M. S., Marshall, R. D., Neuberger, A. 1974. A protein immunologically similar to Tamm-Horsfall glycoprotein produced by cultured baby hamster kidney cells. Proc. R Soc. Lond. (Biol.) 186: 297-316

7. Wallace A. C., Nairn, R. C. 1971. Tamm-Horsfall protein in kidneys of human embryos and foreign species. Pathol. 3: 303-310

8. Phimister, G., Marshall, R. D. 1982. Tamm-Horsfall glycoprotein in human amniotic fluid. Clin. Chim. Acta 128: 261-269

9. Sikri, K. L., Foster, C. L., Bloomfield, F. J., Marshall, R. D. 1979. Localization by immunofluorescence and by light-and electron-microscopic immunoperoxidase techniques of Tamm-Horsfall glycoprotein in adult hamster kidney. Biochem. J. 181: 525-532

10. Hoyer, J. R., Sisson, S. P., Vernier, R. L. 1979. Tamm-Horsfall glycoprotein. Ultrastructural immunoperoxidase localization in rat kidney. Lab. Invest. 41: 168-173

11. Stevenson, F. K., Kent, P. W. 1970. Subunits of Tamm-Horsfall glycoprotein. Biochem. J. 116: 791-796

12. Fletcher, A. P., Neuberger, A., Ratcliffe, W. A. 1970. Tamm-Horsfall urinary glycoprotein: The chemical composition. Biochem. J. 120: 417-424

13. Greven, J., Kölling, B. 1982. Effects of muzolimine in microperfusion studies of loops of Henle in rats. In: Proceedings of the Second International Edrul[R] Symposium, Sorrento, page 37-45, Excerpta Medica, Amsterdam, Geneva, Hong Kong, Princeton, Tokyo.

14. Greven, J. 1983. Studies on the renal receptors of loop diuretics. Clin and Exp. Hyper. Theory and Practice A5: 193-208

15. Schlatter, E., Greger, R., Weidtke, C. 1983. Effect of "high ceiling" diuretics on active salt transport in the cortical thick ascending limb of Henle's loop of rabbit kidney. Pflügers Arch. 396: 210-217

16. De Lean, A, Rodbard, D. 1979. Kinetics of cooperative binding. In: The receptors. A comprehensive treatise, Vol.1, General principles and procedures, Ed.: R. D. O'Brien, Plenum Press, New York - London.

17. Hannafin, J., Kinne-Saffran, E., Friedman, D., Kinne, R. 1983. Presence of a sodim-potassium chloride cotransport system in the rectal gland of Squalus acanthias. J. Membrane Biol. 75: 73-83

18. Forbush, B., Palfrey, H. C. 1982. Bumetanide and benzmetanide binding to membranes from shark rectal gland and canine kidney. Biophys. J. 37: 161a

19. Forbush, B., Palfrey, H. C. 1983. ^{3}H-Bumetanide binding to membranes isolated from dog kidney outer medulla. J. Biol. Chem. 258: 11787-11792

20. Greger, R. 1981. Chloride reabsorption in the rabbit cortical thick asecnding limb of the loop of Henle. A sodium dependent process. Pflügers Arch. 390: 38-43

21. Greger, R. 1981. Coupled transport of Na^{+} and Cl^{-} in the thick ascending limb of Henle's loop of rabbit nephron. Scand. Audiol. (Suppl.) 14: 1-15

22 Greger, R., Schlatter, E. 1981. Presence of luminal K^{+}, a prerequisite for active NaCl transport in the cortical thick ascending limb of Henle's loop of rabbit kidney. Pflügers Arch. 392: 92-94

23. Greger, R., Schlatter, E., Lang, F. 1983. Evidence for electroneutral sodium chloride cotransport in the cortical thick ascending limb of Henle's loop in rabbit kidney. Pflügers Arch. 396: 308-314

24. Greger, R., Schlatter, E. 1983. Properties of the lumen membrane of the cortical thick ascending limb of Henle's loop of rabbit kidney. Pflügers Arch. 396: 315-324

25. Greger, R., Schlatter, E. 1983. Properties of the basolateral membrane of the cortical thick ascending limb of Henle's loop of rabbit kidney. A model of secondary active chloride transport. Pflügers Arch. 396: 325-334

26. Sikri, K. L., Foster, C. L., MacHugh, N., Marshall, R. D. 1981. Localization of Tamm-Horsfall glycoprotein in the human kidney using immuno-fluorescence and immuno-electron microscopical techniques. J. Anat. 132: 597-605

27. Beeuwkes, R., Rosen, S. 1980. Renal Na^{+}-K^{+}-ATPase: Localization and quantitation by means of its K^{+}-dependent phosphatase activity. Current Topics in Membranes and Transport, Vol. 13, 343-354

28. Velaquez, H., Good, D. W., Wright, F. S. 1981. Mutual dependence of sodium and chloride absorption by renal distal tubule. Fed. Proc. 40: 395 (Abstr.)

29. Velaquez, H., Wright, F. S. 1982. Distal potassium secretion is enhanced by low lumen chloride despite adverse voltage change, and is not increased by luminal furosemide. Kidney Int. 21: 290 (Abstr.)

30. Velaquez, H., Wright, F. S. Good, D. W. 1982. Luminal influences on potassium secretion: Chloride replacement with sulfate. Am J. Physiol. 242 (Renal Fluid Electrol Physiol 11): F46-F55

31. McKenzie, J. K., Patel, R., McQueen, E. G. 1964. The excretion rate of Tamm-Horsfall urinary mucoprotein in normals and in patients with renal disease. Aust. Ann. Med. 13: 32-39

32. Grant, A. M., Baker, L. R. I., Neuberger, A. 1973. Urinary Tamm-Horsfall glycoprotein in certain kidney diseases and its content in renal and bladder calculi. Clin. Sci. 44: 377-384

33. Grant, A. M. S., Neuberger, A. 1973. The turnover rate of rabbit urinary Tamm-Horsfall glycoprotein. Biochem. J. 136: 659-668

34. Hartmann, L., Delaunay, J., Ollier-Hartmann, M.P., Bringuier, A. F., Richet, G. 1981. Tamm-Horsfall Protein and erythrocyte ghosts immunologically cross-react. Biomed. 35: 1-3

Cellular Mechanism of Action of Furosemide-Like Diuretics in the Thick Ascending Limb of the Loop of Henle.*

Rainer Greger, Eberhard Schlatter, and Monika Wittner
Max Planck Institut für Biophysik, Kennedyallee 70, D-6000 Frankfurt/Main 70, West Germany

ABSTRACT

The present contribution reviews briefly the cellular events occuring in the thick ascending limb (TAL) segment when a furosemide related compound is added to the luminal perfusate. The diuretic interferes with the $Na^+2Cl^-K^+$ cotransport system present in the lumen membrane of these cells. This step probably involves the interaction of the anionic site ($-COO^-$, $-SO_3^-$, etc) of the furosemide related compound with one of the Cl^--binding sites of the carrier. The consequences of the diuretic-carrier interaction comprise: 1) Fall in cell Cl^- to values not distinguishable from passive distribution. 2) A fall in cell Na^+ to the minimal value achieved by the (Na^++K^+)-pump. 3) A hyperpolarization of both cell membranes until the membrane PDs approximate the chemical PD for K^+. 4) A decrease of the Cl^--conductance of the basolateral membrane as a result of the fall in cell Cl^- with the consequence of a trans-epithelial resistance increase. The transition towards this state takes less than a sec in a TAL cell. Since cellular Cl^- and K^+ are close to equilibrium after this transition, and since the (Na^++K^+)-ATPase turn-over is minimal, this state is stable and little or no energy is required to sustain it. Thus, pretreatment with furosemide related diuretics protects completely against the depolarization and cell swelling observed usually after exposure to ouabain or after removal of metabolic fuels. The effects of furosemide related diuretics are easily and completely reversible. As soon as the diuretic is washed off, the above equilibrium distribution of Cl^- and K^+ is restored rapidly and the lumen positive PD reappears.

INTRODUCTION

Some 11 years ago the nephron site of the action of furosemide, namely the thick ascending limb of the loop of Henle (TAL), and the mechanism of action, i.e. inhibition of active NaCl reabsorption, have been shown unequivocally (1). The concept of NaCl reabsorption suggested then (2,3) had to be revised since it was shown that the reabsorption of Cl^- is strictly dependent on the presence of luminal Na^+ (4) and of luminal K^+ (5). From these, and further studies (6,7,8,9) it was concluded that the reabsorption of Cl^- is secondarily active and occurs via a $Na^+2Cl^-K^+$ co-transport system (cf. Fig. 1). The energy for the carrier mediated uptake is provided by the basolateral (Na^++K^+)-pump (i.e. the (Na^++K^+)-ATPase) keeping low the intracellular Na^+ activity. Part of the Na^+ is reabsorbed passively across the paracellular pathway. This concept, based on trans-epithelial and intracellular PD measurements has meanwhile been confirmed with ion selective microelectrodes (10,11). Also it has been shown that an

* Supported by Deutsche Forschungsgemeinschaft Gr 480/4-7

Diuretics, Jules B. Puschett, Editor

almost identical mechanism serves to reabsorb NaCl in the diluting segment of the amphibian kidney (12,13,14,15), and in the flounder intestine (16). Furthermore, several epithelia such as the trachea (17,18) the colon (19), the cornea (20), and the shark rectal gland (21,22) apparently secrete NaCl by a mechanism comparable to that present in the TAL cell. In the secretory epithelia the same individual components prevail but are localized in the opposite membrane. In the following a brief description of the mechanism of NaCl reabsorption will be provided. This will be followed by a discussion of the molecular characteristics of the furosemide related diuretics. Then the cellular events occuring after luminal application of these diuretics will be described.

MECHANISM OF NaCl REABSORPTION IN THE TAL SEGMENT

A simplified scheme is presented in Fig. 1. The (Na^+/K^+)-pump consumes ATP to keep low cell Na^+ (≈ 12 $mmol \cdot l^{-1}$)(13,no measurement available thus far for the isolated perfused TAL segment), and to keep high cell K^+ (110 $mmol \cdot l^{-1}$)(11). The chemical potentials for Na^+ and Cl^- across the apical cell membrane: ≈ 60 mV, and $2x \approx 45$ mV, respectively, serve to compensate the chemical potential for K^+ ≈ 95 mV. Thus, the $Na^+2Cl^-K^+$ co-transporter has a driving force of ≈ 55 mV to drive all four ions from the lumen into the cell. Both K^+ and Cl^- are above equilirium in the TAL cell: The apical membrane PD is 80 mV, yet the chemical potential for K^+ $(\Delta\mu/F)_{K^+}$ is 95 mV resulting in an electrochemical PD $(\Delta\tilde{\mu}/F)_{K^+}$ of 15 mV. The basolateral membrane PD is -72 mV and the chemical potential for Cl^- $(\Delta\mu/F)_{Cl^-}$ is -45 mV, resulting in an electrochemical PD $(\Delta\tilde{\mu}/F)_{Cl^-}$ of -27 mV. Since the two cell membranes are in fact K^+, and Cl^--conductive (8,9) respectively, K^+ recycling occurs across the apical cell membrane and Cl^- leaves the cell across the basolateral cell membrane. The transcellular K^+ and Cl^- current across the respective cell membranes is responsible for the lumen positive PD of some 5-10 mV. This PD drives Na^+ across the para-cellular cation selective shunt pathway (23) from the lumen to the peritubule side. The basolateral cell membrane has little if any K^+-conductance (9). K^+ recycles across this cell membrane in conjunction with Cl^- (KCl-exit). In terms of quantitation this electroneutral KCl-exit mechanism apparently comprises only some 35% of total Cl^- exit, i.e. 65% occur via the Cl^--conductance. This concept of NaCl reabsorption shown here is almost twice as economical as would be the electroneutral transcellular NaCl-reabsorption (24) since (cf. Fig 1) close to one equivalent of Na^+ is moved passively across the shunt pathway for each equivalent transported actively via the (Na^+/K^+)-pump.

DIURETICS RELATED TO FUROSEMIDE

Diuretic and saluretic substances are usually classified according to their site of action in the nephron. In this classification the so called loop diuretics comprise a heterogenous group including substances such as: mercurials, phenoxyacetic acids, muzolimine, MK447, L-ozolinone, tizolemide, the substances related to furosemide, and others. It has been shown recently (25) that out of this heterogenous collection, the substances related to furosemide comprise a subgroup with several typical features: a) They act from the lumen ($IC_{50,lumen} \approx 0.005\ IC_{50,bath}$). b) They act completely reversibly. c) They share in common a Hill coefficient of close to 1 in the dose response curve. d) Since they all interfere with the $Na^+2Cl^-K^+$ cotransporter their cellular effects are identical. The other loop diuretics act differently, some, in fact,are completely ineffective in doses up to 10^{-4} $mol \cdot l^{-1}$ from either epithelial side. Others act from the bath side (L-ozoline) or almost equally well from either side (ethacrynic acid, indacrinone). Some are poorly reversible and lead to cell depolarization (ethacrynic acid). It was concluded that a molecular structure related to that of furosemide is a prerequisite for the interaction of a loop diuretic with the $Na^{+}2Cl^{-}K^{+}$ cotransporter. Furthermore, comparison of the IC_{50} values for the different relatives of furosemide included in this study allowed the following general conclusions: a) For the interaction an acidic group ($-COO^{-}$ in furosemide) is needed. In case of position 2 (-furfurylamine) substituted compounds the $-COO^{-}$-group (of position 1) can be replaced by $-SO_3^{-}$ or -tetrazole^{-}. In case of position 3-substituted compounds (-butylamine, in case of bumetanide) position 1 must be a carboxylate group. b) Position 2 (-furfurylamine, in case of furosemide) tolerates little if any alterations. c) Position 3 ($-NH_2$-R) can be modified: Cf e.g. bumetanide and piretanide. d) Position 4 is open to large variations. In fact, the -Cl, as in furosemide, is a poor substituent. e) Position 5, the sulfonamide group, is again open to considerable variation without marked changes in the IC_{50} value. From these data it appears that the acidic group (position 1) is the most likely site of the molecule to interact with the (one) Cl^{-}-binding site of the carrier. Obviously, the restrictions on this site (position 1) and in close neighbourhood are most marked (positions 2 and 3).

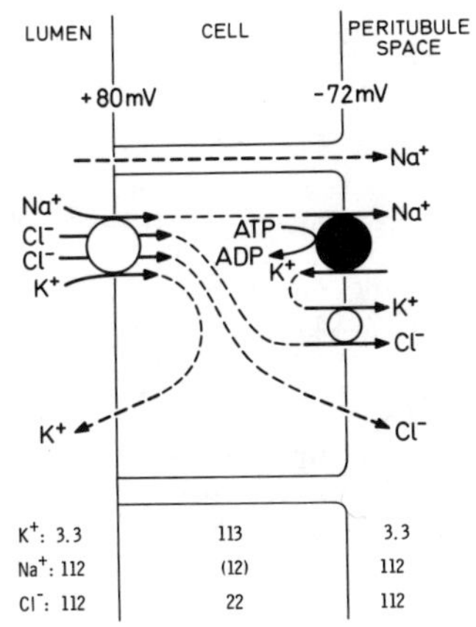

Fig.1: A cell model for the TAL-segment. ---▸ diffusion, carrier mediated transport, $(Na^{+}+K^{+})$-ATPase. The numbers at the bottom denote the cellular activities. The cellular activity for Na^{+} is taken from Oberleithner et al. 1983 (13).

The "fingerprinting" of a Cl^{-} cotransport system by means of its sensitivity towards different relatives of this group of diuretics eg. bumetanide, piretanide, furosemide has become a powerful method. For the $Na^{+}2Cl^{-}K^{+}$ carrier a sequence of the IC_{50} values of bumetanide < piretanide < furosemide with a total span of a factor of 20-50 is typical. Also the IC_{50} for furosemide is generally $< 10^{-4}$ mol$\cdot$l^{-1}. On the other hand, furosemide seems to inhibit the Cl^{-}/OH^{-} antiporter at $> 10^{-4}$ mol$\cdot$l^{-1} (26), and at even higher doses furosemide apparently blocks the KCl symport in red cells (27). Thus, it is insufficient to use but one concentration of these diuretics and to conclude from any observed inhibitory effects that the $Na^{+}2Cl^{-}K^{+}$ carrier present in these cells.

Recent affinity binding studies with radiolabelled relatives of furosemide have lead to conclusions similar to the one cited above. First it was shown in membranes prepared from the rectal gland (21) that Na^+ and K^+ must be present to achieve binding of the diuretic, thus, indicating that the diuretic binds to the Cl^--site of the carrier. Similarly, it was shown that diuretic binding to membranes of the renal medulla required the presence of Na^+, K^+, and low concentrations of Cl^- (28). Finally, for the red cell which also possesses this cotransport system, it was reported recently that the diuretic binding is competitive to that of Cl^- (29). With respect to the possible role of the Tamm Horsfall protein as a furosemide binding site, the reader is referred to the article by Greven in the same volume. To conclude this section it seems clear today that the compounds related to furosemide bind specifically to the $Na^+2Cl^-K^+$ carrier. At high doses, however, these compounds do also exert "nonspecific" effects.

THE TAL SEGMENT IN THE PRESENCE OF FUROSEMIDE

Table 1 summarizes the observations made when furosemide was added ($5 \cdot 10^{-5}$ $mol \cdot l^{-1}$) to the lumen perfusate. These alterations take only the fraction of 1 sec to up to a few sec to occur (7). The lumen positive PD (PD_{te}) collapses. The transepithelial resistance (R_{te}) increases moderately. The equivalent short circuit current ($I_{sc}=PD_{te}/R_{te}$) is abolished by furosemide. The cell hyperpolarizes: the apical membrane from 69 to 73 mV, and the basolateral membrane from -62 to -73 mV. The fractional resistance of the basolateral membrane doubles. Cellular Cl^--activity falls from 22 to 7 $mmol \cdot l^{-1}$, and cellular K^+ activity stays constant.

In the following, on the basis of Fig. 1, these findings will be explained. furosemide "locks" the carrier. Therefore, cell Cl^- has to fall towards equilibrium. Cell Na^+ will decline since the (Na^++K^+)-pump will keep pumping out Na^+ until a minimal activity is achieved. Only then the pump will stand still and no more ATP will be consumed. During the transition period K^+ will leak out of the cell across the apical cell membrane following the driving force across the conductive pathway. Simultaneously, some K^+ will still enter the cell via the (Na^++K^+)-pump. The two opposing fluxes lead to little change in cell K^+. Eventually, also K^+ will be close to equilibrium after this transition period. Then, $(\Delta\mu/F)_{K^+}$ becomes equal to PD_l and $(\Delta\mu/F)_{Cl^-}$ becomes equal to PD_{bl}, and PD_l will be equal (opposite in sign) to PD_{bl}. Now PD_{te} as well as I_{sc} are zero. In this state, K^+ and Cl^- are passively distributed, the (Na^++K^+)-ATPase is put at rest and also Na^+ is in equilibrium across the paracellular shunt pathway.

The fall in transepithelial and basolateral membrane conductance observed after application of furosemide, can be explained by a reduction in the Cl^--conductance of the basolateral membrane (30). A reduction in Cl^--conductance after furosemide has also been noted in the rectal gland tubule cell (33) and in the cornea (31). In the latter report, this effect of the diuretic was claimed to be the primary mechanism by which NaCl secretion is inhibited. This conclusion apparently does not hold true for the rectal gland tubule nor for the TAL segment. In both preparations reduction of cell Cl^- irrespective by what mechanism (Cl^--removal, Na^+-removal, furosemide addition) is the cause for the observed fall in Cl^--conductance. The Goldman constant field equation, provided it is applicable to the process of Cl^--diffusion out of the cell, predicts even quantitatively the observed fall in Cl^--conductance (32,33). In terms of the driving force of the carrier, a maximum value is built up in the presence of furosemide: $(\Delta\mu/F)_{Na^+} \approx 70$ mV, $(\Delta\mu/F)_{Cl^-} \approx -70$ (x2),

$(\Delta\mu/F)_{K^+} \approx -95$ mV. Leading to a $(\Delta\mu/F)_{carrier}$ of ≈ 115 mV. As soon as furosemide is removed, the carrier serves to reload the cell with Cl^- and K^+. The cell depolarizes (mainly at the basolateral membrane) and the transepithelial lumen positive PD as well as the equivalent short circuit reappear. This recovery is complete within a few sec.

Table 1: Effects of furosemide (5 10^{-5} mol l^{-1}, lumen) in the rabbit cTAL segment.

	PD_{te}	R_{te}	I_{sc}	PD_{bl}	FR_{bl}	$a^{cell}_{Cl^-}$	$a^{cell}_{K^+}$
	(mV)	(Ωcm^2)	(μAcm^{-2})	(mV)		(mmol.l^{-1})	
control	+7 $\pm$1	34 $\pm$2	210 $\pm$30	-62 $\pm$2	0.32 $\pm$0.02	22 $\pm$2	113 $\pm$8
furosemide	$\approx$0 $\pm$1	42 $\pm$2	$\approx$0	-73 $\pm$2	0.5 $\pm$0.02	7 $\pm$2	117 $\pm$9
n	30	11	11	12	31	25	20
references	4,38,7,11		38	7	30	10	11

Abbreviations: PD_{te}: transepithelial PD, referenced to grounded bath; R_{te}: transepithelial resistance; I_{sc}: equivalent short circuit current=PD_{te}/R_{te}, referenced to grounded bath; PD_{bl}: basolateral membrane PD, referenced to grounded bath; FR_{bl}: fractional resistance of the basolateral membrane = current induced voltage deflection across the basolateral membrane divided by that across the epithelium. $a^{cell}_{Cl^-}$, $a^{cell}_{K^+}$: cellular activity of Cl^- and K^+, activity coefficient used for extracellular space 0.75.

THE FUROSEMIDE TREATED TAL CELL A "RESTING CELL"

The above description characterized the TAL cell in the presence of furosemide as a cell at or close to equilibrium with no need to consume ATP. This point has been examined recently by applying (Na^++K^+)-ATPase inhibitors (phloretin, ouabain) to furosemide treated segments. It was shown that these inhibitors were devoid of effects on cell PD and cell volume as long as furosemide was present, but that the cells started to depolarize and to swell immediately upon the removal of furosemide (30). Similar observations have been made in the amphibian diluting segment (34) and in the rectal gland tubule (33). Obviously, inhibition of the (Na^++K^+)-ATPase by ouabain is a rather unlikely event under in vivo conditions. On the other hand, inhibition of the (Na^++K^+)-pump by a shortage in ATP supply may occur in real life. Fig. 2 is an example of an experiment where PD_{bl} in a TAL cell was monitored while furosemide was present and while all metabolic fuels were removed. It is apparent that the cell stays hyperpolarized. After furosemide removal, however, PD_{bl} depolarizes with a delay of some 3 min. Readmission of D-glucose "cures" this cell. Thus, the TAL cells are characterized not only by a high substrate turnover, due to the high rates of NaCl-reabsorption, they also have little reserves to live on and are threatened by shortages in O_2 or fuel supply (35). The present data clearly indicate that furosemide desensitizes TAL cells towards the hazzards of O_2 or fuel shortage. This observation should be one rationale to use furosemide in states of threatening renal failure (30).

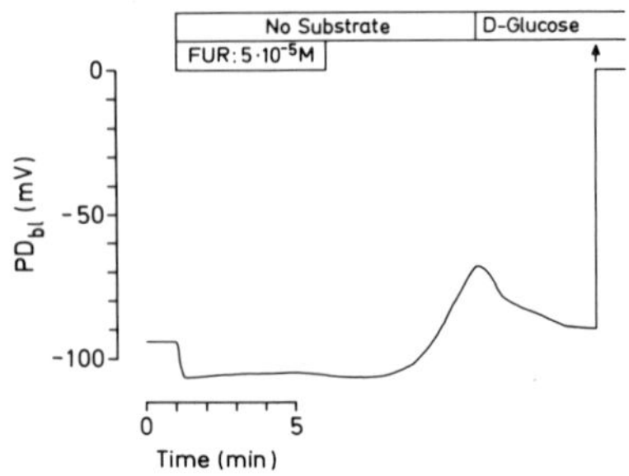

Fig. 2: Effect of removal of substrate on PD_{bl} in an isolated perfused cTAL segment. Substrate (D-glucose, 5 mmol · l^{-1},bath) was removed and simultaneously furosemide was added to the lumen perfusate. This causes a hyperpolarization of PD_{bl}. The PD is sustained until furosemide is removed. Then, with a delay of 2-3 min PD_{bl} starts to depolarizes. Readmission of D-glucose (bath, 5 mmol ·l^{-1}) leads to a hyperpolarization of PD_{bl} back to the control value. This experiment indicates that substrate removal is devoid of effects on PD_{bl} (and cell volume, not shown) as long as furosemide is present.

Turning back to the model of Fig. 1, the present data indicate that the TAL cell has no other significant pathways for Na^+. Otherwise a depolarization should have been observed in the presence of furosemide when the (Na^++K^+)-ATPase was inhibited or when substrates were removed. This conlusion is in accordance with the previous observtions that the TAL cells are insensitive towards amiloride (36) and that they do not possess Na^+-dependent carrier systems in the apical cell membrane for organic compounds (37)

CONCLUSION

Our understanding of the cellular mechanism of action of furosemide like diuretics has progressed rapidly during the last few years. It seems clear today that these diuretics inhibit a specific cotransport system, the $Na^+2Cl^-K^+$ carrier. As a consequence the Cl^--entry into the TAL cell is blocked and transepithelial NaCl-reabsorption ceases. the furosemide type of diuretics have served to analyse the cellular mechanism of NaCl-reabsorption in the TAL segment. They, probably, will be also powerful tools in the purification of the cotransporter molecule.

REFERENCES

1. M.B. Burg, L. Stoner, J. Cardinal, N. Green, Am J Physiol 225 (1): 119-124 (1973)
2. M.B. Burg and N. Green, Am J Physiol 224 (3): 659-668 (1973)
3. A.S. Rocha and J.P. Kokko, J Clin Invest 52:612-623 (1973)
4. R. Greger, Pflügers Arch 390:38-43 (1981)
5. R. Greger and E. Schlatter, Pflügers Arch 392:92-94 (1981)

6. R. Greger, Scand Audiol (Suppl) 14:1-15 (1981)
7. R. Greger, E. Schlatter, F. Lang, Pflügers Arch 396:308-314 (1983)
8. R. Greger and E. Schlatter, Pflügers Arch 396:315-324 (1983)
9. R. Greger, and E. Schlatter, Pflügers Arch 396:325-334 (1983)
10. R. Greger, H. Oberleithner, E. Schlatter, A.C. Cassola, Pflügers Arch 399:29-34 (1983)
11. R. Greger, C. Weidtke, E. Schlatter, M. Wittner, B. Gebler, Pflügers Arch in press (1984)
12. H. Oberleithner, W. Guggino, G. Giebisch, Am J Physiol 242:F331-F339 (1982)
13. H. Oberleithner, G. Giebisch, F. Lang, W. Wang, Klin Wochenschr 60: 1173- 1179 (1982)
14. H. Oberleithner, W. Guggino, G. Giebisch, Pflügers Arch 396:27-33 (1983)
15. H. Oberleithner, F. Lang, R. Greger, W. Wang, G. Giebisch, Pflügers Arch 396:34-40 (1983)
16. M.W. Musch, S.A. Orellana, L.S. Kimberg, M. Field. D.R. Halm, E.J. Krasny Jr., R.A. Frizzell, Nature 300:351-353 (1982)
17. M.J. Welsh, J Clin Invest 71:1392-1401 (1983)
18. S.R. Shorofsky, M. Field, H.A. Fozzard, Phil Trans R Soc Lond B 299: 597-607 (1982)
19. M.J. Welsh, P.L. Smith, M. Fromm, R.A. Frizzell, Science 218:1219-1221 (1982)
20. L. Reuss, P. Reinach, S.A. Weinman, T.P. Grady, Am J Physiol 244: C336-C347 (1983)
21. J. Hannafin, E. Kinne-Saffran, D. Friedmann, R. Kinne, J Membrane Biol 75:73-83 (1983)

22. R. Greger and E. Schlatter, Pflügers Arch submitted (1984)
23. R. Greger, Pflügers Arch 390:30-37 (1981)
24. R.A. Frizzel, M. Field, S.G. Schultz, Am J Physiol 236:F1-F8 (1979)
25. E. Schlatter, R. Greger, C. Weidtke, Pflügers Arch 396:210-217 (1983)
26. P.S. Aronson, In: D.G. Warnock, R. Greger, P.B. Dunham, R.A.Frizzel, M. Field, K.R. Spring, H.E. Ives, P.S. Aronson, J. Seifer. Symposium: Ion transport processes in apical membranes of epithelia. Fed Proc in press (1984)
27. P.B. Dunham, In: D.G. Warnock, R. Greger, P.B. Dunham, R.A. Frizzel, M. Field, K.R. Spring, H.E. Ives, P.S. Aronson, J. Sefier. Symposium: Ion transport processes in apical membranes of epithelia. Fed Proc in press (1984)
28. B. Forbusch III and H.C. Palfrey, J Biol Chem 258:11787-11792 (1983)
29. M. Haas and T. J. McManus, Am J Physiol 245:C235-C240 (1983)
30. R. Greger and E. Schlatter, Klin Wochenschr 61:1019-1027 (1983)
31. O.A. Candia, In: Anion Proton Trans. (Ann N Y Acad Sci 1980) pp. 117-124
32. R. Greger, M. Wittner, E. Schlatter, A. Di Stefano, In: Coupled transport in Nephron, T.Hoshi ed. (Miura Foundation, Tokyo 1984)in press
33. R. Greger and E. Schlatter, Pflügers Arch submitted (1984)
34. W.B. Guggino, H. Oberleithner, G. Giebisch, J Gen Physiol submitted (1984)
35. M. Wittner, C. Weidtke, E. Schlatter, A. Di Stefano, R. Greger, Pflügers Arch submitted (1984)
36. R. Greger, E. Schlatter, C. Weidtke, Wittner M, Pflügers Arch 394:65 (1982)
37. E. Schlatter and R. Greger, Pflügers Arch 394:64 (1982)
38. R. Greger and E. Frömter, In: Kidney and Body Fluids, L. Takacs, ed. (Adv Physiol Sci, Pergamon Press, Budapest, Vol 11) pp. 375-379 (1981)

SITE AND MODE OF DIURETIC ACTION

PETER DEETJEN
Institute of Physiology, University of Innsbruck,
Fritz-Pregl-Str. 3, A-6010 Innsbruck, Austria

Tested in experiments in vitro a diuretic substance like Furosemide is able to inhibit ionic transfer through the membranes of many cell types like gall bladder, intestinum, renal tubule, sweat and salivary glands, frog skin, Ehrlich ascites tumor cells or erythrocytes. However, in vivo only diuresis becomes apparent. Thus, only the solute and water flux across the tubular epithelium is markedly inhibited. Even at doses with maximal diuretic effect, the function of all other cells remains apparently nearly uninfluenced. Therefore, a mechanism must be operative that concentrates the action of diuretic substances solely on the kidney.

Almost all of the modern saluretic substances like Hydrochlorothiazide and its derivatives or the high ceiling diuretics such as Furosemide are all weak organic electrolytes. As such they undergo a very special handling in the kidney. Due to a certain binding affinity to plasma albumen their filtration may be rather restricted. In the case of Furosemide this binding is in the range between 20 and 95% [1,3,8], depending on the analyzing conditions and the animal species. However, like many other organic acids Furosemide undergoes a rather effective tubular secretion.

We have measured the kinetics using the technique of continuous microperfusion of rat proximal tubules in vivo et situ [6]. When perfused with a steady-state solution, which garantees a volume constant flow, the secretion rate of a tested substance can be measured under controlled conditions (Fig. 1). With increasing plasma concentration of Furosemide the proximal tubular

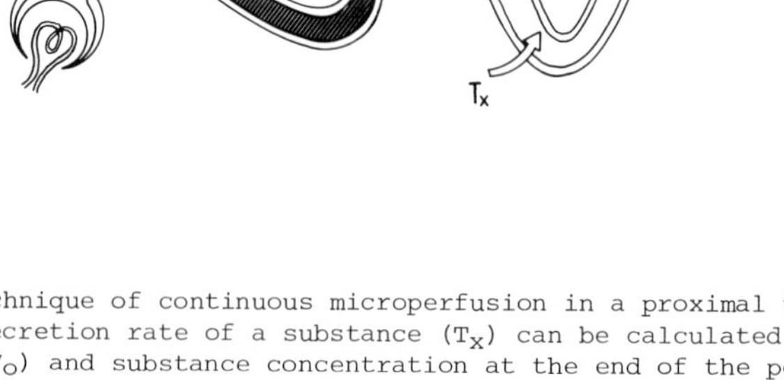

FIG. 1. Technique of continuous microperfusion in a proximal tubular segment. The secretion rate of a substance (T_x) can be calculated from perfusion rate ($\dot{V}_o$) and substance concentration at the end of the perfusion distance (C_x).

Diuretics, Jules B. Puschett, Editor

fluid concentration increases to an approximately 5 times higher concentration due to tubular secretion untill a maximal concentration of about 2 mmol/l is reached (Fig. 2). A further increase in plasma concentration apparently leads to self depression of the secretory mechanism and does not augment the Furosemide concentration of the tubular fluid any more under these conditions of volume constant perfusion.

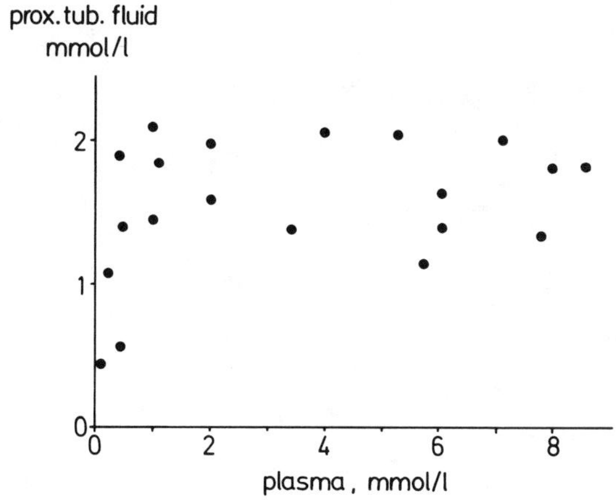

FIG. 2. Secretion of Furosemide in single proximal tubules of rat kidneys during volume constant perfusion at $2 \cdot 10^{-9}$ l $\cdot$ min^{-1}.

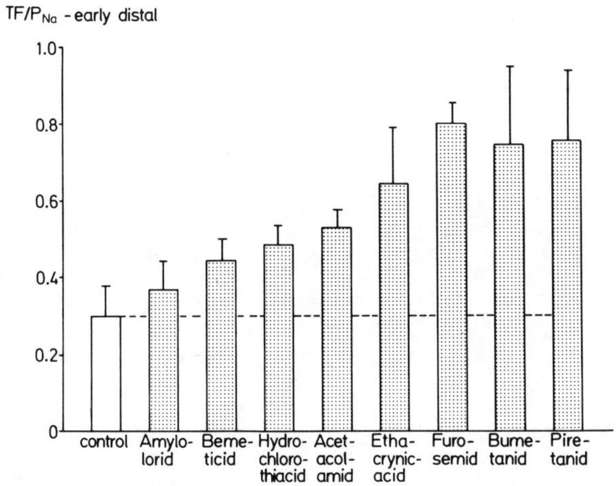

FIG. 3. Ratio of sodium concentration in tubular fluid at the end of Henle's loop during free flow (under control conditions and under the action of several diuretic substances) and of plasma in rat experiments (mean ± SEM).

In this elevated concentration Furosemide arrives at the loop of Henle, where in the luminal membrane of the thick ascending limb of Henle's loop (TAL) a main site of diuretic action is located [2,4,9].

This becomes apparent in simple screening experiments during free flow by sampling early distal tubular fluid and analyzing it for Na^+ or Cl^-. In the normal kidney the reabsorption of NaCl in the TAL and the low water permeability of this nephron segment results in a low NaCl concentration of the tubular fluid of only 1/3 of the plasma concentration (TF/P_{Na} 0.3). During the action of several diuretic substances - always measured at the peak of diuresis - early distal TF/P_{Na} is increased and approaches 1.0 with the so called high ceiling diuretics, indicating a then almost complete blockade of NaCl reabsorption in TAL (Fig. 3).

This effect, however, could at least partially be due to an inhibition of proximal solute and volume reabsorption. Since the capacity of TAL to lower tubular NaCl concentration decreases with increasing flow rate, an augmented load to Henle's loop would result in the same findings [10].

To more directly demonstrate diuretic effects in the loop of Henle, we again applied the technique of continuous microperfusion. From a pipette inserted at the end of the proximal convolution, loops were perfused at a low perfusion rate of 10 nl/min with Ringer's solution containing the diuretic to be tested and H^3-Inulin as a reference substance (Fig. 4).

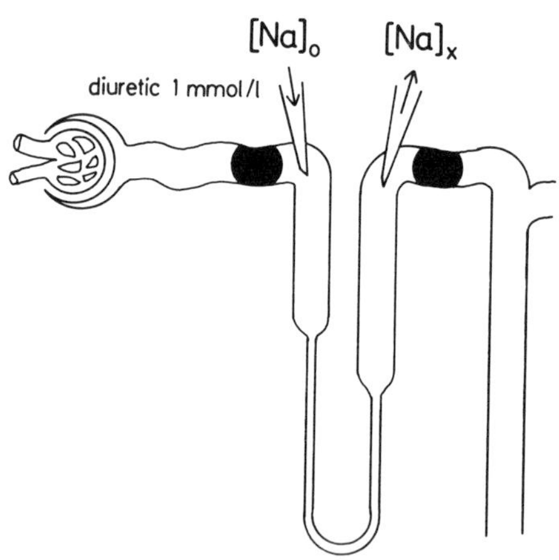

FIG. 4. Technique of continuous microperfusion of a single loop of Henle in vivo et situ.

During control conditions the sodium concentration of 145 mmol/l of the perfusion solution is lowered to about 50 mmol/l at the end of Henle's loop. Fig. 5 demonstrates that all 4 diuretics which we tested inhibited sodium reabsorption considerably. From the differences between control and experimental values it can be calculated that about 75% of sodium reabsorption was inhibited during Furosemide exposure. Interestingly enough this also is true for Bemetizid, which under free flow conditions only exhibited a much smaller effect in the loop of Henle, or with Tizolemide in which fractional Na excretion is only about 1/10 of that of Piretanide. Therefore, the question

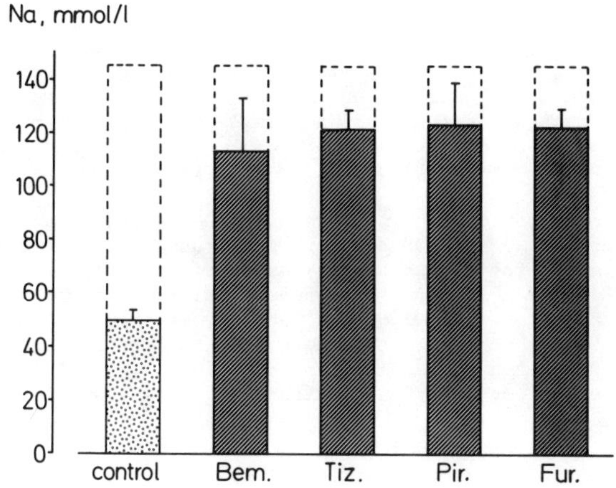

FIG. 5. Sodium concentration in early distal tubular fluid following continuous microperfusion of single loops of Henle with Ringer's solution under control conditions and under the action of several diuretic substances (mean ± SEM).

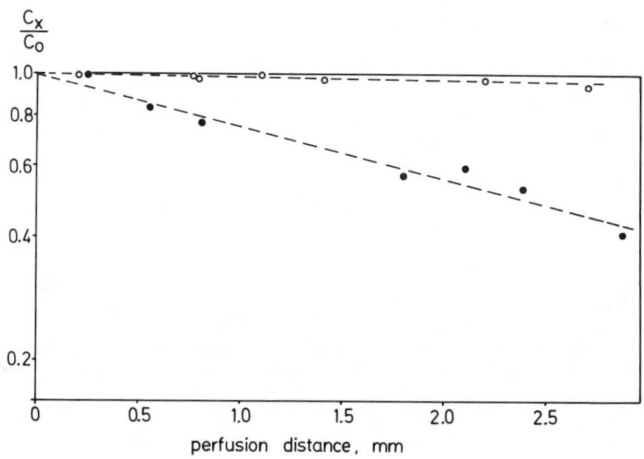

FIG. 6. Permeability of diuretic substances in the proximal convolution of rat kidneys. Microperfusion experiments with C^{14}-labelled Furosemide (⊙) and Bemetizide (●). The ratio of the concentration at the sample site (C_x) and of the perfusion solution (C_o) decreases exponentially. Permeability (P) is calculated by

$$P = \dot{V} \quad \frac{1}{2\pi r} \cdot \frac{1}{x} \cdot \ln \frac{C_x}{C_o}$$

($\dot{V}$: perfusion flow rate, r: radius of the perfused tubular lumen, x: length of the perfused tubular segment).

arises whether the different diuretic substances undergo a different handling in the kidney and as a result come up with different concentrations at the TAL.

As pointed out already, the main route by which weak organic electrolytes get into the tubular fluid is via secretion along the proximal tubule. However, the amount of substance which finally is accumulated there, also depends on the fact whether a substance is leaking back or not. This can be tested by volume constant perfusion of tubular segments when the substance to be tested is isotope-labelled and added in tracer amounts.

Fig. 6 demonstrates that in the proximal convolution almost no Furosemide leaves the tubular fluid. However, in a substance like Bemetizide the concentration along the perfused sections decreases compared to the initial concentration in the perfusate. The concentration decrease has an exponential slope (linear in a semi-log plot) and allows calculation of the tubular permeability of each substance. While the proximal tubule is almost impermeable to Furosemide it has a significant permeability for the other substances under investigation, which is in the range between glucose and urea (Fig. 7).

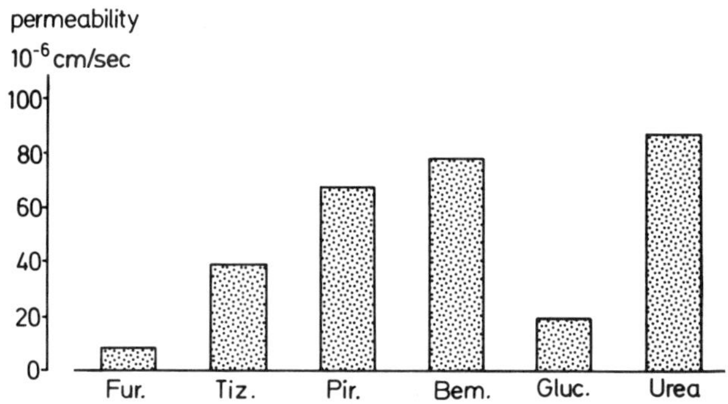

FIG. 7. Permeability constants of several diuretic substances in the proximal tubular epithelium compared to glucose and urea.

A similar type of experiment can be done in the loop of Henle: The loop is perfused with Ringer's solution containing labelled diuretic substances in tracer amounts. The recovery of the substance at an early distal puncture site compared with the initial concentration $(\frac{C_x}{C_o})$ is an approximative measure of loop permeability. Again, the highest leakage is found for Bemetizide (Fig. 8).

A compilation of many such micropuncture and microperfusion experiments offers some model conception where a diuretic is acting and to what extent it becomes available at the site of action [5]. In a drug like Furosemide all the substance that is accumulated in the tubular fluid by filtration and mainly by secretion remains there and is rapidly excreted with the final urine. Since it has no significant effect on proximal reabsorption processes it is further concentrated by solvent reduction and reaches

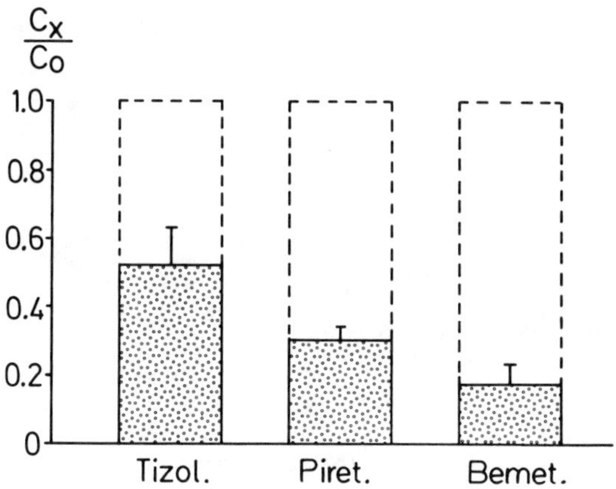

FIG. 8. Activity ratio of C^{14}-labelled diuretic substances in early distal tubular fluid (C_x) and in the perfusion solution (C_o) during continuous microperfusion in vivo et situ of single loops of Henle in rat kidneys.

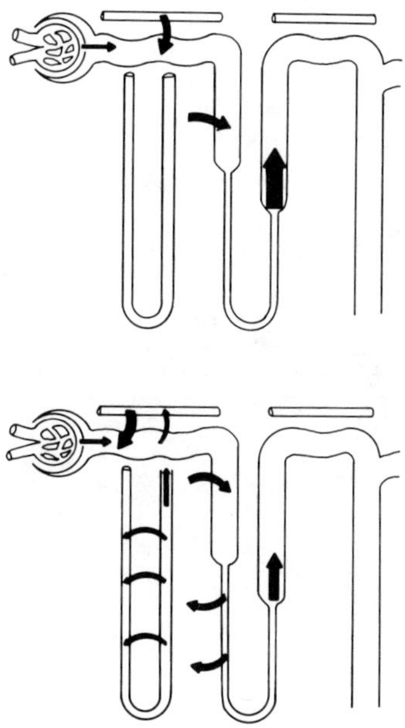

FIG. 9. Nephron scheme illustrating the handling of diuretic substances. Due to some protein binding most of the substances show restricted filtration. They are, however, accumulated by proximal tubular secretion. The highest concentration at the main site of action, the ascending thick ascending limb, is built up when there is no significant back diffusion neither in the proximal tubule nor in the loop of Henle (upper part, e.g. Furosemide). If the substance recirculates in the cortex and/or medulla (lower part, e.g. Bemetizide) effective concentration is kept for a longer periode but on a lower level.

its main site of attack, the TAL, in high concentration. It's strong action there, however, is of relatively short duration (Fig. 9, above). The other extreme of our examples is Bemetizide (Fig. 9, below). It also undergoes proximal tubular secretion but since it possesses a significant proximal permeability it diffuses back following a concentration gradient, which is built up by the secretory process as well as by volume reduction. This substance, therefore, is delivered to Henle's loop and the distal nephron in smaller amounts and a lower concentration. However, due to the recirculation of the substance its elimination is delayed and it, therefore, exerts a moderate but rather prolonged action. Regarding our other examples, the renal handling of Piretanide is similar to that of Furosemide, and therefore resembles its efficacity and relatively short time of action. Tizolemide, on the other hand, is a weak organic base. As such it uses a different transport system by which organic cations are effectively accumulated in the tubular fluid [7]. Since, however, Tizolemide undergoes some back diffusion, it exhibits a lower saluretic potency but of longer duration.

REFERENCES

1. F. Andreasen and P. Jakobsen, Determination of Furosemide in Blood Plasma and its Binding to Proteins in Normal Plasma and in Plasma from Patients with Acute Renal Failure, Acta Pharmacol. Toxic. 35, 49-57 (1977).
2. M. Burg, L. Stoner, J. Cardinal, and N. Green, Furosemide Effect on isolated perfused Tubules, Am. J. Physiol. 225, 119-124 (1973).
3. P. Deetjen, Micropuncture Studies on Site and Mode of Diuretic Action of Furosemide, Ann. N.Y. Acad. Sci. 139, 408-415 (1966).
4. P. Deetjen, The Localization of Transport Processes in the Nephron and their Inhibition by Diuretic Agents as analyzed by Micropuncture Techniques. In: Renal Transport and Diuretics, K. Thurau and J. Jahrmaerker, eds. (Springer, Berlin-Heidelberg-New York 1969) pp. 215-226.
5. P. Deetjen, Der Einfluß des tubulären Transportes von Diuretica auf ihren Wirkungsmechanismus. In: Diuretica II, F. Krück and A. Schrey, eds. (C. Wolf und Sohn, München 1981) pp. 13-18.
6. P. Deetjen and S. Silbernagl, Some new Developments in Continuous Microperfusion Technique, Yale J. Biol. Med. 45, 301-306 (1972).
7. B. Odlind, Renal Tubular Secretion and Effects of the Alcaline Diuretics Amiloride, Tizolemide and MK 447, Naunyn-Schmiedebergs Arch. Pharmacol. 317, 357-363 (1981).
8. B. Odlind, Determinants of Access of Diuretics to their Site of Action, Fed. Proc. 42, 1703-1706 (1983).
9. E. Schlatter, R. Greger, and C. Weidtke, Effect of "High Ceiling" Diuretics on Active Salt Transport in the Cortical Thick Ascending Limb of Henle's Loop of Rabbit Kidney, Pflügers Arch. 396, 210-217 (1983).
10. J. Seely and J. Dirks, Site of Action of Diuretic Drugs, Kidney Int. 11, 1-8 (1977).

STUDY OF DIURETIC SITES AND MECHANISMS OF ACTION IN THE HUMAN SUBJECT.

JULES B. PUSCHETT, M.D., Renal-Electrolyte Division, Department of Medicine, University of Pittsburgh School of Medicine, Pittsburgh, PA 15261 U.S.A.

INTRODUCTION

The investigation of the mode and site of action of diuretics in the nephron has involved five major techniques: 1) The clearance procedure, which can be utilized in both experimental animals and man; 2) The micropuncture technique; 3) The isolated tubule technique, which allows one to study individual defined nephron segments; 4) Cell culture methodology; and 5) Brush border and plasma membrane vesicle techniques. This discussion will involve the application of the clearance technique in the study of diuretic mechanism and locus of action in the human subject, a species in which the other techniques are generally not yet possible.

In assessing diuretic effects on the kidney, we look at principally four features of the drug's action: 1) Its effects on the concentrating and diluting mechanisms, 2) The pattern of anionic excretion it produces, 3) Its effects, if any, on acid excretion, and 4) The alteration in potassium, which accompanies the natriuresis.

Let us discuss first the manner in which we can utilize the physiological principles involved in urinary dilution and concentration to determine drug site of action.

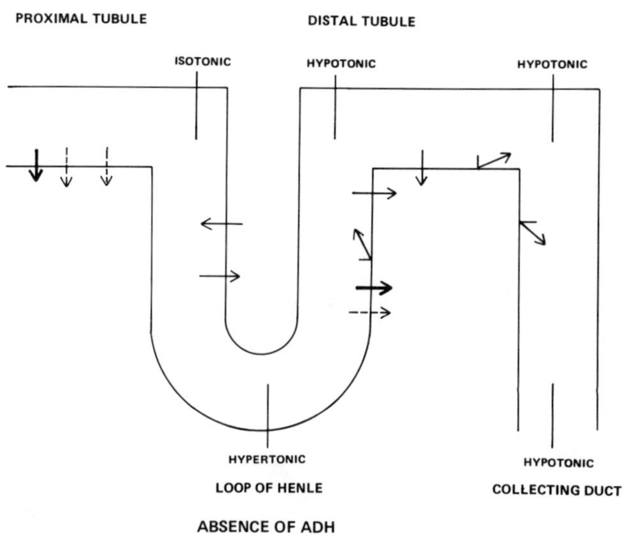

Figure 1. Nephron diagram illustrating the sites of water transport during water diuresis (ADH suppression).

Diuretics, Jules B. Puschett, Editor

In figure 1 is presented a diagram of the nephron to illustrate the situation which exists with regard to water transport when antidiuretic hormone (ADH) is suppressed. Normally, 60-70% of the salt and water is reabsorbed in the proximal nephron, in an isotonic manner. Therefore, the tubular fluid as it leaves the proximal tubule has the same osmolality as it did when first formed in Bowman's space, that is, it is isotonic to plasma. As the fluid traverses the descending limb of the loop of Henle, water is removed and solute is added, such that the fluid at the hairpin turn has become hypertonic to plasma. However, the amount of fluid leaving the segment is small, and need not enter into our subsequent considerations. In the ascending limb of the loop of Henle, sodium chloride is removed from the tubular contents. However, the tubular epithelium behaves as if it is impermeant to water. Accordingly, the process of urinary dilution is accomplished in this nephron segment. That is, the tubular fluid has been freed of some of its solute, the tubular contents have therefore been diluted, and solute-free water has been generated. The symbol for solute-free water is CH_2O. Thus, the fluid which issues from the loop of Henle and enters the distal convoluted tubule is now hypotonic to plasma. Whether the final urine will be concentrated or dilute, now depends crucially upon the presence or absence of ADH. When ADH is absent the dilute tubular contents are excreted, because without ADH, the distal convolution and the collecting duct are likewise essentially impermeant to water [1].

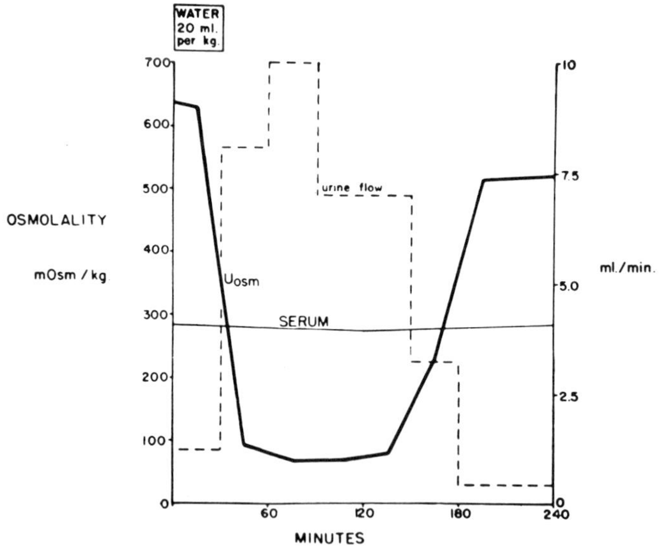

Figure 2. Diagram of the alterations in urinary (Uosm) and serum osmolality and urinary flow rate in a normal subject given an oral water level. Reproduced, with the permission of the editors from Med. Clin. No. Am. 47:915-933, 1963.

If one places a subject in a quiet room, prohibits smoking and asks him or her to drink 20 ml of water per kg of body weight over 30 minutes to one hour, the sequence of events depicted in figure 2, occurs. Serum osmolality falls slightly, causing antidiuretic hormone secretion to be inhibited. Next, urinary osmolality begins to fall as urinary flow rate rises. Most of our subjects have been able to reach a final urinary osmolality below 100 mOsm/kg. If, instead of allowing serum osmolality to rise, one continues to provide water to drink in equivalent amounts each time the subject voids, a state of maximal, sustained water diuresis develops. It is this technique which we have used to assess the actions of various diuretics on the diluting mechanism. That is, we have superimposed administration of the diuretic on sustained water diuresis.

Solute-free water formation or clearance, CH_2O, can be quantified by measuring urinary flow rate, V, and urine as well as plasma osmolality. Since urine flow rate is equal to the clearance of free water (CH_2O) plus solute clearance (Cosm), we can calculate CH_2O by subtracting Cosm from V.

Several important implications result from these physiological principles [2]. First, when ADH is absent, there is a second diluting site located in the early distal convoluted tubule. Here, again, sodium chloride is being transported out of the tubular lumen, but the water stays behind. This site, known as the cortical diluting site, does not generate as much solute-free water as does the loop of Henle, because sodium transport here is only about 5-8% of filtered load, whereas in the loop, it may be as high as 30%. Second, if a drug interferes with sodium chloride reabsorption at either the cortical diluting site or in the ascending limb of the loop of Henle, free water formation, CH_2O, will be decreased, because the drug is interfering with the process of urinary dilution. A minor reduction in CH_2O caused by a diuretic could mean either a major effect on the part of the drug at the cortical diluting site, or a modest interference with transport at the loop of Henle. However, a <u>marked</u> reduction in CH_2O would have to mean an effect of the drug in the loop of Henle, wherever else it might work in the nephron.

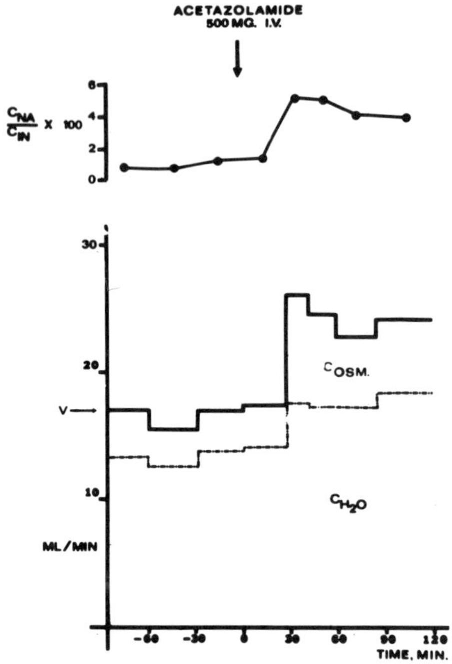

Figure 3. Effects of the administration of acetazolamide (500 mg intravenously, given at the arrow) on the percentage of sodium excreted (C_{Na}/C_{In} x 100), urine flow rate (V), solute clearance (Cosm) and free water clearance (CH_2O). This study was performed in a normal volunteer undergoing maximal steady-state water diuresis.

Alternatively, a drug which inhibits sodium transport in the proximal nephron would present increased amounts of salt and water to the diluting sites. As a consequence, such an agent would be expected to <u>increase</u> CH_2O. Presented in figure 3 is the diagram of a study performed in a normal volunteer undergoing steady-state water diuresis induced by water loading. At the arrow, he was given 500 mg of acetazolamide (Diamox). The percentage of filtered sodium excreted rose rapidly to about 5%. This was accomplished by an increase in urine flow rate, V, an increase in osmolal clearance, Cosm, which largely represents sodium bicarbonate, and an <u>increase</u> in CH_2O. Thus, acetazolamide appears to have a major effect in the <u>proximal</u> nephron.

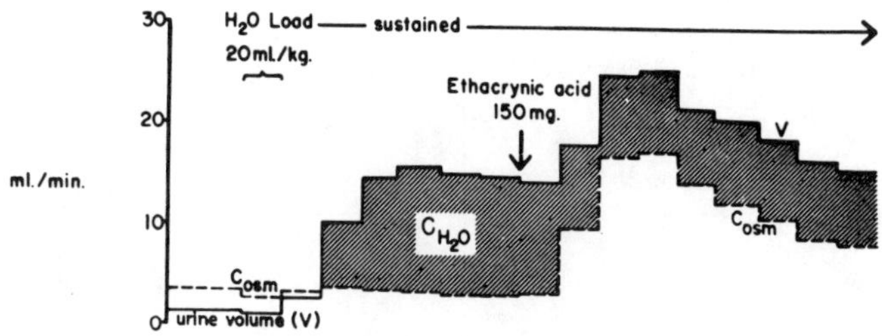

Figure 4. The alteration in free water clearance (CH_2O), urine flow rate (V) and osmolal clearance (Cosm) induced by orally administered ethacrynic acid (given at the arrow) in a water diuretic normal volunteer. Reproduced from Goldberg, et al, J. Clin. Invest. 43:201-216, 1964, with permission.

Shown in figure 4 is another water diuresis study in which the subject received ethacrynic acid, 150 mg by mouth. Shortly after the drug was given, absolute urinary salt excretion rose dramatically. This was associated with a marked reduction in free water clearance, CH_2O. Accordingly, it seemed likely that ethacrynic acid impaired sodium chloride transport in the loop of Henle.

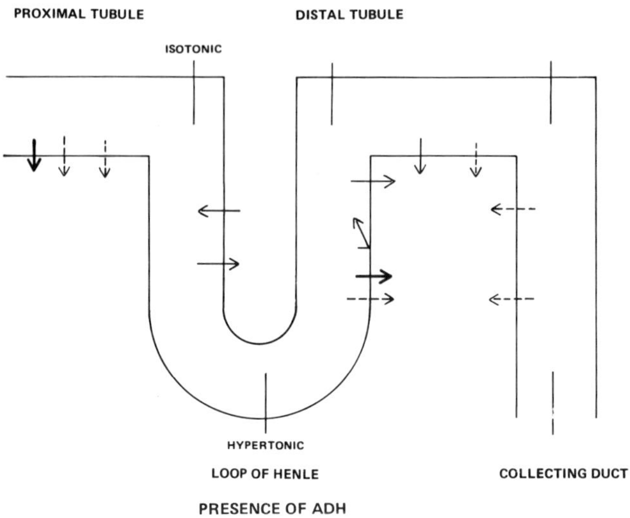

Figure 5. Nephron diagram illustrating the sites of water transport during hydropenia, in which circumstance ADH effect is present.

Let's now consider the opposite situation, that is, the effect on tubular water transport when ADH is present, rather than absent (figure 5). Notice that everything is the same as in figure 1 through the proximal nephron and the loop of Henle. At this point, a difference occurs. When ADH is present, the tubular epithelium of the distal convolution and the collecting duct behave as if they are "leaky", so that water flows back into the hypertonic medullary interstitium. The medulla is hypertonic for two reasons: 1) salt and urea have been deposited there by active transport mechanisms, and 2) the counter-current system has been functioning to increase the tonicity of the medulla as one proceeds from outer to inner portions of this part of the kidney. Since the abstraction of water from the collecting duct depends, therefore, upon normal loop of Henle functioning, a diuretic which interferes with sodium chloride transport in the ascending limb of the loop of Henle would be expected to interfere with water abstraction from the collecting duct, the symbol for which is T^cH_2O [2].

T^cH_2O can also be quantified since it represents negative free water clearance. We can therefore calculate it as equal to solute clearance (Cosm) minus V, urinary flow rate. The measured parameters, as before, are urinary and plasma osmolality, as well as V.

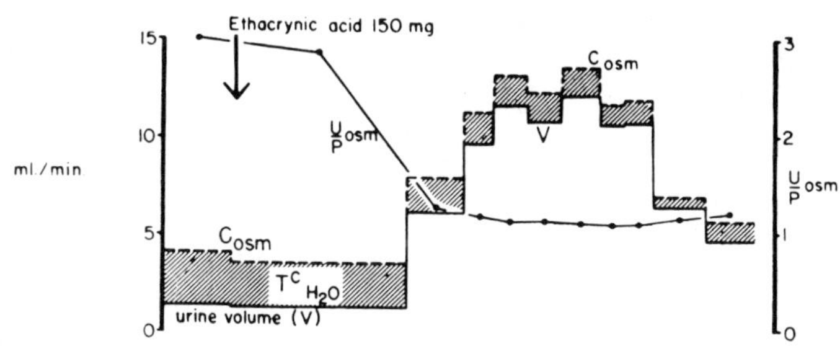

Figure 6. Studies performed in a hydropenic normal volunteer to whom an infusion of hypertonic saline was given to induce an increase in solute clearance (Cosm). The simultaneous effects on Cosm and on the reabsorption of solute free water (T^cH_2O) due to the administration of ethacrynic acid are depicted. Reproduced from Goldberg, et al, J. Clin. Invest. 43:201-216, 1964, with permission.

In the studies shown in figure 6, as opposed to those discussed earlier (figures 3 & 4), the subjects were hydropenic, rather than water diuretic. Hypertonic saline was administered to increase urinary flow rate and solute clearance. In figure 6, solute clearance (Cosm) is plotted on the abscissa vs. water abstraction, T^cH_2O, on the ordinate. In the control study, as Cosm was increased by the infusion of hypertonic saline, T^cH_2O rose progressively, peaking at about 7 ml/min and then declining slightly. The subject was brought back two weeks later and the same protocol was followed, except that when Cosm had increased, ethacrynic acid was given. As noted in figure 6, ethacrynic acid caused a dramatic reduction in T^cH_2O. These data, taken together with the free water findings presented earlier (figure 4), helped the investigators to reach the conclusion that ethacrynic acid is natriuretic largely due to its ability to inhibit sodium chloride reabsorption in the ascending limb of the loop of Henle [3].

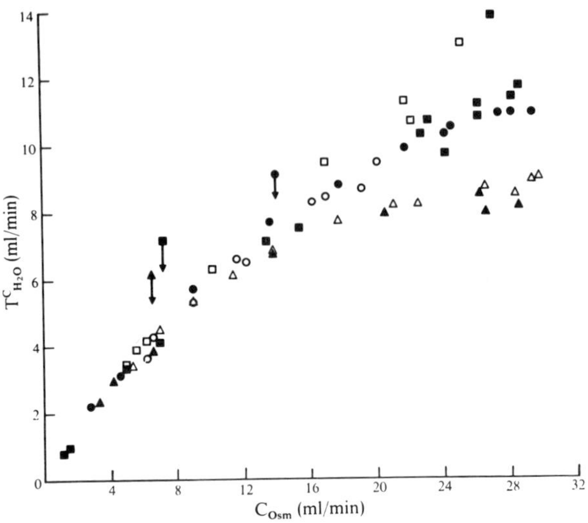

Figure 7. Studies performed in three subjects infused with hypertonic saline only (open symbols) and, in separate experiments, with the addition of metolazone, 1 mg intravenously (closed symbols), given at the arrows. The data for each individual (open vs. closed symbols) are virtually superimposable. From Steinmuller, S.R. and Puschett, J.B. Kidney International, 1:169-181, 1972. Reproduced with permission of the editors.

Shown in figure 7 are the studies of three hydropenic subjects infused with hypertonic saline according to the protocol just described. Experiments in which hypertonic saline alone was administered are presented along with data obtained in the same subjects who were later studied during the addition of the diuretic agent, metolazone, in a dose of 1-3 mg, given intravenously. Again, as in the previous study, $T^{C}H_2O$ increased as solute clearance rose because of the hypertonic saline infusion. In two of the subjects, $T^{C}H_2O$ continued to rise, whereas in one study it appeared to level off. If one compares the control study and that during which the diuretic was administered, the data for each of the three subjects is virtually superimposable. These observations, therefore, allowed us to conclude that wherever in the nephron metolazone works, it is not effective in inhibiting sodium reabsorption in the loop of Henle [4].

Let us move on, now, to a consideration of the means by which one can utilize the pattern of anionic excretion induced by a drug to determine site and mechanism of action. The proximal nephron is a major locus for the reabsorption of both bicarbonate and phosphate. In fact, it has been estimated, based largely on micropuncture data, that 80-90% of the filtered bicarbonate is reabsorbed proximally and that almost all of the phosphate which will be reabsorbed is transported proximally as well. Therefore, if a diuretic causes both a phosphaturia and a bicarbonate diuresis, it seems reasonable to conclude that it works, at least in part, in the proximal nephron [5]. We evaluated this thesis by looking at the effects of three drugs: acetazolamide, furosemide and ethacrynic acid.

Shown in figure 8 are the changes from control levels in the percentage excretion of bicarbonate for the three drugs. Acetazolamide, the prototype carbonic anhydrase inhibitor, was the most bicarbonaturic. Ethacrynic acid was inconsistent in its effects on bicarbonate excretion. Furosemide was significantly bicarbonaturic, although not to the extent demonstrated for acetazolamide.

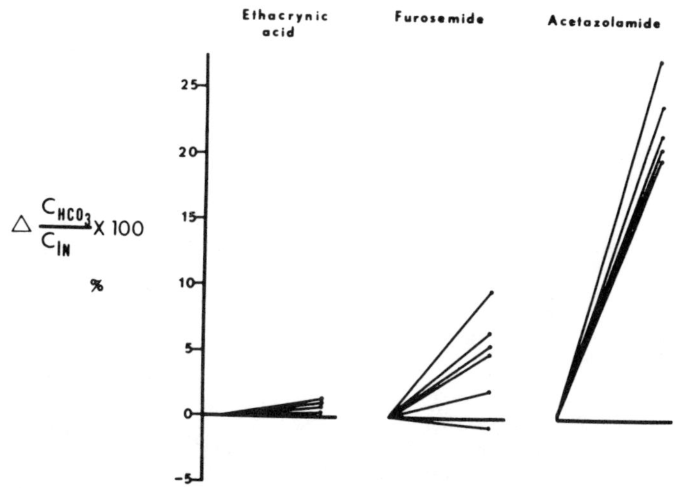

Figure 8. Alterations in the percentage of filtered bicarbonate excreted (C_{HCO_3}/C_{In} x 100) induced by the administration of acetazolamide, furosemide and ethacrynic acid.

Do these observations with regard to bicarbonate excretion reflect the capacity of the drugs to alter proximal transport? If so, their individual actions on phosphate excretion should have been similar.

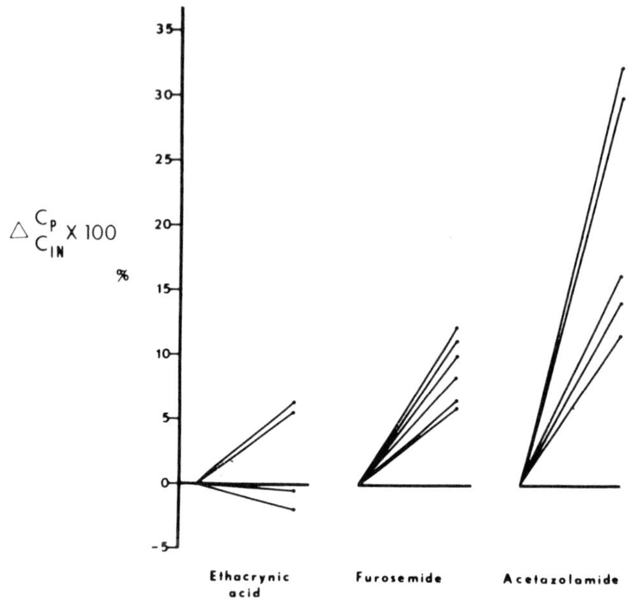

Figure 9. Alterations in the percentage of filtered phosphate excreted (Cp/C_{In} x 100) following the administration of acetazolamide, furosemide and ethacrynic acid.

Alterations in percentage phosphate excretion induced by each of the three agents are depicted in figure 9. Notice that the excretion pattern for phosphate is similar to that just described for bicarbonate. Acetazolamide caused a marked increase in phosphate excretion, ethacrynic acid had little, if any effect, and furosemide, while causing a substantial increase in the excretion of this ion, was not as phosphaturic as acetazolamide. These data, therefore, strongly suggest that both acetazolamide and furosemide have proximal tubular effects, but that ethacrynic acid does not. What might be the basis for these differences? The answer to this question most probably lies in the chemical structures of these agents (figure 10). Both acetazolamide and furosemide have as part of their structures, an unsubstituted SO_2NH2, or sulfonamido, group. This is the grouping recognized as necessary for carbonic anhydrase inhibition. Indeed, these two drugs are effective inhibitors of carbonic anhydrase in vitro [5]. Since, as discussed earlier, the majority of bicarbonate is reabsorbed proximally, it is not surprising that agents capable of carbonic anhydrase inhibition should have a proximal effect. Furthermore, alkalinization of the urine is a very reproducible method for inducing a phosphaturia [6]. Ethacrynic acid, on the other hand, is a derivative of phenoxyacetic acid, has no sulfonamido group, is not a carbonic anhydrase inhibitor, and therefore would not be expected to have proximal activity.

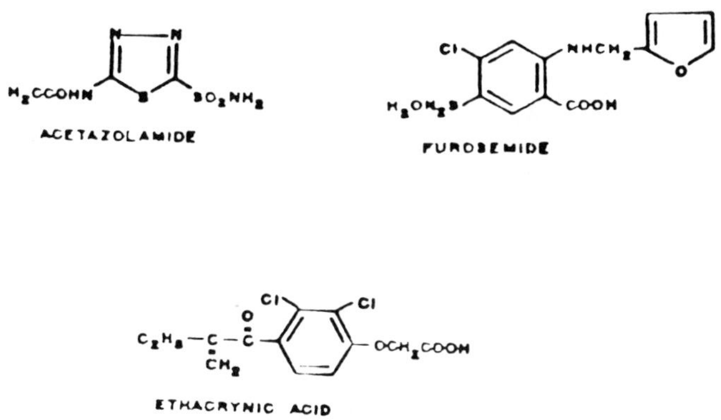

Figure 10. Chemical structure of the diuretic drugs utilized in the studies depicted in figure 9 and 10.

The third item of interest to renal pharmacologists, in their study of the renal tubular actions of diuretic agents, is the effect that the drug has on the parameters of acid excretion. Net acid excretion includes three processes. First, the reabsorption of bicarbonate. Second, the secretion of hydrogen ion into the tubular lumen where it may attach to urinary buffers, such as phosphate, a process called the excretion of titratable acid. Third, the combination of secreted hydrogen ion with ammonia gas to form ammonium ions, which are then excreted. Diuretics could be expected to affect one or more of these processes, depending upon where in the nephron they work, and to what extent. An example of an evaluation of this kind is shown in figure 11.

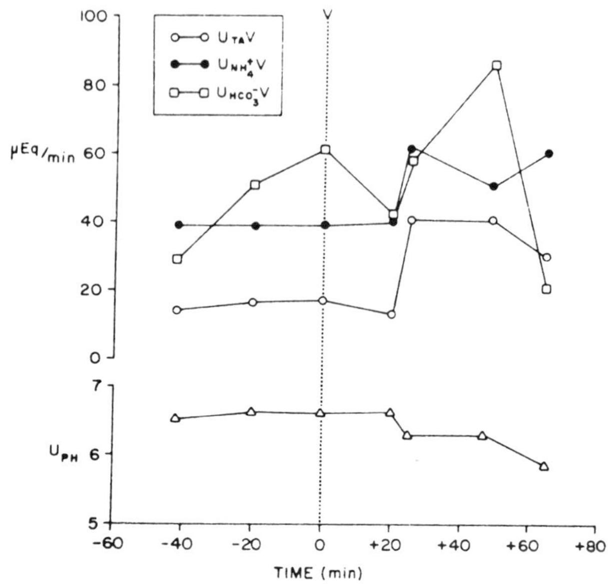

Figure 11. The effect of bumetanide on the acid excretion of a normal volunteer given 1 mg of bumetanide intravenously at time zero. Parameters measured in addition to urinary pH (UpH) included the excretion of titratable acid (UTAV), ammonium ($U_{NH_4^+}V$) and bicarbonate ($U_{HCO_3^-}V$). Reproduced from J. Pharm. Exp. Ther. 201:251-258, 1977, with permission.

In this representative study, the parameters of acid excretion were evaluated before and after administration of bumetanide (Bumex). Bicarbonate excretion rose after the drug was administered. However, so did acid excretion, expressed as titratable acid, and ammonium excretion. The result of these off-setting effects was that urinary pH changed very little. Mean values for 5 such studies showed no change in urinary pH [7].

Finally, it is important to identify the effects of diuretic agents on potassium excretion, both from a physiological as well as a clinical standpoint. My colleagues and I have examined the relationship between sodium and potassium excretion for a number of currently utilized drugs [8]. Shown in figure 12 are the changes from control levels in percentage potassium excretion as a function of the simultaneous increment in percentage sodium excretion for five diuretics. The major point to be made is that, in a general way, the greater the natriuresis, the greater the kaliuresis. Notice, however, that the carbonic anhydrase inhibitor, acetazolamide, was the most kaliuretic agent, causing much greater potassium excretion at equivalent rates of sodium excretion, than any of the other drugs.

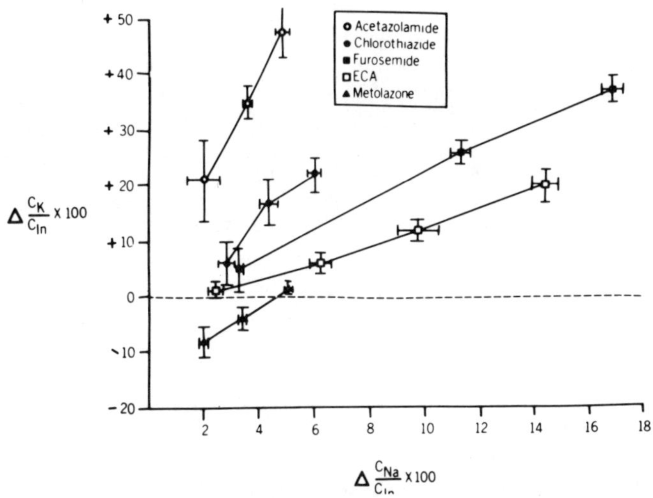

Figure 12. The effects of five diuretic agents on the alteration in the percentage of filtered potassium excreted ($\Delta C_K/C_{In}$ x 100) vs. the simultaneously induced increment in percentage sodium excretion ($\Delta C_{Na}/C_{In}$ x 100). The studies were performed in normal volunteers. Reproduced, with permission of the editors, from Clin. Pharm. Ther. 15:397-405, 1974.

Utilizing the kinds of studies outlined above, it has been possible to compile a list of the relative potencies and sites of action of the currently employed drugs (Table 1). In the moderately potent group are the thiazides and metolazone which act primarily at the cortical diluting site in the early distal tubule, causing a maximal excretion of from 5-8% of filtered sodium load. The loop diuretics, furosemide, bumetanide, ethacrynic acid and the mercurials, are much more potent, resulting in the excretion of up to 25% of filtered sodium. Acetazolamide, which acts largely proximally, is only a modestly potent diuretic, usually causing a sodium excretion of 3-5%. Finally, the special purpose agents, spironolactone, triamterene and amiloride are utilized mainly for their ability to reduce potassium excretion. They are only mildly effective as natriuretic agents, causing the excretion of sodium to increase only to about 2-3% of filtered load.

TABLE I. Relative potencies and sites of action of the currently employed diuretic agents.

Drug	Major Nephron Site of Action	Potency*
acetazolamide	proximal nephron	3-5%
thiazides	early distal tubule	5-8%
metolazone	early distal tubule	5-8%
furosemide	ascending limb, loop of Henle	20-25%
bumetanide	ascending limb, loop of Henle	15-20%
ethacrynic acid	ascending limb, loop of Henle	20-25%
mercurials	ascending limb, loop of Henle	15-20%
spironolactone	late distal tubule and collecting duct	2-3%
triamterene	late distal tubule and collecting duct	2-3%
amiloride	late distal tubule and collecting duct	2-3%

*Expressed as the maximal percentage of filtered sodium which can be delivered into the final urine.

REFERENCES

1. M. Goldberg, Abnormalities in the renal excretion of water. Pathophysiology and differential diagnosis. Med. Clin. No. Am. 47:915-933, 1963.
2. J.B. Puschett, Sites and mechanisms of action of diuretics in the kidney. J. Clin. Pharm. 21:564-574, 1981.
3. M. Goldberg, D.K. McCurdy, E.L. Foltz, and L.W. Bluemle,Jr., Effects of ethacrynic acid (a new saluretic agent) on renal diluting and concentrating mechanisms: evidence for site of action in the loop of Henle. J. Clin. Invest. 43:201-216, 1964.
4. J.B. Puschett, S.R. Steinmuller, A. Rastegar and P. Fernandez, Metolazone: mechanism and site of action, In, Modern Diuretic Therapy in the Treatment of Cardiovascular and Renal Disease. Excerpta Medica Amsterdam, 1973, pp. 168-178.
5. J.B. Puschett and M. Goldberg, The acute effects of furosemide on acid and electrolyte excretion in man. J. Lab. Clin. Med. 71:666-677, 1979.
6. J.B. Puschett and M. Goldberg, The relationship between the renal handling of phosphate and bicarbonate in man. J. Lab. Clin. Med. 73: 956-969, 1969.
7. S. Jayakumar and J.B. Puschett, Study of the sites and mechanisms of action of bumetanide in man. J. Pharm. Exp. Ther. 201:251-258, 1977.
8. J.B. Puschett and A. Rastegar, Comparative study of the effects of metolazone and other diuretics on potassium excretion. Clin. Pharm. Ther. 15:397-405, 1974.

SECTION VI

DIURETIC COMPLICATIONS AND SIDE EFFECTS

DIURETIC COMPLICATIONS AND TOXIC EFFECTS

William M. Bennett, M.D.; Oregon Health Sciences University, 3181 SW Sam Jackson Park Road, Portland, OR 97201 USA.

ABSTRACT

Diuretic drugs when prescribed by competent physicians and used as directed are remarkably safe therapeutic agents considering the number of prescriptions written. However, certain toxicities do exist which the physician needs to keep in mind to maximize the beneficial effects of these agents. This chapter highlights diuretic toxicities, particularly as they affect the kidney.

DIURETIC-ASSOCIATED RENAL DISEASES

Acute Interstitial Nephritis

A clinicopathologic syndrome consisting of varying degrees of renal dysfunction and renal interstitial inflammation has been linked to diuretics. This is most likely a renal hypersensitivity response since there is not a close relationship between the disease and the dose or duration of therapy. This adverse reaction to diuretics must be quite unusual considering the large number of diuretic prescriptions written.

Lyons et al in 1973 first described the association between diuretics and acute interstitial nephritis in four patients with primary glomerular disorders who had deteriorating renal function out of proportion to the usual course of their primary disease.[1] Renal biopsy showed acute interstitial nephritis superimposed on their known glomerular changes. Eosinophilic infiltration of the renal interstitium was noted on biopsy in all four. Three patients had fever and peripheral eosinophilia while two patients had a non-specific skin rash. With the discontinuation of furosemide or thiazide diuretics and institution of corticosteroids, renal failure was rapidly reversible. One of the patients inadvertently had thiazide diuretics reintroduced and again developed biopsy-proven acute interstitial nephritis. Since the thiazides and furosemide are chemical derivatives of sulfonamides, hypersensitivity to this class of agents was suggested. Similar cases have been documented by other authors with other diuretics containing a sulfonamide-like moeity.[2,3,4] A single case of interstitial nephritis related to the chemically unrelated diuretic triamterene was recently described.[5] It is likely that diuretic-associated interstitial nephritis is seriously underdiagnosed. Interestingly, patients with biopsy proven allergic interstitial nephritis allegedly due to allopurinol or ampicillin were also receiving concomitant diuretic therapy.

Most of the clinical features and pathologic findings in acute interstitial nephritis associated with diuretics are identical to cases due to penicillin derivatives. Interstitial nephritis has been described in patients receiving diuretic treatment only for mild hypertension. The duration of diuretic therapy prior to acute deterioration of renal function is variable but is usually weeks to months. In some cases, the drug has already been stopped when symptoms appear. Variably present is the triad of fever, eosinophilia and a maculopapular skin rash. Loin pain, sometimes severe, may occur along with lymphadenopathy, arthralgias and malaise. Urinalysis shows hematuria (gross or microscopic), sterile

Diuretics, Jules B. Puschett, Editor

pyuria and often eosinophiluria. However, absence of eosinophils in the urine does not exclude the diagnosis. Proteinuria when not present as a part of underlying renal disease is usually less than 2 grams per 24 hours. The severity of renal failure may vary with some patients requiring temporary dialysis support. Since the patient usually has good preservation of urine output, renal dysfunction may be overlooked until renal failure is well-established.[6]

The exact immunologic mechanism or mechanisms responsible for this adverse reaction to diuretics is unclear. It is possible that several mechanisms participate perhaps varying from case to case. It is thought that the drug or some portion of it becomes covalently bound to a renal tissue component. Host reactions are then directed at the drug-hapten-host conjugate.[7] No specific data are available from most cases of acute interstitial nephritis associated with diuretics. The presence of plasma cells and eosinophils in the interstitial infiltrate has been used as evidence for an antibody-mediated immunopathogenesis. Only a few cases have been studied for the presence of granular or linear immunofluoresence with antisera to immunoglobulins or complement. With diuretics there is little direct evidence to support cell-mediated mechanisms except perhaps by analogy to other drug-induced interstitial nephritis. In one case where diuretics were possibly implicated, Husby et al demonstrated T cell infiltration of the renal interstitium.[8] Magill has demonstrated interstitial granuloma formation in nine cases of acute interstitial nephritis, eight of which were associated with diuretics, as further evidence for cell-mediated mechanisms.[9] Thus, regardless of the precise mechanisms involved, epidemiologic data suggests that an allergic or immunologic pathogenesis is likely for diuretic-induced acute interstitial nephritis rather than direct toxic damage. The low prevalence relative to the number of individuals exposed to the drug, the lack of a dose-response relationship, the latency period between exposure and clinical disease and the associated allergic manifestations all support this general type of pathophysiology.

Diuretic-Induced Hyperuricemia and Renal Disease

Hyperuricemia is a frequent complication of diuretic treatment and in some series occurs in 75% of patients treated.[10] Most patients remain asymptomatic, however, in some instances, particularly in individuals with past histories of gout, acute attacks of gouty arthritis may supervene.[11] Thiazides and loop diuretics are prone to raise the serum uric acid. Whether parenchymal renal disease or uric acid nephrolithiasis ever results from diuretic-induced hyperuricemia is unknown.[12] It would appear unlikely since asymptomatic hyperuricemia not associated with diuretic therapy is infrequently, if ever, a cause of nephropathy or stones.[13] Furthermore, hyperuricemia associated with chronic diuretic therapy is accompanied by a decrease in urinary uric acid due to enhanced tubular reabsorption rather than the increased uric acid excretion noted with other hyperuricemic states.[14]

Uricosuric Diuretics and Renal Failure

The introduction of ticrynafen, a potent uricosuric diuretic, was widely accepted as a new approach to diuretic treatment of hypertensive patients. Although the drug was withdrawn from the market in the United States primarily because of reports of hepatic toxicity, some other patients developed oliguric acute renal failure during the drug's brief period of general use. It is well to be aware of this complication, since the goal of therapeutically lowering extracellular fluid volume while avoiding hyperuricemia remains a desirable objective. Both ticrynafen and indacrinone, the two uricosuric diuretic agents which have been used in humans, are phenoxyacetic acid derivatives and as such are chemically related to ethacrynic acid.

Uricosuria produced by ticrynafen is maximal in the first few days of treatment and is greater in magnitude than therapeutic doses of probenecid. Ticrynafen also decreases urinary pH and produces an increase in net renal acid excretion.[15] It could be anticipated that intrarenal uric acid deposition might be a problem particularly when hyperuricemic patients were switched to ticrynafen from other diuretics without volume repletion or a suitable washout period. Indacrinone induces uricosuria within the first six hours of its use but thereafter urate excretion is reduced, resulting in no net change in 24-hour urinary urate.[15] It was recommended that patients with a history of renal stones, hyperuricemia, or gout should force fluids and alkalinize the urine during the first few days of therapy to avoid uric acid stones or intrarenal uric acid deposition.[16]

Hypokalemic Nephropathy

Chronic potassium deficiency produced by diuretics may produce, in rare instances, structural changes in the kidney as well as renal dysfunction. The renal lesion is similar to that seen with chronic potassium depletion from other causes. Characteristically there is vacuolization in the proximal convoluted tubule with only occasional lesions in the distal tubule.[17] This vacuolization is not specific for potassium deficiency since similar findings have been reported following the use of osmotic diuretics.[18]

Cremer and Bock documented the clinical course of 21 patients with longstanding potassium deficiency. Chronic tubulointerstitial nephritis with renal failure developed slowly over 5-10 years. Urinalysis findings were non-specific and hypertension was a late finding. At least four of their patients developed chronic renal failure following the prolonged use of diuretics with consequent potassium depletion. Until frank renal failure was noted, metabolic alkalosis with hypochloremia and hyponatremia were present. Urinary tract infection, although frequently present, was felt to be a consequence rather than a cause of interstitial fibrosis.[19] Conn and Johnson reported 80 cases of hypokalemic nephropathy, most of which were due to cathartic and diuretic abuse in which the extent of damage depended on the duration of hypokalemia.[20] Patients who covertly abuse diuretics often have personality disorders such as depression, hypochondriasis and may demonstrate a preoccupation with their body image. Women predominate and often anorexia nervosa is evident. The patient frequently has an occupational association with the medical profession. Screening the urine of a patient for evidence of diuretics may be diagnostically rewarding.

The pathophysiologic mechanism of progressive interstitial damage from potassium depletion is unclear. Prolonged potassium deficiency in man may increase the kidney's susceptibility to other insults such as bacterial infection or toxic damage from rhabdomyolysis.

Tubular functional changes may accompany the structural abnormalities. Impaired concentrating ability and polyuria are frequently noted. A 2- to 4-month negative potassium balance of approximately 400 mEq was associated with inability to maximally concentrate the urine in 17 diuretic treated patients.[21] Potassium deficiency probably induces vasopressin unresponsiveness by causing release of prostaglandins which antagonize the effect of the vasopressin to generate renal tubular cyclic AMP at the level of the collecting tubule.[22]

Nephrolithiasis

Triamterene is relatively insoluble in water. Peak drug excretion occurs within 1 to 2 hours after oral ingestion. In 1979, Ettinger et al reported a patient who passed approximately 50 mustard-colored stones. Mass spectroscopy showed the stone material to be identical with the drug.[23] Triamterene may be found as the nucleus of the stone or it may be deposited with calcium oxalate or uric acid. Hydroxytriamterene, a drug metabolite, may also be a prominent stone component. Ettinger et al identified triamterene in .4% of 50,000 urinary calculi submitted for analysis.[24] Stones were noted in patients taking recommended doses of triamterene or thiazide-triamterene combinations. The authors estimated that the annual incidence of nephrolithiasis is one stone per 1500 users of triamterene-hydrochlorothiazide combinations.[24] Triamterene given to normal subjects without any renal disease may produce casts which are covered with crystals. These casts give a blue fluorescence in ultraviolet light as does triamterene itself. Free crystals or casts could act as a nidus for stone formation.[25]

DIURETIC-INDUCED OTOTOXICITY

High ceiling diuretics acting in the Loop of Henle are known to produce temporary, as well as, permanent hearing loss. The most significant ototoxin is ethyacrynic acid,[26,27] but furosemide is also capable of producing similar changes.[28] Bumetanide has been reported to produce less ototoxicity in experimental animals.[29] The clinical relevance of any differences observed in experimental animals awaits controlled trials. Loss of hearing can be observed with intravenous use after only a short latency period. It now has become widely known that patients wiht renal failure are at particular risk.

The important synergistic interaction between loop diuretics and aminoglycoside antibiotics has been emphasized by Brummett.[30] This drug combination particularly in patients with renal failure often produces irreversible ototoxicity. In patients the onset of acute loss of hearing may be evident 1/2 to 2 hours after intravenous loop diuretics in a patient receiving concomitant aminoglycosides. Brummett et al could not demonstrate any interaction between aminoglycoside antibiotics and other diuretics such as mannitol, hydrochlorothiazide or mercurials.[31] The cancer chemotherapeutic drug cis-platinum can have additive ototoxicity when used with loop diuretics. Clinicians should be alert for this interaction because of the recommended diuresis necessary to prevent cis-platinum nephrotoxicity.

Loop diuretics cause loss of hair cells and a corresponding functional decrease in cochlear electrical potentials. In cochlear sensory hair cells clumping of nuclear chromatin and loss of subsurface cisternae were seen as early as one hour after ethacrynic acid in guinea pigs, particularly when the animals had received prior aminoglycosides.[30] There was also swelling of the stria vascularis. Eventually hair cells in the organ of corti die with resultant permanent hearing loss.[31] Loop diuretics alone produce reversible changes in the stria vascularitis which usually corresponds temporally to the transient hearing loss.

Vestibular symptoms or signs are not generally a feature of diuretic ototoxicity. However, temporary alterations of vestibular function have been reported after the administration of ethacrynic acid.[32] In animals structural changes in the vestibular apparatus have not been noted after large doses of loop diuretics. Loop diuretics, as with other classes of drugs, may produce tinnitus with or without other manifestations of ototoxicity.[31]

REFERENCES

1. H. Lyons, V.W. Pinn, and S. Cortell, N. Engl. J. Med. 288, 124-128 (1973).
2. M.A. Fialk, J. Romankiewicz, F. Perrone, and R.L. Sherman, 81, 403-404 (1974).
3. R.T. McCluskey, and A.K. Bhan in: Nephrotoxic Mechanisms of Drugs and Environmental Toxins, G.A. Porter, ed. (Plenum Press, New York 1982) p. 393-402.
4. A.B. Magil, H.S. Ballon, E.C. Cameron, and A. Rae, Am. J. Med. 69, 939-943 (1980).
5. R.R. Bailey, K.L. Lynn, C.J. Drennan, and G.A. Turner, Lancet 1, 226 (1982).
6. G.B. Appel, and C.L. Kunis in: Tubulo-Interstitial Nephropathies, R.S. Cotran, B.M. Brenner, and J.H. Stein, eds. (Churchill-Livingstone, New York 1983).
7. T.J. Fuller, C.G. Barcenas, and M.G. White, J.A.M.A. 235, 1998-1999 (1976).
8. G. Husby, K.S.K. Tung, and R.C. Williams, Am. J. Med. 70, 31-38 (1981).
9. A. Magill, Human Pathol. 14, 36-41 (1983).
10. F.E. Demartini, E.A. Wheaton, L.A. Healey, and J.H. Laragh, Am. J. Med. 32, 572-577 (1962).
11. D.L. Davies, and G.M. Wilson, Drugs 9, 178-226 (1975).
12. M.W. Johnson, and W.E. Mitch, Drugs 21, 220-225 (1981).
13. M.H. Liang, and J.F. Fries, Ann. Intern. Med. 88, 666-670 (1978).
14. W.J. Fessel, Am. J. Med. 67, 74-82 (1979).
15. B.T. Emmerson, Kidney Internat. 18, 677-685 (1980).
16. E.D. Frohlich, New Engl. J. Med. 301, 1378-1382 (1979).
17. A.S. Relman, and W.B. Schwartz, Am. J. Med. 24, 764-773 (1958).
18. R.E. Cronin, and J.P. Knochel in: Acid-Base and Potassium Homeostasis, B.M. Brenner, and J.H. Stein, eds. (Churchill-Livingstone, New York 1978).
19. W. Cremer, and K.D. Bock, Clin. Nephrol. 7, 112-119 (1977).
20. J.W. Conn, and R.D. Johnson, Am. J. Clin. Nutr. 4, 523-528 (1956).
21. J.J. Healy, T.J. McKenna, B. Canning, T.G. Brien, G.J. Duffy, and F.P. Muldowney, Brit. Med. J. 1, 716-719 (1970).
22. O.G. Galvez, W.H. Bay, B.W. Roberts, and T.F. Ferris, Circ. Rsch. 40, 1-11 (1977).
23. B. Ettinger, E. Weil, N.S. Mandel, and S. Darling, Ann. Intern. Med. 91, 745-746 (1979).
24. B. Ettinger, N.O. Oldroyd, and F. Sorgel, J.A.M.A. 244, 2443-2444 (1980).
25. K.F. Fairley, D.F. Birch, and I. Haines, Lancet 1, 421-422 (1983).
26. V.K. Pillay, F.D. Schwartz, K. Ami, and R.M. Kark, Lancet 1, 77-79 (1969).
27. W.J. Schneider, and E.L. Becker, Arch. Intern. Med. 117, 715 (1966).
28. G.H. Schwartz, D.S. David, R.R. Riggio, K.H. Stenzel, and A.L. Rubin, 282, 1413-1414 (1970).
29. R.E. Brummett, T. Bendrick, and D. Himes, J. Clin. Pharmacol. 21, 628-636 (1981).
30. R.E. Brummett in: Nephrotoxicity and Ototoxicity of Drugs, P. Fillastre, ed. (University of Rouen Press, Rouen, France 1982) p. 359-376.

31. R.E. Brummett, Drugs 19, 412-428 (1980).
32. R.M. Levinson, Annals of Otology, Rhinology and Laryngology 83, 223-229 (1974).

DOSE-DEPENDENT METABOLIC PERTURBATIONS BY HYDROCHLOROTHIAZIDE AND PROPRANOLOL

B.J. MATERSON, E.D. FREIS, D. REDA, AND THE VETERANS ADMINISTRATION COOPERATIVE STUDY GROUP ON ANTIHYPERTENSIVE AGENTS, Medical and Research Services, VA Medical Center, Miami, FL 33125, Washington, DC and Hines, IL.

INTRODUCTION

We had studied 683 men with mild to moderate hypertension (seated diastolic blood pressure 95-114mmHg) in a randomized, double-blind protocol in which they were treated with either hydrochlorothiazide (50 to 200mg) or propranolol (80 to 640mg) until diastolic blood pressure (DBP) was less than 90mmHg or the maximum drug dose was reached [1]. The 394 patients who completed the short-term titration phase and had two consecutive visits with DBP less than 100mmHg and at least 6mmHg below baseline were continued on treatment for one year [2]. The data were analysed to determine whether treatment associated metabolic changes were related to drug dose or race.

METHODS

Data were retrieved from the computer files for laboratory tests done on patients receiving either hydrochlorothiazide or propranolol. Patients who received oral potassium supplementation were not separately identified. The P values in Tables II and IV indicate whether the magnitude of the difference between dose groups is significant.

RESULTS

Short-term changes from baseline were as anticipated (Table I), but there were differences with respect to lipids in the long-term pattern.

Table I. Short and long-term trends in laboratory values after treatment with hydrochlorothiazide (mean±S.D.).

	Baseline N=310	10 Weeks N=274	1 Year N=170
Potassium[a)]	4.26± 0.70	-0.68± 0.87	-0.67± 0.53
Uric Acid	6.53± 1.45	1.48± 1.40	1.38± 1.35
BUN	14.0± 3.87	2.77± 4.37	2.47± 4.49
Creatinine	1.16± 0.21	0.07± 0.25	0.03± 0.21
Glucose	100 ± 24.9	4.0 ± 22.9	5.2 ± 28.7
Cholesterol	225 ± 47.7	8.8 ± 39.1	-3.0 ± 41.0
Triglyceride (W)	215 ± 168	56.4 ± 325	9.3 ± 184
Triglyceride (B)	156 ± 193	14.7 ± 251	-16.7± 243

a) mmol/L. All other values are mg/dL. W=white; B=black.

Diuretics, Jules B. Puschett, Editor

Potassium

Changes in serum potassium were a function of dose of hydrochlorothiazide, race and time (Table II). After one year, white patients had a greater percentage decline in serum potassium than did blacks (-18.5 vs -12.7%; P<.001). The major decrement in potassium for white patients was at 200mg and was significantly different from 50 and 100mg. For black patients, the potassium decrements with 100 and 200mg were significantly greater than at 50mg.

Table II. Serum potassium changes in hydrochlorothiazide-treated patients (mean±S.D.). Numbers in parenthesis = N for each subgroup.[a)]

Time	Race	50mg	100mg	200mg	P
A	W	-0.54±0.51(21)	-0.64±0.59(23)	-1.03±1.26(83)	.09
A	B	-0.31±0.47(60)	-0.40±0.63(30)	-0.75±0.56(57)	.0001
B	W	-0.50±0.36(18)	-0.91±0.24(12)	-0.90±0.58(52)	.014
B	B	-0.35±0.40(37)	-0.69±0.48(23)	-0.67±0.56(28)	.007

a) All values in mmol/L; A=10 weeks; B=1 year; W=whites; B=blacks.

In general, hypokalemia (<3.3 mmol/L) was more frequent at the higher doses and in whites (Table III). Serum potassium increased 4.0% after one year of propranolol therapy. There was no racial effect.

Table III. Serum potassium after 1 year of hydrochlorothiazide.[a)]

	50mg		100mg		200mg	
	W	B	W	B	W	B
Number in group	13	27	9	11	31	11
% Serum K^+ <3.0 mmol/L	7.7	0	0	0	6.4	9.1
% Serum K^+ <3.3 mmol/L	30.8	3.7	22.2	36.4	54.9	27.3
% Serum K^+ <3.5 mmol/L	38.5	22.2	55.5	45.5	71.1	45.5
% Serum K^+ <4.0	84.7	66.6	77.7	81.9	100.0	91.0

a) W=white; B=black; N=number in group.

Uric Acid

At 10 weeks, white patients had a dose-related increase in uric acid (50mg = 0.72; 100mg = 0.83; 200mg = 1.64 mg/dL; p=.01), but not at one year (50mg = 1.01; 100mg = 1.43; 200mg = 1.17 mg/dL). Black patients had greater, but not clearly dose-related increases (50mg = 1.49; 100mg = 1.53; 200mg = 1.74 mg/dL) at 10 weeks and at one year (50mg = 1.60; 100mg =1.69; 200mg = 1.42 mg/dL). There were no changes associated with propranolol.

Glucose

Changes in true fasting glucose associated with hydrochlorothiazide were related to time, dose and race (Table IV). The best dose-response correlation occurred in black patients at one year. The changes associated with propranolol were similar to hydrochlorothiazide (baseline = 98.7; 10 weeks = 102.3; 1 year = 105.9), but there was no dose-response or racial effect.

Table IV. True fasting glucose in hydrochlorothiazide-treated patients.

Time	Race	50mg	100mg	200mg	P
A	W	5.2 ±15.7(21)	-10.3±45.1(23)	7.3 ±23.5(83)	.03
A	B	3.0 ±14.8(61)	5.3±13.9(30)	4.9 ±20.9(56)	NS
B	W	1.7 ±21.5(18)	-12.9±60.5(12)	5.4 ±23.6(51)	NS
B	B	-0.5 ±21.3(38)	15.7±28.7(23)	14.1 ±26.2(28)	.02

Cholesterol and Triglyceride

There were no dose-response relationships associated with hydrochlorothiazide although there were racial differences in triglyceride. With propranolol, there was a trivial decrease in cholesterol (baseline = 221; 10 weeks = 217; 1 year = 215 mg/dL), but triglyceride increased (baseline = 164; 10 weeks = 191; 1 year = 209 mg/dL). White patients accounted for most of this change (baseline = 202; 10 weeks = 234; 1 year = 258 mg/dL).

BUN and Creatinine

These values increased in patients taking hydrochlorothiazide, but there was no dose-response relationship. Although not statistically significant, blacks had a lower baseline BUN (13.0 vs. 15.2 mg/dL) and had a greater increase at one year (3.44 vs. 1.41 mg/dL). There were no changes associated with propranolol.

COMMENT AND CONCLUSIONS

It is possible that the lesser reduction of serum potassium in black patients is owing to their initial low renin-aldosterone activity [3]. Some of the acute metabolic changes corrected to or toward normal with long-term treatment. These data suggest that some, but not all metabolic perturbations associated with hydrochlorothiazide therapy can be minimized by using the lowest effective dose.

REFERENCES

1. Veterans Administration Cooperative Study Group on Antihypertensive Agents: Comparison of propranolol and hydrochlorothiazide for the initial treatment of hypertension. I. Results of short-term titration with emphasis on racial differences in response. J. Amer. Med. Assoc. 248, 1996-2003 (1982).
2. Veterans Administration Cooperative Study Group on Antihypertensive Agents: Comparison of propranolol and hydrochlorothiazide for the initial treatment of hypertension. II. Results of long-term therapy. J. Amer. Med. Assoc. 248, 2004-2011 (1982).
3. Freis E, Materson BJ, Flamenbaum W, and the Veterans Administration Cooperative Study Group on Antihypertensive Agents: Comparison of propranolol or hydrochlorothiazide alone for treatment of hypertension III. Evaluation of the renin-aldosterone system. Amer. J. Med. 74, 1029-1041 (1983).

MAINTENANCE OF DIURETIC-INDUCED METABOLIC ALKALOSIS

Allen M. Kaufman, Claudine Brod-Miller, Marvin F. Levitt and Thomas Kahn. Bronx Veterans Administration Medical Center, Mount Sinai Hospital and Mount Sinai School of Medicine of the City University of New York, NY, USA.

The repeated administration of a diuretic may increase plasma bicarbonate consequent in part to an increase in net acid excretion [1,2]. Diuretics may have a direct effect to stimulate hydrogen secretion [3]. The state of electrolyte balance provoked by the diuretic rather than the diuretic itself is probably also a major determinant of net acid excretion and plasma bicarbonate. Indeed, one study in dogs receiving a low chloride intake noted that net acid excretion and plasma bicarbonate actually increased more after the discontinuation of furosemide than during the administration of the drug [4]. In our preliminary studies, following the administration of furosemide to rats receiving a low chloride intake, net acid excretion was also noted to remain higher than baseline when the diuretic was discontinued. Plasma bicarbonate, however, did not increase in the post-diuretic period. The failure of plasma bicarbonate to rise could have been due to excretion of base in a form other than bicarbonate. One such bicarbonate equivalent is citrate which, when metabolized to carbon dioxide and water, yields bicarbonate. Citrate excretion is known to increase with sodium bicarbonate feeding [5] but decrease in potassium depletion alkalosis [6]. The present studies were performed to evaluate whether alterations in base excretion in the form of citrate modify acid-base balance in rats with diuretic-induced metabolic alkalosis, and what factors may determine the level of net acid excretion in this state.

METHODS

Studies were performed on male 300g Sprague-Dawley rats housed in metabolic cages, receiving water ad libitum. All rats consumed 13 grams of a normal diet low in sodium chloride to which 4000 uEq per day sodium was added with sulfate (12 rats) or neutral phosphate (8 rats). Following adaptation to the diet 3 experimental periods were recorded: 4 days baseline, 3 days of furosemide administration (1.75mg bid), and 4 days post-furosemide administration. Urine was collected daily in flasks containing mineral oil and thymol and analyzed by standard methods [2]. Urine citrate was measured by an enzymatic method and organic anion by titration [7]. Blood was drawn by cardiac puncture with ether anesthesia during baseline, and at the end of the furosemide and post-furosemide periods. Plasma aldosterone was measured by radioimmunoassay.

RESULTS

In rats fed sodium sulfate, the administration of furosemide resulted in a daily increase in chloride and potassium excretion. Potassium excretion remained above baseline levels post-furosemide and cumulative potassium loss increased while cumulative chloride loss remained essentially stable (Table). Sodium excretion increased on day 1 of furosemide administration, returned to baseline levels on day 2 and fell sufficiently below baseline on day 3 so that there was no cumulative sodium loss during this period. Post-furosemide sodium excretion fell significantly below baseline levels, resulting in progressive sodium retention (Table). Net acid excretion increased during furosemide administration and remained higher than baseline each day post-furosemide. Plasma bicarbonate increased to 33.8 mEq/l after 3 days of furosemide. Post-furosemide, plasma bicarbonate remained elevated but fell from peak values despite the persistent increment of net acid excretion above baseline levels (Table). Citrate excretion increased during furosemide and was higher post-furosemide. The increment in organic anion excretion was greater than the increment in urinary citrate. Plasma

Diuretics, Jules B. Puschett, Editor

aldosterone averaged 45.5ng/100 ml in the baseline period, and decreased to 17.1ng/100ml and 22.9ng/100ml at the end of the furosemide and post-furosemide periods respectively.

Electrolyte excretion in rats fed sodium neutral phosphate was similar in the baseline period to the sodium sulfate group. The pattern of chloride, potassium and sodium loss during and after furosemide administration was also similar as were the changes in plasma bicarbonate (Table). Baseline net acid excretion, however, was significantly greater than in the sulfate group primarily due to an increase in titratable acidity. Baseline citrate excretion was also significantly higher than in the sulfate group and may, in part, explain the stability of plasma bicarbonate despite higher net acid excretion under basal conditions. During furosemide administration net acid excretion increased as did citrate excretion. Post-furosemide the increase in net acid and citrate excretion above baseline was markedly greater than in the sulfate group (Table). As in the sulfate group, the increment in organic anion excretion was greater than the increment in citrate excretion.

	Urine					
	Na	K	Cl	NAE	Citrate	P_{HCO_3}
Sulfate Group		uEq/24 hr				mEq/l
Baseline	3520±65	956±22	67±10	1192±38	64±6	21.4±0.6
Furosemide	3513±71	1714*±39	921*±57	1662*±47	173*±17	33.8*±0.9
Post-furosemide	3010*±132	1154*±43	27*±10	1647*±58	293*±40	29.9*±0.8
Phosphate Group						
Baseline	3260±67	1027±29	97±5	1570±46	185±14	23.1±0.7
Furosemide	3150±104	1732*±58	896*±72	2023*±72	510*±33	36.6*±0.6
Post-furosemide	2925*±200	1247*±102	19*±108	2329*±108	717*±63	35.8*±0.7

Urinary mean daily values ± SEM are shown for baseline, 3 days furosemide administration and 4 days post-furosemide. NAE = net acid excretion = $U_{NH_4}V+U_{TA}V-U_{HCO_3}V$. An asterisk (*) indicates values significantly different from baseline with P less than 0.05.

DISCUSSION

In these studies metabolic alkalosis was produced by furosemide administration and sustained after the discontinuation of furosemide. Post-furosemide net acid excretion was persistently greater than baseline net acid excretion but did not result in a further rise in plasma bicarbonate. Moreover, plasma bicarbonate was stable post-furosemide despite a greater increment in net acid excretion in the phosphate as compared to sulfate group. Thus adaptive mechanisms may function to stabilize plasma bicarbonate during metabolic alkalosis.

Alterations in base excretion in the form of citrate appears to be of major importance in stabilizing plasma bicarbonate. Increases in net acid excretion were associated with increases in citrate excretion which, in turn, mitigated the rise in plasma bicarbonate that would be predicted to occur. The increment in citrate excretion, however, did not fully explain the failure of plasma bicarbonate to rise post-furosemide. The increase in organic anion excretion was greater than the increase in citrate excretion, suggesting that excretion of other base precursors or release of organic acids may also increase in metabolic alkalosis and play a role in modifying acid-base balance.

It is generally thought that citrate excretion increases with renal cellular alkalosis and decreases with renal cellular acidosis [8]. In the metabolic alkalosis associated with predominant potassium depletion decreased citrate excretion has been observed [6], and other studies have documented intracellular acidosis [9]. It has been suggested that this intracellular acidosis may be the factor that maintains acid excretion in the face of elevated bicarbonate concentrations in the plasma. In our studies the increase in citrate excretion suggests an increase in intracellular pH and/or bicarbonate and implies that the higher level of net acid excretion in the post-furosemide period cannot be explained by intracellular acidosis. The maintenance of increased levels of net acid excretion post-furosemide may, in part, be consequent to decreased luminal chloride availability as a result of the low chloride diet and chloride depletion coupled with enhanced avidity for sodium reabsorption [10]. Sodium depletion, however, was not promoting sodium avidity as both groups were actually in positive sodium balance. Since plasma aldosterone fell below baseline values, an increase in aldosterone was not promoting the increase in net acid excretion. Analysis of the daily data post-furosemide demonstrated a tendency for net acid excretion to decrease while potassium depletion increased, suggesting that potassium depletion was not primarily responsible for increasing net acid excretion. Whatever the primary stimulus for increased net acid excretion, the greater increase in net acid excretion in the phosphate group despite similar electrolyte excretion as the sulfate group suggests that net acid excretion under these circumstances can be modified by the buffer capacity of the urinary anion.

The present studies suggest that altered handling of organic anions, especially citrate, may play an important role in modifying the metabolic alkalosis induced by diuretics.

REFERENCES

1. JP Bosch, MH Goldstein, MF Levitt, T Kahn. Am. J. Physiol. 232: F397-F404 (1977).
2. T Kahn, AM Kaufman, F MacMoune. Clin. Sci. 64:565-572 (1983).
3. PD Lief, BF Mutz, N Bank. J. Clin. Invest. 65:1095-1103 (1980).
4. C Van Ypersele de Strihou, J Morales-Barria. Clin. Sci. 37:859-871 (1969).
5. BM Evans, EI MacIntyre, CR MacPherson, MD Milne. Clin. Sci. 16:53-65 (1957).
6. S Adler, B Zett, B Anderson. J. Lab. Clin. Med. 84:307-316 (1974).
7. DD Van Slyke, WW Palmer. J. Biol. Chem. 41:567-585 (1920).
8. D Simpson. Am. J. Physiol. 244:F223-F234 (1983).
9. S Adler, DS Fraley. Kid. Intl. 11:433-442 (1977).
10. WB Schwartz, JJ Cohen. Am. J. Med. 64:417-428 (1978).

Acknowledgements: We thank Dr. Lester Gabrilove for his measurement of plasma aldosterone in his laboratory. We also thank Bernice Middleton for technical assistance and Evelyn Shapiro for secretarial assistance. The work was supported by the New York State Health Research Council and the General Medical Research Service of the Veterans Administration.

Correspondence: Dr. Allen Kaufman, Renal Section, Room 9A-07, Veterans Administration Medical Center, 130 W. Kingsbridge Road, Bronx, NY 10468 USA.

PATHOGENESIS OF CARDIAC ARRHYTHMIAS INDUCED BY DIURETICS

A. J. REYES,* W. P. LEARY,** AND K. VAN DER BYL**
*Departamento de Investigación Cardiovascular, Fundación Procardias, Montevideo, Uruguay; **Department of Clinical Pharmacology, University of Natal, Durban, South Africa

ABSTRACT

Chronic administration of loop or thiazide-type diuretics may lead to somatic depletion of Mg. As a result, there is an increase in cytosolic K, primarily due to the hyperkaliuresis these drugs induce. These changes destabilise the myocardium electrically and are the main cause of arrhythmias ascribed to diuretics.

INTRODUCTION

Cardiac arrhythmias due to diuretics have hitherto been ascribed to K depletion secondary to hyperkaliuresis [1]. However, recent evidence indicates Mg depletion due to hypermagnesiuresis is a more important determinant [2,3]. The objective of the present study was to describe the pathogenesis of diuretic-induced cardiac arrhythmias adopting the renal excretory actions of diuretics as points of departure.

METHODS

Data compiled by the authors from personal and other sources were processed through an unconventional system analysis, where differential equations or statistical relationships represented the links between variables.

RESULTS AND CONCLUSIONS

Urinary Mg excretion is increased by common loop or thiazide-type diuretics given at standard doses, and is not significantly changed by K-retaining diuretics. Protracted treatment with these drugs, particularly when other factors associated with Mg deficiency are present, leads to a decrease in the intramyocardial concentration of the ion. Thus, the activity of the Mg dependent Na^+,K^+-ATPase, responsible for active transport of K into the cell and Na extrusion from it, is reduced. As a result, the intracellular concentration of K decreases. The hyperkaliuresis caused by diuretics may result in clinically significant K depletion and further reduction in intracellular K, particularly when treatment is prolonged or other factors promoting a negative K balance are present.

Decreased Na^+,K^+-ATPase activity at the cell membrane due to lack of Mg not only affects K balance but also promotes intracellular Na accumulation and increased transmitochondrial interchange between Na and Ca, Na passing to the mitochondria and Ca into the cytosol. There is also a reduction in the activity of the Mg-dependent Ca^{2+}-ATPase which incorporates Ca into the endoplasmic reticulum; cytosolic Ca is further increased as a result. In addition, extracellular Ca enters the cytosol as a

Diuretics, Jules B. Puschett, Editor

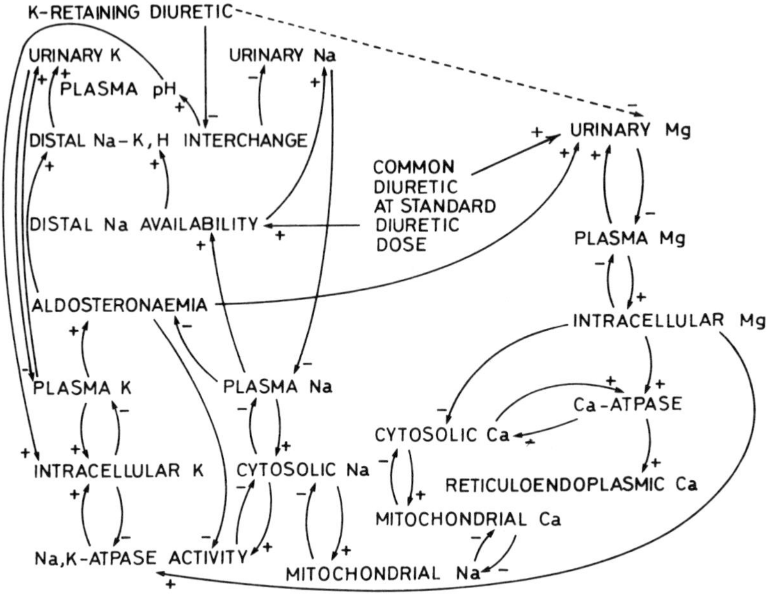

FIG. 1. Causal diagram of the principal mechanisms whereby diuretics alter the intramyocardial concentrations of Mg, K, Ca and Na. The diagram depicts changes (+: augmentation; -: diminution) resulting from increases in the variables from where arrows depart (system dynamics notation). The dotted line indicates an effect which becomes clinically relevant only at doses above those generally prescribed in practice. Adapted from Reyes [4], by courtesy of La Prensa Médica Argentina.

consequence of reduced environmental Mg (FIG. 1). Magnesium depletion resulting from hypermagnesiuresis causes an increase in catecholamine release by the nerve endings and the suprarenal glands. The haemodynamic effects of diuretics, including falls in plasma volume and cardiac output, cause increased sympathetic activity. This increases the activity of adenylate cyclase, whose effect is reinforced by some diuretics which inhibit phosphodiesterase, thereby decreasing the catalysis of cyclic adenosine monophosphate (cAMP).

Raised cAMP levels result in the activation of triglyceride lipase, lipolysis and an increase in free fatty acid (FFA) production. Cyclic AMP-mediated changes in glycolysis cause a further increase in FFA which combine with Mg in plasma reducing the amount available for transfer to the cell and aggravating the intramyocardial Mg deficiency. Raised FFA levels also further reduce the activity of Na^+,K^+-ATPase, potentiating pre-existing intramyocardial electrolyte imbalances.

Increased cAMP activates protein kinase, increasing the sarcolemmal permeability to ions in favour of their electrochemical gradients, thus leading to further increases in cytosolic Ca and Na and decreases in K and Mg (FIG. 2). These alterations

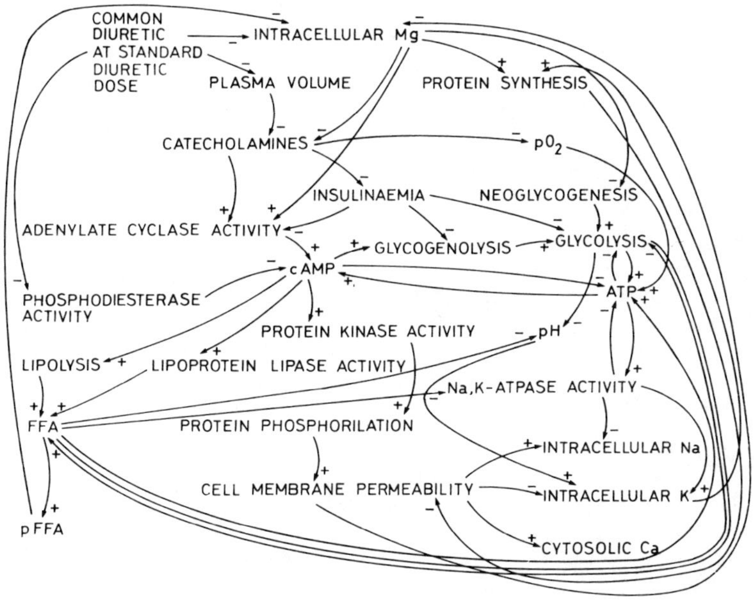

FIG. 2. Causal diagram of the complementary mechanisms whereby diuretics alter the intramyocardial concentrations of Mg, K, Ca and Na. The diagram depicts changes (+: augmentation; -: diminution) resulting from increases in the variables at which arrows start (system dynamics notation). p: plasma; FFA: free fatty acids. Adapted from Reyes [4], by courtesy of La Prensa Médica Argentina.

destabilise the myocardium electrically and induce cardiac arrhythmias.

The coadministration of hydrochlorothiazide and amiloride, which spares K and does not increase Mg renal excretion, does not prevent the occurrence of hypomagnesaemia upon prolonged administration.

REFERENCES

1. T.O. Morgan, Drugs 18, 218-225 (1979).
2. T. Dyckner, and P.O. Wester, Amer. Heart J. 97, 12-18 (1979).
3. J. Sheehan, and A. White, Br. Med. J. 285, 1157-1159 (1982).
4. A.J. Reyes, Pren. Méd. Argent. 70, 448-456 (1983).

CHLORTHALIDONE MEDIATED CHANGES IN SERUM AND ERYTHROCYTES POTASSIUM IN UREMIC HEMODIALYZED PATIENTS.

DOMENICO SCHINELLA,GIACOMO PANARELLO,GEMMA CATTAPAN(¨),ANTONINO RAIMONDI, EMANUELA VACCHER,FRANCO TESIO
Division of Nephrology and Dialysis;(¨)Chemical Chemistry Department- Ospedale Civile di Pordenone - Pordenone,Italy.

INTRODUCTION

The serum potassium concentration can be a major problem in managing patients with renal failure since it may occasionally increase to cardiotoxic levels(1). Potassium homeostasis is maintained in uremic patients through a combination of dietary restriction, increased fecal potassium excretion and dialysis. Occasionally exchange resins must be administered. Neverthless hyperkalemia is a leading cause of death in dialyzed patients (2). Jones and Narna reported that Chlorothiazide 0.5 gm twice a day induced a serum potassium decrease in hypertensive patients with severe renal failure, without significant changes in renal potassium excretion(3). Moreover a single dose of Chlorothiazide has been reported to acutely lower kalemia in anuric chronic hemodialyzed patients(4). The purpose of this study was to evaluate the steady state effects of Chlorthalidone administration on hyperkalemia in uremic hemodialyzed patients. The renal effect of Chlorthalidone was obviated by enrolling in the study functionally anephric subjects.

PATIENTS AND METHODS

12 uremic patients undergoing chronic hemodialysis from 13 to 61 months (mean time 23) were enrolled in the study because of their known tendency to usual hyperkalemia(predialytic K serum levels graeter than 5 mEq/L). There were 5 males and 7 females, mean age 49 years (range 21-63), none of whom had edema, diabetes mellitus or any sign of cardiac decompensation.
7 of 12 patients were anuric, 5 maintained daily urine output less than 500 ml and showed creatinine clearances less than 2.5 ml/min/1.73 m^2.
4½-5 hours of hemodialysis was performed three times a week with hollow fibers cuprophan dialyzers and dialysis fluid containing 2 mEq/L of potassium. Between dialysis the patients were maintained on a diet providing 45-55 mEq of potassium per day. Eight patients were receiving $1,25(OH)_2$ vitamin D_3, all patients were receiving vitamin supplements and aluminum hydroxide. Chlorthalidone 25 mg once a day was given orally for 15 days to each patient. At day 0 and day 15 of Chlorthalidone treatment the serum levels of K (SK),Na,Cl,Ca,Mg,glucose,BUN,uric acid,albumin,standard HCO_3, arterial pH,hematocrit,and erythrocyte K (EK) were determined.
SK and EK were measured also at day 7 of Chlorthalidone administration and 15 days after Chlorthalidone withdrawal. Urinary excretions of Na,K,Cl were assessed on day 0 and day 2 and 4 in oliguric patients.
Electrolytes,BUN,glucose,uric acid, and albumin were determined by Technicon autoanalyzer (SMA 20), hematocrit by a microcentrifuge, arterial pH by

Diuretics, Jules B. Puschett, Editor

a calibrated blood gasautoanalyzer technique. Standard bicarbonate was determined by Siggard-Andersen method. EK was measured by flame photometry in 1 ml whole blood diluted into 10 ml of distilled water after centrifugation at 1200 g for 15 minutes. Correction for plasma concentration was done. Data are shown as mean±standard deviation for all indexes. Statistical analysis was done using the two tailed paired Student's test.

RESULTS

The results are summarized in table I.

TABLE I. Biochemical data.

	day 0	15	30
SK mmol/L	6.41±.69	5.81±.89*	6.59±.94
EK mmol/L	93.7±18.1	112.9±23.2*	95.9±30.3
Na mmol/L	139.7±3.8	140.8±4.1	
Cl mmol/L	101.6±2.7	102.5±5.3	
Ca mg%	9.8 ±.71	9.75±.72	
Mg mg%	2.34±.38	2.42±.34	
pH	7.29±.04	7.30±.03	
HCO_3 mmol/L	15.4±1.7	16.8±2.4	
BUN mg%	87 ±19	85 ±13	
Uric acid mg%	8.2 ±.88	8.4 ±.82	
Glucose mg%	98 ±11	96 ±17	
Albumin g%	3.9 ±.22	3.8 ±.20	
Hematocrit %	29.6±6.9	29.2±7.7	

*p=.01

A decrease in SK and an increase in EK levels were found after Chlorthalidone treatment. No changes were detected in all other investigated biochemical indexes. Urinary electrolytes excretion patterns showed no differences during Chlorthalidone administration (table II).

TABLE II. Urinary electrolytes daily excretion

	day 0	2	4
U_{Na} mmol/L	62.5±22.1	64.6±16.1	65.4±21.7
U_K mmol/L	9.3±6.2	8.8±7.1	7.9±6.6
U_{Cl} mmol/L	61.6±16.1	65.2±24.8	63.6±12.1

15 days after Chlorthalidone withdrawal, SK rose to prestudy levels, and EK concentrations were found to decrease toward starting values.

DISCUSSION

Since renal excretion is the major determinant of steady-state serum potassium, in uremic hemodialyzed patients without residual renal function, serum potassium rises between dialysis with time. In our patients a less marked rise was found during Chlorthalidone treatment. Renal effect of Chlorthalidone was obviated because we enrolled only functionally anephric subjects. Moreover, in oliguric patients kalemia decrease was not associated with any change in urinary electrolytes excretion patterns.

Of the extrarenal factors known to affect serum potassium concentrations, changes in extracellular volume and acid-base balance can be ruled out in our patients. Aldosterone serum concentrations were not assessed because prestudy levels resulted higher than upper limit of our method in many of enrolled patients. The disposal of an acute potassium load has been reported affected by endogenous insulin(5) and cathecolamines(6) serum levels. Whether these hormones played a role in steady-state balance of potassium in our patients, we cannot clarify in this study protocol.

Although the erythrocyte is a highly specialized cell which may not be representative of cells at large, concurrent SK fall and EK rise might involve, in our opinion, Chlorthalidone promoted cellular uptake of potassium. Furthermore, a cell membrane defect thiazides responsive has been postulated for pathogenesis of a recently discovered hereditary disorder involving hyperpotassemia(7). Analysis of feces to exclude Chlorthalidone-induced increased intestinal loss of potassium was not carried out in this study. Neverthless, Hayes et al. reported(8) that fecal potassium in chronic renal failure was independent of thiazides administration.

In conclusion, Chlorthalidone administration induced a steady-state decrease in serum potassium levels in functionally anephric hemodialyzed patients. Chlorthalidone-mediated changes in potassium diffusion through the cellular wall might offer alternate explanations for the releaved variations in serum and erythrocyte potassium levels.

REFERENCES

1. W.E. Mitch and S. Wilcox, Am. J. Med. 72, 536-550 (1982).
2. Combined Report on Regular Dialysis and Transplantation in Europe, X, 1979, in: Proc. EDTA, 17, B.H.B. Robinson and J.B. Hawkins eds.(Pitman Medical, London, 1980), p.36.
3. B. Jones and R.S. Nanra, Lancet 2, 1258-1260 (1979).
4. D. Ezra, A. Iaina, S. Kapuler et al., Min. Electr. Metab. 7, 285-291 (1982).
5. R.H. Sterns, P.U. Feig, M. Pring, J. Guzzo and I. Singer, Kidney Int. 15, 651-660 (1979).
6. R. Rosa, P. Silva, J.B. Young et al., N. Eng. J. Med. 302, 431-434 (1980).
7. Z. Farfel, A. Iaina, J. Levi and J. Gafni, Arch. Intern. Med. 138, 1837-1840 (1978).
8. C.P. Hayes, M.E. McLeod and R.R. Robinson, Trans. Assoc. Am. Physns. 58, 207-216 (1967).

ENALAPRIL ATTENUATES HYDROCHLOROTHIAZIDE-INDUCED HYPOKALEMIA, HYPERGLYCEMIA, HYPERURICEMIA AND HYPERCHOLESTEROLEMIA

H.J. GOMEZ, J.F. WALKER, F. MONCLOA, V.J. CIRILLO, J.A. SROMOVSKY AND M. GABRIEL. Merck Sharp & Dohme Research Laboratories, Rahway, N.J. and West Point, PA., USA

Research in the last decade has been aimed at evaluating the clinical importance of the undesirable metabolic side effects of current diuretics in relation to their well known beneficial antihypertensive effects. Hypokalemia, which develops in 10-50% of the patients treated with diuretics [1], seems to enhance the risk of serious cardiac arrhythmias and sudden death [2,3]. Long-term diuretic treatment impairs glucose tolerance [4], probably as a result of hypokalemia which has been associated with a decrease in insulin secretion [5]. Diabetes is frequently aggravated or precipitated by diuretics, presumably by the same mechanism [6]. In addition to precipitating gout and urolithiasis, diuretics induce hyperuricemia which has been identified as a risk factor for cardiovascular disease [7]. There is concern that long-term use of thiazides raises serum lipoprotein, triglyceride and total cholesterol concentrations, and reduces HDL-cholesterol, increasing the risk of coronary heart disease [8,9].

Enalapril (EN), an angiotensin-converting-enzyme inhibitor [10], has been shown to be effective in the treatment of essential and renovascular hypertension and congestive heart failure without producing any of these undesirable metabolic side effects [11,12,13]. We report on the metabolic effects of EN, propranolol (P) and atenolol (A), alone and in combination with hydrochlorothiazide (H), in patients with essential hypertension.

METHODS

EN was compared to H, P and A in three multicenter studies. Study A was a double-blind, randomized, parallel trial in which 546 patients with mild to moderate essential hypertension were treated for 8 weeks with EN (20 mg/day), H (50 mg/day) or EN/H (20/50 mg/day). The dose was doubled at the end of 4 weeks if the supine diastolic blood pressure (SDBP) was >90 mmHg. Study B was a double-blind, randomized, parallel trial in 485 patients with mild to moderate essential hypertension who received either EN (10-40 mg/day) or P (80-240 mg/day) for a 12 week titration period. H (25-50 mg/day) was added to the monotherapy for an additional 14 weeks if the SDBP was >90 mmHg. Study C was an open, randomized, parallel study in 176 patients with moderate to severe hypertension who received EN 20 mg/day or A 50 mg/day. Titration was done by first doubling the dose of test drug, followed by sequentially adding H 25-100 mg/day. Patients were treated for 16 weeks. Patients were seen at 2-4 week intervals in each study.

RESULTS

All treatments produced a significant reduction in BP ($p < 0.01$). The addition of H to EN, P or A produced a greater antihypertensive response (Table I). Eighty-five to 96 percent of the patients with EN/H had their SDBP controlled (<90 mmHg and/or a decrease ≥10 mmHg).

Diuretics, Jules B. Puschett, Editor

TABLE I. Pretreatment SDBP and mean changes after therapy (mmHg)

	STUDY A			STUDY B				STUDY C			
	EN	H	EN/H	EN	P	EN/H	P/H	EN	A	EN/H	A/H
n	176	189	90	183	184	97	99	92	81	62	52
Pre	105	105	104	104	104	104	104	114	113	116	116
Change*	-12	-13	-21	-13	-11	-19	-16	-14	-15	-21	-23

*All changes from pretreatment were significant, $p < 0.01$

Serum Potassium - EN, P, and A did not affect K^+. H decreased K^+, and this effect was attenuated by the addition of EN (Table II). K^+ decreased in the β-blocker/H groups but not in the EN/H group ($p < 0.01$ vs A/H).

Serum Glucose - EN, P and A did not affect glucose. H increased glucose and this effect was attenuated when EN was coadministered. There were slight increases in the P/H and A/H groups (Table II).

Serum Urate - Neither EN nor the β-blockers produced significant changes in urate; H elevated urate. EN/H produced a smaller increase in urate ($p < 0.05$) than that produced by A/H (Table II).

Serum Cholesterol - EN, P and A did not affect cholesterol; H increased it. Levels were significantly higher with A/H than with EN/H (Table II).

TABLE II. Serum potassium, glucose, uric acid and cholesterol after mono- and combination therapy.

	STUDY A			STUDY B				STUDY C			
	EN	H	EN/H	EN	P	EN/H	P/H	EN	A	EN/H	A/H
					K^+ (mEq/l)						
n	190	187	94	174	163	49	63	70	60	59	45
Pre	4.1	4.1	4.1	4.2	4.1	4.1	4.1	4.1	4.0	4.0	4.0
Post	4.2	3.4[d]	3.9[b]	4.3	4.3	4.1	3.9[d]	4.3	4.2	4.0	3.7[d]
					Glucose (mg/dl)						
n	190	188	94	159	154	44	50	25	30	39	30
Pre	111	107	108	90	89	89	88	92	91	93	95
Post	110	118[d]	112[a]	88	88	86	93[d]	90	95	96	98
					Urate (mg/dl)						
n	190	188	94	163	151	47	53	35	37	42	34
Pre	6.3	6.2	6.3	5.6	5.4	5.3	5.8	5.7	6.0	5.8	6.5
Post	6.3	7.7[d]	7.4[b]	5.8	5.8	6.0[d]	6.5[d]	5.7	6.0	6.9[d]	7.9[d]
					Cholesterol (mg/dl)						
n	190	188	94	157	146	40	47	19	22	36	30
Pre	218	220	222	241	227	230	238	232	244	235	231
Post	218	232[d]	232[d]	236	229	235	237	230	234	239	248[c]

a,b Significantly different from H, $p < 0.05$, $p < 0.01$
c,d Significant change from pretreatment, $p < 0.05$, $p < 0.01$

Adverse Experiences - EN and EN/H were associated with a low incidence of clinical and laboratory adverse experiences. Of note was the absence of taste loss, proteinuria and neutropenia. There were a few cases of skin rash distributed evenly among the treatment groups. The safety profile of EN and EN/H has recently been reviewed [14].

DISCUSSION

This report confirms the effects of H on serum K^+, glucose, urate and cholesterol, and demonstrates that EN does not adversely affect these parameters. When combined, EN appears to attenuate the H-induced changes. Similar results have been reported for captopril [15], suggesting that these may be general properties of converting enzyme inhibitors. Also, EN has recently been shown to reverse the hypokalemia associated with primary and secondary hyperaldosteronism [16].

In conclusion, EN is an effective antihypertensive agent which does not cause hypokalemia, hyperglycemia, hyperuricemia or hypercholesterolemia. Its combination with H results in more efficacious therapy while ameliorating diuretic-induced side effects.

REFERENCES

1. F.G. McMahon, Management of Essential Hypertension (Futura Publishing Co., New York 1978), pp. 21-54.
2. J.W. Hollifield and P.E. Slaton. Acta. Med. Scand. Suppl. 647, 67-73 (1980).
3. O.B. Holland, J.V. Nixon and L. Kuhnert. Am. J. Med. 70, 762-768 (1981).
4. M.B. Murphy, P.J. Lewis, E. Kohner, B. Schumer and C.T. Dollery. Lancet 2, 1293-1295 (1982).
5. J.H. Helderman, D. Elahi, D.K. Andersen, et al. Diabetes 32, 106-111 (1983).
6. C. Grunfeld and D.A. Chappell. Am. J. Med. 75, 553-554 (1983).
7. W.J. Fesel, Am. J. Med. 68, 401-404 (1980).
8. D. Maclean and G.R. Tudhope, Br. Med. J. 286, 1419-1422 (1983).
9. R.P. Ames, Am. Heart J. 106, 1207-1214 (1983).
10. H.J. Gomez, V.J. Cirillo and K.H. Jones. J. Hypertens. 1 (Suppl. 1), 65-70 (1983).
11. J. Biollaz, H.R. Brunner, J. Gavras, B. Waeber and H. Gavras, J. Cardiovas. Pharmacol. 4, 966-972 (1982).
12. G.P. Hodsman, J.J. Brown, A.M.M. Cumming, et al. J. Hypertens. 1 (Suppl. 1), 109-117 (1983).
13. D. Fitzpatrick, M.G. Nicholls, H. Ikram and E.A. Espiner. J. Hypertens. 1 (Suppl. 1), 147-153 (1983).
14. R.O. Davies. Am. J. Med. (1984), in press.
15. M.H. Weinberger. Hypertension 5 (Supp. III), 132-138 (1983).
16. G.T. Griffing and J.C.Melby. Clin. Exp. Hyper. Theory Practice A5(6), 779-801 (1983).

THERAPY OF MILD HYPOKALEMIA IS INDICATED.

A. FERNANDEZ-CRUZ M.D., M. LUQUE OTERO M.D., C. FERNANDEZ-PINILLA M.D., M. RUIZ-TOVAR M.D., N. MARTELL CLAROS M.D., L. REINARES M.D., J. ALCAZAR M.D., J. RAMON M.D., J. PESO M.D. and F. PEREZ-CASAR M.D.
Hypertension, Diabetes and Obesity Center. Department of Medicine. Hospital Clínico San Carlos. Complutense University. Madrid - Spain.

In this paper we will review the adverse consequences of potassium deficiency induced by diuretics. Three leading articles were chosen as guide lines based on occasional review (1,2,3).

The critical biological role of potassium was recognized at the turn of the century, but concern among clinicians about potassium deficiency was initiated by observations made 30 years ago, shortly after accurate measurements of serum potassium concentration became readily available. Weakness and ileus in surgical patients, arrhythmias in patients receiving digitalis, and disturbances in kidney function were attributed to potassium depletion, and these manifestations were often corrected when potassium salts were added to the therapeutic regime (4). At about the same time Schwartz and Wallace showed that physiologic effect of mercurial diuretics included a substantial renal potassium wastage as patients lost salt and water and recovered from their edematous states (5). In those early years the correlation between the extent of potassium deficit and the severity of clinical manifestations attributable to such a deficit was not clearly defined: it was simply assumed that it was not particularly healthy to be depleted of potassium. Thus concern about the adverse consequences of potassium deficiency was part of the "background noise" when oral diuretics were introduced 25 years ago (3).

Reduction in the plasma potassium concentration occurs commonly in patients taking diuretics, and hypokalemia may develop within a few weeks of begining treatment (1). On all the available cross-sectional data, maximum fall in the serum potassium value after the thiazides or chlorthalidone had happened by the end of the first week of treatment and that there was little further fall thereafter. A similar pattern was seen in most of the longitudinal studies, even those that lasted two years (6,7).

In contrast, when the diuretics are stopped the serum potassium value takes several weeks to return to normal. If this delay is the time taken to replete the body potassium then it is surprisingly long, as the deficit of body potassium is small. The dose-response curve is flat. There are however major differences among various diuretics; in particular frusemide causes a much smaller fall in serum potassium concentration than do the thiazides in the commonly used doses as reported in individual studies (1,8). Bumetanide probably causes a similar fall in serum-potassium value to frusemide, although there are few, if any, studies with bumetanide or ethacrinic acid in which no potassium supplements were given (9).

Diuretics have been used to treat symptoms of hypertension, congestive heart failure, renal disease and cirrhosis.

The use of thiazide diuretics in hypertension has steadily increased over the past 20 years, and the effect of recent publications may be to accelerate this trend. On the other hand considering congestive heart failure as the inability of the heart to pump adequate amounts of blood to meet the metabolic needs of the body, this pump failure results in an increase in left ventricular filling pressure by expansion of the intravascular volume. Diuretics have been used to treat symptoms of pulmonary congestion seen in heart failure by reducing the volume overload.

Published 1984 by Elsevier Science Publishing Co., Inc.
Diuretics, Jules B. Puschett, Editor

Morgan and Davidson (1) studied an analysis of publications on the effects of thiazides and frusemide only in cases of heart failure and hypertension. The data shows that the diuretics caused the same average fall in the serum potassium concentration in heart failure as in hypertension. The serum potassium concentration before treatment, however, was higher in the patients with heart failure than in those with hypertension.

The frequency of hypokalemia after diuretics depends on the initial value as well as the fall in serum potassium concentration. The frequency of hypokalemia is less in patients with heart failure than in the patients with hypertension, because the patients with heart failure have higher serum potassium concentration before treatment.

In order to evaluate the effect of antihypertensive therapy on serum electrolyte concentration we studied 121 essential hypertensive patients. Table 1 shows their clinical characteristics.

TABLE 1.- CLINICAL CHARACTERISTICS OF ESSENTIAL HYPERTENSIVE PATIENTS

Age Range: 23-67 years
Sex: 72 F. 49 M.
WHO STAGE
- I - 37 patients
- II - 60 "
- III - 24 "

TREATMENT OF HYPERTENSION

- Sodium-restricted diet	9 patients
- Chlorthalidone	20 "
- Tienilic acid	20 "
- Atenolol	32 "
- Chlorthalidone and Atenolol	23 "
- Chlorthalidone, Atenolol and Hydralazine Retard	17 "

The results of a sodium-restricted diet of 2.000 cal; 46% carbohydrates, 20% proteins, 34% fat (ratio of polyunsaturated to saturated = 0.3); 80 mmol of sodium, 80 mmol of potassium and 750 mg of calcium content, is illustrated in Table 2.

TABLE 2.- BLOOD PRESSURE, BODY WEIGHT, ELECTROLYTE CONCENTRATION, SERUM GLUCOSE AND URINARY EXCRETION OF SODIUM AND POTASSIUM BEFORE (B) AND AFTER ONE YEAR (1 Y) OF SODIUM-RESTRICTED DIET (mean $\pm$ SEM)

	B	1Y
Weight (Kg)	73.9 $\pm$ 3.7	69.2 $\pm$ 3.6
SBP (mm Hg)	145 $\pm$ 6.3	130 $\pm$ 4.5*
DBP (mm Hg)	95 $\pm$ 1.6	87 $\pm$ 3.2*
Urinary Na^+ (mmol/24h)	184 $\pm$ 21	100 $\pm$ 18*
Urinary K^+ (mmol/24h)	62 $\pm$ 11	120 $\pm$ 18*
Serum Na^+ (mmol/l)	148 $\pm$ 1.6	141 $\pm$ 1.7*
Serum K^+ (mmol/l)	4.6 $\pm$ 0.1	4.2 $\pm$ 0.1*
Glucose (mg/dl)	102 $\pm$ 3.6	96 $\pm$ 5

*$p < 0.05$

These data clearly indicate that while blood pressure was controlled a significant decrease in urinary sodium excretion was observed. In addition, urinary potassium excretion increased significantly, Conversely, the results demonstrate that both serum potassium and sodium concentration fell significantly within the normal range.

As can be seen in Table 3 serum sodium, potassium and glucose were not affected either under chlorthalidone therapy (over 2 years) or tienilic acid therapy (over one year).

Table 4 given the sodium, potassium and glucose concentration in hypertensive patients under combined atenolol and chlorthalidone therapy. The results again indicate no significant changes associated with this type of therapeutic regime.

Table 4 also shows that when a vasodilator (Hydralazine Retard) was added to obtain the control of blood pressure, the serum potassium levels significantly fells from 3.9 $\pm$ 0.1 to 3.6 $\pm$ 0.1 mmol/l, p 0.05.

TABLE 3.- BLOOD PRESSURE ELECTROLYTE CONCENTRATION AND SERUM GLUCOSE BEFORE (B) AND AFTER ONE YEAR (1 Y) OF CHLORTHALIDONE OR TIENILIC ACID THERAPY, AND TWO YEARS (2 Y) OF CHLORTHALIDONE THERAPY (mean ± SEM)

		SBP mm Hg	DBP mm Hg	SERUM Na mmol/l	SERUM K mmol/l	GLUCOSE mg/dl
CHLORTHALIDONE n = 20	B	167 ± 7	107 ± 3	146 ± 2	4.1 ± 0.1	99 ± 10
	1Y	131 ± 6*	86 ± 3*	143 ± 1.5	3.9 ± 0.1	95 ± 4
	2Y	134 ± 2*	86 ± 2*	143 ± 1.5	4.1 ± 0.1	90 ± 1.5
TIENILIC ACID n = 20	B	168 ± 3	103 ± 1.5	143 ± 0.7	4.2 ± 0.1	105 ± 2.4
	1Y	142 ±2*	91 ±1.4*	148 ± 1.1	4.2 ± 0.1	107 ± 2.9

* p 0.05

TABLE 4.- BLOOD PRESSURE, ELECTROLYTE CONCENTRATION AND SERUM GLUCOSE BEFORE (B) AND AFTER ONE YEAR (1 Y) OF DIURETIC AND BETA-BLOCKER, OR TRIPLE THERAPY (mean ± SEM)

		SBP mm Hg	DBP mm Hg	SERUM Na mmol/l	SERUM K mmol/l	GLUCOSE mg/dl
CHLORTHALIDONE AND ATENOLOL n = 23	B	199 ± 5	117 ± 3	142 ± 0.9	4 ± 0.1	112 ± 6
	1Y	143 ± 4^{+}	90 ± 2^{+}	140 ± 3	3.7 ± 0.2	115 ± 5
DIURETIC, β-BLOCKER AND HYDRALAZINE R n = 17	B	180 ± 7	108 ± 2	142 ± 1.7	3.9 ± 0.1	104 ± 4
	1Y	145 ± 4^{+}	89 ± 1^{+}	145 ± 1.7	3.6 ± 0.1*	107 ± 6

* $p < 0.05$ $^{+}p < 0.001$

In conclusion, our results seem to indicate minor differences between various therapeutic regimen for the treatment of hypertension. In addition, the fall in serum potassium possibly depends on the initial value: the lower the initial level of potassium the greater the decrease of serum potassium induce by the treatment.

An association between severe hypokalemia, whatever the cause, and arrhythmias has long been recognised (10). Arrhythmias are also common in digitalised patients with mild hipokalemia, and an association between hipokalemia and arrhythmias after acute myocardial infarction has been observed (13). Holland et al (11) and Hollified et al (12) have reported an association between thiazide induced changes in serum potassium concentrations and premature ventricular contractions during treatment for essential hypertension. Holland et al have also reported a striking decrease in the frequency of ventricular extrasystoles after the administration of potassium sparing agent (11).

The arrhythmogenic potential of hypokalemia is a matter of considerable controversy. Based on extensive studies of hypokalemic patients, some investigators have concluded that hypokalemia in itself only rarely produces life-threatening cardiac arrhythmias (14). In addition in the principal studies, no firm temporal relationship was established between the level of serum potassium and the observation of ventricular ectopic activity. Similarly, in the reports of hypokalemia associated with acute myocardial infarction serum potassium was frequently measured from 12 to 24 hours after an episode of ventricular ectopic activity, often following protacted cardiopulmonary resuscitation (15). Because resuscitative events include some factors that lower serum potassium and some that increase serum potassium, it is difficult under these circunstances to determine what the serum potassium concentration was before the event (3).

Secondly, although two studies have demonstrated a reduction in ventricular ectopic activity in hypokalemic patients after serum potassium was restored to normal, neither study employed multiple 24-hour recordings, both before and after potassium repletion to differentiate a therapeutic response related to potassium replacement from spontaneous variation in ventricular ectopic activity (11,16). In regard to the arrhythmogenic potential of hypokalemia Harrington (3) concludes that despite evidence that benign forms of ventricular ectopic activity are increased in the presence of hypokalemia, a critical review of the published experience discloses no evidence that fatal ventricular ectopic activity results from hypokalemia per se. The evidence that hypokalemia decreases the threshold for malignant arrhythmias in patients with acute myocardial infarction is limited and circunstantial. Finally malignant ventricular ectopic activity related to hypokalemia has been adequeately documented only in hypokalemic patients receiving digitals.

We decided to study patients in the acute phase of chronic heart failure. 15 patients, 5 F and 10 M, aged 53.8 $\pm$ 2.3 years were studied. The diagnosis was dilated cardiomiopathy in 8 patients, valvular heart disease in 4 and ischemic heart disease in 3. The treatment prior the admission was digitalis in 10 patients, diuretics in 10 and miscellaneous (including prazosin, quinidine, beta blockers, nifedipine, captopril, etc., in 9 patients. The treatment received by this patients on admission was: digitalis (loading dose 0.25 mg) 14 patients, Diuretics (bumetanide, 2-8 mg daily, 7 patients; frusemide 40-320 mg daily 8 patients), Vasodilators (prazosin, 1-10 mg daily 4 patients; captopril 50-75 mg daily 3 patients; nitrates 30 mg daily e patients and hydralazine 30 mg daily, 1 patient) and Miscellaneous (verapamil 1 patient and amiodarone 1 patient). Table 5 shows the effect of the standard treatment on body weight, serum sodium, chloride potassium and glucose over a three week periods. The data cleartly indicate a mild decrease of serum potassium over the first two weeks of treatment. During the third week the serum potassium returned to the admission level.

TABLE 5.- EFFECT OF THE TREATMENT OF ACUTE HEART FAILURE ON BODY WEIGHT, ELECTROLYTE CONCENTRATION AND SERUM GLUCOSE (mean ± SEM)

	BASELINE	1 WEEK	2 WEEK	3 WEEK
Weight (Kg)	59 ± 3	58 ± 3	59 ± 3	57 ± 2
Serum K^+ mmol/l	4.3 ± 0.2	3.9 ± 0.1	3.9 ± 0.1	4.4 ± 0.2
Serum Na^+ mmol/l	138 ± 1.9	136 ± 1.5	140 ± 2	137 ± 2.2
Serum Cl^- mmol/l	98 ± 2.7	101 ± 1.2	102 ± 1.6	100 ± 1.7
Glucose mg/dl	104 ± 13	135 ± 24	109 ± 17	128 ± 19

In order to examine the arrhythmogenic potencial of hypokalemia in our patients we performed an electrochardiogram concomitantly with the measurement of serum potassium over the three week period. The data clearly indicate that we like many others investigators, did not find any relationship between serum potassium and cardiac arrhythmias in these patients.

We made a further study of the ECG pattern in 43 patients with chronic renal failure and under dyalisis. The purpose of this was to examine the question of whether or not changes in electrolytes generate a typical ECG pattern. The coefficient of lineal correlation shows that we were unable to find any correlation between serum potassium (mean 4.1 ± 0.1 mmol/l, range 7.1-2) or serum calcium (mean 4 ± 0.08 mg/dl, range 5.6-1.9) and some ECG patterns (heart rate, p duration, PR interval, QRS axis, QRS duration, QT corrected and T wave voltage). However must be pointed out that our patients exhibits and abnormal range both of serum potassium and calcium. Therefore, our data only permits us to draw conclusion about this particular group and not to make any broader generalisation.

This survey of publications, analysis of published data and our own results supports long-held beliefs about the mild effect of diuretics-induced potassium depletion. In cirrhosis the published data (17,18) supports that the serum potassium value tends to be low even before treatment and the frequency of hypokalemia in patients who are taking diuretics is therefore probably much greater than in patients with hypertension or heart failure. In fact potassium salts or potassium sparing diuretics should be given prophylacticaly to those patients. In renal failure however the frequency of hypokalemia caused by diuretics would be less because of a relatively high serum potassium concentration before treatment.

In regard to the arrythmogenic potential of hypokalemia the analysis of the data allow us to conclude that only rarely produces life-threatening cardiac arrythmias. Our analysis of our own data will not even allow us to conclude that this is major problem in those patients with chronic heart failure receiving digitalis and diuretics.

However there is a body of evidence to support that mild diuretic-induced magnessium depletion is arrythmogenic in patients with heart failure. In addition several reports relates magnessium levels and cardiac digitalis intoxication (19,20). Until more data are available those results will not be conclusive. Finally the involvement of prostaglandins in hypertension (21), congestive heart failure (22) and mechanism of action of diuretics (23) is, with the adrenergic control of serum potassium (24) an important factor recently involved in potassium homeostasis.

From the practical point of view the risks of appreciable hipokalemia on most patients who are given diuretics are small, and the need for routine potassium suplements is not clear. However when a patient has plasma potassium concentration value low enough (say less than 3.0 mmol/l) potassium supplements or potassium sparing diuretic is indicated.

In patients with heart failure under digitalis and diuretics with or without miocardial infarction we conclude that mild diuretic-induced potassium depletion is arrhythmogenic so again potassium supplements would be justified only if the benefit of treatment exceeded the risks. In elderly people, diabetic patients and impaired renal function dangerous hyperkalemia has been reported in connection with the use of spironolactone and potassium suplementation (3).

In our opinion until more data are available we continue to recommend dietary recommendations and potassium salts or potassium sparing diuretics will be indicated for severe potassium depletion or for clinical manifestations related to hypokalemia.

REFERENCES

1. B. Morgan and C. Davidson: Hypokalaemia and diuretics: an analysis of publications. Br. Med. J. 280, 905-908 (1980).
2. Medical Research Council Working Party on Mild to Moderate Hypertension: Ventricular extrasystoles during thiazide treatment: substudy of MRC muld hypertension trial. Br. Med. J. 287, 1249-53 (1983).
3. J.T. Harrington, J.M. Isner and J.P. Kassirer: Our National obsesion with potassium. Am. J. Med. 73, 155-59 (1982).
4. L.G. Welt, W. Hollander Jr. and W.B. Blythe: The consequences of potassium depletion. J. Chron. Dis. 11, 213 (1960).
5. W.B. Schwartz and W.M. Wallace: Electrolyte equilibrium during mercurial diuresis. J. Clin. Invest. 30, 1089 (1951).
6. C. Bartorelli, N. Argano and G. Lecnetti: Potassium loss and potassium replacement during long-term diuretic treatment in hypertension in: Antihypertensive therapy-principles and practice. F. Gross ed. (Springer-Verlag, Berlin, 1966).
7. A.J. Marshall, D.W. Barritt, J. Pocock and S.T. Heaton: Evaluation of beta blockade bendrofluazide and prazosin in severe hypertension. Lancet i, 271-4 (1977).
8. J. Anderson, B.E. Godfrey, D.M. Hill, A.D. Munro-Faure and J. Sheldon: A comparison of the effects of hydrochlorothiazide and of frusemide in the treatment of hypertensive patients. Q. J. Med. 160, 541-60 (1971).

9. L.E. Murchison and P.D. Bewsher: Lack of effect of bumetanide on body potassium content in hypertension. Br. J. Clin. Pharmacol. 2, 87-91 (1975).
10. J.W. Hollifield and P.E. Slaton: Thiazide diuretics, hypokalemia, and cardiac arrhythmias, in "Potassium, the Heart and Hypertension", Symposium Proceedings (Rome, Italy, 1981).
11. O.B. Holland, J.V. Nixon and L. Kuhnert: Diuretic-induced ventricular ectopic activity. Amer. J. Med. 70, 762-68 (1981).
12. J.W. Hollifield and P.E. Slaton: Cardiac arrhythmias associated with diuretic-induced hypokalemia and hypomagnesaemia. Royal Society of Medicine International Congress and Symposium Series 44, 17-26 (1980).
13. T. Dyckner, C. Helmers, T. Lundman and P.O. Wester: Initial serum potassium level in relation to early complications and prognosis in patients with acute myocardial infarction. Acta Med. Scand. 197, 207-10 (1975).
14. T. Dyckner and P.O. Wester: Ventricular extrasystoles and intracellular electrolytes before and after potassium and magnesium infusions in patients on diuretic treatment. Am. Heart J. 97, 12 (1979).
15. J. Hulting: In-hospital ventricular fibrilation and its relation to serum potassium. Acta Med. Scand. S647, 109 (1981).
16. J. Morganroth, E.L. Michelson, L.N. Horowitz, M.E. Josephson, A.S. Pearlman and W.B. Dunkman: Limitations of routine long-term electrocardiographic monitoring to assess ventricular ectopic frequency. Circulation 58, 408 (1978).
17. D.S. Amatuzia, F. Stutzman, N. Shrifter and S. Nesbitt: A study of serum electrolytes in patients with severely, descompensated portal cirrhosis of the liver. J. Lab. Clin. Med. 39, 26-9 (1952).
18. E.L. Artman and R.A. Wise: Hypokalemia in liver cell failure. Am. J. Med. 15, 459-67 (1953).
19. R.P.C. Bigg, and R. Chia: Magnesium deficiency. Role in arrhythmias complicating acute myocardial infarction?. Med. J. Aust. 1, 346-48 (1981).
20. L. Cohen and R. Kitzes: Magnesium sulfate and digitalis-toxic arrhythmias. J. Amer. Med. Assoc. 249, 2808-10 (1983).
21. S.Y. Tan, P. Sweet and P.J. Mulrow: Impaired renal production of prostaglandin E: A newly identified lesion. Prostaglandins. 15, 139-49 (1978).
22. V.J. Dzau, M. Packer, L.S. Lilly, S.L. Swartz, N.K. Hollenberg and G.H. Williams: Prostaglandins in severe congestive heart failure. N. Engl. J. Med. 310, 347-52 (1984).
23. J. Webster, C.T. Dollery and C.N. Hensby: Circulating prostacyclin concentrations may be increased by bendrofluazide in patients with essential hypertension. Clin. Sci. 59, 125s-28s (1980).
24. F.H. Epstein and R.M. Rosa: Adrenergic control of serum potassium. N. Engl. J. Med. 309, 1450-51 (1983).

SECTION VII

DIURETIC PHARMACOLOGY AND PHARMACOKINETICS

INTERACTION BETWEEN NON-STEROIDAL ANTIINFLAMMATORY DRUGS AND DIURETICS

D. CRAIG BRATER, M.D.
Associate Professor of Pharmacology and Internal Medicine
The University of Texas Health Science Center at Dallas
Departments of Pharmacology and Internal Medicine
5323 Harry Hines Blvd.
Dallas, TX 75235

INTRODUCTION

Early studies showing inhibition by non-steroidal anti-inflammatory drugs (NSAID's) of diuretic, natriuretic and renal vasodilating effects of loop diuretics were interpreted to mean that prostaglandins (PG's) were important mediators of response to these diuretics. Subsequent studies showing increases in urinary PG's concomitant with maximal diuretic or natriuretic effects supported this notion. More recent studies have addressed the mechanisms of diuretic-NSAID interactions with the objective of gaining insight into pharmacologic mechanisms of action and into the physiological role of renal prostaglandins. These latter studies will serve as the focus of this review with the major focus on furosemide as the prototype loop diuretic. It does not appear that other loop diuretics differ from furosemide in the context of the current subject.

Because of the known effects of loop diuretics and the sites within the kidney at which PG's may have an important physiological role, a number of possible mechanisms of interaction could be proposed as illustrated schematically in Figure 1.

Loop diuretics such as furosemide increase renal blood flow which in itself, by decreasing filtration fraction, can cause a diuresis and natriuresis [1-4]. Consequently, the inhibiting effect of NSAID's such as indomethacin could occur by blocking this hemodynamic effect.

At the proximal tubule, furosemide is actively secreted into the tubular lumen by the organic acid transport pathway from which it is carried with the luminal fluid to its tubular site of action at the thick ascending limb of the loop of Henle (stippled area in Figure 1). Since NSAID's are organic acids, they could conceivably block access of loop diuretics to their lumen site of action, thereby diminishing response. This interaction, then, would be purely pharmacokinetic in nature and any effect on PG's would represent an epiphenomenon.

At the thick ascending limb of the loop of Henle, two options are possible. First, if the effect of loop diuretics to block chloride reabsorption is mediated by PG's, their inhibition would blunt the effect of the diuretics. A second possible mechanism would involve separate effects of loop diuretics and of PG's on chloride reabsorption. If PG's exerted a tonic inhibition of chloride reabsorption, their removal would allow increased reabsorption. If this occurred in the face of administration of a loop diuretic, the net effect of the diuretic to decrease reabsorption might be less, and overall diuresis would be blunted.

Diuretics, Jules B. Puschett, Editor

Lastly, PG's have been implicated to decrease sodium reabsorption at the cortical collecting tubule [5,6]. Though loop diuretics do not affect this site, inhibition of PG's with consequent increased sodium reabsorption could cause a net decrease in response to loop diuretics if response were assessed as total volume or solute excretion as opposed to increase in excretion relative to the appropriate control; i.e. NSAID alone versus NSAID plus the loop diuretic.

Since NSAID's are able to blunt the incremental response to loop diuretics, it appears that this last potential mechanism can be discounted. Studies have addressed each of the other possibilities. First, consider data concerning a pharmacokinetic drug interaction.

EFFECT OF NSAID'S ON THE PHARMACOKINETICS OF LOOP DIURETICS

Studies *in vivo* in animals and *in vitro* had demonstrated that organic acid diuretics reached their site of action from the lumen as opposed to the peritubular side of the nephron [7-9]. Our laboratory performed studies in man using probenecid to permute the relationship between amounts of furosemide in serum and in urine to demonstrate that these prior data could be extrapolated to man [10]. Hence, when assessing response to diuretics, one must examine amounts of diuretic in urine rather than in serum. Moreover, these and other studies showed that the kinetic determinants of response to a loop diuretic are not only the total amount of diuretic entering the urine but also the time course of its delivery into the urinary site of action [10,11].

Indomethacin had no effect on either parameter in normal subjects after 20 and 40 mg doses of intravenous furosemide [12]. Figure 2 shows the time course of excretion of furosemide after a 40 mg dose indicating no effect (left panel). In contrast, the rate of sodium excretion was clearly decreased by indomethacin (right panel). The interaction, then, is purely pharmacodynamic and not pharmacokinetic. This concept is best illustrated by the depiction in Figure 3 which relates urinary furosemide excretion ("dose") to response as sodium excretion. Indomethacin clearly decreases maximal response without affecting other parameters of the dose-response curve [12].

Interestingly, we have recently found similar results; i.e., no kinetic interaction but a pharmacodynamic effect, in normal volunteers administered furosemide plus ibuprofen, naproxen, or sulindac [13]. Consequently, it appears that all NSAID's are able to blunt the response to furosemide. Since similar data have been observed with bumetanide in animals and in man [14,15], the phenomenon is probably also common to all loop diuretics.

If the interaction is pharmacodynamic, the obvious question is what is its mechanism.

PHARMACODYNAMIC MECHANISMS OF THE NSAID-LOOP DIURETIC INTERACTION

Effects on Renal Hemodynamics

The initial studies describing the interaction of NSAID's with diuretics used anesthetized dogs instrumented with electromagnetic flow probes around the renal artery. They showed that ethacrynic acid and furosemide increased renal blood flow and that this effect could be blocked by indomethacin [16-20]. Numerous studies have ensued probing the mechanisms of this effect.

Important concomitant observations in the prostaglandin area were the discovery of prostacyclin, PGI_2, and its probable ability to serve as a locally synthesized vasodilator in many tissues. Wilson et al then showed in dogs that small intravenous doses (0.1 mg/kg) of furosemide caused a natriuresis without affecting urinary excretion of 6-keto-$PGF_{1\alpha}$, the degradation product of PGI_2 [21]. Higher doses (1.0 mg/kg) caused a predictably greater natriuresis but also increased renal blood flow, plasma renin activity and urinary 6-keto-$PGF_{1\alpha}$. Renal blood flow correlated significantly ($r=0.81$, $P<0.001$) with 6-keto-$PGF_{1\alpha}$ while there was no correlation of sodium excretion with this PG metabolite. Importantly, secretin increased renal blood flow without affecting urinary 6-keto-$PGF_{1\alpha}$, implying that the change in hemodynamics was not causal of changes in PG's. These data, then, supported the concept that furosemide caused local synthesis of PGI_2, in turn causing increased renal blood flow and also renin release. Clearly, then NSAID's, by inhibiting renal synthesis of PGI_2, could block this hemodynamic component of furosemide's overall effect. Net natriuresis might then be decreased and represent solely the tubular component of furosemide's pharmacologic effects.

Further support for this hypothesis was garnered by Nies et al [22]. They and others had noted that renal PG's seem to be physiologically important in maintaining renal perfusion in various "stress" states such as sodium depletion, anesthesia, surgery, hemorrhage, heart failure and cirrhosis [23]. In these conditions, inhibition of PG synthesis with NSAID's can cause profound decrements in renal blood flow by removing the vasodilating effect of PG's and allowing the unopposed vasoconstriction of circulating catecholamines and angiotensin [23]. They reasoned that in a state in which endogenous PG's were diminished, such as sodium repletion, administration of loop diuretics should have little or no effect to increase renal blood flow. Consequently, if the mechanism of the NSAID-loop diuretic interaction is via an effect on hemodynamics, no interaction would occur in the sodium replete state while it would still be observed in a state in which perfusion was more dependent on renal synthesis of PG's.

To test their hypothesis, these investigators assessed the effects of indomethacin on the response to 1 mg/kg of intravenous furosemide in dogs [22]. In sodium depleted animals, furosemide increased renal blood flow 35% and indomethacin pretreatment blocked this effect with a concomitant decrease in natriuresis of 40-50%. In contrast, in sodium loaded animals, neither furosemide nor indomethacin affected renal blood flow or sodium excretion.

These data support the hypothesis that NSAID's block the renal hemodynamic component of the overall natriuretic effects of loop diuretics, and that this hemodynamic effect is mediated by prostaglandins, most likely PGI_2. However, an additional component of the interaction could also involve effects at the tubular site of action of loop diuretics.

Effects at the Thick Ascending Limb of the Loop of Henle

Studies employing microperfusion of isolated nephron segments and micropuncture techniques had shown that renal PG's at the tubular level could be physiologically important modulators of solute reabsorption by the medullary segment of the thick ascending limb of the loop of Henle [24,25]. Consequently, if PG's exerted a tonic inhibitory effect on solute reabsorption, their inhibition would result in increased reabsorption and decreased urinary excretion of solute. If this transport pathway were identical to that affected by loop diuretics its interuption could account at least in part for the NSAID interaction.

To address this possibility, our laboratory performed clearance studies in man to assess the nephron site of effect of NSAID's [26]. During water diuresis, we found a decrease in generation of free water but a parallel decrease in delivery of solute to the diluting segment. Free water clearance corrected for this delivery was unaffected by inhibition of PG synthesis. Therefore, solute transport at the diluting segment was not affected whereas more proximal sites were. During hydropenia, indomethacin caused an increase in free water reabsorption relative to osmolar clearance. These data are consistent with the hypothesis that in man NSAID's increased solute reabsorption at the medullary segment of the thick ascending limb of the loop of Henle, consistent with *in vitro* and animal data. These results also imply that PG's *are* physiologically important in solute homeostasis at this nephron segment. However, the quantitative importance of this PG influence is unknown. Similarly, in the NSAID-loop diuretic interaction, the relative contribution of this effect of NSAID's compared to effects on renal hemodynamics is unclear. It would appear that the tubular component is of a relatively minor magnitude, and that the major mechanism of the interaction is the effect of NSAID's to inhibit the PG-mediated renal vasodilating effect of loop diuretics [22].

SUMMARY AND CONCLUSIONS

Sorting out the implications and mechanisms of the NSAID-loop diuretic interaction has provided important insight into mechanisms of pharmacological effects of diuretics and of NSAID's and has allowed better understanding of the physiological role of renal prostaglandins. There are no effects of NSAID's on the pharmacokinetics of loop diuretics. Instead, they change the pharmacodynamics of response predominantly by blocking the renal hemodynamic effects of these diuretics. Presumably further pursuit of the mechanisms of these and other similar drug interactions will prove as fruitful and enlightening as it has in the past.

REFERENCES

1. L.E. Earley, R.M. Friedler. J. Clin. Invest. 44, 1857 (1965).
2. J.E. Lewy, E.E. Windhager. Am. J. Physiol. 214, 943 (1968).

3. B.M. Brenner, K.H. Falchuk, R.I. Kiemowitz, R.W. Berliner. J. Clin. Invest. 48, 1519 (1969).
4. B.M. Brenner, J.L. Troy. J. Clin. Invest. 50, 336 (1971).
5. J.B. Stokes, J.P. Kokko. J. Clin. Invest. 59, 1099 (1977).
6. U. Iino, M. Imai. Pflugers Arch. 373, 125 (1978).
7. B. Odlind. J. Pharmacol. Exp. Ther. 208, 515 (1979).
8. B. Odlind. J. Pharmacol. Exp. Ther. 211, 238 (1979).
9. M.B. Burg. Kidney Int. 9, 189 (1976).
10. P. Chennavasin, R. Seiwell, D.C. Brater, W.M.M. Liang. Kidney Int. 16, 187 (1979).
11. S. Kaojarern, B. Day, D.C. Brater. Kidney Int. 22, 69 (1982).
12. P. Chennavasin, R. Seiwell, D.C. Brater. J. Pharmacol. Exp. Ther. 215, 77 (1980).
13. D.C. Brater, S. Anderson, B. Baird, W.B. Campbell. Clin. Res. 31:868A, abstract (1984).
14. D.E. Smith, H.S.H. Lau. J. Pharm. Sci. 72, 1298 (1983).
15. D.C. Brater, P. Chennavasin. Clin. Pharmacol. Ther. 27, 421 (1980).
16. H.E. Williamson, W.A. Bourland, G.R. Marchand. Prostaglandins 25, 297 (1974).
17. M.D. Bailie, J.A. Barbour, J.B. Hook. Proc. Soc. Exp. Biol. Med. 148, 1173 (1975).
18. H.E. Williamson, W.A. Bourland, G.R. Marchand. Proc. Soc. Exp. Biol. Med. 148, 164 (1975).
19. H.E. Williamson, G.R. Gaffney, W.A. Bourland, D.B. Farley, D.E. VanOrden. J. Pharmacol. Exp. Ther. 204, 130 (1978).
20. M.D. Bailie, K. Crosslan, J.B. Hook. J. Pharmacol. Exp. Ther. 199, 469 (1976).
21. T.W. Wilson, C.B. Loadholt, P.J. Privitera, P.V. Halushka. Hypertension 4, 634 (1982).
22. A.S. Nies, J. Gal, S. Fadul, J.G. Gerber. J. Pharmacol. Exp. Ther. 226, 27 (1983).
23. J.G. Gerber, R.J. Anderson, R.W. Schrier, A.S. Nies in: Prostaglandins and the Cardiovascular System, J.A. Oates, ed. (Raven Press, New York 1982) pgs. 227-254.
24. E. Higashihara, J.B. Stokes, J.P. Kokko, W.B. Campbell. J. Clin. Invest. 64, 1277 (1979).
25. J.B. Stokes. J. Clin. Invest. 64, 495 (1979).
26. S. Kaojarern, P. Chennavasin, S. Anderson, D.C. Brater. Am. J. Physiol. 244, 134 (1983).

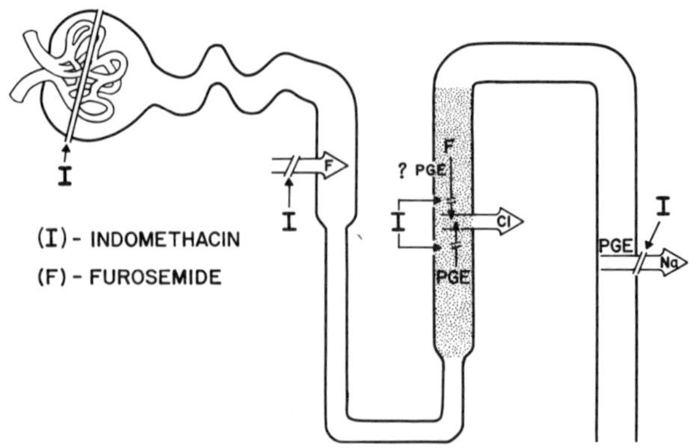

FIG. 1. Schematized nephron showing possible sites of interaction between NSAID's and diuretics.

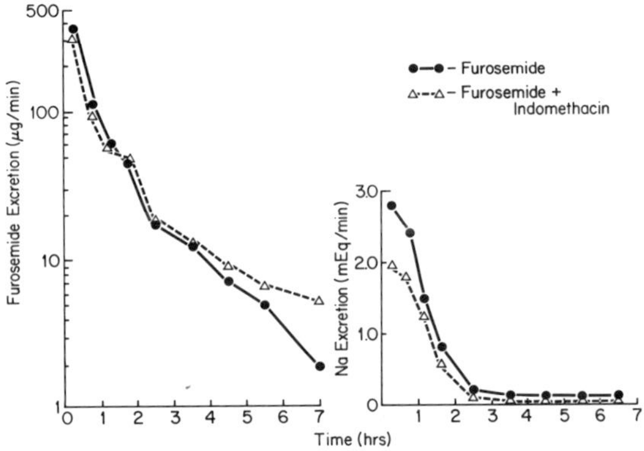

FIG. 2. Effect of inaomethacin on the time course of excretion of furosemide (left panel) and of sodium (right panel).

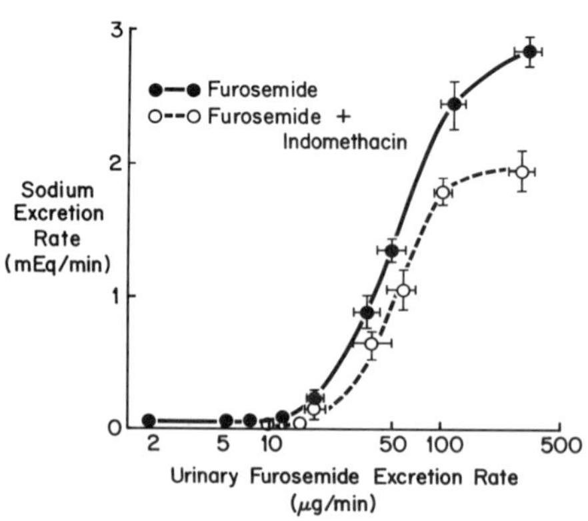

FIG. 3. Dose-response curves to furosemide with and without pretreatment with indomethacin.

EFFECT OF INDOMETHACIN PRETREATMENT ON DIURETIC-INDUCED SALIDIURESIS, RENIN RELEASE, AND THE PHARMACOKINETICS OF DIURETICS IN DOGS

MAX HROPOT,* FRITZ SÖRGEL,** WOLFRAM P. GLUTH,** and ERIK KLAUS*
*Hoechst AG, Postfach 80 03 20, 6230 Frankfurt/M. 80;
**Carl-Korth-Institute for Cardiovascular Research, Div. of Clinical Pharmacology, and Institut für Rechtsmedizin, University of Erlangen, 8520 Erlangen, FRG

ABSTRACT

The oral pretreatment of indomethacin twice i.e. 17 hours and 1 hour before the intravenous administration of furosemide (1.56, 6.25, and 25 mg/kg) and of hydroflumethiazide (3.12 and 12.5 mg/kg) to dogs reduced the natriuretic response as compared to diuretics alone and did not alter the urine excretion. The furosemide-induced increase in plasma renin activity was also significantly diminished by indomethacin pretreatment. The administration of hydroflumethiazide caused only a moderate increase in plasma renin activity. However, the 24 hour values of plasma renin activity were not affected by indomethacin pretreatment and were increased after both diuretics. There was a positive correlation between sodium excretion and plasma renin activity irrespective of whether the dogs were treated with indomethacin or not. The pretreatment with indomethacin did not influence the urinary excretion of furosemide, but the total clearance and plasma clearance of furosemide were reduced by about 20 - 30 %. In summary it can be said that pretreatment with indomethacin reduced the natriuretic response to furosemide and hydroflumethiazide and did not alter the excretion of urine and furosemide. Pharmacokinetics data do not support the thesis that inhibition of tubular secretion is the mechanism of indomethacin interaction with diuretics.

INTRODUCTION

There are discrepancies in reports concerning the effect of indomethacin on the pharmacodynamic and pharmacokinetic response to diuretics. It has been shown that indomethacin attenuates the natriuretic response to diuretics by competing for tubular secretion and/or by inhibition of prostaglandin synthesis [1, 2, 3].

On the other hand it has been demonstrated that the effect of indomethacin differed with the respective dose of furosemide and implies a dose-dependent interaction [4]. Other authors have shown that prostaglandins are not a major factor in mediating the diuretic response to furosemide in the dog and that diuretic response to furosemide is independent of changes in magnitude or distribution of renal blood flow [5]. Brater reported that indomethacin may also attenuate the natriuretic response to chlorothiazide [6], whereas other authors did not observe any significant influence of indomethacin either on the pharmacokinetics of hydrochlorothiazide or the pharmacodynamic response to this diuretic [7]. The purpose of this study was, therefore, to determine whether the pharmacological effect or pharmacokinetics of furosemide and hydroflumethiazide were altered by simultaneous administration of indomethacin.

Diuretics, Jules B. Puschett, Editor

METHODS

The experiments were performed in 20 male conscious beagle dogs with a mean body weight of 17.3 ± 1.4 kg. Food was withdrawn 24 hours prior to the experiments and the animals received only water ad libitum. The dogs were compared intra-individually, thus in the first series of experiments the dogs received diuretics alone. Furosemide in doses of 1.56, 6.25, and 25 mg/kg as well as hydroflumethiazide in doses of 3.12 and 12.5 mg/kg were injected intravenously. Urine and blood samples were then collected up to 24 hours. Urine was collected at the following intervals: 15, 30, 45, 60, 90, 120, 180, 240, 300, 360, and 420 minutes and 7 - 24 hours after administration of diuretics, whereas blood samples were obtained at 0, 5, 10, 20, 30, 60, 90, 120, 180, 240, 300, 360, and 420 minutes as well as at 24 hours after administration of diuretics.

The second series of experiments were performed in the same dogs two weeks later. Indomethacin was administered orally in a dose of 12.5 mg/kg 17 hours and 1 hour before the second treatment with the diuretics in the abovementioned doses. Urine and blood samples were collected at the same intervals as before. Sodium, potassium, calcium, magnesium and chloride as well as osmolality were measured in urine and plasma. Plasma renin activity was determined in plasma, whereas furosemide and hydroflumethiazide were assayed in urine and plasma by high performance liquid chromatography [8]. The pharmacodynamic data were compared with Student's paired t-test.

RESULTS

After intravenous administration of furosemide, a dose-dependent increase in urine and sodium excretion has been observed (Fig. 1 and 2). Pretreatment with indomethacin (I) had little influence on urine excretion but decreased sodium excretion significantly. As is already known hydroflumethiazide is less effective in dogs and shows a poor dose-dependent natriuretic effect, whereas the urine excretion is moderate. After pretreatment with indomethacin, sodium excretion was diminished but not significantly so. Urine excretion increased moderately after intravenous administration of hydroflumethiazide, but pretreatment with indomethacin did not alter this (Fig. 1).

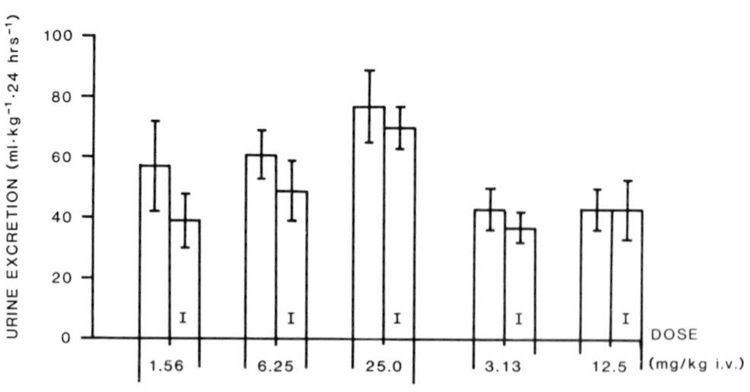

Fig. 1. Urine excretion over a period of 24 hours after intravenous administration of furosemide and hydroflumethiazide either with or without indomethacin ($\bar{x}$ ± SD, n = 4).

In Fig. 3, the plasma renin activity is plotted over the observation time of 24 hours. After intravenous administration of furosemide, the plasma renin activity already increased significantly 5 minutes after administration and reached a plateau at 60 minutes. Pretreatment with indomethacin significantly diminished furosemide-induced renin release, but 24 hour plasma renin activity values increased again and were quite comparable with values after furosemide alone. Administration of hydroflumethiazide caused only a moderate increase in plasma renin activity up to 90 minutes, and was slightly diminished by pretreatment with indomethacin. However, 24 hours after administration of hydroflumethiazide either with or without indomethacin, plasma renin activity was increased considerably.

A linear dose-dependent increase in plasma renin activity after administration of diuretics could not be established. However, there was a positive correlation between sodium excretion and renin release irrespective of whether the dogs were pretreated with indomethacin or not (Fig. 4). The regression lines were calculated for both diuretics and all doses used either with or without indomethacin pretreatment and showed no difference in steepness of slopes.

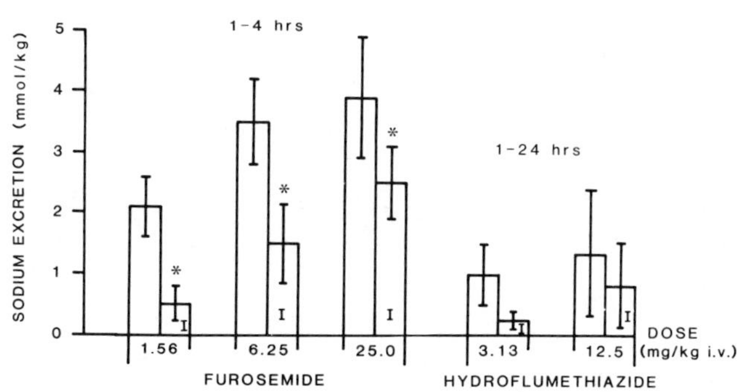

Fig. 2. Sodium excretion over periods of 1 - 4 and 1 - 24 hours after intravenous administration of furosemide and hydroflumethiazide either with or without indomethacin ($\bar{x} \pm SD$, n = 4).

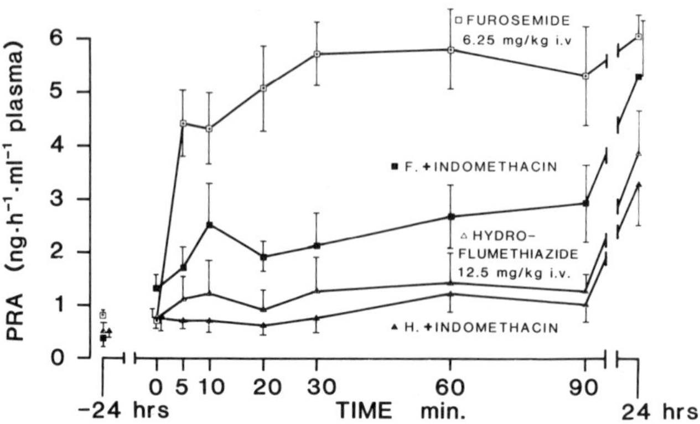

Fig. 3. Plasma renin activity (PRA) over a period of 24 hours before and after intravenous administration of furosemide and hydroflumethiazide either with or without indomethacin ($\bar{x} \pm$ SEM, n = 4).

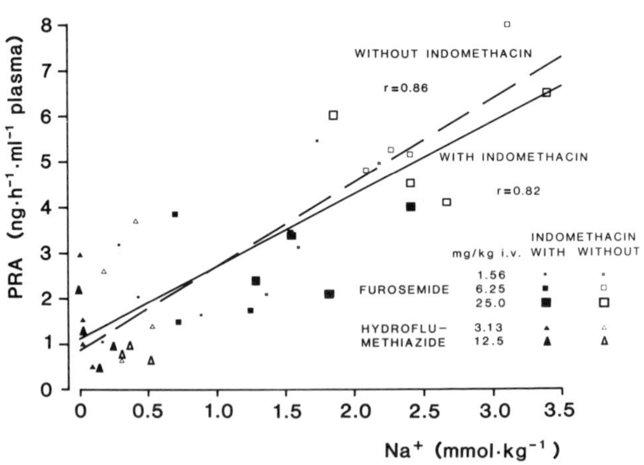

Fig. 4. Relationship between plasma renin activity and sodium excretion 1 hour after administration of diuretics. The regression lines represent both the dogs treated with diuretics alone and with diuretics plus indomethacin.

In Fig. 5 and 6, it becomes clearly evident that the urinary excretion of furosemide is virtually unchanged in dogs irrespective of whether the dogs were pretreated with indomethacin or not. Although there is some variation at different collection periods in the two representative dogs shown, the overall elimination is unchanged. Moreover, when plasma levels are compared (Fig. 7 and 8), the pretreatment with indomethacin caused distinctly higher plasma levels of furosemide resulting in a decrease of total and renal clearance by about 20 - 30 %. Again a variation between different dogs was observed. Indomethacin pretreatment did not effect the renal excretion of furosemide and hydroflumethiazide at any dose used (results not shown here).

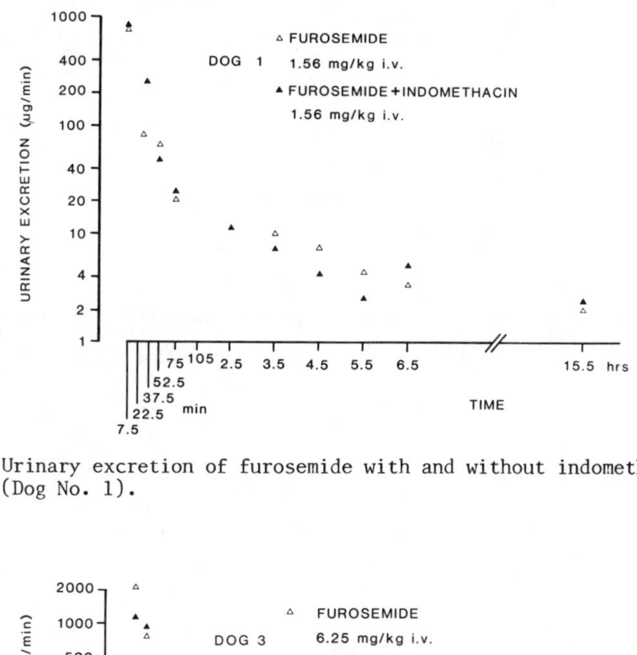

Fig. 5. Urinary excretion of furosemide with and without indomethacin (Dog No. 1).

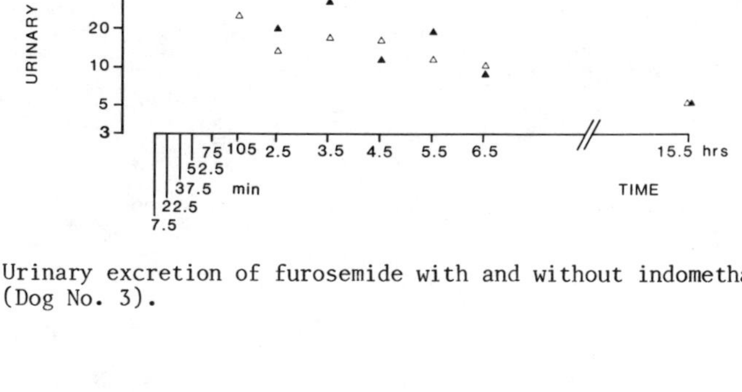

Fig. 6. Urinary excretion of furosemide with and without indomethacin (Dog No. 3).

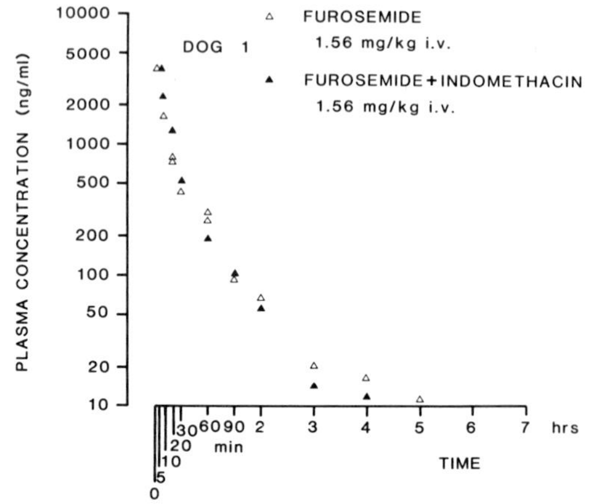

Fig. 7. Plasma concentration of furosemide with and without indomethacin (Dog No. 1).

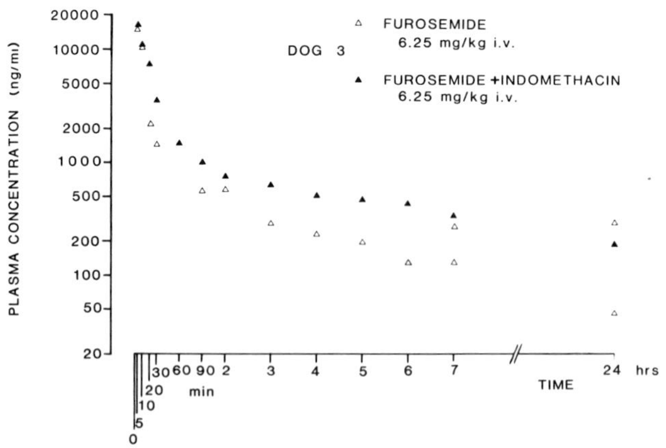

Fig. 8. Plasma concentration of furosemide with and without indomethacin (Dog No. 3).

DISCUSSION

Indomethacin possesses different pharmacodynamic effects among which the inhibition of prostaglandin synthesis via the cyclooxygenase enzyme system and the competition with other organic acids for the renal anion secretory transport mechanisms are well understood. In the present study, the pretreatment with indomethacin has little influence on furosemide-induced urine excretion, but it decreased furosemide-induced natriuresis significantly. Thus, there seems to be a dissociation of diuretic and natriuretic response to furosemide after pretreatment with indomethacin. Several reports have documented that indomethacin attenuates many of the intra- and extrarenal actions of furosemide and other loop diuretics [1, 2, 3, 9].

The hydroflumethiazide-induced natriuresis was also distinctly decreased after pretreatment with indomethacin, although the differences were not statistically significant. Moreover, the urine excretion was not changed at all. These findings are in part contrary to Williams' et al. [7] who reported no influence of indomethacin on the pharmacodynamic response to hydrochlorothiazide in man.

Pretreatment with indomethacin significantly reduced the furosemide-induced increase in plasma renin activity up to 7 hours (not shown in Fig. 3) and had no influence on 24 hour values, which were again increased even after both diuretics. Electrolyte losses might be responsible for this prolonged effect on renin release. Moreover, a positive correlation between urinary sodium and plasma renin activity was observed indicating a sensitivity of macula densa cells for luminal sodium. In addition, our data clearly demonstrate that the renal delivery of furosemide into urine is not changed by indomethacin pretreatment. Some other mechanisms such as renin-angiotensin-aldosterone response to diuretics but not the interaction at tubular level might be responsible for diminished saluresis. The reasons for the decreased total clearance as well as renal clearance observed in this study are not quite clear but are in agreement with the results of Data et al. [5] who found a reduction of these parameters of almost the same magnitude.

It can be concluded from this study that in the dog indomethacin reduced the natriuresis caused by furosemide to a higher extent than that of hydroflumethiazide. Since the delivery of furosemide into urine was not changed by indomethacin, prostaglandins might be involved in the mechanism of furosemide-induced saluresis.

REFERENCES

1. E. Oliw, G. Kover, C. Larsson, and E. Angaard, Pharmacol. 38, 95-100 (1976).
2. U.B. Olsen, Pharmacol. Toxicol. 27, 65-78 (1975).
3. R.B. Patak, B.K. Mookerjee, C.J. Bentzel, P.E. Hysert, M. Babey, and J.B. Lee, Prostaglandins 10, 649-659 (1975).
4. D.C. Brater, J. Pharmacol. exp. Ther. 210, 386-390 (1979).
5. J.L. Data, A. Rane, J. Gerkens, G.R. Wilkinson, A.S. Nies, and R.A. Branch, J. Pharmacol. exp. Ther. 206, 431-439 (1978).
6. D.C. Brater, Clin. Res. 24, 2680 (1977).
7. R.L. Williams, R.O. Davies, R.S. Bermann, G.I. Holmes, P. Huber, Winnie Liang Gee, E.T. Lin, and L.Z. Bennet, J. Clin. Pharmacol. 22, 22-32 (1982).
8. W.P. Gluth, W. Hetz, and M. Geldmacher von Mallinckrodt, Naunyn-Schmiedeberg's Arch. Pharmacol., Supplement Vol. 322, Abstract 36 (1983).
9. A.S. Nies, J. Gal, S. Fadul, and J.G. Gerber, J. Pharmacol. exp. Ther. 226, 27-32 (1983).

PHARMACOKINETICS OF POTASSIUM RETAINING DIURETICS

ERNST MUTSCHLER* AND HEINRICH KNAUF**
*Institute of Pharmacology, University of Frankfurt, D-6000 Frankfurt/Main
**Department of Medicine, University of Freiburg, D-7800 Freiburg, W.-Germany

ABSTRACT

The pharmacokinetic properties of the potassium retaining diuretics spironolactone, triamterene and amiloride in healthy volunteers and patients with liver and renal diseases as well as in the elderly are described.

INTRODUCTION

The potent loop diuretics as well as the thiazides cause a natriuresis associated with kaliuresis. Only those diuretics whose site of action is the late distal tubule and the collecting duct retain potassium. They are therefore called potassium sparing or better potassium retaining diuretics. The main representatives are the aldosterone antagonist spironolactone and the two cycloamidine derivatives triamterene and amiloride [FIG. 1]. The

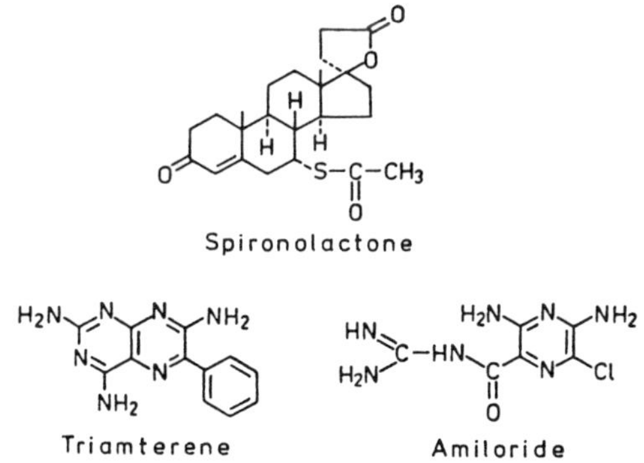

FIG. 1. Potassium retaining diuretics.

following pharmacokinetic description of the antikaliuretics includes the invasion and elimination characteristics in healthy volunteers and in patients with liver and kidney diseases.

Absorption

Spironolactone is rapidly and almost completely absorbed from the gastrointestinal tract. Its bioavailability, refered to the main active metabolite, canrenone, is only 70 % due to the significant first-pass effect [1]. It is however noteworthy that other metabolites are also biologically active.
In contrast to literature [2] triamterene is absorbed to at least 80 %.

Published 1984 by Elsevier Science Publishing Co., Inc.
Diuretics, Jules B. Puschett, Editor

Similar to spironolactone, triamterene undergoes a marked first-pass effect, its bioavailability, therefore, is only about 50 %. In this context it has to be noted that the main metabolite of triamterene has also an antikaliuretic effect.
So far no data are available about the absolute bioavailability of amiloride. This is because the agent can not be administered intravenously because of the risk of histamine release. According to data of urinary recovery the absorption of amiloride was estimated to amount to about 50 %. In the fasted state more amiloride is absorbed than after meals.

Distribution

As far as distribution is concerned protein binding of an agent plays an important role since only the free part is biologically active. Protein binding of spironolactone has been reported to amount to 98 %. For native triamterene it is only about 55 % and for its active phase-II metabolite it is 96 %. The lowest protein binding is reported for amiloride with only 40 %.

Biotransformation

With respect to metabolism of the antikaliuretics important results have recently been put forward. This is due to the improvement of analytical technics.
Spironolactone has been found to be completely degraded. No native spironolactone is recovered in the urine. Until now more than twenty metabolites have been identified. Formerly canrenone was regarded as the main active substance after application of spironolactone. However, it makes up only 1/10 to 1/4 of the antimineralocorticoid effect of spironolactone dependent on the mode of application that is single dose or repetitive dosage [3].
As first shown by Lehmann [4] triamterene is quickly transformed to hydroxy-triamterene which is immediately conjugated to the hydroxy-triamterene sulfuric acid ester [FIG. 2]. This phase-II metabolite is biologically active and contributes to the action of triamterene [5].

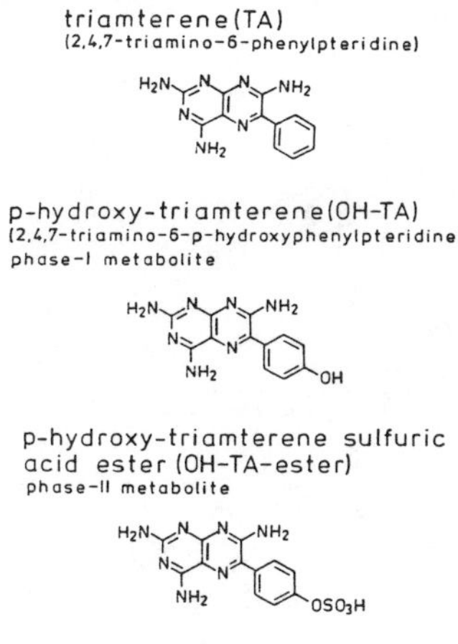

FIG. 2. Metabolic pathway of triamterene [2].

Amiloride has been reported in literature not to be degraded [6]. Our own experiments provide evidence in favour of some biotransformation. As shown in figure 3, we found that amiloride is metabolized to a small extent to the corresponding amide. So far this metabolite has only been identified in plasma but not in urine. We do not know whether this metabolite contributes to the diuretic and potassium retaining effect of the agent.

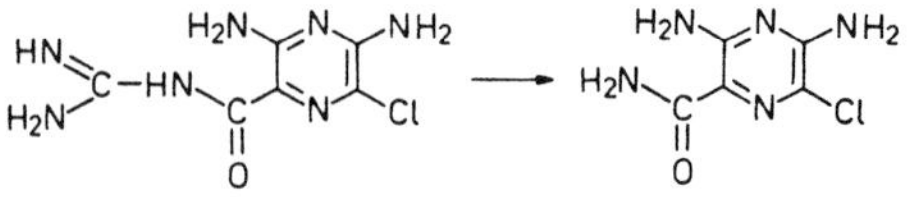

FIG. 3. Putative metabolization of amiloride [7].

Excretion

Healthy control persons excrete about 45 % of the radioactivity of labelled spironolactone through the kidney and about 35 % by biliary excretion. Triamterene is also excreted via the kidneys and the bile, the biliary excretion exceeding the renal excretion. With respect to amiloride only urinary excretion has been studied until now.
So far the methods used for the analysis of triamterene and its metabolites were not satisfactory. We therefore developed a new method which permits a simple and accurate determination of both the native triamterene and its main metabolites [8]. By this way, the i.v. kinetics of triamterene could first be determined in human beings [9]. Figure 4 shows the plasma level time curves of triamterene and hydroxy-triamterene sulfuric acid ester after i.v. administration of 10 mg triamterene. It is noteworthy that already early in the beginning of the ten minutes infusion period the plas-

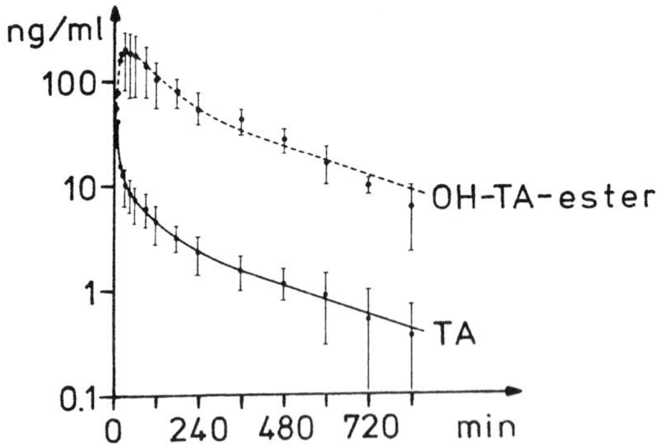

FIG. 4. Plasma level time curves of triamterene and hydroxy-triamterene sulfuric acid ester after intravenous application of 10 mg triamterene during 10 min [9].

ma levels of the ester exceed by far those of the native drug. The maximum plasma level of the ester was significantly higher than that of native triamterene. According to the rapid biotransformation of triamterene the total plasma clearance of triamterene was 4.5 l/min and thus exceeding the rate of liver perfusion which is assumed to be 1.5 l/min. Elimination half life of triamterene and its main metabolite was determined to be 3 hours. Figure 5 illustrates the corresponding data obtained after oral administra-

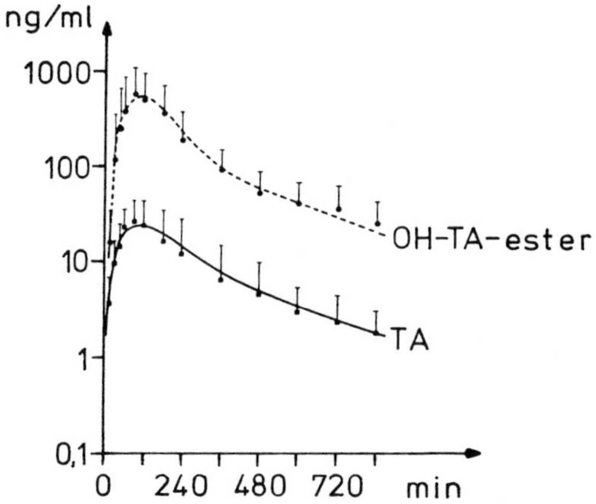

FIG. 5. Plasma level time curves of triamterene and hydroxy-triamterene sulfuric acid ester after oral application of 50 mg triamterene [2].

tion of 50 mg triamterene. This figure again stresses the high plasma levels of the phase-II metabolite as compared to those of native triamterene. The ratio of the concentrations of native triamterene and its sulfuric acid ester was nearly constant throughout the experimental period.

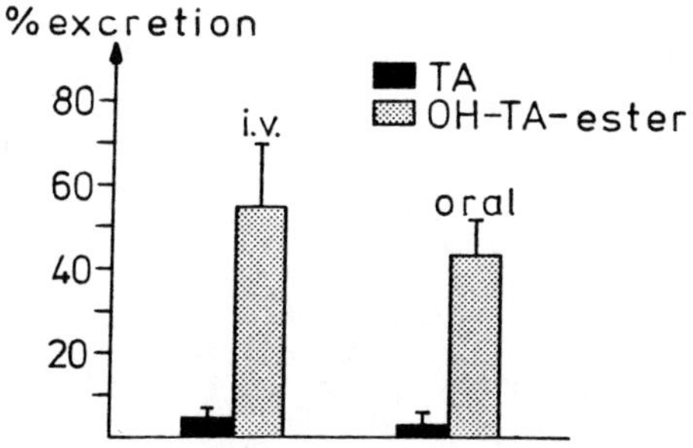

FIG. 6. Urinary excretion rate of triamterene and hydroxy-triamterene sulfuric acid ester after intravenous infusion of 10 mg triamterene during 10 min and oral application of 50 mg [2].

Figure 6 depicts the cumulative urinary excretion of triamterene and the phase-II metabolite. The figure clearly shows that the sulfuric acid ester makes up the main part of urinary recovery as compared to the portion of the native drug. By comparing the i.v. data with those after oral application it is obvious that urinary recovery after i.v. and oral administration do not differ significantly from each other. It can therefore be concluded that about 80 % of the given triamterene are absorbed. Studies on pharmacokinetics of amiloride in humans have so far only been carried out with labelled drug. We therefore developed a new analytical method [10]. Figure 7 illustrates our results on amiloride determination in plasma of healthy volunteers after administration of 10 mg of amiloride.

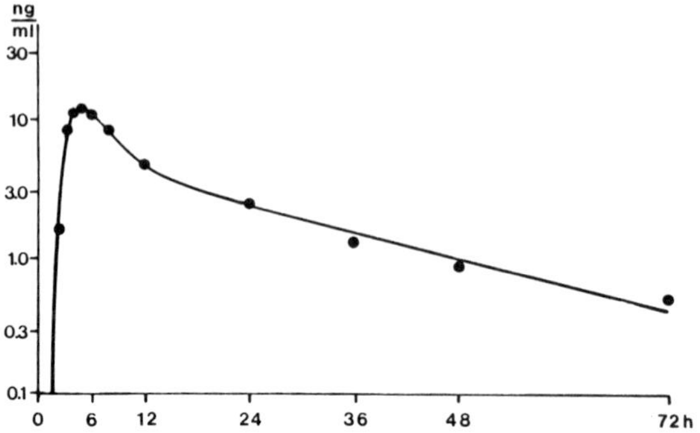

FIG. 7. Plasma level time curve of amiloride after oral application of 10 mg amiloride hydrochloride to a healthy volunteer [7].

The curve can be described by a two-compartment open model. This is at variance with data from literature which attribute a one-compartment model to the amiloride plasma level curve. Furthermore, the elimination half life of amiloride has been reported to be in the range of 6 to 12 hours. However, our data provide evidence in favour of an elimination half life of 17 to 24 hours. This has been corroborated by comparing the measured plasma levels after repetitive dosage with computer simulated data on the basis of the single dose half life. The measured data agree well with the calculated data. About 40 % of given amiloride were recovered in the native form in the urine.

Kinetics in liver diseases and chronic renal failure

For clinical use it is of particular relevance to know the kinetics of kaliuretic drugs in patients with liver and kidney diseases since these drugs are used in patients with liver cirrhosis and in elderly hypertensives with compromised kidney function.

It has been considered a striking finding that the elimination characteristics of spironolactone studied in patients with decompensated cirrhosis of the liver did not significantly deviate from the data obtained in healthy controls [11]. An explanation for this finding may be that this agent is metabolized more by hydrolysis than by oxidative processes. Hydrolytic cleavage is maintained to a sufficient extent also in severely compromised liver function.

On the other hand, the influence of liver function on plasma kinetics of triamterene is very evident. In figure 8 the plasma level time curves of triamterene and its sulfuric acid ester of a healthy volunteer can be compared with the data obtained in a patient with liver cirrhosis. The plasma levels of the ester are significantly lower in hepatic cirrhosis than in the healthy control. In the control, the maximum plasma levels of triamterene reach only about 1/8 of those of the phase-II metabolite.

However, in the patient with liver cirrhosis the plasma levels of triamter-

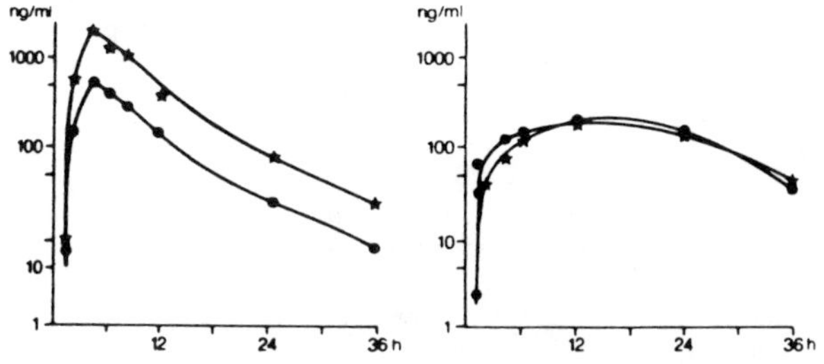

FIG. 8. Plasma level time curves of triamterene and hydroxy-triamterene sulfuric acid ester after oral application of 300 mg triamterene to a volunteer (left side) and to a patient with liver cirrhosis (right side) [2].

ene are increased and the levels of the phase-II metabolite are significantly decreased resulting in almost equal levels of the native drug and the metabolite. Furthermore, the elimination of triamterene is significantly retarded in hepatic cirrhosis of the liver. In these patients $t_{1/2}$ of triamterene is about 4 times longer than in healthy controls. The elimination half life of the sulfuric acid ester is not changed as compared to the control. These alterations clearly illustrate how much biotransformation of triamterene is impaired in patients with hepatic cirrhosis.
In patients suffering from hepatitis (no indication for the drug but a good pharmacokinetic model) the most striking finding was the increase in urinary excretion of native triamterene as well as its phase-II metabolite. Whereas only 25 to 40 % of given dose are recovered in the urine of healthy controls the urinary recovery of triamterene and its metabolites rises to about 80 % in patients with hepatitis [FIG. 9]. This means, that normally

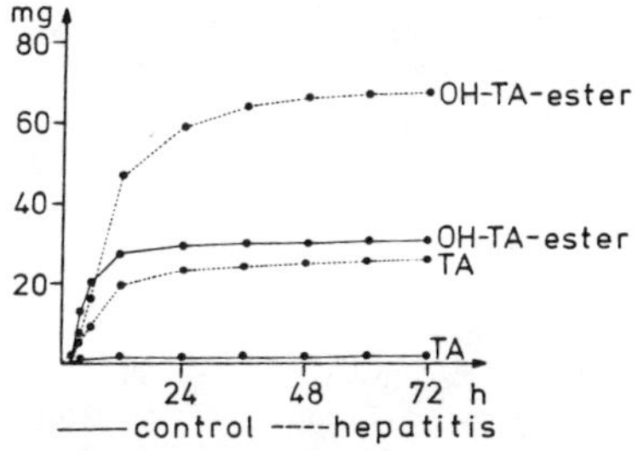

FIG. 9. Cumulative urinary excretion of triamterene and hydroxy-triamterene sulfuric acid ester after oral application of 100 mg triamterene and 50 mg hydrochlorothiazide to healthy volunteers and patients with hepatitis [12].

there is a significant biliary excretion of the drug and this biliary excretion is markedly impaired in patients with hepatitis. Obviously, in the state of hepatitis the liver cell is no more capable to eliminate the phase-II metabolite via the bile. It is furthermore noteworthy that after restitution of the clinical parameters - that is when the patient is considered to have fully recovered from hepatitis - the kinetics of triamterene continue to deviate from healthy controls. This means, that the laboratory tests we use in the clinic, are not sensitive enough to detect

completely the underlying impairments of hepato-cellular metabolism. It may thus be speculated that pharmacokinetic studies on hepatic handling of drug metabolization may provide deeper insight into liver function and they may tell us whether there has already been achieved complete recovery from liver disease. Respective studies are under investigation.
To our knowledge, amiloride has not been studied so far in patients with liver diseases. As degradation of amiloride may be considered to be very small, it can be concluded that the influence of liver diseases on amiloride kinetics is not very important.

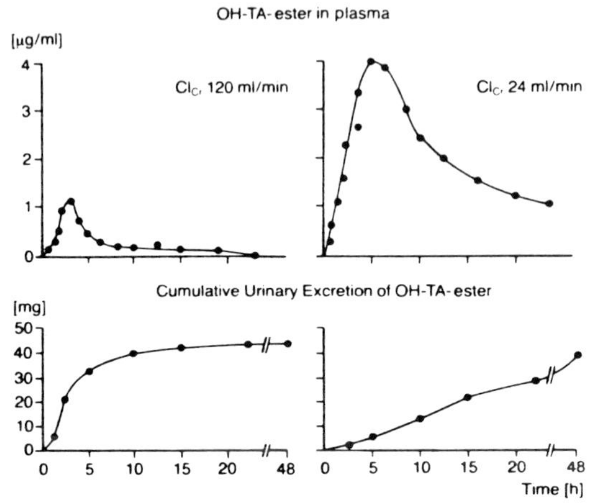

FIG. 10. Plasma level time curves and urinary excretion of hydroxy-triamterene sulfuric acid ester after a oral dose of 100 mg triamterene. Left: Normal renal function. Right: Impaired renal function.
Bottom: Cumulative urinary excretion of the active metabolite OH-TA-ester in a control (left) and in a patient with reduced creatinine clearance (right) [2].

In chronic renal failure the pharmacokinetics of the potassium retaining diuretics change significantly. In figure 10 the plasma levels of the main metabolite of triamterene as well as its cumulative urinary excretion are illustrated. In the patient with chronic renal failure the plasma levels of the sulfuric acid ester are significantly increased as compared to the control data and in turn urinary excretion of the metabolite is retarded [13]. Concerning amiloride, the influence of kidney function on plasma data and urinary recovery is even much more pronounced as depicted in figure 11. In a patient with a creatinine clearance of 20 ml/min the plasma levels decrease only very slowly. Elimination half life of amiloride increases from 20 hours in controls to more than 70 hours in patients with creatinine clearance of 20-30 ml/min. The cumulative urinary excretion of amiloride decreases at the same time from 40 to 17 % [FIG. 11]. The elimination rate constant decreases in proportion with the creatinine clearance [FIG. 12]. Due to predominantly renal elimination of amiloride, the drug accumulates in chronic renal failure. From these data it must be postulated that the administration of amiloride in patients with a creatinine clearance of 30 ml/min and less is contraindicated because of drastic accumulation of the drug [14].

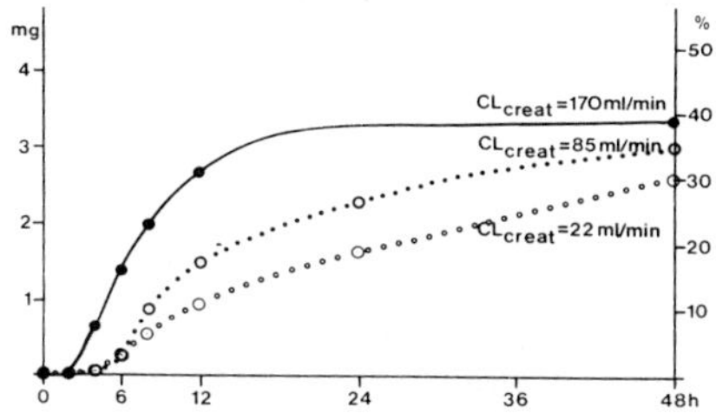

FIG. 11. Cumulative urinary excretion of amiloride in patients with different creatinine clearance after an oral dose of 10 mg amiloride [7].

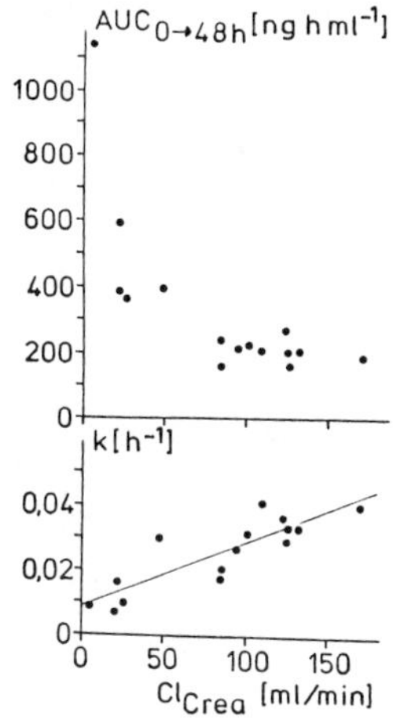

FIG. 12. The area under the plasma level time curve (AUC), top, and the elimination rate constant in relation to the creatinine clearance of the patients after an oral dose of 10 mg amiloride.

Kinetics of antikaliuretics in the elderly

It is well known that the pharmacokinetics of drugs are changed in the elderly. Platt and coworkers [15] have reported that in patients above 70 the peak and the mean plasma levels of canrenone following a single dose of 100 mg spironolactone are about twice as high as the data in healthy controls. Furthermore, the pattern of metabolization of spironolactone significantly differs from that in controls. In collaboration with Platt and coworkers we studied the pharmacokinetics of triamterene in the elderly [16]. t_{max} was not changed which indicates a normal rate of absorption of the agent in the elderly. However, C_{max} was found to be 5 times greater in the elderly as compared to the controls. On the other hand t_{max} of the ester was significantly prolonged which indicates the reduction of metabolic clearance of triamterene at the age above 70.
Corresponding information about amiloride is not available so far. It may, however, be expected due to reduced glomerular filtration rate in this age

that a similar retardation of elimination of the drug occurs in the elderly. Thus it can be concluded for clinical use that the dosis regimen of antikaliuretics has to be reduced to about 1/2 in patients of the age of 65 years.

Concluding remarks

In contrast to amiloride, the antikaliuretics spironolactone and triamterene are mainly eliminated via biotransformation. It is particularly noteworthy that the metabolites of spironolactone as well as those of triamterene contribute to the pharmacological effect of the drug. This fact has to be taken into account when considering the pharmacokinetic characteristics of these drugs. In cirrhosis of the liver the degradation rate of spironolactone is not changed whereas biotransformation of triamterene is significantly retarded in these patients. Thus, when triamterene is used in cirrhosis the usual dosage regimen has to be adapted. Below a creatinine clearance of 30 ml/min the antikaliuretics have to be avoided.

REFERENCES

1. A. Karim in: Aldosterone Antagonists in Clinical Medicine, Excerpta Medica, G.M. Addison, N. Wirenfeldt Asmussen, eds. (Amsterdam-Oxford 1978).
2. E. Mutschler, H.J. Gilfrich, H. Knauf, W. Möhrke and K.D. Völger, Clin. Exp. Hypertens. A5, 249-269 (1983).
3. U. Abshagen, E. Besenfelder, R. Endele, K. Koch and B. Neubert, Eur. J. Clin. Pharmacol. 16, 255-262 (1979).
4. K. Lehmann, Drug Res. 15, 812-816 (1965).
5. H. Knauf, E. Mutschler, K.D. Völger and U. Wais, Drug Res. 28II, 1417-1420 (1978).
6. M.F. Grayson, A.J. Smith and R.N. Smith, Br. J. Pharmacol. 43, 473-474 (1971).
7. K. Reuter, H. Knauf and E. Mutschler, Publication in preparation.
8. B. Grebian, H.E. Geißler and E. Mutschler, Drug Res. 26, 2125-2127 (1976).
9. H.J. Gilfrich, G. Kremer, W. Möhrke, E. Mutschler and K.D. Völger, (in press).
10. K. Reuter, H. Knauf and E. Mutschler, J. Chromatogr. 233, 432-436 (1982).
11. U. Abshagen, H. Rennekamp and G. Luszpinski, Eur. J. Clin. Pharmacol. 11, 169-176 (1977).
12. K.H. Antonin, C. Antonin, W. Möhrke, E. Mutschler and K.D. Völger, Therapiewoche 32, 3909-3917 (1982).
13. B. Grebian, H.E. Geißler, H. Knauf, E. Mutschler, I. Schnippenkoetter, K.D. Völger and U. Wais, Drug Res. 28II, 1420-1425 (1978).
14. L. Dettli, Klin. Pharmacokin. 1, 126-134 (1976).
15. U. Abshagen, D. Platt and H.J. Horn, Klin. Wochenschr. 59, 909-910 (1981).
16. W. Möhrke, E. Mutschler, K.D. Völger, W. Mühlberg and D. Platt, Publication in preparation.

PHARMACOKINETICS OF ACIDIC AND BASIC TRIAMTERENE ANALOGUES

HELGA KRAFT AND ERNST MUTSCHLER
Pharmacological Institute, University of Frankfurt, Theodor-Stern-Kai 7, 6000 Frankfurt 70, W.-Germany

INTRODUCTION

The potassium retaining drug triamterene (TA) is widely used in the therapy of edema and hypertension, mainly in combination with thiazides and loop diuretics. But the very low water solubility of triamterene causes several problems, thus the drug is not available for parenteral application and kidney stones, containing TA, have been found [1].

Therefore we synthesized better water soluble TA-derivatives, i.e. ethers of hydroxytriamterene with basic and acidic groups in the side chain [2]. The most promising compounds - as found in screening experiments in rats - were 4-carboxybutoxytriamterene (Val-O-TA) and dimethylaminohydroxypropoxy-triamterene (RPH 2823) (Fig.1).

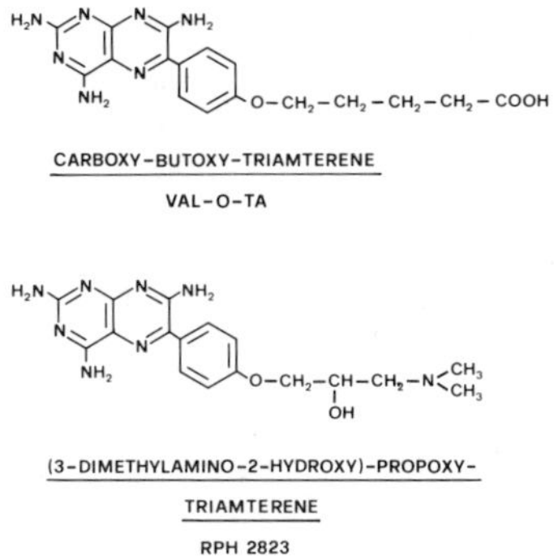

FIG. 1.

Both substances have the same or an even better natriuretic and potassium retaining effect than TA. After these first, encouraging results we investigated the pharmacokinetic behaviour of the two new diuretics in female Wistar rats.

METHODS

During a short ether anaesthesia the substances were injected in one of the caudal veins. At about 10 different times after injection blood samples were obtained from the veins of the retroorbital plexus. Furthermore urine samples were collected in 7 fractions for four days. The concentrations of Val-O-TA and its metabolites and of RPH 2823 in plasma and urine were determined using thin-layer chromatography [3]: the samples were diluted with methanol and centrifuged; an aliquot of the supernatant

Diuretics, Jules B. Puschett, Editor

was applied to thin-layer plates; after development the fluorescence of the spots was measured directly on the TLC-plates.

PHARMACOKINETICS OF VAL-O-TA

The rat metabolizes Val-O-TA to a large extent, four biotransformation products could be identified: the ether bond is dealkylated oxidatively and hydroxytriamterene is formed, which then is conjugated to hydroxytriamterene sulfuric acid ester. In addition, hydroxytriamterene can be conjugated with glucuronic acid. Furthermore, the aliphatic side chain is decomposed by ß-oxidation and carboxyethoxytriamterene is formed. As could be shown, the metabolites carboxyethoxytriamterene and hydroxytriamterene sulfuric acid ester are active as potassium retaining diuretics [2,4] and therefore contribute to the effect of Val-O-TA.

The plasma concentration time curve of Val-O-TA after application of 10 mg/kg can be described with a two compartment open model: the elimination half-life of the α-phase was calculated to be 3 min, for the ß-phase it is 18 min. Val-O-TA is metabolized very quickly, already 3 min after application the two main metabolites can be found in the plasma samples. The ß-oxidation runs faster than the decomposition of the ether bond and the following conjugation: carboxyethoxytriamterene has its highest plasma levels 8-15 min after injection, the hydroxytriamterene sulfuric acid ester reaches its maximum concentration not before 20-40 min after application.

On an average, 15% of the given dose are excreted with urine, but only 3% are unchanged Val-O-TA. Additional 3 % are eliminated as hydroxytriamterene and as hydroxytriamterene sulfuric acid ester, resp. The greatest portion of the administered dose, 5,6%, is excreted renally as carboxyethoxytriamterene. This low renal excretion rate indicates that Val-O-TA is eliminated mainly through bile and faeces; this could be confirmed by investigations with radioactively labelled Val-O-TA: 60% of the administered radioactivity were excreted with the faeces.

Further experiments in female mongrel dogs showed that Val-O-TA has natriuretic and potassium retaining properties in this species, too. Therefore we conducted experiments in which renal clearance and pharmacokinetic data were obtained simultaneously. Val-O-TA was administered i.v. in three different doses - 0,5, 5 and 10 mg/kg - and also in combination with furosemide, probenecid and para-aminohippuric acid.

The rate constant of the terminal phase of elimination λ_z is independent of the applied dose and is not affected by the combination with furosemide, probenecid or para-aminohippuric acid; the terminal elimination half-life is 28 min.

On the other hand the urinary excretion rate is dose dependent: after i.v. administration of 0,5 and 5 mg/kg 17% and 20% of the dose, resp., are eliminated by the kidneys within 2 hours. After 10 mg/kg the renal excretion decreases to 6% of the dose; the simultaneous infusion of furosemide can prevent this decrease, the excretion rate remains 21% of the dose. Probenecid, too, reduces the rate of renal elimination to 8% of the dose. After application of Val-O-TA alone and together with para-aminohippuric acid no difference in the amount of renal excretion can be observed, in either case 21% of the dose are eliminated with urine.

The mean values of the renal clearance of Val-O-TA and of the glomerular filtration rate are shown in fig.2. Except in the combination with probenecid the renal clearance of Val-O-TA is 50% of the GFR. If the diuretic and probenecid are given simultaneously, the renal clearance of Val-O-TA decreases to 20% of the GFR. Obviously probenecid obstructs the secre-tion of Val-O-TA into the proximal tubule and only the amount which is filtered appears in the urine, i.e. 8% of the dose.

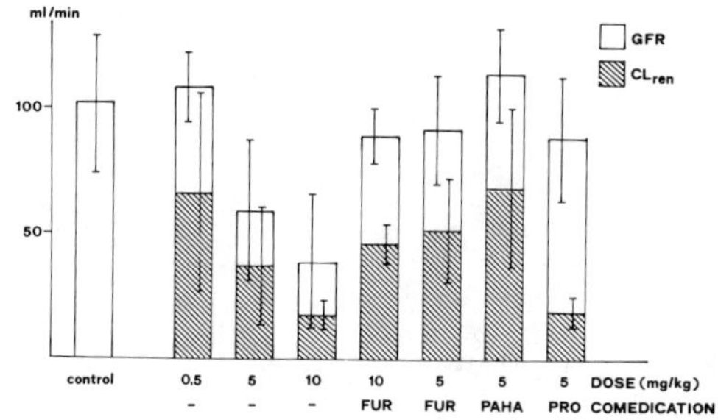

FIG. 2: Renal clearance of Val-O-TA and glomerular filtration rate after i.v.-application of Val-O-TA to dogs.

PHARMACOKINETICS OF RPH 2823

In contrast to Val-O-TA, the basic triamterene derivative RPH 2823 is not metabolized by rats.

After i.v.-application of 1 and 5 mg/kg the plasma concentration time curves can be described with a three compartment open model; the elimination half-life of the α-phase is 5 min; the elimination half-life of the ß-phase is 0,6 hours and the terminal elimination half-life was calculated to be 3 hours.

Compared with Val-O-TA, RPH 2823 is excreted renally to a larger extent: after i.v.-application of 1 and 5 mg/kg 49% and 44% of the dose, resp., were found in urine within 60 hours.

SUMMARY

The acidic triamterene derivative Val-O-TA is a potassium retaining diuretic with a short elimination half-life in rats and dogs; it is strongly metabolized. Because of its acidic structure it should be possible to combine it with loop diuretics like furosemide in the same ampoule.

RPH 2823, a basic triamterene ether with an even higher antikaliuretic potency, has a longer terminal elimination half-life of about 3 hours in rats, but is not metabolized by this species.

REFERENCES

1. Ettinger,B., N.O. Oldroyd, F. Sörgel, J.Am.Med.Assoc. 244 (21), 2442 (1980)
2. Vollmer,G., dissertation (Dep. of Pharmacol., Univ. Frankfurt) 1980
3. Kraft, H., dissertation (Dep. of Pharmacol., Univ. Frankfurt) 1982
4. Leilich, G., H. Knauf, E. Mutschler, K.-D. Völger, Drug Res. 30, 949 (1980)

EFFECT OF RENAL FAILURE ON THE PHARMACOKINETICS OF BUMETANIDE

P. J. PENTIKÄINEN,[1] A. PASTERNACK,[2] E. LAMPAINEN,[3] P. J. NEUVONEN[4] AND A. PENTTILÄ[5]
[1]Third Department of Medicine, University of Helsinki, Helsinki, [2]Department of Medicine, University of Tampere, Tampere,[3]Department of Medicine, University of Kuopio, Kuopio, [4]Department of Clinical Pharmacology, University of Helsinki, Helsinki, [5]Research Laboratories of Medica Pharmaceutical Company Ltd., Helsinki, Finland

INTRODUCTION

Bumetanide is a high ceiling loop diuretic which resembles furosemide in its diuretic action but is 40-60 times more natriuretic and relatively less kaliuretic than furosemide on a weight basis. Its pharmacokinetics in healthy volunteers is characterized by practically complete gastrointestinal absorption, small volume of distribution, high degree of plasma protein binding and rapid elimination by both metabolism and excretion of unchanged drug into urine (1, 2). Bumetanide is often used in high doses in patients with renal failure, but its pharmacokinetics in these patients is little known. Recently, impaired total plasma clearance and renal clearance as well as prolonged elimination half life of bumetanide in six renal patients was reported (3). We have studied the pharmacokinetics in healthy volunteers and in 22 patients with variable degree of renal failure and correlated the pharmacokinetic changes with parameters of renal function.

PATIENTS AND METHODS

The control group (Group I) consisted of six healthy volunteers. The results of their liver and renal function tests were normal. The renal group consisted of 22 patients with chronic renal failure. Six patients had slight renal failure with serum creatinine 115-300 µmol/l (Group II) eight had moderate renal failure with serum creatinine 301-800 µmol/l (Group III) and eight patients had severe renal failure with serum creatinine exceeding 800 µmol/l (Group IV). Group II-IV refers to the pooled renal group. Three patients underwent haemodialysis therapy, two of them were anephric. Their haemodynamic status was stabile and serum transaminase levels were within the normal range. An informed consent was obtained from the volunteers and patients prior to the study. The protocol of the study was accepted by the ethical committees of the hospitals where this study was performed.

^{14}C-bumetanide with a specific activity of 1.45 mCi/mmol and radiochemical purity exceeding 99 % was synthetized. Single intravenous doses of 1 mg/3.08 µCi were administered as bolus injections. Timed blood samples were collected up to 12 h after the dose and all urine was collected in fractions over two days after the dose. Faeces was collected in some subjects up to one week following the drug administration. Total ^{14}C in plasma, urine and faeces samples was determined by liquid scintillation counting. ^{14}C-bumetanide was extracted several times with benzene at pH 3.2. The recovery of ^{14}C-bumetanide was practically complete and no metabolites were extracted.

The plasma concentration-time curves of total ^{14}C and ^{14}C-bumetanide were two-exponential and a two-compartment open model was used to describe the kinetics of both total ^{14}C and ^{14}C-bumetanide. Curve fitting was performed by the nonlinear least squares program NONLIN (4). The parameters of the two-compartment model and model independent pharmacokinetic parameters were calculated by standard formulas. Plasma protein binding of ^{14}C-bumetanide was determined by the equilibrium dialysis method (5) in plasma sample obtained 15 min after the dose.

Simple linear regressions were calculated for serum creatinine and creatinine clearance values and pharmacokinetic variables of ^{14}C-bumetanide. Student's t-test was used to compare the results in renal patients with those in healthy volunteers.

Diuretics, Jules B. Puschett, Editor

RESULTS

The plasma concentrations of ^{14}C-bumetanide and total ^{14}C are presented in FIG.1. and 2. and the pharmacokinetic variables are listed in TABLE I.

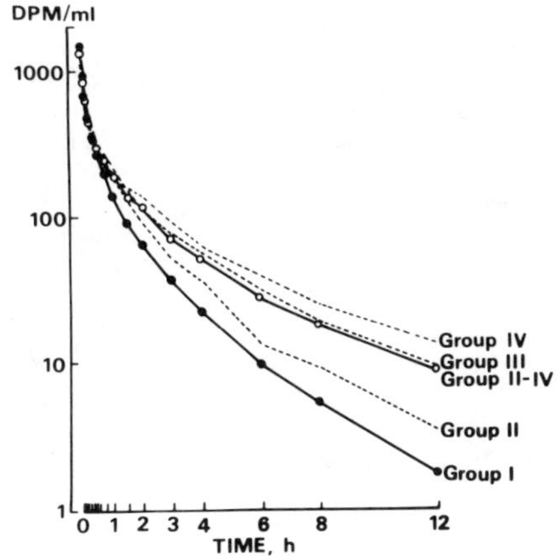

FIG.1. Plasma concentrations of ^{14}C-bumetanide in different groups.

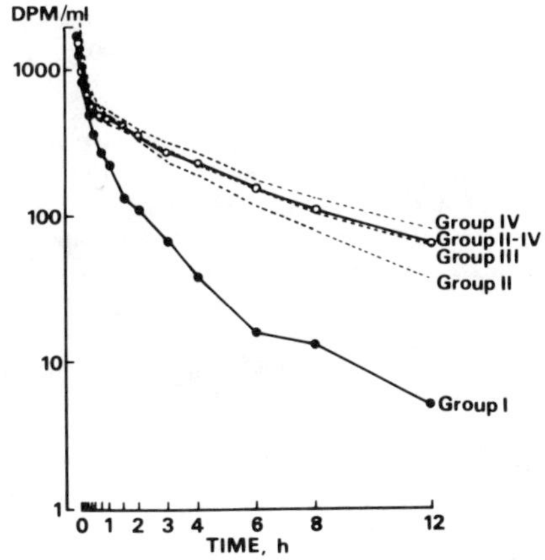

FIG.2. Plasma concentrations of total ^{14}C in different groups.

TABLE I. Pharmacokinetic parameters of ^{14}C-bumetanide in healthy volunteers and renal patients. Means±SE.

Parameter		Group I	Group II	Group III	Group IV	Group II-IV
V_c	l	5.30±0.59	4.73±0.40	6.09±0.66	5.00±0.61	5.34±0.35
Vd_{ss}	l	16.9±1.0	18.9±2.5	27.1±2.7[b]	19.2±2.1	22.1±1.6[b]
$T_{1/2\alpha}$	h	0.14±0.04	0.09±0.01	0.06±0.01	0.07±0.01	0.07±0.01
$T_{1/2\beta}$	h	1.44±0.12	1.53±0.21	2.19±0.24[a]	1.98±0.26	1.93±0.15[a]
Cl_P	ml/min	189±15	200±27	156±23	142±20	163±14
Cl_R	ml/min	90.1±12.8	26.3±6.7[b]	7.6±2.6[c]	1.5±0.6[c]	10.5±2.7[c]
Cl_{NR}	ml/min	99±6	174±31[a]	149±23	140±20	153±14[b]
K_{10}	h^{-1}	2.32±0.34	2.6±0.35	1.73±0.33	1.77±0.16	1.99±0.18
Au[d]	% of dose	46.8±3.2	15.2±4.0	5.0±1.7	1.2±0.4[c]	6.4±1.7[c]
Free fraction	%	4.3±1.0	7.7±1.7	6.6±1.6	7.2±1.0[a]	7.2±0.7[b]

[a]$p<0.05$, [b]$p<0.01$, [c]$p<0.001$ as compared with group I.
[d]Au = recovery in urine in 48 h after the dose.

The pharmacokinetic changes of total ^{14}C were similar to but more profound than those of bumetanide.

The recovery of total ^{14}C in faeces was 13 % and 14 % of the dose, respectively, in two healthy volunteers, whereas it averaged 39±10 % of the dose in ten renal patients.

Both the serum creatinine level and creatinine clearance correlated significantly ($p<0.05$) with K_{el}, Cl_R and $T_{1/2\beta}$ of ^{14}C-bumetanide. The plasma albumin level showed significant ($p<0.05$) correlations with Cl_R, Vd_{ss} and the free fraction of ^{14}C-bumetanide.

DISCUSSION

The results show that the renal clearance of bumetanide decreases with failing renal function. At the same time there is an increase in nonrenal clearance of bumetanide. As a result of these opposite changes the total plasma clearance of bumetanide remains almost unchanged. The steady state volume of distribution of bumetanide is increased in renal patients and the half life of elimination, $T_{1/2\beta}$ is prolonged.

The pharmacokinetics of bumetanide could be adequately described by a two-compartment model. However, the urinary excretion rate data disclosed a slow terminal phase of bumetanide elimination not apparent from the plasma data. Like $T_{1/2\beta}$ the half life of this phase was prolonged in renal patients (3.0 ± 0.3 h vs 6.9 ± 1.3 h, $p < 0.001$). The rate of distribution of bumetanide was not altered in the renal patients nor was the volume of the central compartment, but the steady state volume of distribution showed a significant increase in the pooled renal group. This contrasts with the findings of Marcantonio et al. who reported a significant increase of V_c but not of Vd_{ss} in patients with renal failure (3). In the present study the prolongation of $T_{1/2\beta}$ is mainly a consequence of the increase in Vd_{ss} since the total plasma clearance did not show significant change. The mechanism behind the increase of Vd_{ss} is probably the observed decrease in plasma protein binding of bumetanide. This could also well explain the increase in the nonrenal clearance of bumetanide in the renal patients. The nonrenal clearance of bumetanide is most probably hepatic metabolism and biliary excretion. The high recovery of bumetanide in faeces of renal patients suggests that their biliary excretion of bumetanide is increased.

Thus, the two basic changes in the pharmacokinetics of bumetanide in renal patients seem to be the decrease in renal clearance and the reduced protein binding. The decrease in protein binding results in an increase in the volume of distribution with a subsequent prolongation of the elimination half life. The decrease in protein binding can also explain the increase in nonrenal clearance of bumetanide.

REFERENCES

1. P. J. Pentikäinen, P.J. Neuvonen, M. Kekki, and A. Penttilä , J. Pharmacol. Biopharm. 8, 219-228 (1980)
2. L.A. Marcantonio, W.H.R. Auld, G.G. Skellern, C.A. Howes, W.R. Murdoch, and R. Purohit, J. Pharmacol. Biopharm. 10, 393-409 (1982)
3. L.A. Marcantonio, W.H.R. Auld, W.R. Murdoch R. Purohit, G.G. Skellern, and C.A. Howes, Br. J. Clin. Pharmacol. 15, 245-252 (1983)
4. C.M. Metzler, G.L. Elfring, and A.J. McEven, Biometrics 30, 562 (1974)
5. M. Ehrnebo, S. Avrell, B. Jalling, and L.O. Boreus, Eur. J. Clin. Pharmacol. 3, 189-193 (1971)

COMBINED EFFECTS OF BUMETANIDE AND METOLAZONE IN NORMAL VOLUNTEERS

A. GREENBERG, R. WALLIA, AND J. B. PUSCHETT
Renal-Electrolyte Division, Department of Medicine,
University of Pittsburgh School of Medicine, Pittsburgh
Pennsylvania, USA

INTRODUCTION

It is a well-established principle that diuretics act at circumscribed sites within the nephron (1). Thiazide-type diuretics act in the early distal tubule, loop active agents in the thick ascending limb of the loop of Henle and carbonic acid inhibitors in the proximal tubule. Theoretically, the inhibition of sodium reabsorption at a given site will fail to induce a comparable natriuresis if sodium reabsorption at nephron sites more distal to the inhibited site is augmented. Distal micropuncture studies with furosemide provide support for this hypothesis as a cause for diuretic resistance (2). Clinical studies show an enhanced natriuresis when patients receiving a maximal dose of a loop-active agent are given an agent with activity at a separate sodium resorptive site (3, 4).

Metolazone is active primarily in the early distal convoluted tubule. Studies in this laboratory have shown it to have an additional inhibitory effect in the proximal tubule where it blocks phosphate-linked sodium reabsorption (5). The goal of the present study was to determine whether simultaneous blockade of these two sites by metolazone combined with blockade of loop chloride-linked sodium reabsorption with bumetanide would lead to augmented natriuresis. In particular, the study was designed to show whether this combination of drugs would have a supra-additive effect.

METHODS

Six normal subjects were admitted to a metabolic ward. After a dietary history was obtained, the subjects were placed on a fixed 125-200 mEq sodium diet simulating intake prior to the study. Water intake was allowed ad libitum. After balance was achieved, defined as maintenance of constant weight and 24-hour sodium excretion equal to dietary intake, the subjects were randomized to receive either bumetanide 1-2 mg or metolazone 2.5 mg by mouth. Urinary sodium collections were continued and losses above the balance value replaced with salt tablets. After balance was re-established, each subject received the other drug. Urinary sodium losses were again replaced, and after balance was re-achieved, both drugs were given together.

Clinical laboratory tests were carried out in our laboratory or in the laboratory of the Presbyterian-University Hospital using standard techniques. All data are expressed as mean ± S.E.M. The Student's t-test for paired variables was used for statistical comparisons. When present, statistical significance with $p < 0.05$ or better is indicated by the superscript c for comparisons with the control group, b for comparisons with the bumetanide group, and m for comparisons with the metolazone group.

RESULTS

Diuretic-induced changes in weight and fluid and electrolyte excretion are listed in the table. Administration of either drug alone led to a significant fall in weight. Weight fell by a mean of 1.1 kg after bumetanide and

Diuretics, Jules B. Puschett, Editor

1.2 kg after metolazone. The magnitude of the weight loss after combined treatment was 2.1 kg. Weight fell to a level significantly lower than the levels after either drug alone.

TABLE I. Effects of Treatment with Bumetanide, Metolazone or Both Drugs Together.

	control	bumetanide	metolazone	both
Weight, kg	74.6 ± 5.6	73.5 ± 5.5^{c}	73.4 ± 5.7^{c}	72.5 ± 5.4^{c,b,m}
Volume, ml	1886 ± 231	3584 ± 431^{c}	3037 ± 300^{c}	4509 ± 712^{c}
$U_{Na}V$, mEq	165 ± 12	285 ± 24^{c}	319 ± 28^{c}	381 ± 49^{c}
$U_{K}V$, mEq	79 ± 4	110 ± 9^{c}	106 ± 7^{c}	148 ± 13^{c,b,m}

mean ± S.E.M.

c: $p < 0.05$ vs control
b: $p < 0.05$ vs bumetanide
m: $p < 0.05$ vs metolazone

Urine volume increased approximately 1700 ml after bumetanide, 1140 ml after metolazone and 2600 ml after both drugs together. Volumes after one or both drugs were significantly greater than after control. Although the volume after both drugs together was fully 1½ times the volume after metolazone alone, this trend did not reach statistical significance because of the small number of subjects and the large standard errors.

The sodium excretion pattern was similar to that for urine volume. Excretion after bumetanide was 120 mEq greater than control while excretion after metolazone increased by more than 150 mEq and after both drugs by 215 mEq, to a value more than twice control. Changes in fractional sodium excretion (data not shown) were of similar magnitude.

Both drugs and the combination were highly kaliuretic. Bumetanide and metolazone alone each increased potassium excretion by approximately 30 mEq. Excretion after combined therapy was 69 mEq higher than basal excretion and was significantly higher than excretion after either drug alone.

The change in urine volume during the 24 hours after administration of drug was expressed as a percentage of control urine volume using the formula:

$$100 \times [(\text{volume after drug(s)} - \text{control volume}) \div \text{control volume}].$$

Similar formulae were used to calculate changes in 24 hour urine sodium excretion and potassium excretion.

Bumetanide treatment led to a 95 ± 15% increase in urine volume, metolazone to a 66 ± 16% increase and combined therapy a 147 ± 33% increase. These percentage changes were all statistically different from zero but not from each other. The sum of the increases in volume on the days bumetanide and metolazone were given alone was not statistically different from the increase in volume the day of combined therapy. This indicates that administration of the two drugs together had an additive but not supra-additive effect.

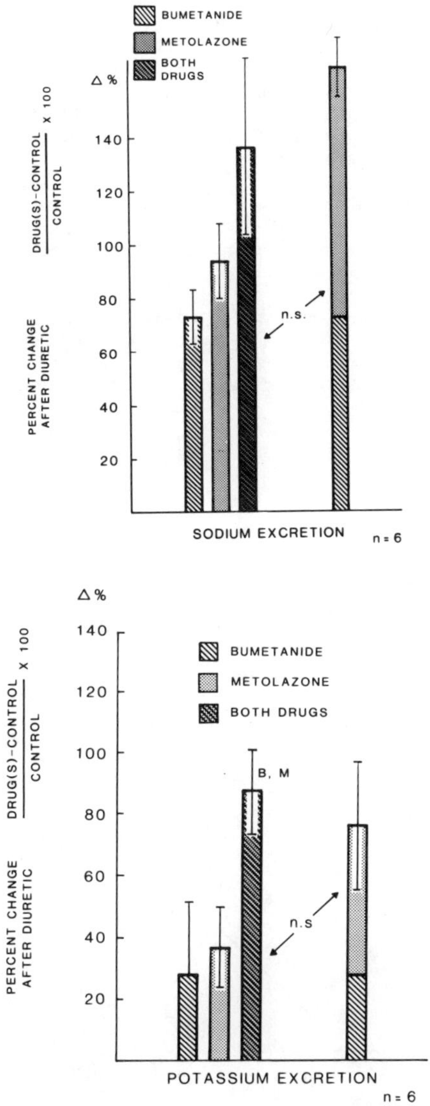

FIG. 1. Sodium excretion (upper panel) and potassium excretion (lower panel) after diuretic administration. Hatched bars show changes after bumetanide alone, dotted bars after metolazone alone and hatched-dotted bars after combined treatment. In both panels, all three changes were statistically different from zero. Symbol b or m, if present, indicates significant differences between combined treatment day and bumetanide alone or metolazone alone, respectively. Fourth bar represents sum of excretion on the two single drug treatment days. In neither panel was this different from excretion on combined treatment day.

The percentage changes for sodium excretion are depicted in figure 1, upper panel. The increments after bumetanide, after metolazone, and after both drugs together, were significantly different from zero but not from each other. The increase in excretion after combined therapy was nearly twice that after bumetanide alone but this difference did not reach statistical significance. Here again, the effects were additive but not supra-additive as the effect of both drugs given together was similar to that of the sum of the increments after each was given alone.

The data for potassium excretion are shown in figure 1, lower panel. They indicate that combined treatment was significantly more kaliuretic than either bumetanide or metolazone. Again, the effect was additive but not supra-additive.

The augmented kaliuresis seen after combined therapy did not appear to be a specific effect of the drugs. Rather, it was in proportion to the augmented natriuresis. In figure 2, the percentage change in potassium excretion, $\Delta U_K V$, is plotted as a function of percentage change in sodium excretion, $\Delta U_{Na} V$. $\Delta U_K V$ appeared to be a linear function of $\Delta U_{Na} V$.

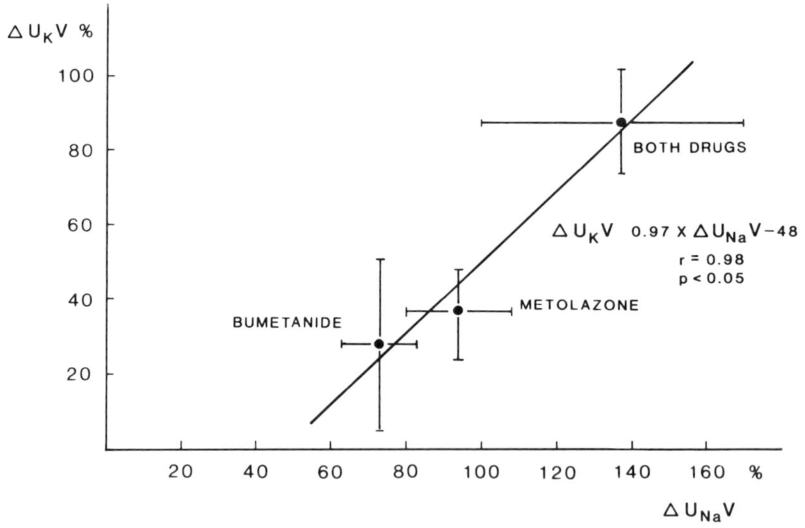

FIG. 2. Percentage change in potassium excretion, $\Delta U_K V$, plotted as a function of $\Delta U_{Na} V$.

DISCUSSION

The reason for the failure to show a supra-additive effect is uncertain. The explanation could in part be methodologic as we had only a small number of subjects and the large standard errors made it hard to show a statistical significance. Sigurd et al (6) demonstrated that the combination of bumetanide and bendroflumethiazide had a supra-additive natriuretic effect when given to subjects with congestive heart failure. A major difference between their study and ours is that their subjects would be expected to have an augmentation of nephron sodium avidity because of their congestive heart failure. The presence of increased nephron sodium avidity was also likely in the subjects in those clinical studies (3, 4) that have previously suggested a supra-additive effect of segmental nephron diuretic blockade. Whether a supra-additive effect occurs only in the presence of a disease state that augments basal sodium avidity is a hypothesis requiring further testing.

SUMMARY

In this study, six normal subjects were treated with bumetanide, metolazone, or both drugs together. All three treatment regimens led to a significant weight loss and increased urine volume and sodium and potassium excretion. Sodium excretion and urine volume tended to be higher after combined treatment than after treatment with either drug alone, but these differences were not statistically significant.

Weight loss and potassium excretion were greater after combined treatment than after treatment with either drug alone. The rise in potassium excretion seen with each drug and with the combination appeared to be in proportion to the increased natriuresis. Combined drug treatment did not have a demonstrable supra-additive effect.

REFERENCES

1. J.B. Puschett. J. Clin Pharmacol. 21, 564 (1981).
2. C.G. Duarte, F. Chomety, and G. Giebisch. Amer. J. Physio. 221, 632 (1971).
3. M. Epstein, B.A. Lepp, D.S. Hoffman, and R. Levinson. Current Therap. Res. 21, 656 (1977).
4. A.W. Asscher. Clin. Trials J. 11, 134 (1974).
5. J.B. Puschett, S.R. Steinmuller, A. Rastegar, and P. Fernandez in: Modern Diuretic Therapy in the Treatment of Cardiovascular and Renal Disease, A.F. Lant and G.M. Wilson, eds. (Exerpta Medica, Amsterdam 1973) pp. 168-175.
6. B. Sigurd, K.H. Olesen, and A. Wennevold. Amer. Heart J. 89, 163 (1975).

SECTION VIII

DIURETICS: IN VIVO AND IN VITRO STUDIES

RED CELL CHLORIDE TRANSPORT IN RELATION TO THE ACTION OF DIURETICS

ARIEL LANT
Department of Clinical Pharmacology and Therapeutics, Westminster Hospital, London, SW1P 2AP, England.

SUMMARY

We have become accustomed to using the term 'loop' diuretics' to encompass all those compounds possessing short-lived high-ceiling effects which act primarily in the thick ascending limb of Henle's loop (TAL). Yet, chemically, it is clear that loop diuretics represent a heterogeneous group whose actions at a cellular level may not be the same. Just as experience with clearance methodology has shown subtle and distinct differences between, for example, phenoxyacetic acid (POA) diuretics and sulphamoylbenzoates, so there appear to be clear differences in the way these compounds interfere with transport of ions across cell membranes.

Use of the red cell model has permitted a number of clearly defined transport pathways to be explored separately and independently from the sodium pump. Two Cl-dependent cation co-transport systems and the band-3 Cl-exchange system can all be inhibited in a specific and reversible manner by various loop diuretics. The Na,K,2Cl co-transport system has a high affinity for sulphamoylbenzoates whilst the Cl self-exchange system has a high affinity for POA derivatives.

Whilst recognising the limitations imposed by model systems, the parallelisms that have been observed between the behaviour of diuretics in red cell membranes and the TAL of the nephron raise the hope that each of these approaches may help to unravel the molecular mechanisms involved in the action of different types of loop diuretics.

INTRODUCTION

The pioneering work of Ussing with frog skin [40], Skou with crab nerve [39] and Leaf with toad bladder [24], set the scene for an extraordinary intensity of investigative work on transport mechanisms in epithelia that has flourished over the past twenty five years. Characterization of the ion movements mediated by the sodium pump and study of the ways in which the pump utilises energy from ATP hydrolysis to perform osmotic and electric work emphasised the primacy of sodium in epithelial transport whilst relegating chloride to the secondary role of a passive partner.

It was therefore not surprising that when the task came of trying to work out the mechanism of action of oral diuretics discovered and brought into widespread clinical use over this same period of time, the major thrust of research in the field up until ten years ago, was directed to the effects which these drugs exerted on the Na,K-ATPase that constitutes the sodium pump. A few lone voices that raised the possible importance of chloride ion [2] were quickly overwhelmed by the abundance of published work which sought to relate the high concentrations of Na,K-ATPase in transporting tissues to the inhibitory effects of diuretics on transport [15;37]. Anomalies emerged, however, which could not be explained.

Diuretics, Jules B. Puschett, Editor

For example, the concentrations of diuretic needed to block Na,K-ATPase in vitro were considerably in excess of those likely to be attained in vivo within the relevant segments of the nephron [29]. Certain groups of diuretics such as the benzothiadiazines or potassium-sparing diuretics did not have significant direct inhibitory effects on the sodium pump. Indeed, whilst the molecular mechanism of action of the former still remains totally obscure, the primary action of the latter drugs like amiloride and triamterene is clearly directed to blocking passive luminal sodium entry mechanisms [3;5;13].

SECONDARY ACTIVE CHLORIDE TRANSPORT

The finding by Burg, Kokko and their colleagues [10;32] that the epithelium of the perfused TAL possessed a luminally-orientated positive PD together with specificity for chloride movement that was blocked by low concentrations of 10^{-5}M frusemide, gave an enormous upsurge in interest in the relevance of transepithelial movement of Cl in relation to the action of diuretics.

Evidence quickly mounted for the presence in a variety of animal tissues of chloride transport mechanisms that were coupled to sodium, inhibited by low doses of loop diuretics like frusemide as well as by low doses of ouabain. Obvious parallelisms can thus be seen between the chloride secretory mechanisms of the amphibian cornea [26], rabbit colon [16] teleost operculum [25] or intestine [18], elasmobranch rectal gland [38] and the TAL of the mammalian nephron [21]. To date, however, no epithelial chloride transporting mechanism has been identified that is energised by direct coupling to the flow of a metabolic reaction in the manner that primary cation transport is energised by ATP hydrolysis via the Na,K-ATPase of the sodium pump. 'Active' chloride transport can best be viewed as an example of secondary active transport driven by the Na and K gradients generated within cells by the action of Na,K-ATPase. [17;20] In keeping with this working hypothesis, a number of observations have shown that there is a requirement for both Na and K to the loop diuretic-sensitive cellular uptake of chloride. Thus the membrane carrier responsible appears to move all three ion species in an electroneutral manner. Electroneutral cation-linked chloride transport which is sensitive to inhibition by loop diuretics has been identified not only in the mammalian TAL [36] but also in teleost intestine [41], human red cells [12], squid giant axons [35], Ehrlich ascites tumour cells [19] and HeLa carcinoma cells [1].

Many might feel that transport systems identified in such diverse tissues across the animal kingdom has little relevance of a direct nature to the processes in the human kidney that are involved in the actions of diuretic drugs. However, the remarkable similarities that have been noted between the behaviour of various transporting epithelia have more than justified the development and application of these simpler tissue models to the problem of trying to isolate the components of the mechanisms involved in drug inhibition. There remain undoubted limitations in using model systems in different species to study the action of diuretics. Extra - polation of observed effects to the functional operation of the kidney may not always be valid. Yet, amphibian epithelia (toad bladder and frog skin) have paid off handsomely as model tissues mimicking the distal nephron and have allowed detailed examination of the molecular mechanisms involved in the action of amiloride and triamterene on membrane sodium channels [5].

Even where study has been undertaken of the natural target tissue, as with microperfusion of TAL tubules of rabbit kidney, a clear lack of homogeneity in action amongst loop diuretics emerges at a cellular level. Thus whereas sulphamoylbenzoate compounds related to frusemide have a high affinity for the electroneutral Na,K, 2Cl co-transport mechanism, other loop diuretics of differing structure like muzolimine, MK-447 or etozoline, leave this transport mechanism unaffected [36].

RED CELL CHLORIDE TRANSPORT SYSTEMS

Three chloride transporting systems in red cells have been used as models which each possess some of the characteristics of renal tubular epithelial cells sensitive to the action of certain diuretics.

1. Electroneutral Na,K, 2Cl Co-transport

The red cell Na, K co-transport system appears to be an example of the generally distributed Cl-dependent cation-linked transporter system [12].

Sulphamoylbenzoate compounds inhibit this system with high affinity and the relative inhibitory effectiveness of the commonly available members of the series: bumetanide > piretanide > frusemide = 56: 8: 1 [14] agrees with equivalent estimates for in vivo saluretic potency for these compounds in man [33]. The concentrations (I_{50}) giving half-maximal inhibition of the human red cell co-transport system for these three sulphamoylbenzoates are shown in Table I:

Compound	I_{50} (M) [a]
Bumetanide	1.6×10^{-7}
Piretanide	1.2×10^{-6}
Frusemide	9.0×10^{-6}

[a] from Ellory and Stewart [14].

Ethacrynic acid is a poor inhibitor in this system (I_{50} = 10^{-7}M) whereas ethacrynic acid-cysteine is effective at an I_{50} of 4.0 x10^{-7}M. The potassium-sparing agents, triamterene and amiloride, as well as benzothiadiazine analogues, chlorothiazide and metolazone, are inactive at concentrations of 10^{-4}M.

2. Hormone-stimulated Cl-dependent Cation Co-transport

This system was first reported in duck erythrocytes and has been extensively studied in turkey erythrocytes [4;23]. Palfrey et al [30] reported the effects of a large series of 3-aminobenzoic acid derivatives in turkey and human red cells. The Cl-dependent Na,K co-transport, independent of the sodium pump, is activated by catecholamine β -agonists or cyclic AMP, and is subject to reversible inhibition by a number of sulphamoylbenzoates as shown in Table II:

Compound	I_{50} (M) [a]
I [b]	4.6×10^{-8}
Bumetanide	2.5×10^{-7}
Piretanide	2.8×10^{-6}
Frusemide	2.3×10^{-5}
XI (HH594) [c]	3.9×10^{-5}

[a] from Palfrey et al. [30] [b] 3-benzylamino-4-phenylthio-5-sulphamoylbenzoic acid

[c] 3-N-n-butylamino-4-chloro-5-sulphamoylbenzoic acid

By comparing the co-trasnport blocking activities of a number of compounds with different substitutents at position 1 in the molecule, it is clear that the anionic function at C_1 is essential for expression of inhibitory activity. Palfrey et al. [30] found the most active compound in their series was compound I and they noted further a positive correlation between inhibition of co-transport in the turkey red cell and the natriuretic activity evoked by these same derivatives in vivo in the dog.

It is noteworthy that benzothiadiazines are inactive as inhibitors of this system up to concentrations of 10^{-3}M.

3. Cl-Self-Exchange or Band 3 Anion Transport

For over one hundred years it has been known that the human red cell possesses a very rapid anion exchange system which physiologically permits the exchange of Cl^- for HCO_3^- and thereby increases the CO_2-carrying capacity of blood (the chloride or Hamburger shift) [28]. This transport system is highly specialized and has a $t_{\frac{1}{2}}$ for chloride exchange of the order of 50 msec at 38°C. Ligand and chemical probe studies have identified the transport protein with a 93-95 k-dalton intrinsic membrane glycoprotein called band 3, a portion of which serves as the translocating carrier [22;34]. The anion exhcange system is inhibited by disulphonic stilbenes such as DIDS or SITS which bind selectively to the band 3 carrier but leave the slower cation fluxes mediated by the sodium pump unaffected.

Chloride flux through this mechanism is an electrically silent obligatory one for one exchange. Segments of the band 3 protein can exist in two conformations, one facing outwards and the other inwards, conformational changes occurring only when anion is bound to the substrate (transport) site. [31]

At concentrations up to 10^{-4}M, ouabain and potassium-sparing diuretics like triamterene and amiloride, are without effect on this system whilst benzothiadiazines cause substantial inhibition [7].

When the inhibitory activities of various sulphamoyl-benzoates upon the band 3 anion transport system are compared with either of the two Cl-dependent co-transport systems considered above, it is clear that the affinity of these compounds for the former system is about two orders of magnitude (in log.units) less [6 ; 7]. Certain anomalies emerge, as for example, the finding that compound I (Table II), which was the most active of all derivatives tested in the avian co-transport system by Palfrey et al.[30], is hardly active at all in respect of inhibiting band 3 chloride exchange.

The concentrations (I_{50}) giving half-maximal inhibition of band 3 chloride transport in human red cells of a number of sulphamoyl-benzoates are given in Table III. In this series, piretanide > bumetanide > frusemide, a relationship which also correlates with the relative lipophilicity of the compounds determined as log P [8].

POA derivatives based on the prototype, ethacrynic acid, also inhibit band 3 chloride transport. Using ox red cells, Moutais and Cousin [27] found a high potency effect which was instantaneous and reversible. It did not appear to relate to reactivity with membrane thiol groups since dihydroethacrynic acid, which lacks SH-binding capacity, had an I_{50} of 9.0×10^{-6}M, of the same order as ethacrynic acid (7.0×10^{-6}M). The relative inhibitory activities of the various POA derivatives studied was highly correlated with their lipophilicity [27].

TABLE III. Half-maximal inhibitory concentrations (I_{50}) for the human red cell band 3 chloride transport system and liposolubility characteristics (log P) of selected sulphamoylbenzoate derivatives. [a)]

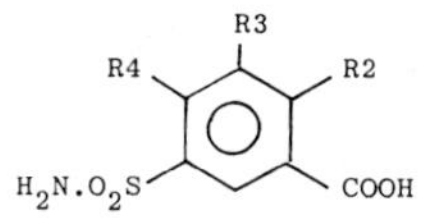

Compound	R4	R3	R2	I_{50}(M)	LogP [b)]
Frusemide	Cl	H	-NH - CH_2 - 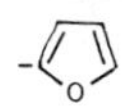	3.6×10^{-4}	1.45
Bumetanide	- O 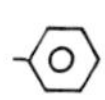	- NH - C_4H_9	H	9.0×10^{-4}	2.01
Piretanide	- O 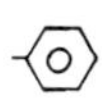	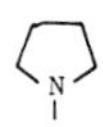	H	8.1×10^{-5}	3.21
HH 594	Cl	- NH - C_4H_9	H	3.0×10^{-3}	2.21
711	- O 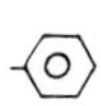	H	-NH - C_4H_9	8.0×10^{-5}	3.48

a) from Brooks and Lant [8]
b) Log P determined by reversed phase HPLC.

We have found that other POA derivatives such as tienilic acid and the separated enantiomers of indacrinone, which have distinctive actions within the nephron in vivo [9], display a high degree of inhibitory activity upon the human red cell chloride exchange system. Half-maximal inhibitory concentrations (I_{50}) are shown in Table V:

Compound	I_{50} (M) [a)]
Racemic indacrinone (MK196)	3.3×10^{-6}
(-) indacrinone	1.4×10^{-6}
(+) indacrinone	1.0×10^{-5}
Tienilic acid	$2.9 \times 10{-5}$

a) from Brooks and Lant [8]

It is of interest to compare the relative I_{50} values for these POA derivatives with the I_{50} values obtained by Schlatter et al [36] for inhibition of the Na,K,2Cl co-transport system in isolated TAL segments of rabbit kidney. Racemic indacrinone yielded a luminal I_{50} of 1.2×10^{-5}M as compared with 5.1×10^{-6}M for ethacrynic acid-cysteine. Tienilic acid was poorly active in the rabbit kidney preparation with a luminal I_{50} of $>10^{-4}$M and a bath I_{50} of 4.1×10^{-4}M . Schlatter et al [36] did not include the separated enantiomers of indacrinone in their study.

IN VITRO INHIBITION OF Cl TRANSPORT vs. IN VIVO SALURETIC ACTIVITY

A number of attempts have been made to try and correlate inhibitory effects of various sulphamoylbenzoates or POA derivatives upon in vitro co-transport or band 3 chloride exchange with in vivo saluretic efficacy in the dog or in man [8;30]. Unfortunately apart from species differences which may impose their own independent changes (as, for example, the extensive metabolic degradation of bumetanide in rats), such comparisons become exceedingly difficult when so little is known about the kinetics, metabolism or renal handling of the individual compounds under study other than those agents that have been developed as diuretics for clinical use.

Study of red cell chloride transport systems has made it clear, however, that distinct differences exist in the molecular mechanisms of action of drugs which appear to act similarly in the TAL and have earned the composite label of loop diuretics. Evidence from the various red cell systems discussed in this paper together with the findings from isolated TAL segments of rabbit kidney [9;36] emphasises that loop diuretics are not only chemically but also functionally heterogeneous with respect to their effects on transepithelial transport of chloride.

Whilst there are obvious similarities between the effects of various loop diuretics on the co-transport systems defined in both human and avian erythrocytes, the question arises as to what is the renal counterpart of the band 3 chloride transport system. Since the selective stilbene inhibitors leave Na,K, 2Cl co-transport in both the red cell and TAL unaffected, but exert clearcut inhibitory effects upon more proximal tubular transport pathways [11], the striking effects seen with certain loop diuretics on band 3 chloride exchange may reflect interference with a luminal Cl transport mechanism proximal to the TAL rather than an alternative chloride transport pathway operative in the TAL. Whether the same holds true for other loop diuretics lacking effects on Na,K, 2Cl co-transport, remains to be clarified.

REFERENCES

1. Aiton, J.F., Chipperfield, A.R., Lamb, J.F., Ogden, P. and Simmons, N.L. Biochim. Biophys. Acta, 646, 389-398 (1981)
2. Axelrod, D.R. and Pitts, R.F. J. Clin. Invest., 31, 171-179 (1952)
3. Baba, W.I., Lant, A.F., Smith, A.J., Townshend, M.M. and Wilson, G.M. Clin. Pharmacol. Ther. 9, 318-327 (1968)
4. Bakker-Grunwald, T. Biochim. Biophys. Acta, 641, 427-431 (1981)
5. Benos, D.J. Amer. J. Physiol., 242, C131-C145 (1982)
6. Brazy, P.C. and Gunn, R.B. J. gen. Physiol., 68, 583-599 (1976)
7. Brooks, B.A. and Lant, A.F. Clin. Sci. Mol. Med., 54, 679-683 (1978)
8. Brooks, B.A. and Lant, A.F. Submitted for publication (1984)
9. Brooks, B.A., Lant, A.F., McNabb, W.R. and Noormohamed, F.H. Renal Physiology, 7, In Press (1984)
10. Burg, M., Stoner, L., Cardinal, J. and Green, N. Amer. J. Physiol. 225, 119-124 (1973)
11. Dantzler, W.H. and Bentley, S.K. Amer. J. Physiol. 238,F16-F25 (1980)
12. Dunham, P.B., Stewart, G.W. and Ellory, J.C. Proc. natl. Acad. Sci. 77, 1711-1715 (1980)
13. Ehrlich, E.N. and Crabbé, J. Pflügers Arch., 302, 79-96 (1968)
14. Ellory, J.C. and Stewart, G.W. Brit. J. Pharmacol. 75,183-188 (1982)
15. Epstein, F.H. in: Modern Diuretic Therapy in the Treatment of Cardiovascular and Renal Disease, eds. Lant, A.F. and Wilson, G.M. (Amsterdam, Excerpta Medica 1973), pp. 188-193.
16. Frizzell, R.A. J. Membrane Biol., 35, 175-187 (1977)
17. Frizzell, R.A., Field, M. and Schultz, S.G. Amer. J. Physiol., 236, F1 - F8 (1979)

18. Frizzell, R.A., Smith, P.L., Vosburgh, E. and Field, M. J. Membrane Biol. 46, 27-39 (1979)
19. Geck, P., Pietrzyk, C., Burckhardt, B.C., Pfeiffer, B. and Heinz, E. Biochim. Biophys. Acta, 600, 432-447 (1980)
20. Greger, R. and Schlatter, E. Pflügers Arch., 396, 325-334 (1983)
21. Greger, R., Schlatter, E. and Lang, F. Pflügers Arch., 396, 308-314 (1983)
22. Knauf, P.A. and Grinstein, S. in: Chloride Transport in Biological Membranes. ed. Zadunaisky, J.A. (New York, Academic Press, 1982), pp. 61-90.
23. Kregenow, F.M. in; Membrane Transport in Red Cells. eds. Ellory, J.C. and Lew, V.L. (New York, Academic Press, 1977), pp. 383-426.
24. Leaf, A. J. gen. Physiol., 43, 175-189 (1960).
25. Maetz, J. Phil Trans. roy. Soc. Lond., B, 262, 209-249 (1971).
26. McGahan, M.C., Yorio, T. and Bentley, P.J. J. Pharmacol. exp. Ther. 203, 97-102 (1977)
27. Moutais, R. and Cousin, J.L. Amer. J. Physiol., 231, 1485-1489 (1976).
28. Nasse, H. Arch. gesamte Physiol., 16, 604-634 (1878).
29. Nechay, B.R., Palmer, R.F., Chinoy, D.A. and Posey, V.A. J. Pharmacol. exp. Ther. 157, 599-617 (1967)
30. Palfrey, H.C., Feit, P.W. and Greengard, P. Amer. J. Physiol., 238, C139-C148 (1980).
31. Passow, H., Fasold, H., Gärtner, E.M., Legrum, B., Ruffing, W. and Zaki, L. Ann. N. Y. Acad. Sci., 341, 361-383 (1980)
32. Rocha, A.S. and Kokko, J.P. J. clin. Invest., 52, 612-623 (1973).
33. Roberts, C.J.C., Homeida, M., Roberts, F. and Bogie, W. Brit. J. clin. Pharmacol., 6, 129-133 (1978)
34. Rothstein, A., Cabantchik, Z.I. and Knauf, P. Fed. Proc. 35, 3-10 (1976).
35. Russell, J.M. J. gen. Physiol., 73, 801-818 (1979).
36. Schlatter, E., Greger, R. and Weidtke, C. Pflügers Arch., 396, 210-217 (1983).
37. Schmidt, U. and Dubach, U.C. Nephron, 7, 447-458 (1970).
38. Silva, P., Stoff, J., Field, M., Fine, L., Forrest, J.N. and Epstein, F.H. Amer. J. Physiol., 233, F298-F306 (1977).
39. Skou, J.C. Biochim. Biophys. Acta, 42, 6-23 (1960).
40. Ussing, H. H. and Zerahn, K. Acta Physiol. Scand. 23, 110-127 (1951).
41. Zeuthen, T., Ramos, M. and Ellory, J.C. Nature, Lond., 273, 678-680 (1978).

EFFECT OF DIURETICS (FUROSEMIDE) ON OXIDATIVE PHOSPHORYLATION

Y. ORITA, Y. FUKUHARA, M. YANASE, T. NAKANISHI, M. HORIO, A. ANDO, AND H. ABE
Department of Medicine, Osaka University Medical School,
1-1-50 Fukushima, Fukushima-ku, Osaka 553, JAPAN

ABSTRACT

The effects of furosemide on the mitochondrial electron transport system and on oxidative phosphorylation were investigated.

Furosemide above $2x10^{-3}M$ was found to inhibit state 3 respiration of mitochondria from the rat liver, renal cortex and renal medulla. Furosemide above $5x10^{-6}M$ inhibited the respiration of rat liver mitochondria released by SF 6847. This fact exactly indicated the electron transport system in mitochondria was inhibited by furosemide. Furosemide above $4x10^{-3}M$ inhibited the activities of NADH-cytochrome c reductase and succinate-cytochrome c reductase in sonicated mitochondrial subparticles from beef heart. The inhibitory site of the electron transport was identified as being between cytochrome b and cytochrome $c+c_1$ by spectroscopy of the redox state of the electron transport system in the rat liver.

ATP content in the kidney of furosemide-infused rats was decreased about 20%. However, no decrease in that of the liver could be seen. Decrease in ATP content in the kidney was also confirmed by ^{31}P-NMR spectra using TMR-32 in furosemide-infused rabbit in vivo. On the contrary, CSA had no effect on mitochondrial respiration. It could be concluded that the inhibitory effect of furosemide on oxidative phophorylation seems to be the fundamental effect on a part of diuretic action of furosemide.

However, the membrane permeability of furosemide, the mode and the rate of metabolism of furosemide are important properties to cause diuresis in the kidney.

INTRODUCTION

Biochemical properties of furosemide still remain unclear, although there have been some reports on inhibitory effect on several enzymes (1,2,3).

The present authors have used quantum chemical calculation employing iterated Hückel's Molecular Orbital Method (4) indicating that furosemide might have an elctron accepting nature.

In the present study, we investigated the effect of the electron accepting nature of furosemide on the mitochondrial electron transport system in vitro by determining oxygen consumption, then to identify the site of inhibition by determining furosemide-sensitive enzymes, and by the spectroscopy on the redox state of cytochromes. The results were compared with those of 4-chloro-5-sulfamoyl-anthranilic acid (CSA), one of the important metabolites of furosemide (5,6,7,8,9,10) which does not exhibit a remarkable diuretic activity in the rat (10). Further, the effect of furosemide on ATP content in the kidney and the liver from furosemide-infused rats was determined by the freeze clamping and a high performance liquid chromatography (HPLC). In addition, the change in ATP content in the

Diuretics, Jules B. Puschett, Editor

kidney of furosemide-infused rabbits was measured by ^{31}P-NMR spectra using topical magnetic resonance (TMR) in vivo.

MATERIALS AND METHODS

1. Preparation of mitochondria and mitochondrial subparticles

Male S.D. rats weighing 200-250 g were killed by decapitation and the kidneys and the liver were immediately excised and immersed in an ice-cold preparation medium (0.25 M sucrose, 0.2 mM EDTA and 10 mM Tris-HCl). The kidneys was divided macroscopically into cortex and medulla. Mitochonria were prepared from the liver, renal cortex and renal medulla by modified Weinbach's method (11).

Mitochondrial subparticles were isolated from freshly slaughtered beef heart by Azzone's method (12). The protein concentration of mitochondria isolated from the rat was determined by the Lowry's method(13), and that of beef heart mitochondrial subparticles was determined by the biuret method (14). Adjustment due to the optical absorbance of sucrose, Tris buffer and cytochrome C was done.

2. Determination of oxygen consumption

Mitochondrial oxygen consumption was determined with a galvanic elctrode (Kyusui Chem., Tokyo) in a 25°C incubation medium (0.3 mM mannitol, 0.25 mM EDTA, 2.5 mM $MgCl_2$, 10 mM KCl and 5 mM potassium phosphate buffer). A mixture of 5 mM glutamate and 5 mM malate was used as a substrate. Oxygen consumption of rat liver mitochondria pretreated with 3,5-di-tert-butyl-4-hydroxy-benzylidenemalononitrile (SF 6847) was determined (15). P/O ratio was calculated by the method of Chance and Williams (16).

3. Determination of enzyme activities of the electron transport system

Frozen beef heart mitochondria were thawed and sonicated by Azzone's method (12). The obtained subparticles were assayed for enzyme activities of NADH-DCIP reductase, NADH-cytochrome c reductase, succinate dehydrogenase and succinate-cytochrome c reductase at 25°C. Activities of these enzymes were determined according to the methods of Kagawa and Asano (17).
A Cary 17 autorecording spectrometer was used to monitor the spectrum during the initial 1 min after the addition of NADH or succinate. Measurement was done at 600 nm for DCIP and 550 nm for cytochrome c.

4. Spectroscopic determination of the redox state of cytochrome b and cytochrome $c+c_1$

Mitochondria from rat liver were suspended at the final concentration of 1mg protein/ml in a medium containing 0.3 mM mannitol, 25 mM $MgCl_2$, 0.25 mM EDTA and 5 mM potassium phosphate buffer. The reduction rate of cytochomes was monitored with a dual wave autorecording spectrometer (Hitachi 556) by the method of Higuchi and Muraoka (18).

5. Determination of adenine nucleotides content in the kidney and the liver of furosemide-infused rat by freeze clamping and HPLC (19)

Male S.D. rats weighing 200-250 g were anesthesized with sodium pentobarbiturate (25 mg/kg body weight). PE 50 catheter attached to a motor driven syringe containing furosemide was introduced into the external jugular vein. Furosemide was delivered at a rate of 0.1, 3, 10 and 20 mg/kg body weight/h and 0.9% saline containing furosemide was administered at a rate of 100 μl/min intravenously.

The abdomen was opened and the right kidney was rapidly excised. The liver samples, less than 100 mg, were excised serially. The sample was squashed with tongs which were precooled in a liquid nitrogen and then lyophilized overnight. The lyophilized sample was homogenized with Potter-Elvehjem homogenizer. The homogenate was centrifuged for 5 min at 3000 r.p.m. and the supernatant was neutralized with 5 N potassium hydroxide. The precipitate was removed by centrifugation and the supernatant was used for assay of adenine nucleotides.

ATP, ADP and AMP were determined by HPLC using an anion exchange column

(IEX 540, 4x300 mm, Toyo Soda Co.) equilibrated with 0.1 M Tris buffer (pH 7.6) containing 190 mM Cl. Effluent rate was 1.0 ml/min and the eluate was continuously monitored at 260 nm. A 10 μl aliquot of extracts was injected on this column and developed with the same buffer as above at a rate of 1.0 ml/min. The method was sensitive enough to measure adenine nucleotides in about 1 mg of tissue (19).

6. Measurement of ATP in the kidney of furosemide-infused rabbit by ^{31}P-NMR spectra using TMR in vivo.

Male albino rabbit weighing 1.5 kg was anesthesized by sodium pentobarbiturate (the initial dose=30 mg/kg/h, then 15 mg/kg/h) infused from the right ear vein. The back was incised, the left kidney was placed at the suitable surface coil on the frame made by resin. The operated rabbit was secured in a cradle of the magnet. NMR spectra was recorded with TMR-32 (Oxford) (20). Prior to each experiment, the field homogeneity was adjusted. After confirming the spectra of sugar phosphate and ATP for 30 min (control period), furosemide was infused from the left ear vein at a rate of 40 mg/kg/h. Contents of sugar phosphate and β-ATP were estimated by their heights of the spectra. Intracellular pH was derived from chemical shift of inorganic phosphate. Since creatine phosphate is absent in the kidney, the intracellular pH is assumed as 7.2 according to Radda (21).

7. Chemicals

NADH, cytochrome c (type III), antimycin A, rotenone and ADP were obtained from Sigma Co. (U.S.A.). DCIP was obtained from Wako Pure Chem. Co. (Japan). Furosemide and CSA were obtained from Hoechst (Japan). Other chemicals were of highest purity available from commercial sources.

RESULTS

1. Respiration of rat mitochondria

The oxygen consumption rate of state 3 respiration, that of state 4 respiration, P/O ratio and respiration control indices of mitochondria from rat liver, rat renal cortex and medulla in control experiments were all the same as those previously reported by the present authors (21). These values agreed with those of other reports (22,23,24).

2. Effect of furosemide and CSA on the mitochondrial respiration

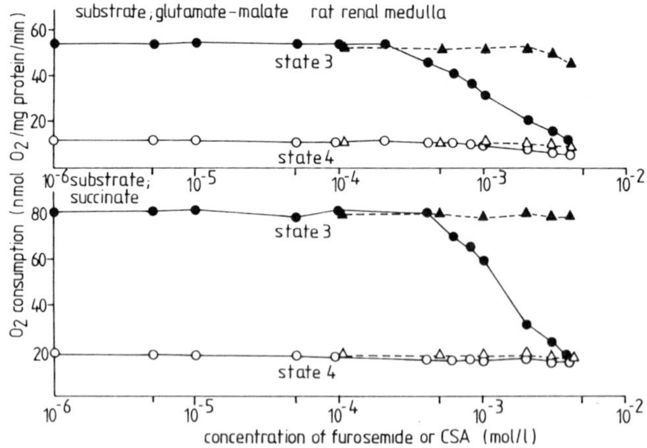

Fig.1 Effects of furosemide (closed circle and open circle) and CSA (closed triangle and open triangle) on respiration of rat renal medulla mitochondria using two different substrates. All values represent the mean of four experiments. In all cases, standard error was less than the radius of the symbol.

Fig.1 shows furosemide above $5x10^{-3}M$ inhibited state 3 respiration in the renal medullary mitochondria when substrate was succinate or glutamate-malate. State 4 respiration was unchanged by furosemide up to $5x10^{-2}M$. Neither state 3 nor state 4 respiration was changed by CSA up to $5x10^{-2}M$. The same results were obtained in the liver and the renal cortex. With regard to the effect of furosemide on state 4 respiration released by SF 6847 ($10^{-7}M$), in glutamate-malate oxidation, the reduction rate of oxygen consumption was significantly affected above the furosemide concentration of $7.5x10^{-6}M$. In succinate oxidation, the same effect was also observed above the furosemide concentration of $5x10^{-6}M$.

3. Effect of furosemide on enzyme activities of the electron transport system

Table 1 shows the effects of furosemide on enzyme activities of sonicated mitochondrial subparticles from beef heart. Furosemide of $4x10^{-3}M$ significantly inhibited the activitities of NADH-cytochrome c reductase and of succinate-cytochrome c reductase. On the other hand, the activity of NADH-DCIP reductase or succinate dehydrogenase was not inhibited by furosemide.

Table 1 Effects of furosemide on enzyme activities of beef heart submitochondrial particles.

	control	n	furosemide 4 mM	n	% inhibition	
NADH-DCIP reductase*	149.9±2.0	4	144.2±6.3	4	3.8	n.s.
NADH-cytochrome c reductase**	351.8±4.2	4	76.6±8.0	4	78.2	p<0.001
succinate dehydrogenase*	114.1±9.8	4	99.9±0.7	4	12.4	n.s.
succinate cytochrome c reductase**	252.4±9.1	4	52.4±4.1	4	79.2	p<0.001

* Data expressed as nmoles DCIP reduced/mg protein/min.
** Data expressed as nmoles cytochrome c reduced/mg protein/min. n.s. : not significant

4. Effect of furosemide on the redox states of cytochrome b and cytochrome $c+c_1$

Figs.2 and 3 show the effect of the final furosemide concentration of 2 mM on the percent reduction of cytochrome b (Fig.2) and cytochrome $c+c_1$ (Fig.3). The state of complete oxidation (state 4) was obtained by the

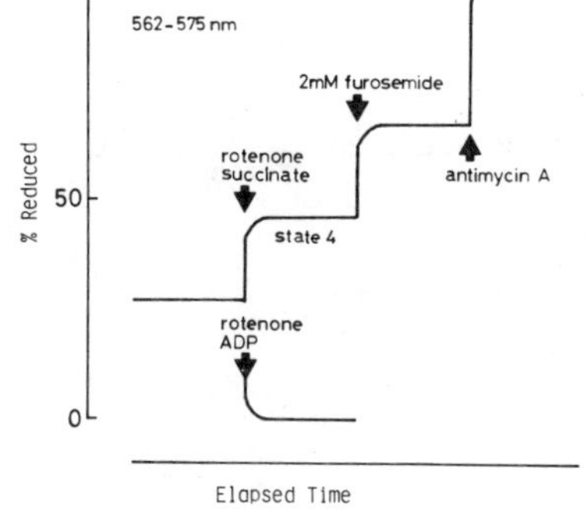

Fig.2 Effect of 2 mM furosemide on the redox state of rat liver mitochondrial cytochrome b.

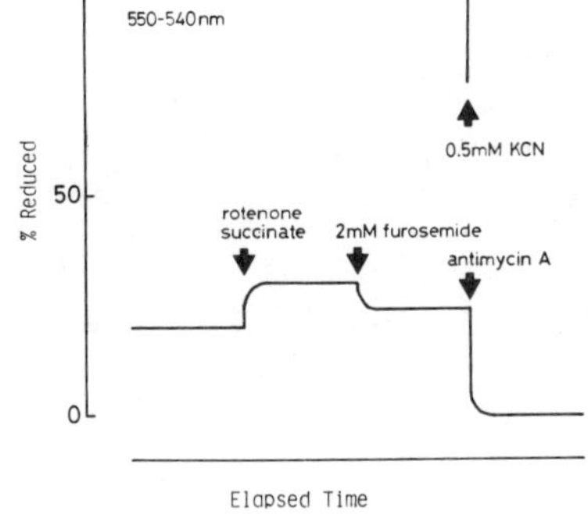

Fig.3 Effect of 2 mM furosemide on the redox state of rat liver mitochondrial cytochrome $c+c_1$.

addition of rotenone and ADP at the final concentration of 2.5 μM and 200 μM, respectively. When the furosemide at the final concentration of 2 mM was added to mitochondria pretreated with rotenone and succinate, the percent reduction of cytochrome b was significantly increased from 46% to 67%. Simultaneously, the percent reduction of cytochrome $c+c_1$ was significantly decreased from 29% to 24%. The effects of furosemide on the percent oxidation reduction of cytochrome b and the percent oxidation of cytochrome $c+c_1$ were dose-dependent.

5. Adenine nucleotides content in the kidney and the liver of furosemide-infused rats measured by the freeze clamping and HPLC

Fig.4(A,B) shows the chromatogram of the kidney from control rat (A) and that from furosemide-infused rat (B, 10mg/kg body weight/h for 60 min). A satisfactory separation could be obtained among AMP, ADP and ATP.

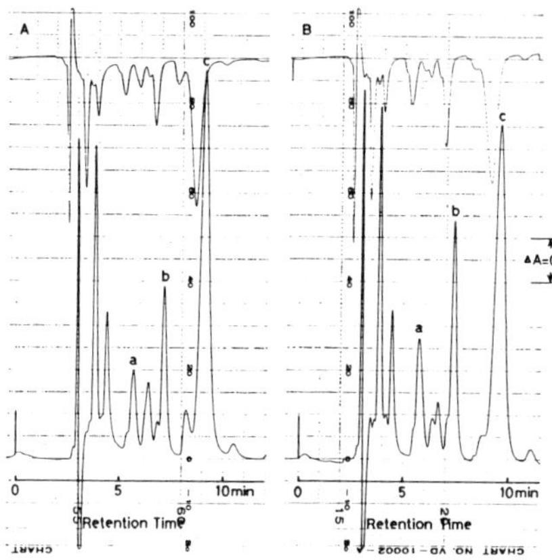

Fig. 4 High pressure liquid chromatograms of adenine nucleotides from normal (A) and furosemide-treated (B) rat kidneys.

a; AMP
b; ADP
c; ATP

Fig.5(A,B) shows the time course of change in ATP, ADP and AMP in the kidney (A) and the liver (B) of furosemide-infused rats (0.1. 3.0, 10.0 and 20.0

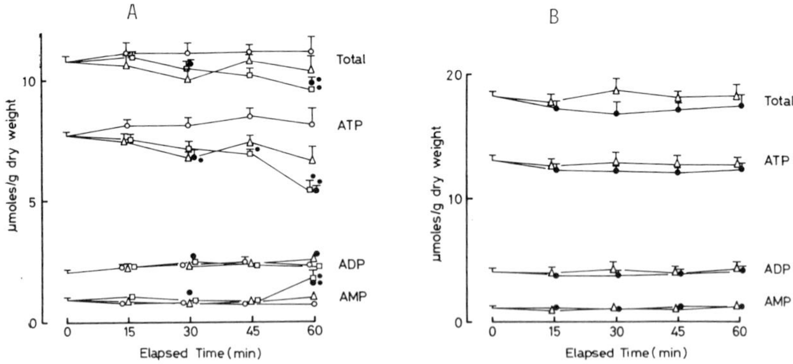

Fig. 5 Changes in cellular contents of adenine nucleotides in furosemide - infused rat kidneys (A) and rat livers (B). All values represent mean±S.E.M. (n=4).
dose of furosemide : —○— 0.1mg/kg B.W./hr, —△— 3mg/kg B.W./hr
—□— 10 mg/kg B.W./hr, —●— 20mg/kg B.W./hr
* $p<0.05$

mg/kg body weight/h, respectively). ATP content in the kidney from furosemide-infused rat (10 and 20 mg/kg body weight/h, respectively) was significantly reduced ($p<0.05$) comparing to that from control rat, while AMP content was increased. On the other hand, in the liver, no significant change in content of adenine nucleotides could be observed by the furosemide infusion up to 20 mg/kg body weight/h.

6. Measurement of ATP in the kidney of furosemide-infused rabbit by ^{31}P-NMR spectra using TMR in vivo

Fig.6 shows ^{31}P-NMR spectra recorded by TMR-32 (Oxford). Thick line indicates ^{31}P-NMR spectra of the left kidney of control period (without furosemide infusion, urine volume=0.1 ml/15 min). These spectra are composed of sugar phosphate, inorganic phosphate, α-, β-, γ-phosphate of ATP, α-, β-phosphate of ADP and unknown peak. Signal of creatine phosphate could not be seen. This finding confirms that spectra are obtained selectively from the kidney. Dashed line indicates ^{31}P-NMR of the left kidney of rat in the period of furosemide infusion at a rate of 40 mg/kg body weight/h for 30 min. Urine volume of this period was 8 ml/15 min. The height of the peak of β-ATP is decreased about 20%. Thin line indicates ^{31}P-NMR spectra of the kidney after continuous infusion of furosemide at the same rate as above for 90 min. Urine volume was 13 ml/15 min. Decreases in ATP and sugar phosphate were almost the same degree as those of the period for 30 min. Contents of ATP and sugar phosphate were gradually recovered but could not reach to the level of control period after the cessation of furosemide infusion (data not shown). Estimated decrease in intracellular pH was 0.6–1.2.

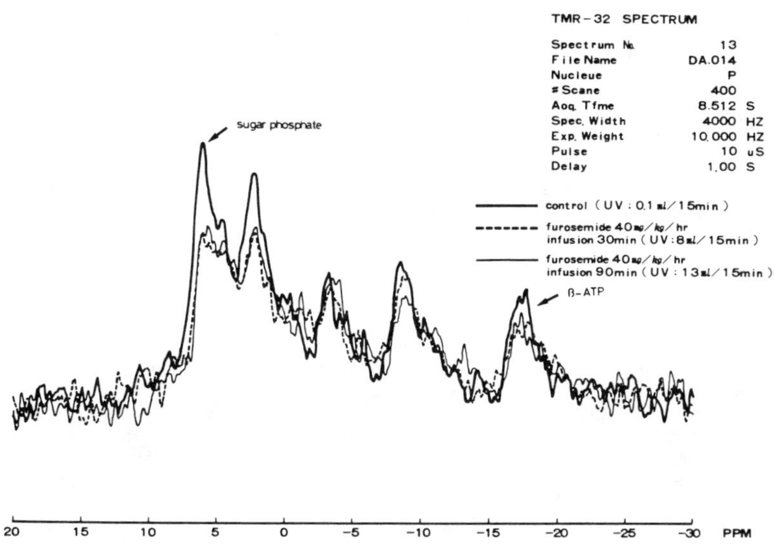

Fig. 6 ^{31}P-NMR spectra of the kidneys in control period and in furosemide infusion period recorded by TMR-32.

DISCUSSION

The present study aimed at confirming our quantum chemical prediction (4) and biochemical properties of furosemide previously reported (22,23,24,25), further at pursuing the inhibitory effect of furosemide on electron transport system and oxidative phosphorylation in mitochondria. The inhibition of the electron transport system in mitochondria might result in decrease of sodium reabsorption in the tubules with decline of energy production. The result showed that furosemide above $2x10^{-3}$M decreased the oxygen consumption of state 3 respiration of rat renal cortex, renal medulla and the liver mitochondria (substrate either glutamate-malate or succinate). This result agrees with those by Sawa et al. (23) and Ekynoyan et al. (24). We tried to obtain more direct evidence for the inhibitory effect of furosemide on the electron transport system. As the most powerful and stable uncoupler, SF 6847 (15) was employed to release the respiration of rat liver mitochondria to state 4. Furosemide above $7.5x10^{-6}$M (substrate: glutamate-malate) or $5.0x10^{-6}$M(substrate: succinate) inhibited state 4 respiration in a dose-dependent manner. This fact exactly indicates that furosemide inhibited the electron transport system in mitochondria. Since it is generally accepted that inhibitors of the electron transport system affect all mitochondria, regardless of the species or tissue, in the same manner(25), furosemide might inhibit the electron transport system in the kidney.

The present study focused on identifying the inhibitory sites in the electron transport system of mitochondria by furosemide. Enzymatic studies in the electron transport system have usually been done using beef heart mitochondrial subparticles (12). Our results show that NADH-cytochrome c reductase and succinate-cytochrome c reductase were furosemide-sensitive and the electron transport could be inhibited at these sites. In order to clarify the exact site of the electron transport inhibition, the redox states of cytochrome b and cytochrome $c+c_1$ were spectroscopically determined using rat liver mitochondria. The inhibitory site was identified as being between cytochrome b and cytochrome $c+c_1$ (18). Manuel et al. (26) reported that the site of the electron transport inhibition of furosemide was between flavoprotein and cytochrome b. This discrepancy might be caused by different experimental conditions or the possibility that their spectroscopic observation included flavoprotein and nonhem iron. Maneul et al. (27) and Quintanilla et al. (28) reported that furosemide inhibited adenine nucleotide translocase of mitochondria from rat and dog kidneys at the concentration above 10^{-4}M. This finding agrees well with our experimental result in which state 3 respiration was inhibited by furosemide.

The biochemical action of furosemide was compared with that of CSA. Recently, the biotransformation of furosemide was well investigated. CSA was considered as one of the important metabolites of furosemide in human, dog and rat (5,6,7,8,9,10). CSA has no remarkable diuretic activity in the rat (10). CSA has no inhibitory effect on state 3 or 4 respiration of rat liver, renal cortex or renal medulla mitochondria up to the concentration of 10^{-3}M. This difference might well be related to the pharmacological action of furosemide.

However, the question was raised whether inhibition of oxidative phosphorylation could be related to diuretic activity of furosemide, because furosemide affected liver mitochondria as well as kidney mitiochondria. To answer this question, we determined adenine nucleotides content in the kidney and the liver using freeze clamping and HPLC in furosemide-infused rats. By this device, it was clearly shown that ATP content in the kidney was decreased, while no significant change in adenine nucleotides content could be seen in the liver. Decrease in ATP content in the kiney was paralleled to urine volume (data not shown). This result suggests that the inhibition of oxidative phosphorylation alone could not be related to diuretic activity of furosemide. Difference in permeability of cellular membrane in the kidney and the liver seems to be important to diuretic action of furosemide besides the biochemical action of furosemide. Twenty % decrease in ATP content is smaller than those by ischemia or some drugs (24, 25). However, since the maximal diuresis attained by furosemide can not exceed about 20% of filtered sodium, the present result might correspond to a rather mild action of diuretics.

Although our method can obtain a good separation of adenine nucleotides, there are some reports with respect to the reliability of freeze clamping method (29). The present result should be confirmed by other method. In addition, in freeze clamping method, by the removal of kidney, a serial result in the same animal could not be obtained. Then, use of TMR is very useful because we can observe serial changes in content of ATP and other substances in the kidney in vivo. We observed the decrease in content of β-ATP and sugar phosphate accompanying diuresis by furosemide infusion. In this experimental condition, change of body fluid was corrected by 0.9% saline infusion. About 20-30% decrease of β-ATP was well agreed with the result obtained by freeze clamping and HPLC.

ACKNOWLEDGEMENTS

The authors heartily thank to Prof. K. Tagawa, Department of Molecular Physiological Chemistry, Osaka University Medical School, for freeze clamping and HPLC, and to Prof. H. Watari, National Institute of Physiology, Okazaki, for the use of TMR-32.

REFERENCES

1. H. W. Radtke, G. Rumrich, E. Kinne-Saffran, and K. J. Ullrich, Kidney Int. 1, 100-105 (1972).
2. G. Senft, K. Munske, G. Schultz, and M. Hoffman, Naunyn-Schmidevergs, Arch. Pharm. 259, 344-359 (1968).
3. J. H. Stein, C. B. Wilson, and W. M. Kirkendall, J. Lab. Clin. Med. 71, 654-665 (1968).
4. Y. Orita, A. Ando, D. Shirai, Y. Takamitsu, S. Urakabe, T. Furukawa, and H. Abe, Jpn. Circ. J. 32, 547-554 (1968).
5. A. Hajdu and A. Haussler, Arzneim. Forsch. 14,709-710 (1964).
6. A. Haussler and H. Wicha, Arzneim. Forsch. 15, 81-83 (1965).
7. S. Seno, S. M. Shaw, and J. E. Christian, J. Pharma. Sci. 58, 935-938 (1969).
8. J. D. Wallin, P. Ryals, and N. Kalplowitz, J. Pharmacol. Exp. Ther. 200, 52-57 (1976).
9. G. J. Yakatan, D. D. Maness, J. Scholler, W. M. J. Novick, and J. T. Doluisio, J. Pharm. Sci. 65, 1456-1460 (1976).
10. T. Miwa, Jap. J. Nephrol. 22, 1125-1140 (1980).
11. E. C. Weinbach, Anal. Biochem. 2, 335-343 (1961).
12. G. F. Azzone, R. Colonna, and B. Ziche. Methods in Enzymology 55. 46-50 (1979).
13. R. J. Randall, J. Biol. Chem. 193, 265-275 (1951).
14. A. G. Gornall, J. Barawille, and M. M. David, J. Biol. Chem. 177, 751-766 (1949).
15. S. Muraoka, H. Terada, and T. Takaya, FEBS Letters 54, 53-56 (1975).
16. B. Chance and C. R. Williams, Adv. Enzym. 17, 65-134 (1956).
17. Y. Kagawa and A. Asano in :Experimental Methods in Biochemistry Jap. Soc. Biochem. ed. (Tokyo Kagaku Dojin, Tokyo 1976) pp.215-255.
18. T. Higuchi and S. Muraoka in :Methods in Biomembrane M. Akamatsu, A. Asano, Y. Anraku, T. Omura, M. Fujita, and S. Mizushima, eds. (Protein, Nucleic Acid and Enzyme Suppl., Tokyo 1974) pp.5-23.
19. W. Kamiike, F. Watanabe, T. Hashimoto, K. Tagawa, Y. Ikeda, K. Nakao,

and Y. Kawashima, J. Biochem. 91, 1349-1356 (1982).
20. R. S. Balaban, D. G. Gadian, and G. K. Radda, Kidney Int. 20, 575-579 (1981).
21. G. K. Radda, J. J. H. Ackerman, B. P. Sehr, and G. G. Wrong, Brit. J. Biochem. 12, 277-281 (1980).
22. A. Yoshida, T. Yamada, and S. Koshikawa, Biochem. Pharmacol. 21, 1933-1942 (1971).
23. H. Sawa, E. J. Weinman, S. E. Hyde, and G. Ekynoyan, Biochem. Pharmacol. 25, 2649-2655 (1967).
24. G. Ekynoyan, H. Sawa, S. Hyde, J. M. Wood, A. Schwartz, and W. Suki, J. Pharmacol. Exp. Ther. 194, 614-623 (1975).
25. T. P. Singer, Methods in Enzymology 55, 454-462 (1979).
26. M. A. Manuel and M. W. Weiner, J. Pharmacol. Exp. Ther. 198, 209-221 (1976).
27. M. A. Manuel and M. W. Weiner, Biochem. Biophys. Acta 460, 445-454 (1977).
28. A. P. Quintanilla, M. L. Levin, C. C. Lastre, H. Yokoo, and N. W. Levin, J. Pharmacol. Exp. Ther. 211, 456-459 (1979).
29. R. H. Kessler, Proc. Soc. Exp. Biol. Med. 134, 1091-1095 (1970).

CONTROL OF AMILORIDE-SENSITIVE SODIUM CHANNELS IN CULTURED RENAL EPITHELIAL CELLS

MAURICE BURG* AND SARAH SARIBAN-SOHRABY**
*National Heart, Lung, and Blood Institute, Bethesda, MD 20205; **Department of Physiology and Biophysics, Harvard Medical School, Boston, MA 02115

Mammalian collecting ducts reabsorb sodium by means of two kinds of transporters in series. One is Na,K-ATPase located in the basolateral membranes of the cells. Na,K-ATPase actively transports sodium out of the cells, lowering intracellular sodium below the level in the tubule fluid. The others are sodium channels located in the apical cell membranes. The sodium channels passively transport sodium into the cells, along the sodium gradient between the tubule fluid and cell interior. The rate of transepithelial sodium transport is regulated by the permeability of the sodium channels. Vasopressin and aldosterone increase the aggregate permeability of the channels and thus increase collecting duct sodium reabsorption. Amiloride blocks the channels, causing a diuresis by reducing sodium reabsorption. In order to learn more about the sodium channels and how amiloride affects them, we have been studying them, starting with cultured renal epithelial cells.

Renal epithelial cells in tissue culture may retain differentiated properties which can then be studied in ways not otherwise possible [1]. In such cultures the cells remain morphologically polarized with their bases against the supporting structure. Special features such as apical microvilli and tight junctions are preserved, and transporters and receptors remain limited to one cell surface or the other. Further, when filters or other porous sheets form the supporting structure, transepithelial transport is demonstrable. We would have preferred to study amiloride-sensitive sodium transport in differentiated tissue culture lines from mammalian collecting ducts. Despite our own efforts and those of others, however, such cultures are not yet available. Therefore, we have used an available line of cultured amphibian kidney cells which has the desired properties.

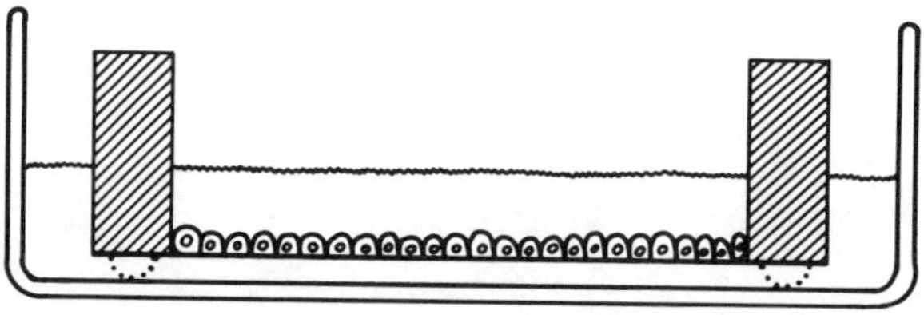

FIG. 1. Porous bottom culture dish (invented by Roderic E. Steele) consists of a millipore (or other) filter cemented to the bottom of a plastic ring. The porous bottom dish sits in a conventional plastic culture dish with medium placed in both dishes. Cells are seeded inside the porous bottom dish, where they can form a confluent epithelial sheet on the filter, as illustrated here. "Feet" cemented to the base of the porous bottom dish elevate it above the plastic dish, allowing access of fluid to the bottom of the filter. The edge of the epithelium seals against the plastic ring. Therefore, transepithelial voltage, short circuit current, sodium fluxes, etc. can be studied directly while the epithelium remains in the porous bottom dish. (Reproduced from [3] with permission)

Diuretics, Jules B. Puschett, Editor

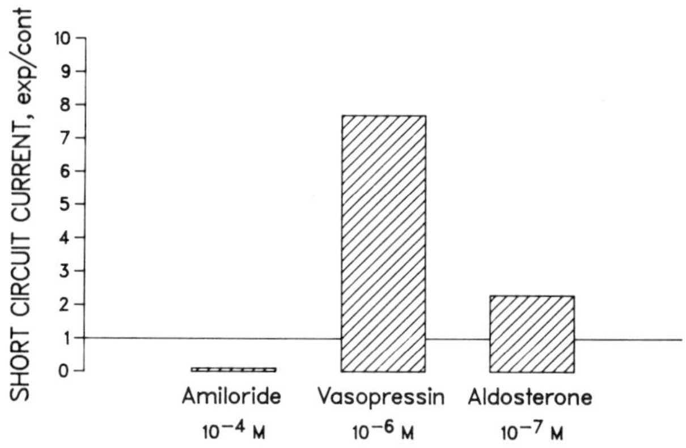

FIG. 2. Effect of amiloride, vasopressin, and aldosterone on short circuit current across A6 epithelia. Short circuit current is equivalent to net sodium transport in this preparation. (Prepared from data in [2] and personal communication from M. Lang and J. Handler.)

Amiloride inhibits transepithelial sodium transport not only in toad bladders but also in lines of cells (TB-M and TB-6c) cultured from toad bladders [1]. Similar results are found in A6 cells derived from toad kidney [2]. When grown on filters (Figure 1), all three of these tissue culture lines form "tight" epithelia that have high transepithelial resistance (approximately 5000 Ω cm^2) and voltage (10 mV or more, apical surface negative). We have chosen to study sodium transport in A6 epithelia. These cells transport sodium from their apical to basal surface, and generate a short circuit current that generally is equal to the sodium transport [2]. Further, their sodium transport is stimulated by aldosterone [2] and vasopressin [4], as well as inhibited by amiloride [2] (Figure 2). In our initial studies we sought to confirm that amiloride and aldosterone affected the sodium permeability of the apical cell surface of A6. When this was established, we isolated vesicles from the apical surface membranes in order to study more directly the effects of amiloride and aldosterone on the sodium channels.

APICAL SODIUM PERMEABILITY OF A6 EPITHELIA [3]

In order to evaluate apical sodium permeability we added ^{22}Na for a short time to the fluid bathing the apical cell surface, then washed with cold non-radioactive "stop solution" to eliminate extracellular ^{22}Na. Initially, the A6 cells were grown on plastic dishes, and the findings were dissapointing. There was no amiloride-sensitive sodium uptake. Eventually we learned, however, that differentiation of A6 cells is limited when they grow on plastic dishes, because then they are exposed to culture medium only at their apical surface [4]. With this in mind we grew the cells in porous bottom dishes which expose the bases of the cells to the medium through the filters. The results were more encouraging. After the cells had became confluent, transepithelial voltage and short circuit current were similar to those reported previously. ^{22}Na uptake was linear for 45 s. We measured it at 30 s for calculation of the rate of sodium uptake. Different

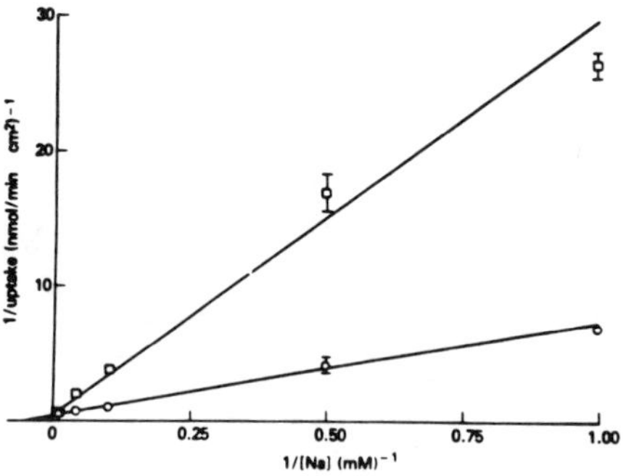

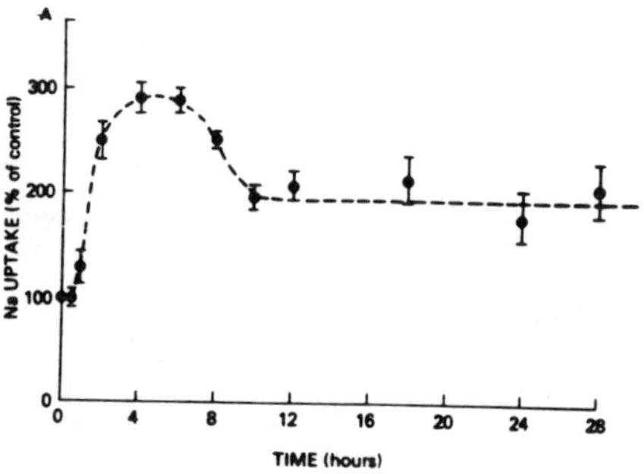

FIG. 3. Kinetics of apical sodium uptake in the presence (o) and absence (□) of 10^{-7}M amiloride. The lines represent fits to the Michaelis-Menton equation with K_m of 18 mM (o) and 74 mM (□). Maximum velocity is the same in both cases. (From [3] with permission.)

FIG. 4. Time course of aldosterone stimulation of initial sodium uptake in A6 epithelia. Epithelia were incubated with 10^{-7}M aldosterone for the times indicated. Fluxes were then measured, and are expressed as a percent of the uptake observed in the absence of aldosterone. (From [3] with permission.)

concentrations of sodium and amiloride were placed in the apical solution (Figure 3). Amiloride competitively inhibited sodium uptake. The K_i was approximately 5 X 10^{-8}M. Further, when 10^{-7}M aldosterone was added to the media in which the cells were grown, sodium uptake increased after a lag of 45 min and, after 4 h, reached a maximum three times the control level (Figure 4). These results confirm that apical sodium permeability in A6 cells is amiloride-sensitive and is stimulated by aldosterone. The studies that followed were aimed at examining more directly the mechanism of sodium permeability and its control.

PREPARATION OF APICAL MEMBRANE VESICLES FROM A6 CELLS [5]

In order to examine the apical amiloride-sensitive sodium channels more directly we prepared vesicles using essentially the same calcium precipitation method previously used to prepare proximal tubule brush border membrane vesicles. The vesicles from the A6 cells were enriched 7-10 times in apical membrane markers, i.e. alkaline phosphatase, γ-glutamyltranspeptidase, and ^{125}I (after direct labeling of the apical surface of the intact epithelium with [^{125}I]-iodosulfanilic acid). We measured equilibrium exchange uptake of ^{22}Na into the vesicles with lmM sodium in the medium. The sodium uptake was osmotically sensitive and was inhibited by low concentrations of amiloride ($K_{0.5}$ = 7 X 10^{-8}M). Further, vesicles prepared from cells treated with 10^{-7}M aldosterone for 4.5 hr showed two-fold enhancement of amiloride-sensitive sodium flux relative to appropriate controls. Thus, the apical amiloride-sensitive sodium transporter was preserved in the vesicle preparation, making it possible to study further the mechanism of aldosterone action.

POSSIBLE INVOLVEMENT OF METHYLATION IN THE ACTION OF ALDOSTERONE [6,7]

Recent experiments demonstrated that aldosterone increased methylation in TB-6c cells and that inhibition of the methylation prevented the increase in sodium transport caused by aldosterone [6]. A possible explanation is that aldosterone acts to increase methylation of the phospholipids surrounding the sodium channels or of some proteins, perhaps the channels themselves, and that methylation increases sodium flux through the channels. Therefore, we tested [7] to see whether methylation of apical membrane vesicles from A6 cells would directly affect sodium transport into them. Since methylating enzymes are associated with membranes, it seemed likely that addition of the methyl donor S-adenosylmethionine (adoMet) would increase methylation. This was demonstrated by adding ^{3}H-adoMet which resulted in labeling of both phospholipids and proteins in the vesicles. The labeling was prevented by deazaAdo, a known inhibitor of transmethylation. Incubation of vesicles from control cells with with adoMet increased the amiloride-sensitive uptake of sodium into the vesicles approximately two-fold. In contrast, when the cells had been incubated with aldosterone, adoMet did not further increase the amiloride-sensitive sodium uptake. In other words, the effects of aldosterone and adoMet were not additive. DeazaAdo prevented the increase in sodium flux with adoMet. Taken together, these observations lead us to suggest that methylation of apical membrane phospholipids or proteins may contribute to the increase in sodium transport that aldosterone causes in cultured amphibian urinary tract epithelia, and presumably in other responsive epithelia, as well.

RECONSTITUTION OF AMILORIDE-SENSITIVE SODIUM CHANNELS INTO PLANAR LIPID BILAYER MEMBRANES [8]

Channels were identified as the route of apical amiloride-sensitive sodium permeability by the observation that addition of amiloride caused electrical noise [9]. The explanation is that amiloride intermittantly blocks the channels, causing rapid fluctuations in sodium current through each individual channel. The channels are then closed so much of the time that fewer sodium ions pass through them, resulting in the observed decrease in macroscopic permeability. In order to characterize directly the individual channels we have incorporated A6 apical membrane vesicles that contain the channels into planar lipid bilayer membranes [8]. Bilayers of phosphatidylethanolamine and phosphatidylserine were formed across a circular aperture approximately 300 μm in diameter. The bilayer separated two aqueous chambers. A chosen voltage was maintained between the chambers, and the resultant current through the bilayer was monitored continuously. After the bilayer was formed, an osmotic gradient was established across the membrane by adding NaCl to the cis side. The osmotic gradient facilitated channel incorporation. NaCl concentrations were typically 200 mM on the cis side and 100 mM on the trans side. Vesicles were added to the cis side and that solution was stirred until current was observed, indicating channel incorporation. Channels incorporated in an unpredictable fashion either in bursts (2-6 channels) or one by one. An example of the current through a single channel is shown in figure 5.

The range of single channel conductance was 4 to 80 pS at 200 mM NaCl with a mean of 35 pS. Both the conductance of any single channel and its opening probability were independent of voltage ($\pm$ 60 mV). The channels spontaneously fluctuated both rapidly and slowly between an open and closed state. The mean residence time of the long-lived closed state was 5 s and was independent of voltage. The mean closed time of the fast state was less than 200 ms. With NaCl solutions only sodium passed through the channels,

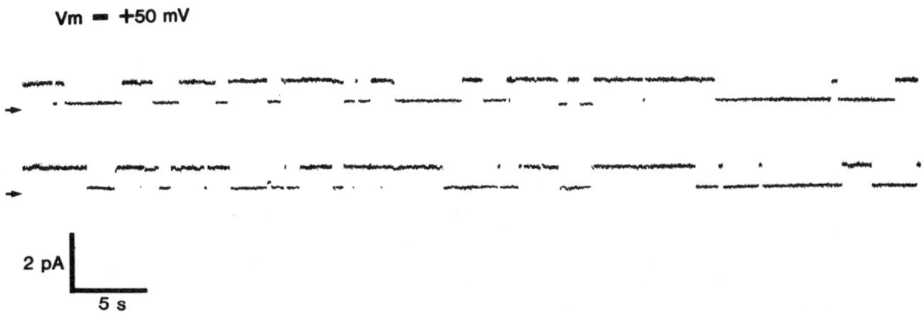

FIG. 5. Current fluctuation through a single sodium channel. Upwards deflection indicates that the channel is open. For the recordings shown here, the holding potential was +50 mV in symmetrical 30 mM NaCl. The arrow indicates zero current level. The average single channel conductance observed in this experiment was 15 pS in symmetrical 30 mM NaCl and 55 pS in 200 mM NaCl. (From [8] with permission.)

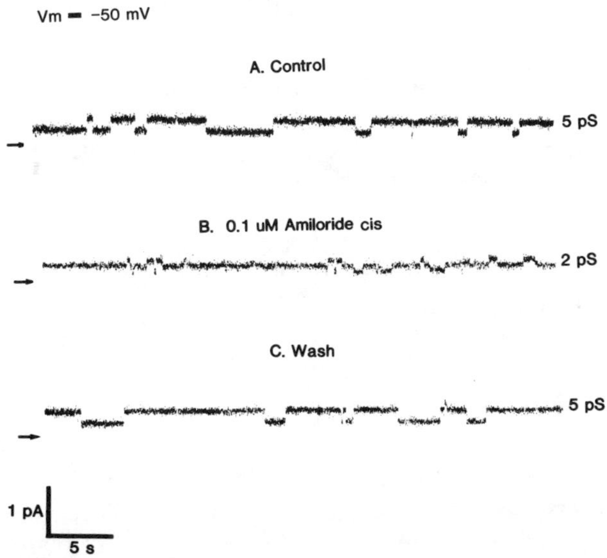

FIG. 6. Inhibition of single channel conductance by amiloride in the cis solution. Symmetrical 10 mM NaCl solutions were present and the voltage was -50 mV. This membrane contained two channels (B), although only one is seen in (A) and (C). (A) prior to the addition of amiloride. (B) After the addition of 10^{-7} M amiloride to the cis side. (C) After amiloride was removed by washing the cis chamber. (From [8] with permission.)

i.e. they were essentially impermeable to chloride. Sodium permeability was 2 to 3-fold greater than potassium permeability.

The effect of amiloride depended on which side the drug was placed. Addition of amiloride to the trans side produced rapid transitions between open and blocked conductance states like those observed by noise analysis in intact epithelia. Cis amiloride, however, did not produce visible fluctuations in the open channel current (Figure 6). Instead, the single channel conductance was reduced in a graded fashion, depending on the concentration of amiloride. The $K_{0.5}$ for amiloride was 10^{-7} M, consistent with the sodium flux data in intact A6 epithelia and vesicles. The results with amiloride demonstrate that the channels are asymmetrical and maintain a consistent orientation. Also, the nature of the cis blockage by amiloride is unexpected in that no visible fluctuation was induced. Taken at face value this could lead to the remarkable conclusion that an amiloride molecule partially blocks a channel to an extent dependent on the concentration of other amiloride molecules in the solution. More likely the cis blockage, like the trans blockage and that observed in frog skins, induces a fluctuation, but the fluctuation is rapid compared to the amplifier response time.

SUMMARY

(1) A6, a continuous tissue culture line derived from toad kidney, expresses amiloride-sensitive sodium channels in its apical cell membranes, but only when the epithelium is grown on filters with access of medium to the base of the cells.

(2) We studied the sodium channels in the intact epithelia, in apical membrane vesicles, and after reconstitution into planar lipid bilayer membranes.

(3) Macroscopic permeability to sodium through the channels is stimulated by aldosterone and vasopressin, and is inhibited by amiloride.

(4) The mechanism of action of aldosterone probably involves methylation of apical membrane phospholipids or proteins.

(5) Single channel conductance, ion selectivity, and response to amiloride were characterized after reconstitution into planar lipid bilayers.

REFERENCES

1. J.S. Handler, F.M. Perkins, and J.P. Johnson. Am. J. Physiol. 238, F1 (1980).
2. F.M. Perkins and J.S. Handler. Am. J. Physiol. 241, C154 (1981).
3. S. Sariban-Sohraby, M.B. Burg, and R.J. Turner. Am. J. Physiol. 245, C167 (1983).
4. J.S. Handler, A.S. Preston, and R.E. Steele. Federation Proc. 43, (1984).
5. S. Sariban-Sohraby, M.B. Burg, and R.J. Turner. Submitted for publication.
6. W.P. Wiesmann, P.K. Chiang, and J.P. Johnson. Clinical Res. 31:445A, (1983).
7. S. Sariban-Sohraby, M. Burg, W.P. Wiesmann, and J.P. Johnson. Submitted for publication.
8. S. Sariban-Sohraby, R. Latorre, M. Burg, L. Olans, and D. Benos. Nature. In press.
9. Lindemann, B. and W. Van Driessche. Science. 195, 292 (1977).

AN EFFECT OF PIRETANIDE ON THE INTRACELLULAR CATIONS OF CULTURED CELLS SUBJECTED TO PARTIAL CHRONIC SODIUM PUMP BLOCKADE BY OUABAIN.

J.F.AITON AND N.L.SIMMONS
Department of Physiology and Pharmacology, University of St.Andrews
St.Andrews, Fife, KY16 9TS, U.K.

ABSTRACT

Cultured cells (HeLa, MDCK and BC_3H1) have been used to study the contribution made by the piretanide-sensitive Na+K+Cl cotransport system to the maintainance of intracellular Na^+ and K^+ contents in normal cells and in cells whose Na-pumps have been subjected to chronic partial inhibition with ouabain. In cells with normally directed cation gradients, piretanide has no significant effect on Na^+ or K^+ contents indicating that the cotransport system is mediating self-exchange. In cells subjected to chronic partial Na-pump inhibition, piretanide causes a significant retardation of K^+ loss and Na^+ gain. This result suggests that under conditions of chronic Na-pump blockade, the Na+K+Cl cotransport system can mediate the exchange of intracellular K^+ for extracellular Na^+.

INTRODUCTION

Loop diuretics,(e.g.piretanide) are capable of inhibiting a large fraction of passive transmembrane cation fluxes in many cell-types by inhibition of an electoneutral Na+K+2Cl cotransport unrelated to other transport systems such as the Na-pump [1,2]. The contribution of this cotransport system to the maintenance of intracellular cations in cells with normal gradients of cations is unclear, though in principle the overall direction of transport through the system is dependent upon the sum of the chemical activity gradients for Na^+,K^+ and Cl^-[2]. There is increasing evidence that a humoral inhibitor of the Na-pump may be important to understanding the aetiology of essential hypertension[3]. Though defects in the cotransport system per se have been suggested, our interest here was to determine the contribution of piretanide-sensitive cotransport to changes in internal cations resulting from partial chronic Na-pump blockade (mimicked here by ouabain)

METHODS

The experimental techniques have been described in detail elsewhere [1,4] and are summarised here. HeLa (human carcinoma), MDCK (epithelial) and BC_3H1 (smooth muscle) cells were maintained in serial culture at 37°C. For experiments, cell monolayers were grown on 60mm petri dishes. Chronic drug applications were made by direct media replacement (all media contained 0.1% serum). Intracellular Na and K contents were measured by flame photometry of cell extracts after washing and removal of extracellular cations in ice-cold sorbitol buffer. Na-pump site number was measured by determining the specific binding of ^{3}H-ouabain. Results are routinely expressed per 10^6 cells, cell number being determined with a Coulter counter from trypsinised cell suspensions.

Diuretics, Jules B. Puschett, Editor

RESULTS AND DISCUSSION

Incubation of cell monolayers in 0.1mM piretanide for up to 24h has no significant effect upon the intracellular Na^+ or K^+ ion contents of HeLa (see fig 1), MDCK [control cell Na^+ and K^+ =28±2,148±3 (±S.D.)mmol/l cell water(n=5), +0.1mM piretanide, Na^+ and K^+=28±1,137±9mmol/l cell water (n=5) respectively], or BC_3H1 cells [control Na^+,K^+ =8±1,152±7 mmol/l cell water(n=3), +0.1mM piretanide, Na^+ and K^+ =8±2,154±8 (n=3) mmol/l cell water respectively]. This indicates that the piretanide-sensitive cotransport is mediating self-exchange of ions in these conditions, and that the sum of the chemical activity gradients for Na, K and Cl is approximately zero [2]

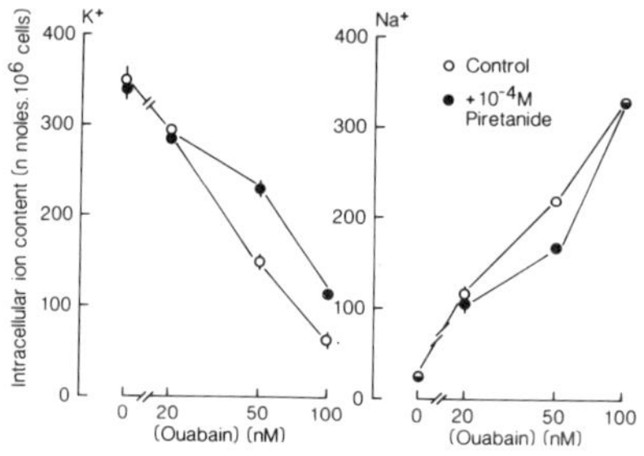

FIG1.Effect of chronic ouabain treatment on intracellular cations of HeLa cells (error bars ± 1 S.D.)

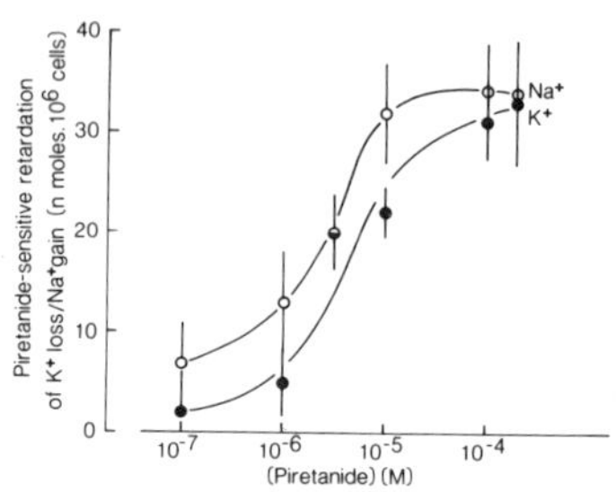

FIG2.Dose-response curve for piretanide action

Fig.1 shows the change in intracellular ion contents of HeLa cells after 24 h chronic growth in increasing concentrations of ouabain. In the range 20-100nM ouabain there is a reciprocal decrease in cell K^+ and increase in Na^+. In these conditions, a 50% reduction in functional Na-pump site number is seen at 10nM ouabain[4]. Changes in intracellular ions are not pronounced (fig.1) due to an increased turnover rate of remaining Na-pump sites [4]. At 50nM ouabain, less than 10% of Na-pump sites are functional. Piretanide (0.1mM) has no direct effect upon ouabain binding to the Na-pump ,so that the piretanide-sensitive retardation of K^+ loss and Na^+ gain observed in 50nM ouabain must reflect a substantial contribution of cotransport to net transmembrane cation movements. The apparent exchange character of Na^+ and K^+ movement in this chronic treatment,would not be expected from the normal operational definition of cotransport where highly coupled fluxes operate in a single transmembrane direction[2]. With moderate change in intracellular cation content (fig.1) no effect of piretanide is seen, though this may be due to the inability of the technique to detect small changes. Fig.2 shows that the effect of piretanide on retardation of K^+ loss and Na^+ gain is of high molar affinity; half-maximal effects being observed at 3-4 μM. The stoichiometry for retardation of K^+ loss and Na^+ gain is 1:1; variations in stoichiometry most probably reflect the apparent variation in stoichiometry seen at different levels of internal ions (fig.1)

Qualitatively identical effects of piretanide upon cellular cations of MDCK cells in conditions of chronic ouabain treatment are observed. Fig.3 shows that the maintanence of intracellular cations is seen not only with piretanide, but also with saturating concentrations of the other loop diuretics, such as bumetanide and furosemide. A substantial effect of piretanide is also observed in the presence of the stilbene, SITS, obviating a general reduction in Cl^- permeability as a likely mechanism for piretanide action.

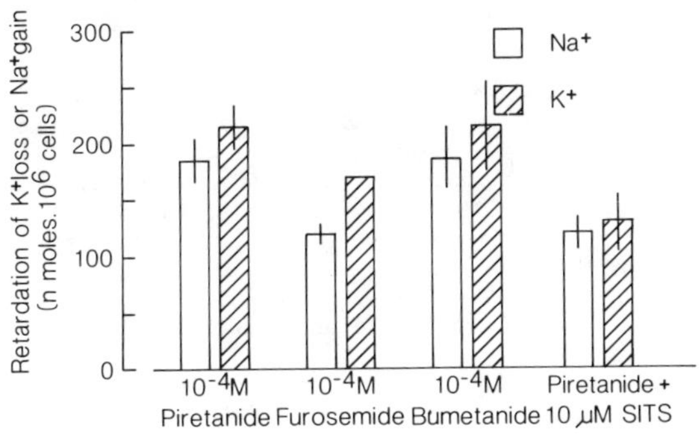

FIG 3.Sensitivity of retardation of K^+ loss and Na^+ gain by diuretics in MDCK cells.

Our data are entirely consistent with the notion that the piretanide-sensitive retardation of K^+ loss and Na^+ gain seen in conditions of chronic partial Na-pump inhibition are the result of blockade of the cotransport system, though our evidence is consistent with an exchange (Na^+ for K^+) mode of operation. Similar effects to those reported here, could be of significance for tissues in vivo. For in vitro smooth muscle preparations where substantial (50%) blockade of Na-pump activity has been seen with hypertensive plasma [3], a substantial ouabain-insensitive K^+ flux component exists [3], which usually indicates cotransport activity. It is possible that cotransport activity could contribute to a reduction in cellular K^+ and increase in Na^+ in these conditions ,which could, in turn, be ameliorated by cotransport blockade. Clearly more work is necessary to define the overall contribution of cotransport activity in these cell types, particually when Na-pump activity is reduced.

ACKNOWLEDGEMENTS

We are grateful to Dr. Chester Osborn of Hoechst U.K. for the kind gifts of furosemide and piretanide.

REFERENCES

1. Aiton J.F.,Chipperfield A.R.,Lamb J.F.,Ogden P. and Simmons N.L.(1981) Biochim et Biophys Acta, 600,432-447
2. Haas M.,Schmidt W.F. and McManus T.J.(1982) J.Gen.Physiol. 180,125-147
3. Haddy F.J. and Pamnani M.B.(1983) Federation Proc. 42,2673-2680
4. Aiton J.F. and Simmons N.L. (1981) Brit. J. Pharmacol.73,333-340

TRANSMEMBRANE POTASSIUM MOVEMENTS, DIURETIC DRUGS AND THE ARACHIDONIC ACID CASCADE: A STUDY WITH CULTURED AORTIC SMOOTH MUSCLE CELLS

P. BRAQUET*, D. DORIAN**, P. BORGEAT***, F.V. DEFEUDIS* and J. LARRUE**
*Institut Henri Beaufour, 17 Avenue Descartes, 92350 Le Plessis Robinson, France; **INSERM U8, Hôp. Cardiologique Haut Lévêque, 33600 Pessac, France; ***Groupe de Recherches sur les Leucotrienes, Université de Laval, 2705 Boulevard Laurier, Québec GIV 4G2, Canada

INTRODUCTION

Diuretic drugs have been shown to increase the release of prostacyclin (PGI_2) from the blood vessel wall (1). The mechanisms of action of these drugs on the arachidonic acid (AA) cascade have never been clarified (2,3). In this report, we describe experiments on cultured aortic smooth muscle cells (ASMC) which have shown that the diuretics, furosemide [Fur], bumetanide [Bum], piretanide [Pir] and cicletanide [Cic], enhanced the production of PGI_2 from exogenously-added AA. Such an effect is not mediated through an inhibition of lipoxygenase (LO) pathways, but seems to be due to a modification of monovalent cation (Na^+/K^+) balance induced by the drugs.

MATERIALS AND METHODS

Preparation of aortic smooth muscle cells

ASMCs were obtained from explants of thoratic aorta of adult male rats, as previously described (4), and grown at 37°C in an atmosphere of 5% CO_2 in air using HAM F10 growth medium supplemented with 10% fetal calf serum (FCS). All experiments were performed on secondary cultures using cells below passage number 7.

Metabolism of exogenous [1-^{14}C] arachidonate by cell homogenates

Cells were scraped with a rubber policeman, suspended in 2 ml of 0.05 M Tris-HCl, 0.15 M NaCl (pH, 7.4) buffer, and homogenized. The reaction mixture had the following composition: cell homogenate (1 mg of protein); [1-^{14} C]AA (50 Ci/mole), 10 nmoles in 10 µl absolute ethanol. The final reaction volume was 1 ml.

Drugs (10 - 100 µM) were added to the incubation mixture 10 min prior to adding AA. Incubations were performed at 37°C for 20 min in the dark with shaking and stopped either by acidification to PH 3.0 with citric acid, or by addition of 1.5 vol of methanol. After extractions, thin-layer chromatography (TLC) or high performance liquid chromatography (HPLC) was performed for determination of AA metabolites using a method that has been previously described (4).

Metabolism of endogenous [1-^{14}C] arachidonate by cell homogenates

Just confluent ASMCs (4.10^{6} cells) were washed twice with fresh medium and incubated for 20 hours in 10 ml HAM F10 medium, containing 2 nmoles of [1^{14} C]AA. After incubation, cells were washed twice to eliminate the unincorporated labelled material. Under these conditions, more than 85% of the starting radioactivity (about 1.3 x 10^{6} cpm) remained associated with the ASMCs and this was found essentially in the phospholipid fraction.

Pre-labelled cells were incubated in 10 ml of modified Krebs Ringer +

Diuretics, Jules B. Puschett, Editor

HEPES buffer. The ionic composition of this medium was: Na^+, 148; Ca^{2+}, 2.5; Mg^2, 1.2; HCO_3^-, 22; Cl^-, 128; $H_2PO_4^-$, 1.2 and SO_4^{2-}, 1.2 mM. Potassium content was adjusted to final concentrations of 0, 5, 10, 50 and 100 mM by substituting different amounts of KCl with corresponding amounts of NaCl; osmolarity was kept constant at 281 ± 0.8 m-OsM. Incubations were performed for 0.5 to 180 min at 37° C in the presence or absence of 5% FCS.

The total radioactivity released into the incubation medium was measured in 100-µl aliquots at different times during the incubation period by scintillation counting. After incubation, media were acidified to pH 3 using HCl (1.0 N), and then extracted twice with 3 vols ethyl acetate. Analyses were performed by TLC or HPLC (4). Concentrations of 6-keto-$PGF_{1}\alpha$ were determined by radioimmunoassay after extraction and purification, using the SEP-PACK elution method (5).

Determination of lipoxygenase inhibition in human leukocytes

After preparation of leukocytes (6), the concentrations of LO products were measured by reversed-phase HPLC (7), in the presence or absence of diuretics.

RESULTS AND DISCUSSION

At concentrations of 1 - 100 µM, the diuretics that were tested produced a significant dose-dependent enhancement of the oxidative transformation of AA, essentially by stimulation of the cyclooxygenase (CO) pathway (Table I), as demonstrated by the significant increase in the release of 6-keto-$PGF_{1}\alpha$ (Table II).

TABLE I. Effects of drugs on the metabolism of exogenous $[^{14}C]$AA by cultured rat aortic smooth muscle cells

Drug	Total transformed	CO pathway	LO pathway	CO/LO
Control (no drug)	17.5 ± 3.6	12.5 ± 3.4	5.0 ± 0.8	1.8
Fur	41.0 ± 8.5	32.3 ± 7.6	6.5 ± 1.2	3.9
Cic	40.0 ± 7.3	32.0 ± 10.1	6.2 ± 1.4	4.3
Bum	48.3 ± 16.2	35.6 ± 12.7	10.5 ± 3.7	2.7
Pir	40.6 ± 11.4	30.5 ± 10.3	8.4 ± 2.1	2.7

Cells were pre-incubated 10 min with the drugs (10^{-5}M) and were incubated for 20 min with $[^{14}C]$AA and analyzed by TLC. Results are expressed as percent of the total radioactivity recovered from the incubation medium (means = ± S.E.M. of 3 experiments with the same cell strain). CO indicates the summation of 6-keto-$PGF_{1}\alpha$, (Rf = 0.11), $PGF_{2}\alpha$, (Rf = 0.25), PGE_2 (Rf = 0.36) and HHT (Rf = 0.74); LO indicates the spot on TLC chromatograms that contained lipoxygenase products, mainly 12-HETE and 15-HETE (Rf = 0.77). All drugs produced significant increases in total $[^{14}C]$AA transformed and in the CO pathway ($p < 0.05$ or $p < 0.01$; Student's t-test; two-tailed), but had no effect on the LO pathway ($p > 0.1$).

TABLE II. Effects of drugs on prostanoid formation by cultured rat aortic smooth muscle cells

Drug	6-Keto-PGF$_1\alpha$	PGF$_2\alpha$	PGE$_2$
Control	9 ± 2.3	1 ± 1.2	1 ± 0.9
Fur	25 ± 6.8	3 ± 2.2	3 ± 1.3
Cic	25 ± 8.4	2 ± 1.4	3 ± 0.6
Bum	23 ± 12.3	5 ± 3.6	4 ± 1.5
Pir	22 ± 4.7	3 ± 2.1	4 ± 0.9

Incubation procedures and expression of results are described in Table I. Note that cells were used at passage n°3.

In contrast, the drugs did not inhibit the LO pathways which, in contrast, seemed to be slightly activated in ASMC. Also, in human leukocytes, no change in the synthesis of LO metabolites was observed. Therefore, the increase in PGI_2 production: (i) seems to be due to a general activation of the AA cascade that is more marked for the CO pathway; (ii) cannot be explained by an inhibition of LO pathways which would result in HPETE production, and subsequent inhibition of PGI_2-synthetase.

As it is well known that diuretic drugs interact with Na^+, K^+ transport systems (8) and as monovalent cation balance has been shown to modulate AA metabolism in a wide variety of tissues (9), we have investigated the influence of changes in Na^+/K^+ balance on AA metabolism in ASMCs.

Increasing $[K^+]_o$ concentrations of the incubation medium from 0 to 100 mM produced a biphasic, time-dependent effect (Table III). Mobilization of intracellular K^+ by the K^+-ionophore valinomycin (10^{-5} M) produced a significant stimulation of icosanoid release. This effect was observed only in the presence of FCS and it was dose-dependently inhibited by increasing $[K^+]_o$ A similar effect was produced when Cic (10^{-5} M) was added in place of valinomycin.

TABLE III. Time course of $[^{14}C]$ icosanoid release into the incubation medium

$[K^+]_o$, mM	Incubation time (min)			
	0.5	15	60	180
0	17.1 ± 5.5	57.2 ± 7.4	146.0 ± 12.0	302.0 ± 21.8
5	27.0 ± 3.9(a)	71.7 ± 3.3(b)	161.0 ± 11.3	181.0 ± 14.4(c)
50	46.5 ± 7.9(b)	85.6 ± 2.4(a)	139.5 ± 10.0	223.0 ± 24.5(d)
100	25.7 ± 5.4(b)	71.3 ± 4.3(b)	128.0 ± 16.3	198.0 ± 16.4(d)

Results (cpm x 10^{-3}) are expressed as means ± S.E.M. of 3 experiments. (a) $p < 0.05$; (b) $p < 0.02$; (c) $p < 0.01$; (d) $p < 0.001$ compared to values obtained at $[K^+]_o = 0$.

In conclusion, the results presented herein have indicated that: (i) diuretics increase PGI_2 synthesis; (ii) this increase appears to be due to a general activation of AA metabolism even though the CO pathway seems to be activated to a greater extent than the LO pathways; (iii) the hypothesis that the increase in PGI_2 formation could be due to a release of the inhibition of PGI_2-synthetase that is produced by HPETE is not supported; (iv) alterations in $[K^+]_o$ induced a modulation of AA metabolism; the K^+-ionophore valinomycin or Cic potentiated the activation of AA release produced by FCS; therefore, diuretics could act by modulating ion transport, particularly K^+ fluxes, thereby leading to changes in membrane potential, phospholipid turnover, and AA metabolism.

REFERENCES

1. S. Moncada, R.J. Gryglewski, S. Bunting and J.R. Vane Nature, 263, 663-8 (1976).
2. G. Hornstra, F. Haddeman and J.A. Don, Thromb. Res., 12, 367 (1978).
3. J.G. Gerber and A.S. Nies, Prostaglandins Med., 6, 135 (1981).
4. J. Larrue, M. Rigaud, D. Daret, J. Demond, J. Durand and H. Bricaud, Nature, 285, 480-482 (1980).
5. W.S. Powell In: Methods in Enzymology, Vol. 87, W.E.N. Lands and W.L. Smith, eds. (Academic Press, New York 1982) pp 467-76.
6. P. Borgeat and B. Samuelsson, Proc. Natl. Acad. Sc. USA, 76, 2148 (1979).
7. P. Borgeat, B. Fruteau de Laclos, H. Rabinovitch, S. Picard, P. Braquet, J. Hebert and M. Laviolette J. Immunol. Aller. Dis. (in press).
8. R.P. Garay, C. Nazaret, J. Diez, P. Hannaert and P. Braquet, Biochem. Pharmacol., In Press.
9. M.R. Knapp, O. Oelz, L.J. Roberts, B.J. Sweetman, J.A. Oates and P.W. Reed, Proc. Natl. Acad. Sci. USA, 74, 4251-4255 (1977).

FUROSEMIDE INHIBITS BASAL AND INSULIN STIMULATED GLUCOSE TRANSPORT IN ADIPOCYTES

D.B. Jacobs, B.K. Mookerjee, and C.Y. Jung.
VA Medical Center and SUNY at Buffalo, NY 14215.

INTRODUCTION

Significant glucose intolerance has been noted clinically during extended Furosemide administration [1]. The exact mechanisms operative in this remain unclear and controversial. Weller and Borodny [2] have shown that incubating of isolated epididymal fat pads with 1mM Furosemide or hydrochlorothiazide resulted in a reduction of their glucose utilization. However, Helderman et al. concluded that thiazides induced glucose intolerance by depletion of body potassium stores [3]. In the present communication, we demonstrate that Furosemide inactivates the glucose transport carrier of adipocytes directly, in a time dependent manner, independent of insulin effect.

MATERIALS AND METHODS

Adipose cells were isolated from the epididymal fat pads of Sprague Dawley (150-180 g) male rats, by the method described by Rodbell [4]. Microsomal and plasma membrane fractions were prepared from isolated adipocytes by the differential centrifugation method described by McKeel and Jarett [5]. 150,000 X g (total particulate fraction) was prepared from isolated fat cells by hypotonic lysis and subsequent centrifugation at 150,000 X g for 1 hr. at 5°C. The resultant pellet was resuspended and stored until used. Cytochalasin B binding assays were carried out by a modification of the centrifugation method described by Jung et al. [6]. Glucose transport in isolated adipocytes was assessed by measuring equilibrium exchange rates of 3-O-methyl glucose (3-O-MG) using (^{3}H)3-O-MG as a tracer and a modification of the oil floatation method. Insulin (7 nM) when used was added to the adipocyte suspensions with incubation for 1 hr. at 37°C.

RESULTS AND DISCUSSION

Equilibrium exchange of 3-O-MG by isolated adipocytes measured at 37°C as a function of sugar concentration showed a simple saturation kinetics with a Km at 5-7 mM. The same batch of isolated adipocytes pretreated with 7 nM insulin for 30 min at 37°C showed a three-fold higher Vmax without significant change in Km (data not shown). Incubation of basal and insulin treated isolated adipocytes with varying concentration of Furosemide for 1 hr. at 37°C inhibited the flux in both in a simple saturable manner (Figures 1, left and right). The apparent Ki was 4-5 mM in either the basal or insulin treated adipocytes for all the 3-O-MG concentrations used. The inhibition was found to be due to a reduction of Vmax without any significant change in the Km value, indicating a noncompetitive mode of inhibition.

Cytochalasin B, a well established specific inhibitor of glucose transport of adipocytes, binds to purified microsomal and plasma membranes of adipocytes (6). Scatchard analyses of these bindings indicate that there are at least two saturated binding components at the ligand concentration range of up to 10^{-5} M. The ligand binding to one of these components is

Diuretics, Jules B. Puschett, Editor

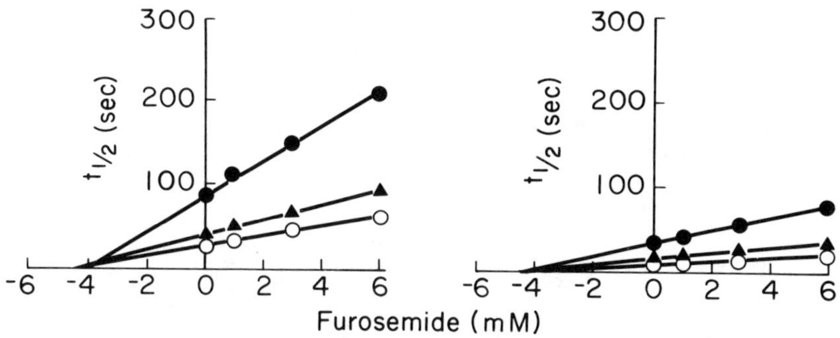

FIGURE 1: Inhibition of the equilibrium exchange by basal (left) and insulin (7 nM) treated (right) adipocytes of 3-0-MG (1( ),5( ) and 20mM ( )), as a function of Furosemide concentration.

displaced specifically by D-glucose, but not by L-glucose. The difference in the ligand bindings observed between these two isomers are taken as the glucose-sensitive binding. There are ample indications that this glucose-sensitive, cytochalasin B binding represents glucose carrier molecules.

The effects of furosemide on this glucose-sensitive, cytochalasin B binding to microsomal and plasma membrane preparations were studied by assaying the ligand binding in the presence of 500 mM L and D glucose. In a series of experiments (pretreatment series) cells were first incubated with a given concentration of furosemide prior to their membrane subfractionation. In other experiments (post-treatment series), the membranes were prepared first, then incubated in the presence of furosemide and its effect on the ligand binding was assessed. Both of the furosemide treatments inhibited the cytochalasin B binding of both the microsomal and plasma membranes equally, regardless of whether they are in basal or insulin-stimulated states. The inhibition is due to a reduction of B_T (total binding capacity) without any change in affinity (or K_D) of the glucose-sensitive binding (Table 1).

PREPARATION	CONTROL		PRETREATMENT		POST-TREATMENT	
	B_T	K_D	B_T	K_D	B_T	K_D
MICROSOMES	35.1	1.98	5.7	1.22	9.7	1.05
(BASAL	35.7	1.41	7.5	1.18	11.1	1.10
	48.1	1.50	5.8	1.22		
MICROSOMES	15.3	1.20	3.6	1.05	5.2	1.05
(INSULIN-TREATED)	17.0	1.41	3.3	1.20	5.3	0.95
	20.8	1.22	3.2	0.95		
PLASMA MEMBRANES	6.6	1.20	2.2	1.15	2.6	0.90
(BASAL)	6.7	1.16				
PLASMA MEMBRANE (INSULIN-TREATED)	23.5	1.26	5.4	0.96	6.5	0.98

TABLE 1. Equilibrium binding parameters B_T (p moles/mg) and K_D (10^{-7}M) of glucose-sensitive, cytochalasin B binding component of microsomal and plasma membrane preparations prior to and after incubation with 6mM furosemide for two hours. The furosemide incubation was done either with intact cells (pretreatment) or with membrane preparations (post-treatment).

This reduction in B_T analysed as a function of furosemide concentration for a fixed incubation time indicates that the effect is saturable with a simple stoichiometry. For a 2 hour-post treatment, the 50% inhibition (K_i) occurred at the furosemide concentration of approximately 3.5 mM and this <u>apparent</u> K_i value was not significantly different between microsomes and plasma membranes. For an 18 hr. post-treatment, the K_i was approximately 0.8 mM for both basal and insulin treated microsomes.

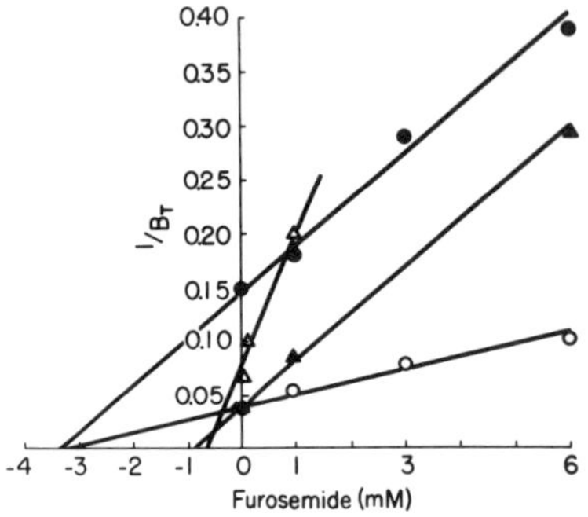

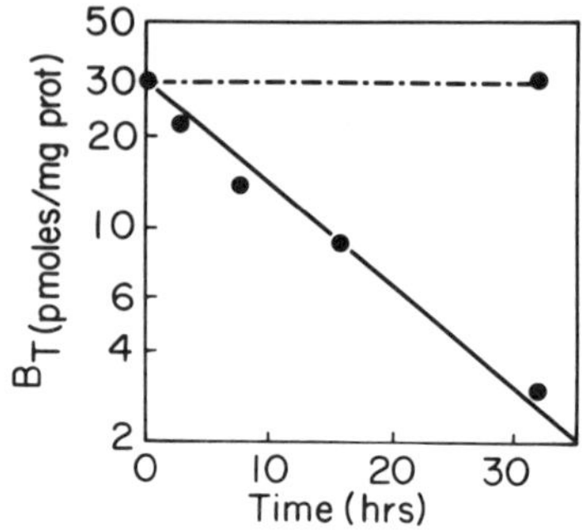

FIGURE 2 (Left): Reduction in B_T (p moles/mg) of the glucose sensitive cytochalasin B binding as a function of furosemide. Preparations are basal plasma membranes ( ) and basal microsomes ( ) after 1 1/2 hr incubation with furosemide, and the basal microsomes ( ) and insulin treated microsomes ( ) each after 18 hr. incubation with furosemide.

FIGURE 3 (Right): Time course of the development of the furosemide (1mM) effect on the glucose sensitive cytocholasin B binding to a 150,000 X g preparation.

Using a total particulate fraction of adipocytes (150,000 X g fraction), the time course of the development of the inhibitory effect on the glucose-sensitive cytochalasin B binding was followed for 32 hours. With the furosemide concentration of 1 mM, the inhibition developed as an exponential function of time with a first order rate constant of approximately 0.12/hour at 4°C (Figure 3).

In conclusion, furosemide inhibits glucose transport in rat adipocytes in a time dependent manner, with a simple stoichiometry, and a noncompetitive mode of inhibition that is independent of whether the adipocytes are in a basal or insulin stimulated state.

REFERENCES

1. P.J. Lewis et al., The Lancet 654-566 (1976).
2. J.M. Weller and M. Barondy, Metabolism <u>16</u>, 532-536 (1967).
3. J.H. Helderman et al., Diabetes <u>32</u>, 106-111 (1983).
4. M. Rodbell, J. Biol. Chem. <u>239</u>, 375-380 (1964).
5. D.W. McKeel and L. Jarett, J. Cell Biol. <u>44</u>, 417-432, 1970).
6. C.Y. Jung and A. Rampal, J. Biol. Chem. <u>252</u>, 5456-5463 (1977).

EFFECTS OF DIURETICS ON SALT TRANSPORT IN MODEL EPITHELIA

ÖRJAN ERIKSSON* AND PER J. WISTRAND**
*Dept. of Pharmacology, National Board of Health and Welfare, Box 607, S-751 25 Uppsala, and **Dept. of Medical Pharmacology, University of Uppsala, Box 573, S-751 23 Uppsala, Sweden

Compared to many other classes of therapeutic agents, relatively little is known about the structure-activity relationship of diuretics. This is largely due to technical difficulties of recording the "intrinsic" activities of the diuretic agents at the different types of tubular cells along the nephron. Thus, it was not until recently that dose-response curves of loop diuretics could be obtained from measurements using either microperfusion techniques in vivo [1] or on isolated tubules [2,3,4] in vitro. However, the use of such techniques to collect the amount of data necessary for studies of structure-activity relationships is unsurmountable for most laboratories. Therefore, the use of model epithelia which have been proven to function analogous to the salt transporting tubular cells of the mammalian nephron would be an attractive alternative for this purpose. We have tested this possibility by studing the effects of various standard types of diuretic agents on the sodium transport across frog (Rana temporaria) skin and the chloride transport across frog (Rana catesbeiana) cornea and killifish (Fundulus heteroclitus) operculum. These epithelia were mounted in an Ussing type of lucite chamber [5] and the transport of sodium and chloride were determined either electrophysiologically by measuring the transepithelial potential difference (PD) the short circuit current (SCC), and the resistance (R), or by measuring transepithelial net ion fluxes.

The frog skin could be used conveniently for the study of drugs which block sodium entry into the cell (amiloride type of drugs) and of inhibitors of Na-K-ATP-ase (oubain and orthovanadate). However, thiazides, carbonic anhydrase inhibitors and loop diuretics had no effect on Na^+-transport when added to either (serosal or pond) side of the skin [6].

The chloride transport of the epithelia of frog cornea and killifish operculum was inhibited only by "loop" diuretics, i.e. by those agents which block chloride transport in the thick ascending loop of Henle (TALH). The relative activities of furosemide (F) piretanide (P) and bumetanide (B), as obtained from parallel dose-response curves, were similar to the activities of these agents in TALH; see TABLE I. The drugs were only active from the chloride import side. Monomethylation of the SO_2NH_2 group of F and B had no effect, whereas dimethylation slightly reduced the effect of these agents. The l-form of indanone (MK-196) was 6 times more active than the d-form; the difference between the l- and d-form of ozolinone was >100 times. A similar difference between the stereo-isomers of these diuretics have been noted in TALH [7] and whole animals [8]. The alkaline agents MK 447 and muzolimine (Bay g 2281) were also active in the opercular skin and the frog cornea, indicating that these drugs should be classified as loop diuretics. In TABLE I is seen how the effects of the standard diuretics F, P and B in TALH compare with the effects in various model systems. "Loop" diuretics are active in a large variety of tissues with chloride transport or chloride exchange mechanisms, and several of these tissues could probably serve as model tissues for screening purposes. If the chloride transport mechanism is sufficiently like that in TALH, practical matters will decide which tissue to use. We would like to suggest the use of killifish operculum since this epithelium is viable and easy to mount for electrophysiological studies, where SCC is a convenient parameter for chloride transport. Moreover the fish is cheap and abundant and can be easily shipped and kept in artificial sea water the year around.

Diuretics, Jules B. Puschett, Editor

Thiazides had no effect on the salt transport in our model tissues. There is an urgent need for a good model tissue for thiazides to enable the study of the mechanism of action of this important type of diuretics.

TABLE I. Comparison of the effects of furosemide (F), piretanide (P) and bumetanide (B) on chloride transport or chloride exchange mechanism in the thick ascending limb of Henle (TALH) and in various model tissues.

Tissue and species	Concentration for 50% effect, μM	Ref.
Microperfusion of TALH, rat	F=10 P=3 B=2	(4)
Isolated TALH		
rabbit	F=3-10 P=1 B=0.2-0.7	(1,3)
rat	F=8-10 B=10	(1,2)
Human red cells	F=160 P<F	(9)
Turkey red cells	F=23 P=2.8 B=0.25	(10)
Amphibian cornea	F=10-37 P=5 B=0.5-0.74	(11,12,13)
Fish opercular skin	F=200 P=90 B=20	Present study

Supported by the Swedish Medical Research Council, grant no. 2874. The following companies generously supplied the tested agents: Merck Sharp & Dohme, USA, MK-196 and MK-447; Hoechst AG, GFR, furosemide and piretanide; Bayer AG, GFR, muzolimine; Gödecke AG, GFR, ozolinone; Lövens Kemiske Fabrik, Denmark, bumetanide.

REFERENCES

1. H.-U. Gutsche, K. Müller-Ott, R. Brunkhorst, and W. Niedermayer, Can. J. Physiol. Pharmacol. 61, 159-165 (1983.
2. M. Imai, Eur. J. Pharmacol. 41, 409-416 (1977).
3. L.C. Stoner and M.E. Trimble, J. Pharmacol. Exp. Ther. 221, 715-720 (1982).
4. E. Schlatter, R. Greger, and C. Weidtke, Pflügers Arch. 396, 210-217 (1983).
5. H.H. Ussing and K. Zerahn, Acta Physiol. Scand. 23, 110-127 (1951).
6. Ö. Eriksson, Acta Physiol. Scand. 128, 1337-1343 (1984).
7. J. Greven, W. Defrain, K. Glaser, K. Meywald, and O. Heidenreich, Pflügers Arch. 384, 57-60 (1980).
8. S.J. deSolms, O.W. Woltersdorf Jr., E.J. Cragoe Jr., L.S. Watson, and G.M. Fanelli Jr., J. Medicinal Chem. 21, 437-443 (1978).
9. B.A. Brooks and F.A. Lant, Clin. Sci. Mol. Med. 54, 679-683 (1978).
10. H.C. Palfrey, P.W. Feit, and P. Greengard, Am. J. Physiol. 238, C139-C147 (1980).
11. M.C. McGahan, T. Yorio, and P.J. Bentley, J. Pharmacol. Exp. Ther. 203, 97-102 (1977).
12. J.R. Schnieders and J. Ludens, Am. J. Physiol. 238, R70-R75 (1980).
13. O.A. Candia, H.F. Schoen, L. Low, and S.M. Podos, Am. J. Physiol. 240, F25-F29 (1981).

THE EFFECT OF AN ALDOSTERONE-ANTAGONIST: CANRENONE ON Na AND K MOVEMENTS ACROSS HUMAN RED CELL MEMBRANES.

JAVIER DIEZ, GEORGES DAGHER, JEAN PIERRE ABITBOL* AND RICARDO GARAY
INSERM U7/CNRS LA 318. Hôpital Necker. Paris 75015 and *Theraplix Lab.,Paris 75013, France.

ABSTRACT

There is indirect experimental evidence that spironolactones may act on transmembrane Na movements. On the other hand, human red cells have been widely used as a model for kinetic studies of ion transport mechanisms. We thus investigated here the effect of the spironolactone active metabolite: canrenone on the different Na and K transport systems of human red cell membranes.

At 0.5 mM, canrenone inhibits by 35±10% the ouabain-sensitive Na efflux without any effect on Na,K cotransport or Na:Na exchange mechanisms. In addition we observed a 45±10% increase in ouabain and bumetanide-resistant K fluxes. A detailed kinetic analysis of the interaction of canrenone with the Na, K-pump showed that this compound may compete with ouabain for a same pump-site. The IC 50% for canrenone was 0.054 mM.

Our results show that canrenone is able to modify Na and K movements across human red cell membranes. In particular, it may compete with endogenous ouabain-like factors that may be in excess in pathological conditions such as essential hypertension.

INTRODUCTION

Spironolactone appears to be rapidly transformed *in vivo* into canrenone which competes with aldosterone for a common cytosolic receptor in distal and collecting tubules of the nephron (1,2). Recently, indirect experimental evidence suggested an additional mechanism of action involving a direct effect on transmembrane Na movements (3,4).

Human red cells are readily accesible to clinical investigation and easy to manipulate. In addition, several Na transport systems have been characterized in these cells (see for instance ref. 5,6). We thus decided to investigate here the effect of canrenone on erythrocyte Na transport systems.

METHODS

Na and K fluxes were determined in fresh and Na-loaded erythrocytes according to previously published methods (5,6). Na,K-pump fluxes are represented by the fraction of total Na efflux in Mg,sucrose medium that is stimulated by 2mM external K and inhibited by 0.1 mM ouabain. Na,K-cotransport fluxes are represented by the fraction of Na and K effluxes in Mg,sucrose, ouabain medium that are inhibited by 0.02 mM bumetanide. The ouabain and bumetanide-resistant fraction of Na efflux that is stimulated by 10mM external Li was considered to represent Na:Li countertransport (a marker of Na:Na exchange).

RESULTS

The effect of canrenone on Na transport systems of human red cells

Table 1 shows that canrenone is a slight inhibitor of the Na,K-pump.Conversely, no effect was observed on the Na,K cotransport or Na,Li counter-

TABLE I. The effect of canrenone on Na and K transport in human red cells*

Condition	Na,K-pump	Na,K-cotransport	Na,Li-countertransport	Ouab+bum-resistant Na efflux	Ouab+bum-resistant K efflux
Control	2220±50	250±25	105±25	110±10	875±40
0.1mM Canrenone	1920±30	255±20	-	115±10	1250±60
0.5mM Canrenone	1350±100	225±20	120±30	140±20	2760±80

* Fluxes are given in μmol/l.cells x h.
Values in this Table are indicated as mean±range. A similar result was obtained in two other experiments.

transport systems (Table 1). It is interesting to note that ouabain and bumetanide-resistant K fluxes are strongly stimulated by canrenone.

Ouabain-sensitive Na efflux is stimulated by the increase in erythrocyte Na content (7). We observed that canrenone inhibits the maximal rate of Na efflux and slightly stimulates the apparent affinity of the pump for internal Na (not showed here).

The interaction of canrenone and ouabain with the erythrocyte Na,K-pump

Ouabain is a well known inhibitor of the Na,K-pump (7). Dose-response curves for the ouabain-effect were obtained at different,constant canrenone concentrations. Figure 1 shows that the increase in canrenone concentration decreases the apparent affinity of the Na,K-pump for ouabain. A kinetic analysis of this effect suggested that canrenone and ouabain may compete for a same pump-site. The IC 50% for canrenone was 0.054 mM. Spironolactone showed no competition with ouabain.

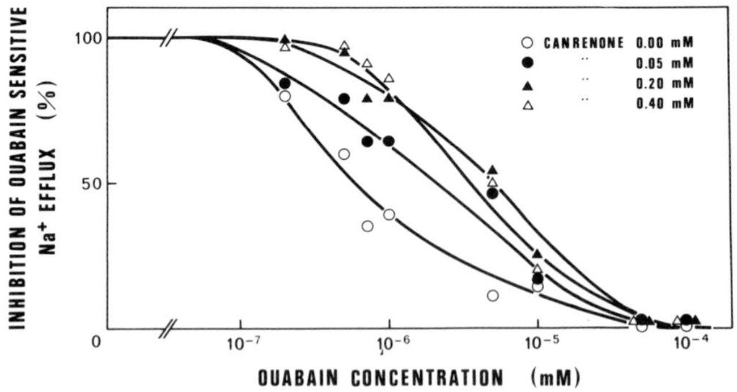

FIG. 1. The effect of canrenone on the percent inhibition of the Na,K-pump by ouabain.

A comparison of the results of Table 1 and Figure 1 shows that canrenone is one order of magnitude more effective to compete with ouabain than to inhibit the Na,K-pump.

DISCUSSION

Antialdosterone drugs appear to counteract digitalis-induced cardiac toxicity in animals and in man (8). In addition, canrenoate was reported to be able to reversal the inhibitory effect of digoxin on basal and furosemide stimulated renin secretion (9). We have observed here that canrenone decreases the ability of ouabain to inhibit the Na,K-pump. These effects may be mediated by a direct competition between canrenone and ouabain for a same pump-site (see Results and ref.4).

It appears that renal Na excretion may be regulated in part by endogenous ouabain-like factors (10). On the other hand the administration of ouabain in resistance vessels increases smooth muscle contractility and reactivity. The observation that endogenous ouabain-like factors are in excess in plasma from some hypertensive patients suggested a role in some forms of essential hypertension.

The above results allowed us to postulate a model for the mechanism of antihypertensive action of canrenone (Figure 2). In this model canrenone may compete with aldosterone receptors and also with endoxine (ouabain-like)-receptors. Further investigation is required in order to elucidate this mode of action.

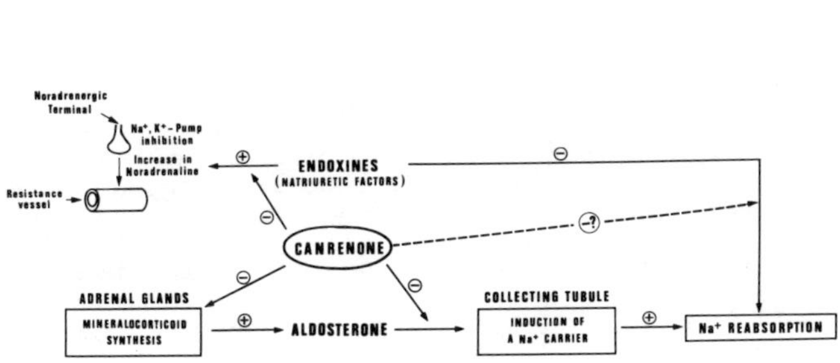

FIG.2. A model for the antihypertensive effect of canrenone.

REFERENCES

1. D.Marver and J.Kokko. Min.Electr.Metab. 9,1 ,(1983)
2. W.Sadeé,M Dagcioglu and R.Schröder.J.Pharm.Exp.Ther. 185,686,(1973)
3. D.Marver. Vitamins and Hormones Vol.18,55 (Acad.Press),(1980)
4. P.Finotti and P.Palatini.J.Pharm.Exp.Ther. 217,784,(1981)
5. R.Garay et.al. Eur.J.Clin.Invest. 13,311,(1983)
6. D.Cusi and R.Garay. Mol.Pharm. 19, 438(1981)
7. R.Garay and P.Garrahan. J.Physiol. 231,297 (1973).
8. B.Yeh,B.Chiang and P.Sung. Am.Heart J. 92,308 (1976)
9. P.Finotti and A.Antonello. Clin.Pharm.Ther. 32,1 (1982).
10.M.Blaustein and J.Hamlyn. Ann.Int.Med. 98(Part 2),785 (1983).

SEPARATE SITES OF ACTION FOR CHLOROTHIAZIDE (CTZ) AND AMILORIDE (AM) IN RAT DISTAL CONVOLUTED TUBULE (DCT)

LINDA S. COSTANZO
Department of Physiology and Biophysics, Medical College of Virginia, Richmond, Virginia, USA

In 1976, we demonstrated that, like thiazide diuretics, amiloride is hypocalciuric in dogs (1). Furthermore, when added to a maximally effective dose of chlorothiazide, amiloride produced further hypocalciuria and dissociation of Ca and Na excretion (1). We recently repeated these experiments in 5 volume expanded rats. Clearance experiments with three phases were performed: a control phase, a phase during which a maximally effective dose of chlorothiazide was infused intravenously and a phase of infusion of chlorothiazide plus amiloride. Chlorothiazide alone (2 mg/kg; 0.25 mg/kg-min) was a potent natriuretic agent, causing fractional Na excretion to increase from 0.078±0.006 to 0.118±0.013, $p < 0.001$. Addition of amiloride (0.02 mg/kg-min) did not further augment the natriuresis. Chlorothiazide alone reduced the Ca clearance ratio by 40%, fractional Ca excretion falling from 0.064±0.006 to 0.040±0.004, $p < 0.001$. In contrast to the results for Na, addition of amiloride to chlorothiazide caused further reduction of fractional Ca excretion to 0.030±0.002, $p < 0.025$. As a consequence, Ca clearance was strongly dissociated from Na clearance in the presence of chlorothiazide and the dissociation was even more pronounced with the drug combination. We also observed the well known kaliuretic effect of chlorothiazide and its amelioration when amiloride was added.

We could not determine from these clearance experiments whether the additive hypocalciuric effects of the two diuretics results from different sites or different mechanisms of action. Recently , _in vivo_ microperfusion of rat distal convoluted tubules has demonstrated that amiloride's hypocalciuric action results from a direct effect on the distal convoluted tubule (2). Specifically, only late distal tubular segments responded to the drug, while early segments did not. It is also known that thiazides are natriuretic and hypocalciuric because of direct effects on epithelial transport in the distal convoluted tubule (3). However, the precise localization of these actions has not yet been determined. Therefore, we performed _in vivo_ microperfusion of early and late rat distal convoluted tubules to localize the thiazide effect and to compare the site of action with that for amiloride.

The technique for microperfusion is as follows. Distal convoluted tubules with two loops on the kidney surface were perfused at 6 nl/min with a solution simulating early distal fluid and containing C-14 inulin to measure water absorption. The tubular segments were classified retrospectively from latex casts as early, first 50%, or late, last 50%. All tubules were perfused sequentially with two solutions: one, control, and the other identical except for the addition of 5×10^{-4} M chlorothiazide. Ca, Na and water reabsorption were measured at constant delivered load and normalized for tubular length. In 8 early distal tubules, Na transport was significantly reduced by chlorothiazide perfusion from 131±12 to 89±10 pmole/min-mm, $p < 0.001$; each early distal tubule responded in qualitatively the same fashion. On the average, chlorothiazide did not affect Na transport in 7 late tubules. The location of thiazide-induced stimulation of distal Ca reabsorption was similar. Chlorothiazide stimulated Ca transport in each of the early distal tubules, with the mean value increasing after drug perfusion from 3.24±0.29 to 4.00±0.18 pmole/min-mm, $p < 0.01$. The late distal tubules, as for Na,were unaffected by the drug. As a consequence

Diuretics, Jules B. Puschett, Editor

of the drug-induced inhibition of Na transport and enhancement of Ca transport in the early distal tubule, the number of Na ions reabsorbed for every Ca ion reabsorbed fell from 42 Na's per Ca to 23 Na's per Ca, $p < 0.025$. In the late tubule, under control conditions, the number of Na's reabsorbed per Ca reabsorbed was the same as in the early tubule. However, late tubules were characterized by a lack of dissociation when chlorothiazide was perfused.

These results, taken together with the earlier data regarding the site of action of amiloride suggest that these two distal diuretics interact with different cell types have different localizations or distributions within the rat distal convoluted tubule. This suggestion is reasonable given the histologic description of the rat distal convolution given by Kaissling (4). She described this segment as having 4 different cell types: the early tubule consists mainly of distal convoluted tubule cells with a few intercalated cells; the late tubule is more heterogeneous, having intercalated cells, connecting tubule cells and principal cells intermingled. There are not sharp borders between any of the cell types in the rat. Thus, it is likely that chlorothiazide inhibits Na transport and enhances Ca transport by interacting with the distal convoluted tubule cell in the early tubule, while amiloride interacts with one of the late distal cell types. If this description is accurate, then a single, long distal convoluted tubule, having both early and late portions should respond to both diuretics. In fact, we were successful in obtaining 2 such tubular segments, 1.65 and 1.74 mm,respectively. Each segment was perfused in sequence with a control solution, followed by 5×10^{-4} M chlorothiazide, and finally with 5×10^{-4}M chlorothiazide plus 10^{-5} M amiloride. The thiazide concentration chosen is one which was demonstrated to maximally inhibit Na absorption and maximally enhance Ca absorption. Upon addition of amiloride, Ca absorption was further enhanced in each tubule. However, there was little additional effect on Na transport with the drug combination. The lack of effect of amiloride on Na absorption when superimposed upon chlorothiazide perfusion may be explained by the increased Na delivery to the late distal tubule caused by the thiazide. The increased Na load would be expected to increase Na reabsorption (3), possibly obscuring any amiloride-induced inhibition.

In summary, chlorothiazide and amiloride are both distal diuretics having natriuretic and hypocalciuric effects. Their respective sites of action within the distal convoluted tubule are different. Thiazides appear to interact with an early distal cell type, whereas amiloride affects electrolyte transport in the terminal portion of the distal tubule. This distinction forms, at least in part, the basis for the additive hypocalciuric actions of these diuretics when administered together and may constitute a rational basis for combined therapy of hypercalciuria.

ACKNOWLEDGEMENTS

Work in the author's laboratory was supported by a grant from N.I.H. (AM-28358). L. Costanzo is an Established Investigator of the American Heart Association.

REFERENCES

(1) L.S. Costanzo and I.M. Weiner. Am.J. Physiol. 239:67-73 (1976).
(2) L.S. Costanzo . Am. J. Physiol. In Press. (1984).
(3) L.S. Costanzo and E.E. Windhager. Am. J. Physiol. 235: F492-F506 (1978).
(4) B. Kaissling. Am. J. Physiol. 243: F221-F226 (1982).

TUBULAR SITES OF ACTION AND RELATIVE POTENCIES OF THE ENANTIOMERS OF INDACRINONE (MK-196)

MICHAEL J. FIELD, NICOLE FOWLER, AND GERHARD GIEBISCH
Department of Physiology, Yale University School of Medicine, New Haven, CT 06510, USA

ABSTRACT

We used the technique of tubular microperfusion, *in vivo*, to study the effects of the enantiomers of indacrinone (MK-196) on sodium and potassium transport in the rat kidney. At the dose used ($5x10^{-4}$M), MK-196(-) was approximately 2-3 times as potent as MK-196(+) at inhibiting Na^+ and K^+ reabsorption by the loop of Henle. In the distal tubule, both enantiomers inhibited Na^+ reabsorption by about 50%, while neither influenced K^+ secretion in this segment. Thus at least two cellular cation transporting mechanisms in the rat nephron are sensitive to this drug.

INTRODUCTION

Indacrinone (MK-196) is a potent indanone diuretic with uricosuric as well as saluretic effects (1). Clearance studies suggest that a key site of the natriuretic action of this agent is the loop of Henle, and *in vitro* microperfusion experiments using isolated thick ascending limb segments are consistent with this proposal (2). Whole animal studies indicate that of the two naturally-occurring enantiomers of MK-196, the (-) enantiomer is significantly more potent as a natriuretic than the (+)(3). Since the two enantiomers have not been studied separately at the tubular level, we undertook *in vivo* microperfusion experiments in the rat kidney to define the differential effects of MK-196(-) and MK-196(+) on monovalent cation transport by the loop of Henle and distal tubule.

METHODS

Male Sprague-Dawley rats were anesthetized with Inactin, prepared for micropuncture using routine methods, and given an intravenous infusion of Ringer solution at 1 ml/100g body weight/hour. Two types of experiments were performed:

Loop of Henle microperfusion, at a rate of 20 nl/min, was performed in 41 nephrons of 11 rats. Fluid was perfused from the last accessible proximal convolution to the corresponding early distal convolution of a given nephron, as previously described (4). The "control" perfusion fluid contained Na^+ 150 mM and K^+ 4 mM, as well as tritiated inulin to act as a water marker. Either MK-196(-) or MK-196(+) was added to separate aliquots of this fluid, at a concentration of $5x10^{-4}$M in each case, and in a given kidney 1-4 loops were perfused with control and either of the drug-containing perfusion fluids.

Distal tubular microperfusion was performed at 13 nl/min in 23 nephrons of 14 rats. Here the perfusion pipette was placed in an early distal convolution, and the collection made from the corresponding late distal segment. The same control and drug-containing perfusion fluids described above were used, although in general, control and drug perfusions in this case were performed in different animals.

From measurements of the rate of fluid collection, the sodium and

Diuretics, Jules B. Puschett, Editor

potassium concentrations, and the inulin counts in perfused and collected fluid samples, it was possible to calculate the net transepithelial fluxes of Na^+, K^+ and fluid in each perfused tubular segment.

RESULTS

Mean data for net transport of sodium (J Na), potassium (J K), and fluid (J v) by the loop of Henle and distal tubule during perfusion with Control, or MK-196(-) or MK-196(+) containing perfusion fluids, are shown in the Table.

	Control	MK-196(-)	MK-196(+)
LOOP OF HENLE			
J Na	2270 ± 200	930 ± 100**	1620 ± 170**
J K	54.7 ± 3.4	-2.1 ± 9.4*	33.3 ± 5.0*
J v	7.8 ± 0.8	5.8 ± 0.2	6.6 ± 0.8
DISTAL TUBULE			
J Na	369 ± 38	159 ± 38**	209 ± 42**
J K	-62.9 ± 16.1	-55.2 ± 13.3	-59.5 ± 11.3
J v	0.5 ± 0.2	0.1 ± 0.2	0.1 ± 0.3

* $p<0.05$, ** $p<0.01$, compared to control

All units are pmol/min, "+" absorption, "-" secretion.

Thus, in the loop of Henle, both drug enantiomers inhibited Na^+ and K^+ reabsorption, but MK-196(-) was about twice as potent as MK-196(+) in regard to Na^+, and three times as potent in regard to K^+, in this segment (see FIG. 1). IN the distal tubule, both enantiomers inhibited Na^+ reabsorption to a similar degree, but neither affected the control levels of K^+ secretion in this segment (FIG. 1). Fluid reabsorption by perfused tubules was not significantly depressed by MK-196 during these experimental protocols.

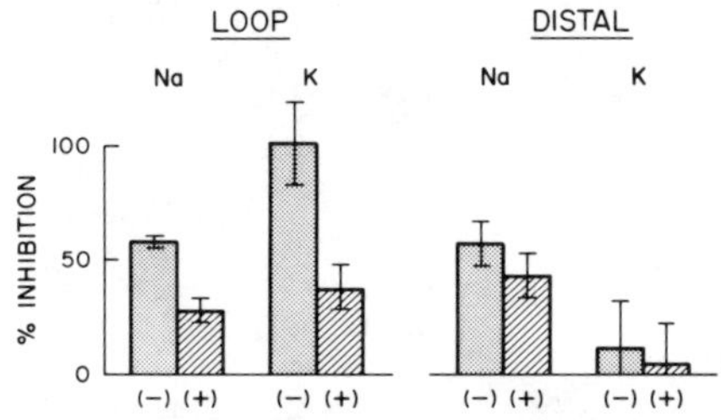

FIG.1. Percent inhibition of control fluxes of Na and K produced by the (-) and (+) enantiomers of MK-196 in the loop of Henle and distal tubule.

DISCUSSION

These studies demonstrate directly that the loop of Henle and the distal tubule are sites of action of MK-196. Since, however, the distal tubule reabsorbs only 1/5 to 1/6 as much sodium as the loop, the overall natriuretic response to the drug is largely due to its action in the loop.

Our transport data in the loop of Henle confirm that the (-) enantiomer is the more potent drug form at this site (3), while a significant difference in potency could not be demonstrated in the distal tubule. Larger differences in effectiveness between the two enantiomers may have been demonstrable, at both tubular sites, at a lower dose of the drug than that used here ($5x10^{-4}$M, a maximally effective dose in *in vitro* systems(2)).

The results of these experiments can be interpreted with reference to recent models for cellular ion transport mechanisms in the two nephron segments studied (see FIG. 2). The action of MK-196(-) in the loop resembles that described for furosemide (4), and probably involves interference with the proposed Na^+:$2Cl^-$:K^+ neutral cotransporter in the luminal cell membrane of thick ascending limb cells (A). Potassium recirculation through a conductive channel in this membrane explains the conversion by the drug of net K^+ reabsorption to net secretion in many individual experiments.

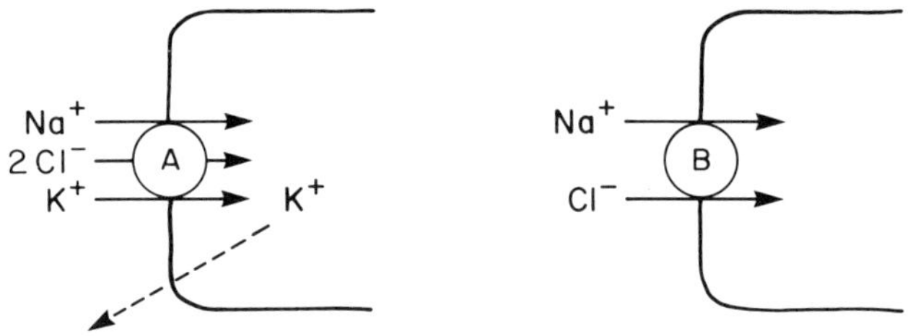

FIG. 2. Possible sites of action of MK-196 on ion cotransport mechanisms in the luminal membrane of cells of the thick ascending limb of Henle's loop (A) and the early distal tubule (B).

Inhibition of distal tubular Na^+ reabsorption by MK-196 also resembles that recently described for furosemide (5). It is likely that this effect is due to partial interaction with the early distal tubular "thiazide" site, at which sodium is cotransported with chloride but without potassium (B). Hence neither thiazides (5) nor typical "loop" diuretics directly affect potassium transport by the distal tubule.

ACKNOWLEDGMENTS

This work was supported by grants from NIH, Merck Inc., and the Postgraduate Medical Foundation, University of Sydney (to MJF).

REFERENCES

1. G.M. Fanelli, Jr, D.L. Bohn, A. Scriabine and K.H. Byer, Jr. J. Pharmacol. Exp. Ther. 200, 402-412 (1977).
2. L.C. Stoner and M.E. Trimble. J. Pharmacol. Exp. Ther. 221, 715-720 (1982).
3. P.H. Vlasses, J.D. Irvin, P.B. Huber, R.B. Lee, R.K. Ferguson, J.J. Schrogie, A.G. Zacchei, R.O. Davies and W.B. Abrams. Clin. Pharmacol. Ther. 29, 798-807 (1981).
4. T. Morgan, M. Tadokoro, D. Martin and R.W. Berliner. Am. J. Physiol. 218, 292-297 (1970).
5. H. Velazquez and F.S. Wright. Kidney Int. 23, 269 (1983).

ACUTE AND CHRONIC EFFECTS OF PIRETANIDE IN CONGESTIVE CARDIAC FAILURE

W.R. McNABB, F.J. NOORMOHAMED, A.F. LANT
Department of Therapeutics, Westminster Hospital, London SW1. ENGLAND

SUMMARY

The sulphamoylbenzoate piretanide was studied in 25 patients in congestive cardiac failure (CCF). After 6mg orally, peak diuresis and saluresis occurred within 4h. Over 0-6h Na^+ and Cl^- losses were 4-fold over control whilst urinary Ca^{2+} and Mg^{2+} doubled. Urinary K^+ increased by 65±16% ($p<0.05$). A significant antidiuretic effect occurred after 6h so that net saluresis over 24h was only 73±14% over control. The net urinary losses of Ca^{2+}, Mg^{2+} and K^+ were insignificant over 0-24h.

Longterm piretanide therapy continued in 15 patients for up to 3 years without addition of other diuretics or potassium supplements. Mean serum K^+ fell from 4.40±0.09 to 4.16±0.16 (n=7, 2 years). Serum urate increased from 0.43±0.02 to 0.47±0.05 ($p<0.01$ at 2 years) whilst 2 patients developed acute gout. Total serum cholesterol significantly increased from 5.80±0.6 to 6.30±0.35 (n=7; 2 years) whilst triglycerides remained unchanged (1.75±0.23 vs 1.41±0.17).

Bioavailability of piretanide was 67±7% (n=3). Mean elimination $t_{\frac{1}{2}}$ was 78±7 mins. Urinary recovery of unchanged drug was 25±1% of the oral dose in the first 24h of which 84±1% was excreted within 0-6h. Total body clearance was 148±24ml min^{-1} compared to a mean value of 150±10 ml min^{-1} in healthy subjects (n=4).

INTRODUCTION

Concern has been expressed about the possible metabolic effects of prolonged diuretic therapy. Diuretics of differing structure may have different sites of action within the renal tubule in addition to varying duration of action. This variability may influence the risk of electrolyte imbalance [1,2]. Piretanide is a sulphamoylbenzoate diuretic which is predominately active in the thick ascending limb of Henle's loop but has additional proximal tubular activity [3]. We set out to study the time course of action and pharmacokinetic profile of piretanide in CCF, to ascertain the long-term efficacy of piretanide, and to monitor the acute and long-term electrolyte balance and metabolic status of patients in chronic heart failure treated with piretanide.

METHODS

A group of 14 patients, 10 male and 4 female, in grade III or IV (NYHA) CCF were studied as in-patients. Mean age (±SEM) was 69±3y. 12 had ischaemic heart disease and 2 a congestive cardiomyopathy. Mean creatinine clearance (±SEM) was 59.5±7 ml/min. They were maintained on a no added salt diet whilst avoiding high salt containing foods. A three day period free of diuretic therapy preceded the first oral 6mg dose of piretanide. Fractional collections of urine were analysed on the day before therapy and compared with the first day on piretanide.

Diuretics, Jules B. Puschett, Editor

In a further 11 patients with grade II or III CCF we compared the acute effects of oral piretanide (6mg) with and without triamterene (50mg). The patients were maintained on a metabolic diet containing 150 mmol Na^+ and 70 mmol K^+.

15 patients with grade III or IV congestive cardiac failure were followed for up to 3 years with 2 monthly clinical assessment and biochemical screening. Piretanide was given on dosages up to 24mg daily without potassium supplements or potassium sparing diuretics.

Piretanide pharmacokinetics were studied in detail in 4 healthy volunteers and in 3 patients with congestive cardiac failure. Each subject remained free of diuretic therapy for 3 days prior to piretanide (6mg) given orally and intravenously on separate occasions. Piretanide was assayed in plasma and urine by a spectrofluorimetric method.

RESULTS

The saluretic effect of piretanide was complete within 6 hours and amounted to 52.8±7.5 mmol Na^+ and 65.4±8.9 mmol Cl^- vs control values of 11.7±3.6 and 11.3±3.0, n=14. Significant increases in potassium, calcium and magnesium were observed over the first 6 hours whilst neither creatinine nor urate clearance changed. Over 24 hours sodium and chloride excretion significantly increased from 53.9±9.5 to 88.6±11.8 mmol ($p<0.001$) and 44.9±9.4 to 89.3±12.2 mmol ($p<0.001$) respectively. Other ion excretion did not change. Thus, for example, potassium excretion was 58.4±7.6 mmol control, and 60.7±7.6 mmol, day 1.

When triamterene was given the kaluretic effect of piretanide alone in the first 6 hours was annulled. Thus potassium excretion was 18.8 ±3.4 mmol control vs 29.4±4.9 mmol after piretanide ($p<0.05$), and 16.9±2.7 mmol control vs 20.6± 3.1 mmol after piretanide plus triamterene. Again after piretanide alone 24 h potassium excretion did not differ from control (61.8±5.4 vs 54.4± 3.9).

The only consistent change in biochemical variables over the 3 year period was a decrease in serum potassium and an increase in total cholesterol with a less significant elevation in uric acid (Fig. 1). The lowest serum K^+ observed was 3.4 mmol/l on one occasion in one patient. Serum magnesium concentration remained unchanged on chronic piretanide therapy. Two patients developed clinical gout when piretanide was increased to 24mg daily. Piretanide was otherwise well tolerated and cardiac failure controlled. Four patients died during follow-up, three with recent myocardial infarction demonstrated at post-mortem and one with a cerebro-vascular accident.

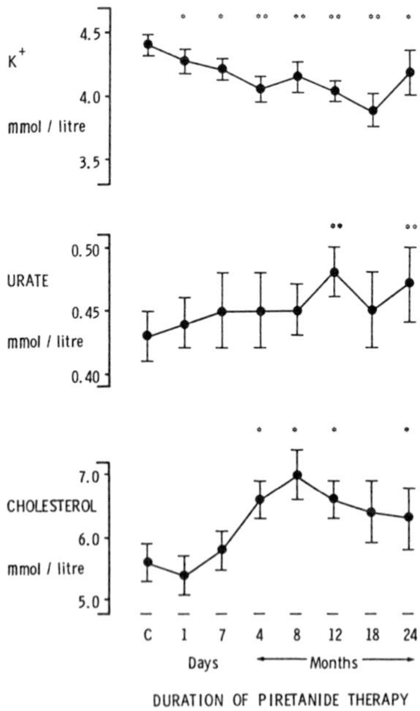

FIG 1. Long-term data in fifteen patients with CCF treated with piretanide for 2 y. (*$p<0.05$;**$p<0.01$)

The pharmacokinetic data are summarized below:

	CREATININE CLEARANCE (ml/min)	TOTAL BODY CLEARANCE (ml/min)	ELIMINATION $t_{\frac{1}{2}}$ (min)	BIOAVAILABILITY (%)	URINARY RECOVERY (%)
HEALTHY VOLUNTEERS (n=4)	120 ± 11	150 ± 10	65 ± 6	79 ± 6	29.4 ± 6.9
C.C.F. (n=3)	62 ± 4	148 ± 24	78 ± 7	67 ± 7	25.4 ± 0.8

DISCUSSION

Few long-term studies with'loop'diuretics have been reported and those that have include the use of potassium retaining diuretics or supplements [4,5]. Our finding that 24 hour potassium loss following piretanide did not differ from control justified the prolonged administration of piretanide without K^+ supplements or K^+ sparing diuretics. Though a significant fall in mean serum potassium occurred, values remained within the normal range. In healthy volunteers total body and intracellular potassium did not change in 6 weeks on piretanide [6,7].

Previous studies in healthy volunteers [3] have demonstrated increased urate clearance at the time of maximal piretanide-induced natriuresis. We were unable to demonstrate any uricosuria following piretanide in our patients. In heart failure sodium retaining mechanisms are already activated and tubular urate handling differs from that in healthy volunteers. The time course of piretanide-induced urate retention in healthy volunteers [8] is post-saluretic suggesting a relation ship to sodium retaining mechanisms rather than to any possible link with tubular secretion of the drug [9].

There is little information available on the long-term effect of 'loop' diuretics on lipid metabolism. In hypertensive patients frusemide [10] and piretanide [11] increased low density lipoproteins. Our data suggest similar changes may occur in congestive cardiac failure but further studies with examination of lipid subfractions are required.

REFERENCES

1. J. Anderson, B.E. Godfrey, D.M. Hill, A.D. Munro-Faure and J. Sheldon, Quart J. Med. 160, 541-560 (1971)
2. R. Gabriel and P. Baylor, Postgrad. med. J. 57, 71-74
3. W.R. McNabb, F.H. Noormohamed, B.A. Brooks and A.F. Lant, Clin. Pharmacol. Ther. 35, 385-392 (1984)
4. K.H. Olesen, B. Sigurd, B. Hesse, E. Steiness and A. Leth, Postgrad. med. J. 51, (suppl 6), 54-63 (1975)
5. M.M. Kubik, E. Bowers and P.N. Underwood, Current Med. Res. & Op, 5, 273-278 (1977)
6. A. Alvestrand and J. Bergstrom, Current Ther. Res. 25, 786-790 (1977)
7. F.O. Muller, B.H. Meyer, A. De Waal, O.R. Van Reenan and H.G. Grigoleit Clin. Pharmacol. Ther. 31, 339-342 (1982)
8. W. Bogie, M. Homeida, C.H.C. Roberts and F. Roberts, Br. J. clin. Pharmacol.4, 392P (1977)
9. B. Odlind, B. Beermann, G. Selen and A.E.G. Persson, J. Pharmacol. exp. Ther. 225, 742-133 (1978)

REFERENCES continued

10. Z. Gluck, G. Baumgartner, P. Weidmann, E. Peheim, C. Bachmann, R. Mordasini, J. Flammer and G. Keusch, Clin. Sci. Mol. Med. 55, 325S-328S (1978)
11. M. Valimaki, K. Harno and E.A. Nikkila, J. cardiovasc. Pharmacol. 5, 525-530 (1983).

SECTION IX

DIURETIC EFFECTS ON THE KIDNEY

IN VIVO MEASUREMENTS OF SEGMENTAL Na AND WATER TRANSPORT BY FUROSEMIDE

BARTOLI E., SATTA A., FAEDDA R., BRANCA G.F., CONTU B.
University Institute of Patologia Medica,Viale San Pietro 12,Sassari(Italy).

ABSTRACT

Na and water resorption by each segment of the human nephron can be measured by a new test based on Furosemide. In previously published data GFR was estimated by creatinine,while in the present experiments it was measured by inulin clearance.The data,expressed as equivalent flows of free water generated per 100 ml of GFR,demonstrate that Henle's Loop (HL) transport is 28.7±7.1,Distal Tubular(DT)transport 11.5±2.4, while solvent back diffusion across collecting ducts(CD)amounts to 22.3±7.4 ml /min/GFR. The data,similar to the previous ones, indicate that the method is reproducible and yields detailed informations on renal function.

INTRODUCTION

The measurements of free water clearance during maximal water diuresis do not account for the volume of water reabsorbed across CD(1)which is larger than in antidiuresis in rats(2).We recently devised a new,improved method, accounting for this volume loss:we measured "true" rates of free water generation and reabsorption across the different nephron segments(3).This method has given details on renal function in a number of clinical conditions(3-8). We deemed it necessary to reproduce our results,previously based on creatinine clearances,by measurements of Inulin clearance.

MATERIALS AND METHODS

Details on the new method and its theoretical background have been given elsewhere.Briefly,we must consider that free-water is formed by HL and DT by salt transport from lumen to interstitium(Fig.1a,1b),forming CH2O-HL and CH2O-DT,the free water clearances of HL and DT. Their sum yields the total amount of solute free water formed,which we call CH2O-T.Therefore,CH2O-HL CH2O-DT = CH2O-T.Fig.1c shows that the free water excreted is less than that formed,since a part is lost by back diffusion across CD.This volume is called CH2O-BD,the free water clearance back-diffusion.During a test of maximal diluting ability,we can obtain measurements of urine flow rate($\dot{V}$)and free water clearance excreted(CH2O)before and after Furosemide injection.Fig.2 shows what happens.Furosemide inhibits salt transport by HL,thus abolishing CH2O-HL. Since the salt pumped into the interstitium makes the medullary tissue hypertonic and drives water reabsorption from CD,Furosemide also abolishes CH2O-BD abstraction.Therefore,the urine flow rate during the action of the diuretic ($\dot{V}f$)increases by an amount equal to CH2O-BD,which is now lost into the urine instead of being reabsorbed.Hence,the difference between $\dot{V}f$ and $\dot{V}$ gives the

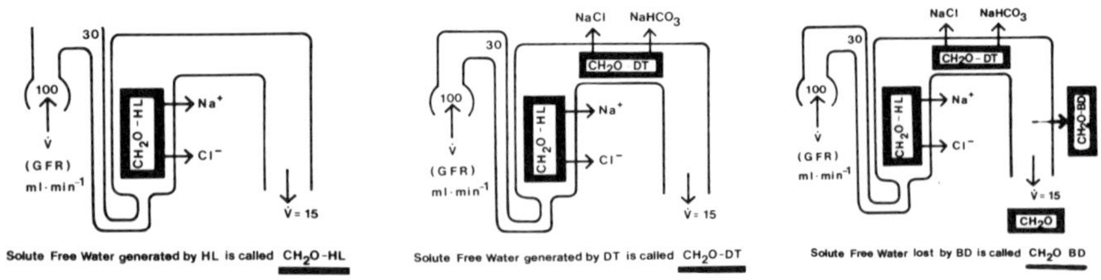

Fig 1. The distilled water generated by salt transport across HL (a) DT (b) is partly lost by back diffusion across CD (c) are shown by the rectangles labeled with their respective symbols.

rate of free water back diffusion directly:CH2O-BD=$\dot{V}$f-$\dot{V}$.This volume of solvent, added to the free water excreted prior to Furosemide(CH2O), yields the total amount of free water formed.CH2O-BD+CH2O=CH2O-T.Finally,we must consider that the free water excreted during Furosemide(CH2Of)can be formed exclusively along DT,since under the action of this drug no free water is generated by the

TABLE I

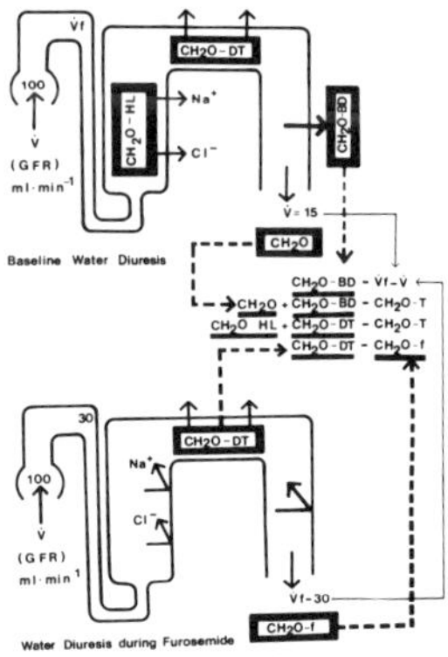

Fig. 2.Nephron before (top) and after (bottom) Furosemide with calculations of free water clearances.

$\dot{V}$ B	$\dot{V}$ A	GFR B	GFR A
22.4± 9.6	52.3± 10 4	91.9± 17.9	126.6± 55.8
$\dot{V}$/GFR B	**$\dot{V}$/GFR A**	**CH2O/GFR**	
23.9± 3.0	46.8± 7.3	17.9± 2.4	
CH2O-T		**CH2O-DT**	
40 3± 7.8		11.5± 2 4	
CH2O-HL		**CH2O-BD**	
28.7± 7.1		22 3± 7.4	

TABLE I. M and se of measurements before (B)and after (A) Furosemide.See text.

HL,nor lost by back diffusion:hence,CH2O-DT=CH2Of.If we substract the calculated CH2O-DT from the total,we obtain the free water clearance of HL: CH2O-T - CH2O-DT=CH2O-HL.Under the assumption that no solvent is being reabsorbed beyond the proximal tubule during Furosemide (9),and that the agent at the dose used does not affect proximal resorption(10)we can calculate fractional proximal resorption as $1-\frac{\dot{V}f}{GFR}$,absolute as GFR-$\dot{V}$f.The studies were performed on 6 normal controls during water diuresis,as already described(3).The only differences were the loading(0.75 mg·Kg^{-1})and maintenance dose (0.02 mg·Kg^{-1}) of Furosemide.Inulin was injected as a bolus injection of 40 mg·Kg^{-1} ,and then by a steady infusion delivered by a Braun pump at a rate of 10 mg·min^{-1} Inulin was measured by the Anthrone method (11).

RESULTS

Table 1 reports the means and standard errors obtained.They are close to those previously reported in normal subjects (3,6).

DISCUSSION

The present data confirm,by Inulin measurements of GFR,the validity and the reproducibility of our technique in measuring segmental nephron transport. The present method has the advantage of measuring a true rate of salt transport and attendant free water generation by the diluting system.In addition it splits this amount into the component of HL and DT.The former accounts for 70% of the total free water formed,and it is almost completely offset by the back diffusion of solvent across CD.Thus,water diuresis and antidiuresis do not basically differ on hydraulic conductivity of CD,since its fall is offset by the increased gradient,which is extremely small during antidiuresis(12).In the latter circumstance water is absorbed by DT,such that the diffusion of a limited amount across CD from a small volume is sufficient to concentrate the solutes.These concepts are compatible with the formulas of concentrating power expressed as ratios between the inflowing volumes at HL and at CD respectively.In conclusion,our method allows us to dissect transport and permeability(3)by each segment of the human nephron and gives results consistent with sophisticated physiologic measurements and with theoretical predictions of the countercurrent system.

REFERENCES

1. Berliner R.W. et al. Am.J.Med. 27,730-744 (1958).
2. Jamison R.L. et al. J.Clin.Invest. 50,2444-2452 (1971).
3. Bartoli E. et al. J.Clin.Pharmacol. 23,56-64 (1983).
4. Satta A. et al. Ital.J.Gastroenterol. 15,10-13 (1983).
5. Zoccali C. et al. Nephron 32,140-148 (1982).
6. Satta A. et al. Renal Physiol.(In press)
7. Satta A. et al. Panminerva Medica (In press).
8. Satta A. et al. Panminerva Medica (In press).
9. Burg M.B. et al. Am.J.Physiol. 224,659-668 (1973).
10. Knox F.G. et al. Am.J.Physiol. 217,192-198 (1969).
11. Führ J. et al. Klin.Wschr. 33,729-730 (1955).
12. Marsh D.L. Am.J.Physiol. 218,824-831 (1970).
13. Berliner R.W. et al. J.Clin.Invest. 38,1416-1427 (1957).
14. Ang G.P. et al. Computers in Biol.and Med. 7,87-111 (1977).

AKNOWLEDGEMENTS. This paper was supported by grants from the Consiglio Nazionale delle Ricerche (CNR) and the Ministero della Pubblica Istruzione (MPI), Rome,Italy.

24 HOUR URINARY ELECTROLYTE PROFILE FOLLOWING FRUSEMIDE, AMILORIDE AND A COMBINATION OF THESE DRUGS, FRUMIL™.

Hamdy R.C.,* Vinson M.,* Robbins A.D.,** Struthers L.P.L.,** Chapman S.F.,** Norris R.J.,** Shaw H.L.**

*St John's Hospital, London, U.K. **Berk Pharmaceuticals Ltd., Eastbourne, U.K.

SUMMARY

Urinary volume and electrolyte excretion were monitored in timed collections over 24 hours in 12 elderly patients with mild congestive heart failure who received single doses of frusemide, amiloride and frusemide/ amiloride (Frumil). The diuresis was similar with frusemide and the combination, but frusemide caused a greater disturbance to the pattern of urine and electrolyte excretion.

INTRODUCTION

The time course of changes in rates of urine and electrolyte excretion have been studied in healthy subjects. With frusemide 80mg, peak urine and potassium output occur in the 3 hours following administration, and urine volume after frusemide is less than in controls in the 6-24 hour period[1,2]. This suggests that a rapid intercompartmental flux of potassium, and reaccumulation of fluid, occur during frusemide therapy. Amiloride significantly reduces potassium excretion, and has an extended, mild, natriuretic effect[3]. This study examines the pattern of urine and electrolyte excretion in hospital in-patients who received single doses of frusemide, amiloride and a combination tablet containing frusemide and amiloride, to establish if these effects are also found under clinical conditions and whether the pattern of diuresis can be favourably modified in a combination agent.

PATIENTS AND METHODS

Twelve, elderly, hospital in-patients with mild congestive heart failure were included in a 3-way crossover study and received single, oral doses of frusemide 40mg, amiloride 5mg and a combination tablet containing frusemide 40mg and amiloride 5mg (Frumil). Each crossover leg consisted of a 24 hour control period of urine collection via an indwelling catheter, from 0-3, 3-6, 6-9, 9-12 and 12-24 hours, immediately followed by diuretic and a further 24 hour collection. The three study legs were separated by one week and treatments were randomly allocated according to a Latin Square design. No other diuretics were taken for 6 days preceding, or during, the study. Fluid intake and diet were in accordance with the normal discipline of the ward but a balance chart was not kept. Patients were excluded from the study if they required additional diuretic or were suffering from other serious disease. The volume and specific gravity of urine collected over each timed interval were measured, and aliquots were frozen for subsequent analysis of sodium, potassium, calcium and magnesium.

RESULTS

Eight female and 4 male patients completed the study, with a mean age and weight of 81 years and 56.5kg respectively. The urine volume and the urinary excretion rate for sodium and potassium during the various time-points are displayed in Tables 1-3. In addition, the cumulative excretion of calcium and magnesium are given in Table 4.

DISCUSSION

The cumulative urine volumes in the 24 hours following administration of frusemide and frusemide/amiloride were not significantly different. Both therapies produced a greater mean diuresis than amiloride alone ($p<0.01$). During the first 3 hours, both frusemide and frusemide/amiloride induced large increases in urine volume. However, from 12-24 hours the urine volume was less than on control days, and significantly less than after amiloride ($p<0.05$). Similar results have previously been described in healthy subjects[1,2].

Published 1984 by Elsevier Science Publishing Co., Inc.

Diuretics, Jules B. Puschett, Editor

Table 1

Timed Urine Volumes (ml)

COLLECTION PERIOD (hours)		FRUSEMIDE 40mg		FRUSEMIDE 40mg/ AMILORIDE 5mg		AMILORIDE 5mg	
		CONTROL	TEST	CONTROL	TEST	CONTROL	TEST
0-3	Mean	120.00	624.17	151.00	529.17	119.75	184.58
	S.D.	94.48	437.81	178.15	331.29	82.84	113.37
3-6	Mean	65.83	281.25	66.25	315.00	76.83	92.75
	S.D.	40.83	180.61	49.96	193.46	89.17	50.65
6-9	Mean	74.17	152.50	80.00	192.92	83.75	115.83
	S.D.	39.42	72.38	36.18	157.11	45.58	71.41
9-12	Mean	91.25	100.83	119.58	117.50	99.58	128.33
	S.D.	56.89	49.08	73.44	60.32	42.13	84.08
12-24	Mean	645.83	512.08	769.17	637.50	474.17	794.17
	S.D.	430.89	216.96	425.39	314.88	307.05	275.27
0-24	Mean	997.08	1670.83	1186.00	1792.08	854.08	1315.67
	S.D.	514.77	661.43	534.59	571.27	448.50	427.96

Table 2

Excretion rates of Sodium (mmol/hr)

COLLECTION PERIOD (hours)		FRUSEMIDE40mg		FRUSEMIDE 40mg/ AMILORIDE 5mg		AMILORIDE 5mg	
		CONTROL	TEST	CONTROL	TEST	CONTROL	TEST
0-3	Mean	3.33	18.71	3.87	14.48	3.72	5.75
	S.D.	2.69	18.42	3.95	9.22	3.27	4.55
3-6	Mean	1.58	7.38	1.99	8.05	2.10	3.56
	S.D.	1.17	5.34	2.11	4.60	2.66	2.38
6-9	Mean	1.71	2.80	1.65	6.20	1.68	3.39
	S.D.	1.21	1.74	1.54	6.01	1.32	1.91
9-12	Mean	1.70	2.11	3.07	3.56	1.82	3.11
	S.D.	1.49	2.28	2.67	2.22	1.37	1.67
12-24	Mean	3.24	1.90	3.91	4.15	2.21	3.73
	S.D.	2.44	1.32	2.56	3.05	2.41	1.77
0-24	Mean	2.66	4.82	3.28	6.11	2.27	3.84
	S.D.	1.65	3.05	1.77	2.71	1.24	1.72

Table 3

Excretion rates of Potassium (mmol/hr)

COLLECTION PERIOD (hours)		FRUSEMIDE 40mg		FRUSEMIDE 40mg/ AMILORIDE 5mg		AMILORIDE 5mg	
		CONTROL	TEST	CONTROL	TEST	CONTROL	TEST
0-3	Mean	1.28	2.97	1.17	2.14	0.95	1.08
	S.D.	1.00	1.98	1.09	1.18	0.60	0.47
3-6	Mean	0.86	1.67	0.82	1.01	0.96	0.49
	S.D.	0.54	0.86	0.58	0.60	1.16	0.40
6-9	Mean	1.30	1.36	1.30	1.09	1.25	0.46
	S.D.	0.78	0.88	0.91	0.93	0.77	0.23
9-12	Mean	1.25	1.23	1.68	0.88	1.58	0.46
	S.D.	0.83	0.64	1.04	0.59	0.83	0.24
12-24	Mean	1.08	0.84	1.09	1.01	0.95	0.65
	S.D.	0.46	0.37	0.55	0.94	0.50	0.66
0-24	Mean	1.13	1.33	1.16	1.15	1.07	0.63
	S.D.	0.35	0.57	0.51	0.71	0.49	0.40

TABLE 4 Cumulative Urinary Excretion

	COLLECTION PERIOD (hours)		FRUSEMIDE 40mg CONTROL	FRUSEMIDE 40mg TEST	FRUSEMIDE 40mg/ AMILORIDE 5mg CONTROL	FRUSEMIDE 40mg/ AMILORIDE 5mg TEST	AMILORIDE 5mg CONTROL	AMILORIDE 5mg TEST
CALCIUM (mg)	0-12	Mean	17.6	50.5	24.4	46.3	22.2	12.2
		S.D.	18.6	27.5	18.5	31.6	31.0	8.7
	12-24	Mean	20.0	12.1	24.4	17.5	13.8	12.6
		S.D.	13.8	7.7	20.5	11.3	12.7	8.6
	0-24	Mean	37.6	62.6	49.3	63.8	36.0	24.8
		S.D.	27.1	29.8	35.0	35.1	38.1	16.1
MAGNESIUM (mg)	0-12	Mean	6.7	13.9	10.3	17.2	7.9	5.1
		S.D.	7.4	6.1	10.7	10.3	10.4	3.4
	12-24	Mean	7.3	4.9	8.5	5.6	7.8	5.8
		S.D.	6.6	3.2	7.8	5.6	7.4	4.3
	0-24	Mean	14.0	18.8	18.8	22.9	15.7	10.8
		S.D.	12.0	8.2	18.2	13.9	15.7	5.7

Both frusemide and frusemide/amiloride were associated with a significantly greater mean sodium excretion rate than amiloride in the 0-3 and 3-6 hour collection periods ($p<0.05$) although there were no significant differences at other timepoints (Table 2). A difference between frusemide and Frumil was seen from the 6-9 hour period onwards, where mean sodium excretion rates were 2.8 and 6.2mmol/hour respectively. In the 12-24 hour period mean sodium excretion with frusemide was 16mmol less than control, indicating that in addition to water retention, definite sodium retention occurred with frusemide, as in healthy volunteers[1,2]. With Frumil, the mean sodium loss in this period was equivalent to control, while amiloride was still actively natriuretic.

The mean potassium excretion rates in the 0-12 hour period were significantly different for all three drugs, with frusemide producing a potassium loss ($p<0.01$), Frumil being not significantly different from control and amiloride conserving potassium ($p<0.01$) in comparison with Frumil (Table 3). Differences in potassium excretion between frusemide and the combination tablet were particularly evident in the first 6 hours of study, with frusemide resulting in a significant loss in comparison with Frumil during the 0-3 hour ($p<0.01$) and 3-6 hour ($p<0.05$) collection periods. With amiloride, potassium conservation was still evident 24 hours post dose, but in the 12-24 hour period there were no statistically significant differences in potassium excretion for any of the drugs.

Frusemide and Frumil both caused significantly greater magnesium losses in the 0-12 hour period ($p<0.01$), but amiloride conserved magnesium throughout the 24 hour period. Amiloride also tended to conserve calcium, whereas the other two drugs induced significantly ($p<0.01$) greater losses in both the 0-12 and 12-24 hour periods (Table 4).

In conclusion, there are two findings of particular interest. Frusemide used alone was associated with definite salt and water retention after its initial rapid diuresis, which could have clinical implications. This pattern was greatly attenuated with the combination of frusemide 40mg amiloride 5mg. Secondly, as expected, the potassium losses seen with frusemide are favourably modified in the combination agent. Further work is currently being undertaken to clarify and extend these results.

REFERENCES

1. A.J. Reyes and W.P. Leary, Curr. Ther. Res. 32, 406 (1982)
2. W.P. Leary and A J Reyes, S. Afr. Med. J. 61, 398 (1982)
3. W,P, Leary, A.J. Reyes and K. Van Der Byl, Curr. Ther. Res. 34, 205 (1983)

MUZOLIMINE VS FUROSEMIDE IN NEPHROTIC SYNDROME: CLINICAL EVIDENCE OF DIFFERENT CARRIERS FOR ENTERAL ABSORPTION

G. Bazzato, U. Coli, S. Landini, A. Fracasso, F. Righetto, F. Scanferla and P. Morachiello.
Nephrology Dept., Umberto I Hospital, Venice-Mestre, Italy

ABSTRACT

The Authors have compared during 4 weeks study the effects of furosemide (F) by oral route or IV and muzolimine (M)/os in 6 pts with nephrotic syndrome (NS) and normal renal function. A satisfactory diuretic response was observed with IV F (100 mg) and M/os (30-60 mg) respect the basal condition ($P < 0.001$). F/os (100 mg) was not effective like M in these pts ($P < 0.001$). This behaviour may be explained by the different pharmacological properties of M vs F, by gut alterations due to the oedema of moucosa or for loss of some "carriers" operating in intestinal absorption of these 2 high-ceiling diuretics.

INTRODUCTION

Protein loss in NS may cause depletion of important carriers for different substances. Furthermore administration of diuretics by oral route may result in reduced effectiveness, probably for incomplete absorption through the oedematous enteral wall. Thus in this condition high dose of powerful diuretics are needed to obtain clinical results like weight loss, satisfactory urine volume (UV) and natriuresis. We report a clinical experience by treating NS pts with different high-ceiling diuretics and comparing the effects by different route of administration.

PATIENTS AND METHODS

Six pts (5 M and 1 F), mean age 42 ys with NS and normal renal function (mean GFR 101 ml/min) were admitted to the following protocol: A)- during the 1st week of hospitalization the pts were keept under control of fluid and diet without diuretics. B)- the 2nd week the pts were given F IV at the dosage of 100 mg. C)- The 3rd week F was given orally (100 mg). D)- The 4th week M (30-60 mg) was administered by oral route. As additional therapy plasma and albumin were daily infused. The following parameters were monitored: MAP, UV, BW,Ht,plasma(Pt)and urine protein. Blood and daily urine samples also were collected for determination of: Na,K,Ca,PO_4,urea creatinine and uric acid. During the entire period of study protein diet content was 1.2 kg/day and a total daily fluid intake of 0.8-1 L was allowed.

RESULTS

During the 1st period (wash out) (fig. 1) the pts showed a further increase of their BW from Δ6.6$\pm$1.2 to 7.4$\pm$1.5 kg despite fluid restriction, with mean UV 580$\pm$180 ml/24h. The 2nd week was caracterized by decrease of fluid overload (Δ 2$\pm$1.2 Kg) with mean UV of 1803$\pm$327 ml/24h ($P < 0.001$). In the 3rd week we noted a gain in BW (Δ 4$\pm$1.2 Kg) with a decrease of mean UV (1408$\pm$272 ml/24h). The oral administration of M (4th week) brought the pts to their dry BW with a significant increase in UV: 2332$\pm$223 ml/24h ($P < 0.001$). Na excretion showed a similar trend (fig. 2) with a significant increase respect the ba

Diuretics, Jules B. Puschett, Editor

sal period when F was given IV from 40±16 to 187±72 mEq/24h ($P<0.001$). Natriuretic effect was more evident with M than F by oral route with a change from 130±30 to 234±60 mEq/24h ($P<0.001$). Urine K^+ excretion was higher during M administration than F but not significantly. F and M do not affect urinary excretion of urea, creatinine, uric acid, while Ca^{++}, P, Mg^{++} appeared higher in comparison with the basal period (fig. 3). The all blood parameters remained unchanged, except uric acid has increased from 7±1 to 9.5±1.6 mg/dl during M administration. MAP, Ht, Pt changed according to the variations induced in the extracellular and intravascular compartments and by the amount of plasma and albumin administrations.

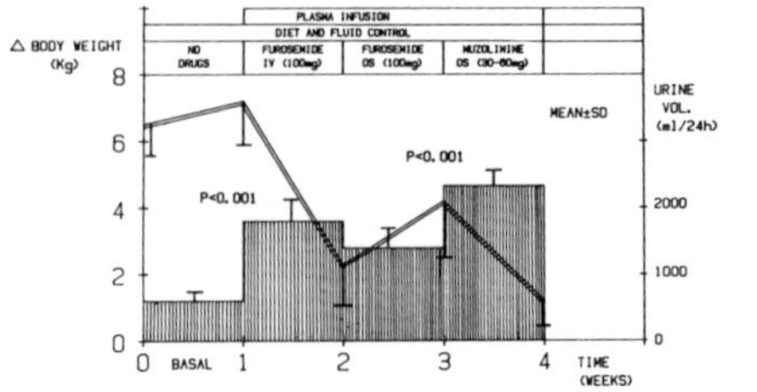

FIG. 1 Weight loss and UV during F and M administration in 6 pts with NS.

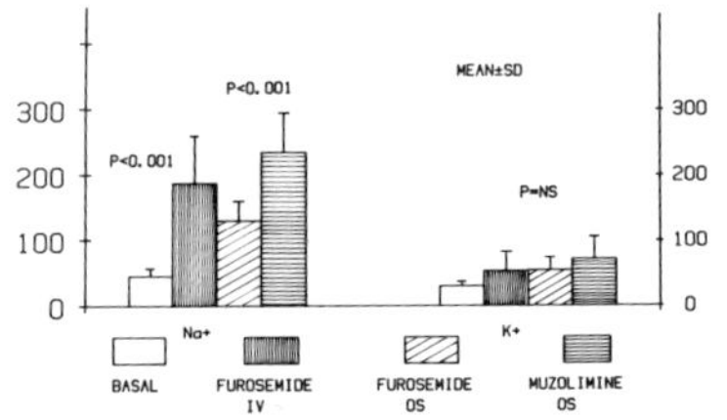

FIG. 2 Urine electrolytes excretion (mEq/24h) before and during diuretic therapy in 6 pts with NS.

DISCUSSION

The refractory to high dose diuretics by oral route is not infrequent and well known in the treatment of pts with NS (1). It seems that the oedema of the enteral mucosa may impair drug absorption. A beneficial effect of M respect F in this pathological condition, is reported by some AA (2,3,4). Our results show a satisfactory diuretic response after F IV and M/os administrations. Oral F, also at high dosage in our study, doesn't manifest the same diuretic effect of M on UV and Na excretion. M indeed manifests different pharmacological properties respect F (5) with complete and quick absorption, 100% of bioavailability longer half-life, less plasma protein binding (60%), minimal urine excretion, mostly after metabolic transformation, no phenomenon of accumulation and different site of actions in the Henle's loop. All these pharmacological aspects probably may account for the better response of M at lower dosage in NS pts than F by oral route. On the other hand similar diuretic effects of M and F, by IV administration, were evident in our pts, that suggests that some intestinal alterations of GI tract mucosa may decrease F absorption when orally given: gut oedema acts probably as a important barrier for F rather than M. Perhaps protein depletion as consequence of NS, may cause a impairment or loss of hypothetical intestinal "carriers" operating in F absorption, which seem different from the M ones. The main laboratoy findings didn't change during the whole study period, while only uric acid increased during M treatment. Regarding this matter several AA reported conflicting results (2,3,4); Hyperuricaemia may related to a tubular reabsorption or to a direct competitive effect of this drug on tubular transport.

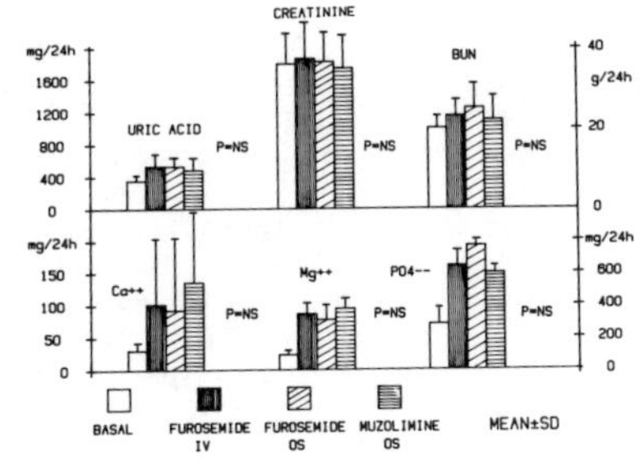

FIG. 3 Solutes excretion on basal condition and during drugs administration in 6 pts with NS.

CONCLUSIONS

Our study carried out in 6 pts NS with normal renal function may suggests some considerations: 1)- F IV administered is equal in diuretic effect to M at lower dosage. 2)- F by oral route is less powerful than M. 3)- This behaviour may be explained by different pharmacological characteristics of M compared to F. 4)- The presence of enteral oedema is probably an important barrier for F absorption but not for M. 5)- Protein loss during NS may deplete F intestinal, renal carrier-s which differs from those of M.

REFERENCES

1. R.P. Wedeen, M. Goldstein and M.F. Levitt, Mechanism of edema and use of diuretics. Pediatr. Clin. North Am. 18, 561 (1971).
2. R. Genova and A. Guerra, Muzolimine in children with renal oedema. A pilot study in: Recent advances in diuretic therapy. Excerpta Medica Proceedings of the Second International Edrul Symposium 269 (1983).
3. A. Dal Canton, D. Russo, R. Gallo, G. Conte and V.E. Andreucci, Effects of muzolimine in patients with renal failure. Clinical Nephrology 19, supplement 1, 54 (1983).
4. A. Röckel, Efficacy of muzolimine in treatment of patients with refractory oedema. Clinical Nephrology 19, supplement 1, 64 (1983).
5. W. Ritter, Pharmacokinetics of muzolimine. Clinical Nephrology 19, supplement 1, 26 (1983).

THE SHORT TERM EFFECT OF POTASSIUM SPARING DIURETICS COMBINED WITH LOOP AND THIAZIDE DIURETICS.

Hamdy R.C.,* Vinson M.,* Robbins A.D.,**
Struthers L.P.L.,** Chapman S.F.,** Norris R.J.,**
Shaw H.L.,**
* St.John's Hospital, London SW11 1SP, U.K.
** Berk Pharmaceuticals Ltd., Eastbourne, U.K.

The effects of administering Frumil TM (frusemide + amiloride, Frusene (frusemide + triamterene) Dyazide (hydrochlorothiazide + triameterene) and Moduretic (hydrochlorothiazide + amiloride) were assessed in 12 elderly patients with mild congestive cardiac failure and indwelling urinary catheters. Urine was collected at the following times: 0, 3, 6, 9, 12 & 24 hours one day before and after the administration of a single dose of each diuretic combination. Six day intervals separated each study period. The urine volume, S.G. as well as sodium, potassium, calcium and magnesium excretion were measured. The mean changes 24 hours post-dose, expressed as difference from control value, are shown in the accompanying table.

MEAN CHANGE (24 hours) FROM CONTROL VALUE

	Frumil	Dyazide	Moduretic	Frusene
Urine volume ml	+606	+450	+413	+401
Na excretion mmol	+68.0	+78.0	+81.6	+52.7
K excretion mmol	-0.5	+1.9	-7.6	-9.1
Ca excretion mg	+18.2	+9.3	+1.2	+7.4
Mg excretion mg	+4.0	+7.0	-1.2	+0.3

The changes in each parameter in each time period following the oral administration of the various diuretic agents are discussed.

Published 1984 by Elsevier Science Publishing Co., Inc.
Diuretics, Jules B. Puschett, Editor

SC-33643, A NEW DIURETIC WITH RENAL VASODILATING PROPERTIES

J.F. WEET,* H.A. WAGNER,* F.M. RADZIALOWSKI* and E.J. CAFRUNY**
*G.D. Searle & Co., Research and Development Division, Departments of Biology and Medicinal Chemistry, Skokie, Illinois 60077 (312)982-8090; **University of Medicine and Dentistry of New Jersey, Newark, New Jersey 07103 USA

ABSTRACT

SC-33643 was studied with respect to its effects on urine flow and electrolyte excretion and on renal function and hemodynamics. Rats were saline loaded and treated i.g. with either SC-33643 or hydrochlorothiazide (HCTZ). No significant differences in diuretic or natriuretic potency were observed over 5 hours. SC-33643 was given i.v. at either 0.3, 1.0 or 3.0 mg/kg to anesthetized dogs to study acute changes in renal function. Urine flow and sodium excretion showed dose related increases of 2.3 to 3.7 fold. Renal blood flow and glomerular filtration rate demonstrated dose related increases of 20 to 83%. SC-33643 is a potent diuretic in the rat and dog and, in addition, possesses marked renal vasodilating activity in the dog. Both the diuretic and renal vasodilating activity last for at least two hours in the dog.

INTRODUCTION

SC-33643 (Fig. 1) is a new diuretic with renal vasodilating properties. It is expected to have utility as an antihypertensive either alone or in combination with other antihypertensive drugs where its properties would offset the fluid retention effects of those drugs and protect the kidney from progressive renal ischemia secondary to the hypertensive disease process [1].

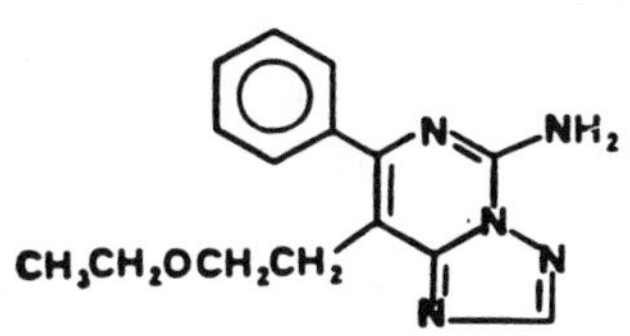

Fig. 1 SC-33643. 8-2(ethoxyethyl)-7-[1,2,4]triazolo[1,5-c]pyrimidine-5-amine

MATERIALS AND METHODS

Charles River rats were volume expanded with 25 ml/kg saline by gavage containing either HCTZ or SC-33643 each at doses of 0.2, 0.6 and 1.8 mg/kg or saline alone [2]. Urinary Na+ and K+ excretion was calculated as mEq/kg/5 hr. Volume excretion was expressed as a percentage of the saline load and relative diuretic potency was calculated.

Anesthetized dogs were prepared for standard renal clearance study [3]. After three 20 minute pretreatment baseline periods, groups of 5 dogs each received an intravenous infusion over 9 minutes of 18 ml 10% ethanol/saline containing either 0.3, 1.0, or 3.0 mg/kg SC-33643. A placebo group received vehicle alone. A 4 ml/min isotonic saline infusion contained inulin and PAH. Glomerular filtration rate (GFR) and renal plasma flow (RPF) were estimated along with volume and Na excretion rates in five 20 minute post-infusion clearance periods. Renal function parameters were monitored for five 20 minute post-infusion clearance periods.

Diuretics, Jules B. Puschett, Editor

RESULTS

The urinary response of the rat to SC-33643 is shown in Table I.

TABLE I. Diuretic Effects of SC-33643 in the Rat

Treatment	Dose mg/kg	N	V % Oral Load	Na_{ex} mEq/kg/5hr	K_{ex} mEq/kg/5hr
Control		4	80.8(4.5)	2.91(0.06)	0.61(0.06)
HCTZ	0.2	4	105.8(3.4)*	3.63(0.19)*	0.92(0.11)
	0.6	4	105.9(3.9)*	4.33(0.08)*	0.78(0.05)
	1.8	4	129.0(4.5)*	5.30(0.07)*	0.91(0.15)
SC-33643	0.2	4	111.3(8.0)*	4.10(0.22)*	0.87(0.10)
	0.6	4	119.0(8.7)*	4.70(0.35)*	0.98(0.10)
	1.8	4	127.5(4.9)*	5.20(0.27)*	1.03(0.10)

$p < .05$ by ANOVA with two sample t tests of treatment-control contrasts

SC-33643 was 1.9 times as potent as HCTZ as a diuretic and 1.5 times as potent as a natriuretic. However these estimates were not significantly greater than unity (95% confidence limits were 0.6-14.2 and 0.8-3.0 respectively.) The effects of SC-33643 and HCTZ on potassium excretion were not statistically significant relative to control animals.

In Table II, the peak diuretic response in dog after 0.3, 1.0 and 3.0 mg/kg SC-33643 occurred at 30 minutes post-infusion and was respectively 2.3, 3.3, and 3.7 times the urine flow observed at pretreatment.

TABLE II. Urine Flow (ml/min) in the Anesthetized Dog with i.v. SC-33643

Treatment Period (min)	N	Placebo	SC-33643 0.3 mg/kg	SC-33643 1.0 mg/kg	SC-33643 3.0 mg/kg
10	5	4.5(0.3)	4.5(0.4)	5.0(0.4)	5.1(0.9)
30	5	4.8(0.3)	4.6(0.3)	5.3(0.5)	5.3(0.8)
50	5	4.9(0.3)	4.7(0.3)	5.4(0.5)	5.4(0.8)
70	5	5.8(0.5)	12.8(1.1)*	18.1(0.9)*	20.5(1.4)*
90	5	6.2(0.7)	15.1(1.3)*	22.1(1.4)*	24.8(1.3)*
110	5	5.8(0.6)	12.7(0.9)*	19.2(1.6)*	21.7(1.8)*
130	5	5.6(0.6)	10.6(0.4)*	15.8(2.1)*	19.2(1.6)*
150	5	5.2(0.4)	9.5(0.5)*	14.1(2.4)*	18.1(1.5)*
170	5	5.1(0.4)	8.6(0.5)*	12.8(2.3)*	17.0(1.6)*

* $p < .05$ by analysis of covariance of the treatment vs. placebo difference using the mean pretreatment baseline as the covariate. (ANOCOVA)

In Table III peak UNa was 2.4, 2.7 and 2.8 times pretreatment.

TABLE III. Na+ Excretion (mEq/min) in the Dog with i.v. SC-33643

Treatment Period (min)	N	Placebo	SC-33643 0.3 mg/kg	SC-33643 1.0 mg/kg	SC-33643 3.0mg/kg
10	5	0.45(0.08)	0.40(0.07)	0.44(0.03)	0.52(0.12)
30	5	0.48(0.07)	0.43(0.06)	0.51(0.06)	0.52(0.11)
50	5	0.54(0.05)	0.48(0.01)	0.52(0.07)	0.56(0.10)
70	4	0.63(0.07)	1.30(0.05)*	1.53(1.12)*	1.68(0.18)*
90	5	0.74(0.11)	1.49(0.09)*	1.80(0.19)*	2.00(0.22)*
110	5	0.68(0.11)	1.28(0.08)*	1.34(0.14)*	1.73(0.15)*
130	5	0.64(0.10)	1.09(0.06)*	1.10(0.15)*	1.51(0.17)*
150	5	0.57(0.07)	0.97(0.05)*	1.01(0.10)*	1.39(0.19)*
170	5	0.55(0.07)	0.84(0.07)	0.88(0.15)	1.39(0.20)*

* $p < .05$ by ANOCOVA

The effect of SC-33643 on renal blood flow is shown in Table IV. The mean increases relative to pretreatment were 41, 61 and 83% for the 0.3, 1.0 and 3.0 mg/kg doses respectively. Over the 2 hour post infusion period, renal blood flow of placebo treated animals fell by more than 35%. Therefore, relative to placebo controls, the renal blood flow for the 0.3 and 3.0 mg/kg dose groups were significantly elevated 2 hours after the infusion started.

TABLE IV. Renal Blood Flow (ml/min) in the Dog with i.v. SC-33643

Treatment Period (min)	N	Placebo	SC-33643 0.3 mg/kg	SC-33643 1.0 mg/kg	SC-33643 3.0 mg/kg
10	5	450(76)	330(48)	343(64)	243(29)
30	5	422(61)	327(54)	363(58)	245(20)
50	5	449(70)	363(92)	343(50)	241(32)
70	5	493(64)	449(61)	500(61)*	434(46)*
90	5	490(68)	478(91)	563(54)*	445(27)
110	5	441(59)	435(60)	478(49)	393(22)
130	5	423(69)	424(56)*	433(45)	360(25)*
150	5	392(69)	424(63)*	400(34)	355(41)*
170	5	358(52)	432(83)	384(12)	374(59)

* p<.05 by ANOCOVA

As shown in Table V, GFR increased 20, 52 and 60% for the 0.3, 1.0 and 3.0 mg/kg doses respectively. Although GFR tended to decrease relative to the peak response, it remained significantly higher than in placebo treated animals.

TABLE V. Glomerular Filtration Rate (ml/min) in the Dog with iv SC-33643

Treatment Period (min)	N	Placebo	SC-33643 0.3 mg/kg	SC-33643 1.0 mg/kg	SC-33643 3.0 mg/kg
10	5	78.4(10.5)	74.8(5.0)	71.0(9.0)	60.4(6.3)
30	5	74.4(8.3)	71.3(7.0)	72.5(9.1)	57.7(4.5)
50	5	74.6(9.5)	68.0(6.6)	66.1(7.8)*	54.2(6.9)*
70	5	80.0(9.1)	85.3(3.8)	91.1(8.3)*	91.6(5.4)*
90	5	79.1(11.4)	82.1(8.7)	106.4(9.6)*	84.7(7.3)*
110	5	71.2(8.9)	79.9(4.5)	98.1(4.2)*	76.8(8.2)*
130	5	69.6(10.4)	81.1(4.9)*	90.6(7.9)*	73.4(8.4)*
150	5	65.4(8.6)	82.2(3.9)*	88.7(3.4)*	72.8(11.4)*
170	5	64.9(7.2)	81.2(3.6)	89.5(3.5)	79.0(14.1)

* p<.05 by ANOCOVA

SUMMARY

1) SC-33643 is a potent diuretic and saliuretic in the rat and in the dog.
2) Renal blood flow, glomerular filtration rate, and urinary excretion rates are enhanced for at least two hours following intravenous administration of SC-33643 relative to placebo in the dog.

REFERENCES

1. Riddiough, M.A. Am. J. Hosp. Pharm. 34, 465-479 (1979).
2. Lipschitz, W.L., Z. Hadidian and A. Kerpesar, J. Pharmacol. Exp. Ther. 79, 97-110 (1943).
3. Smith, H.W., The Structure and Function in Health and Disease, (New York, Oxford University Press 1951) pp 419-421.

SYNTHESIS AND PHARMACOLOGICAL EVALUATION OF ABBOTT(A)-53385: A NEW HIGH CEILING SALIDIURETIC AND URICOSURIC AGENT

P.R. BUNNELL, J.J. PLATTNER, A.K.L. FUNG, R.J. PARIZA AND P.W. DODGE.
Division of Pharmacology and Medicinal Chemistry, Abbott Laboratories, North Chicago, IL 60064

There are an ever increasing number of diuretics described in the literature which provide the physician with a wide scope of therapeutic regimens. The thiazides have a long history of safe, effective control of a major segment of the hypertensive population. In the last twenty years, the (aryloxy)acetic acids, starting with ethacrynic acid **1a** [1] and the sulphamoylbenzoic acids, represented by furosemide [2], provided the potency of mercurial diuretics while significantly reducing their toxicity and side effects. However, the search continues for effective diuretics that are devoid of untoward side effects such as hypokalemia, hyperglycemia and hyperuricemia. The advent of the "potassium sparing" agents exemplified by amiloride and triamterene provided the possibility of combination therapy which can reduce the problems of potassium loss [3]. The development of ticrynafen **1b** [4] presented the advantage of an antihypertensive diuretic with potent uricosuric activity. Before its withdrawal for safety reasons [5], ticrynafen had been enthusiastically received in the market indicating the keen interest in compounds that may reduce the potential risk associated with hyperuricemia as induced by diuretic therapy.

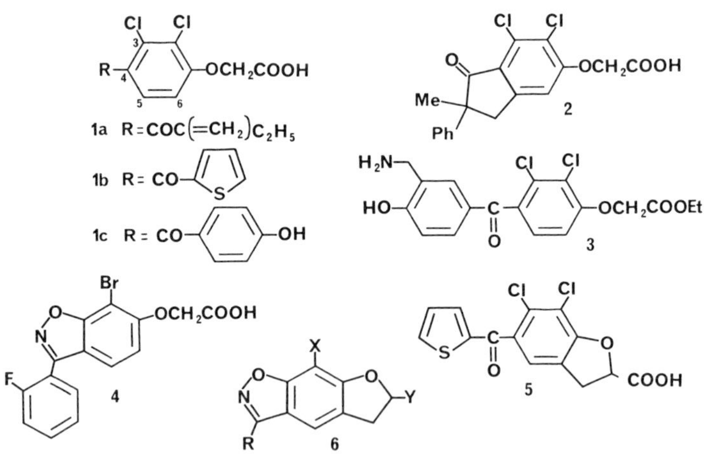

The continued effort toward the development of indacrinone **2**, with several distinctive aspects to its profile, represents another series derived from the (aryloxy)alkanoic acid family. Indacrinone has been shown to be a high ceiling salidiuretic with uricosuric and antihypertensive activity that has been intensively investigated in animals [6] and man [7].

Diuretics, Jules B. Puschett, Editor

In our own laboratories, work on the intriguing variety of pharmacologic profiles associated with modification of the (aryloxy)-acetic acid pharmacophore has produced several series of compounds since we initiated diuretic research in the mid-seventies. Part of this work has been reviewed in another segment of this publication.

The clinical development of two of these series in our own laboratories has produced both a low ceiling uricosuric diuretic, A-46228 **1c** [8], and a high ceiling salidiuretic of considerable potency, A-49816 **3** [9]. The broad range of renotrophic properties within the class of (aryloxy)acetic acids has been expanded by yet another functional class with the preparation of new 5,6-dihydrofuro[3,2-f]-1,2-benzisoxazoles **6** [10], which exhibit potent salidiuretic activity and moderate uricosuria. Herein we report the synthesis, optical resolution and the preclinical pharmacology of a new high ceiling, salidiuretic and uricosuric compound, 8-chloro-3-(2-fluorophenyl)-5,6-dihydrofuro[3,2-f]-1,2-benzisoxazole-6-carboxylic acid, A-53385, **12**.

FIGURE 1: Synthesis of A-53385.

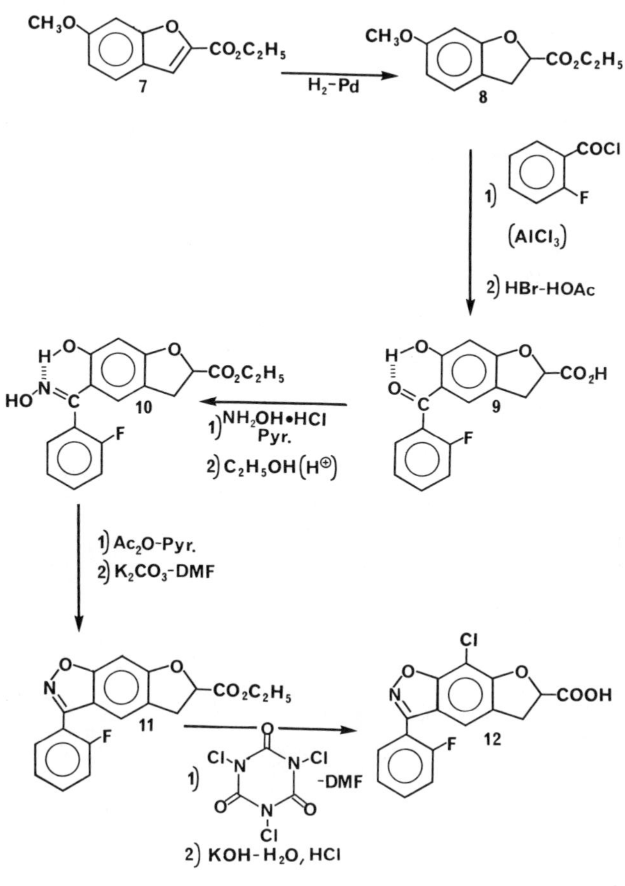

CHEMISTRY

Without exception, we observed that all phenoxyacetic acid diuretics with a high ceiling diuretic and uricosuric profile possess structures which are formally derived by ring annelation procedures. For example, annelation to position 5 of formula **1a** affords the (indanyloxy)acetic acids, as exemplified by indacrinone **2**, while annelation to position 3 leads to the [1,2-benzisoxazole-6-yl)oxy]acetic acids, of which HP-522 **4** [11] is the prototype. The indeno[5,4-b]furan-2-carboxylic acids [12] are derived by annelation at both position 5 and position 6 and represent yet another class of high ceiling diuretics which also display uricosuria. Interestingly, annelation to position 6, as in ticrynafen analog **5** [13], does not alter the uricosuric component of activity but substantially increases the saliuretic potency and once again results in a high ceiling uricosuric profile. We have extended this annelation concept to the preparation of new 5,6-dihydrofuro[3,2-f]-1,2-benzisoxazoles **6** which are tricyclic structures derived formally by simultaneous annelations at positions 3 and 6 of formula **1a**.

The synthetic route used to prepare A-53385 is outlined in FIGURE 1. Catalytic hydrogenation of benzofuran **7** [10] produced high yields of the dihydrobenzofuran **8**, with some contamination of fully saturated material. Use of excess $AlCl_3$ at room temperature during the Friedel-Crafts acylation step cleaves the methyl ether, and treatment of the crude product with HBr in acetic acid gives **9** in 93% overall yield. The oximation reaction requires prolonged heating with excess hydroxylamine hydrochloride, but after esterification of the crude oxime, a 90% yield of **10** is obtained. In the cyclization leading to isoxazole **11**, the presence of pyridine increases the reaction rate, and reduces formation of an oxazole, isomeric with **11**, which apparently occurs from a Beckmann rearrangement with intramolecular capture by the phenol [14]. Treatment of the crude oxime acetate with K_2CO_3 in DMF at 60° gives the isoxazole **11** cleanly, in high yield. The remarkable step in this synthesis is the facile chlorination of **11** with trichloroisocyanuric acid, utilizing all three chlorines from the reagent, leading to pure **12** in nearly quantitative yield.

Optical resolution of **12** was carried out by the sequence outlined below. D(−)-alpha-phenylglycinol was converted to oxazolidone **13** by treatment with dimethylcarbonate/K_2CO_3 in refluxing toluene. The lithio salt of **13**, generated with n-BuLi at −78°C was allowed to react with the acid chloride of **12**, formed by a reaction of **12** with thionyl chloride. The diastereomers of **14** were readily separated by extraction and chromatography, and hydrolyzed to enantiomerically pure **12**. The absolute configuration of (−)**12** as determined from x-ray analysis of the corresponding imide derivative **14** is 2R.

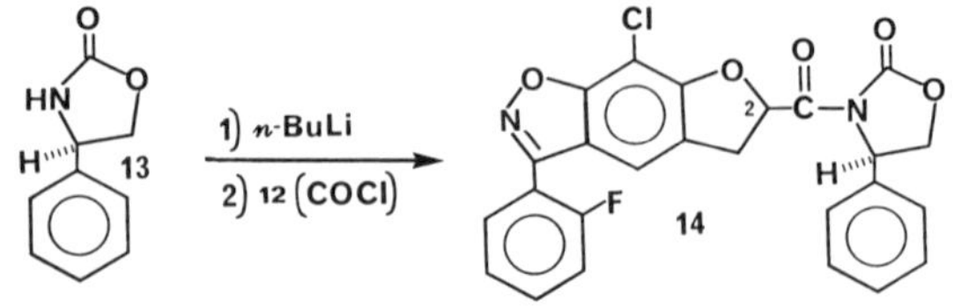

PRECLINICAL PHARMACOLOGY OF A-53385

A-53385 was tested orally (p.o.) in mice, rats, beagle dogs and Cebus monkeys to evaluate its salidiuretic and uricosuric activities. Complete methodologies for these assays are described elsewhere [10]. In order to compare the relative potency of A-53385 to its analogs and to a series of reference compounds with varied saliuretic profiles, we have established the use of EDx values as presented in FIGURES 2-4. An EDx is defined as the p.o. dose (mg/kg) required to produce an excretion of x milliequivalents (mEq) of Na^+ per kilogram of body weight during the relevant observation period. The specific EDx values (e.g., ED6 for mouse, ED2 for rats, and ED5 for dogs) were selected based on 2 criteria: (1) the values represent doses that cause a significant natriuretic effect when compared statistically to control levels of excretion; and, (2) the values represent levels of excretion that are the approximate midpoints of the linear regression of the Na^+ response versus the log of the doses for a family of curves representing the classes and/or relative activities of the compounds in question.

In saline-loaded male mice, A-53385 was equipotent to furosemide and indacrinone (ED6 = 4.2, 5.0 and 4.4 mg/kg, p.o., respectively) and exhibited similar profiles of electrolyte excretion (FIGURE 2). A-53385 was also equipotent to hydrochlorothiazide (ED6 = 4.2 versus 8.6 mg/kg, p.o.), although the thiazide displayed a different salidiuretic profile, typical of a low ceiling diuretic. In addition, A-53385 was significantly more potent than ticrynafen and ethacrynic acid in this assay. Only ticrynafen at the dose of 250 mg/kg, p.o., was significantly uricosuric in this model.

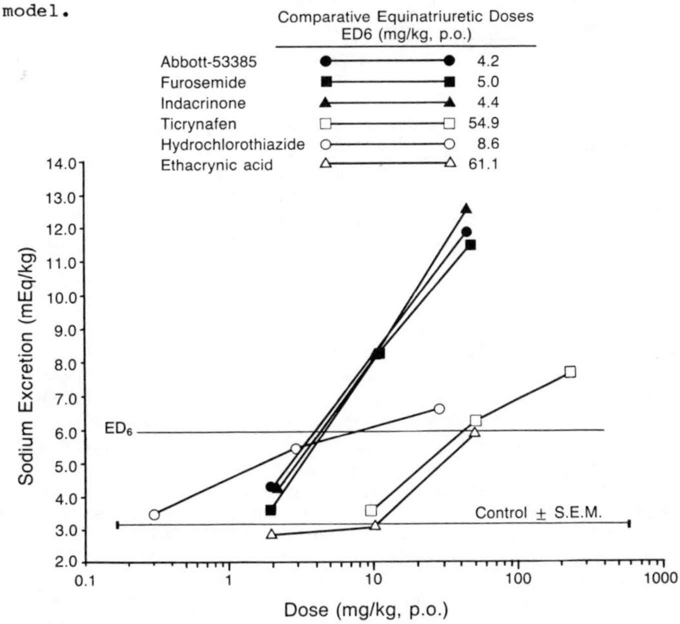

FIGURE 2: Sodium excretion during 4 hour period after p.o. administration of A-53385 and reference diuretics to male saline-loaded mice. Each point is the mean of 4 cages of 5 mice/cage. The area marked represents the excretion level used to calculate the ED6 values.

In our rat model, compounds of this series, including A-53385, were not particularly active in comparison to reference diuretics (FIGURE 3). Furosemide and indacrinone were approximately 4 and 8 times more potent, respectively than A-53385. However, this relatively weak activity in rats has been reported for other similar compounds [11]. No measurement of uric acid excretion was made in this model.

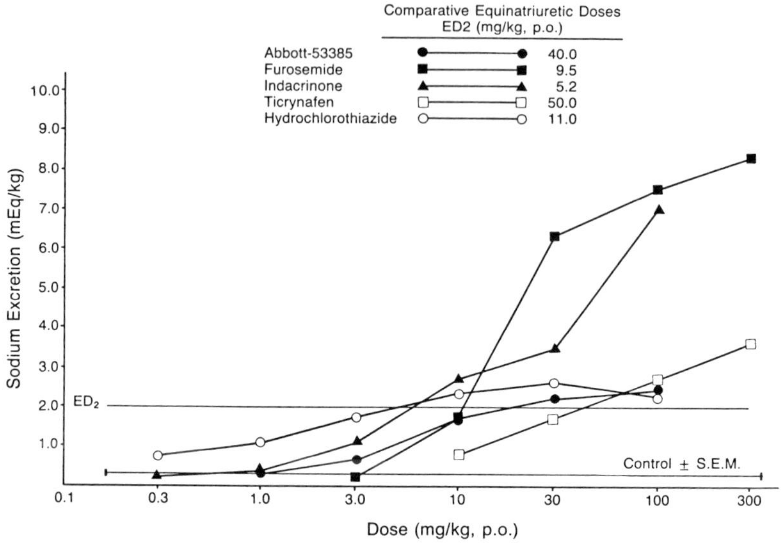

FIGURE 3: Sodium excretion during 4 hours after p.o. administration of A-53385 and reference diuretics to female rats. Rats were fed glucose and water overnight, DOCA pretreatment, 5 mg, s.c., 2 hours prior to dosing. Loaded with isotonic NaCl-KCl (40:60%) to 3% body weight. Each point is the mean of 4 rats dose. The area marked represents the excretion level used to calculate the ED2 values.

In conscious non-loaded female dogs, A-53385 produced a marked salidiuresis that was dose dependent and delayed in onset. The natriuretic potency of A-53385 was approximately 6 times greater than furosemide and significantly more potent than indacrinone, ethacrynic acid, ticrynafen or hydrochlorothiazide (FIGURE 4). Detailed comparison to furosemide showed that there were no significant differences in the net excretion of potassium, chloride, calcium, magnesium, phosphate, urea nitrogen or glucose through 6 hours of observation when compared at equinatriuretic doses. Urine volume was also increased in dose related manner typical of a high ceiling diuretic profile. Urate excretion was significantly increased for A-53385 in this model, but not for furosemide, ticrynafen or indacrinone (TABLE 1). Fractional excretion of urate, based on endogeneous creatinine clearance, demonstrated significantly increase excretion for A-53385 in a dose related fashion, but there was no significant increase due to furosemide. Fractional excretion data also show concomitant increases in both the salidiuretic and the uricosuric activities at lower doses of A-53385 in these conscious female dogs. This profile of A-53385, as a potent "loop type" diuretic and its moderate uricosuric activity indicates two sites of action. Further studies are planned to elucidate these activities and define their relative dose response ratios.

TABLE 1: Comparison of the Natriuretic and Uricosuric Activities of A-53385 and its Enantiomers to Reference Compounds in Conscious Dogs and Cebus Monkeys.

Conscious Female Dogs

3 mg/kg, p.o.

Compound	N[b]	Na^+ Excreted[a] mEq/kg, 0-6 hrs.	Urate Excreted[a] mg/kg, 0-6 hrs.
Vehicle Control	6	0.24 ± 0.07	0.61 ± 0.07
A-53385	6	8.18 ± 0.62[d]	0.82 ± 0.09[d]
Furosemide	6	5.23 ± 0.42[d]	0.70 ± 0.06
Indacrinone	4	1.44 ± 0.32[e]	0.71 ± 0.08
Ticrynafen[c]	6	1.54 ± 0.10[e]	0.80 ± 0.15
(+) Enantiomer	2	7.60 ± C.40[e]	1.32 ± 0.14[e]
(-) Enantiomer	2	0.62 ± 0.09[e]	1.25 ± 0.32[e]

Conscious Cebus Monkeys
Water Loaded
20 mg/kg, p.o.

Compound	N[b]	Na^+ Excreted[a] mEq/kg, 0-6 hrs.	Urate Excreted[a] mg/kg, 0-6 hrs.
Vehicle Control	4	0.75 ± 0.13	3.40 ± 0.54
A-53385	4	1.51 ± 0.23[d]	7.08 ± 1.14[d]
Furosemide	4	1.41 ± 0.38[d]	4.03 ± 1.35
Indacrinone	4	1.24 ± 0.33	9.53 ± 2.31[d]
Ticrynafen	4	1.37 ± 0.26[d]	11.84 ± 3.88[d]
(+) Enantiomer	6	2.95 ± 0.52[e]	8.34 ± 1.75[e]
(-) Enantiomer	6	0.77 ± 0.19	8.32 ± 2.85[e]

[a] Mean values ± S.E.M.
[b] Number of animals.
[c] Ticrynafen dose was 10 mg/kg, p.o. in dogs.
[d] P <0.05, based on analysis of variance and Duncan's Multiple Range Test.
[e] P <0.05, unpaired t-test.

Comparative Equinatriuretic Doses

	ED_2 (mg/kg, p.o.)	ED_5 (mg/kg, p.o.)
☐ Abbott-53385	0.07	0.6
☐ Furosemide	0.70	3.5
☐ Indacrinone	4.82	(>100)
☐ Ticrynafen	28.0	(>300)
☐ Hydrochlorothiazide	2.9	N/A
☐ Ethacrynic acid	1.2	10.5

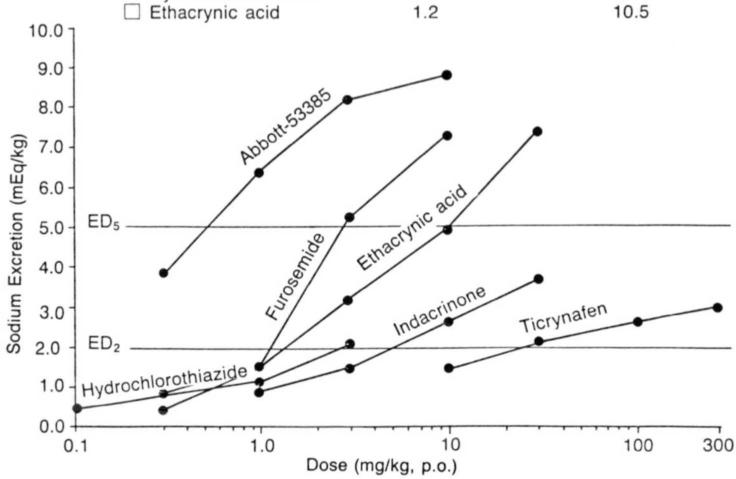

FIGURE 4: Sodium excretion during 6 hour period after p.o. administration of A-53385 and reference diuretics to conscious female dogs. Each point is the mean of at least 4 dogs/dose. The areas marked represent the excretion levels used to calculate the ED values.

Tests in water-loaded conscious Cebus monkeys produced significant uricosuric activity which was equal to indacrinone but less than ticrynafen with single p.o. doses. Furosemide did not increase urate excretion in this assay (TABLE 1).

Intraduodenal administration of equivalent natriuretic doses of A-53385 and furosemide produced similar hemodynamic effects which were related to their potent diuretic activities. Both compounds lowered central venous pressure, maximum left ventricular dP/dt and cardiac output. Pulmonary and systemic vascular resistances were increased by both compounds. Preliminary studies showed no significant central nervous system activity in male mice tested to 30 mg/kg, p.o. The p.o. LD50 in male mice was determined to the 617 mg/kg, giving A-53385 a therapeutic index of 147 [LD50/ED6, p.o., mice]. A-53385 was negative in the Ames test for mutagenicity.

The resolved (+) and (-) enantiomers of A-53385 were tested in mice, dogs and monkeys in comparison to the racemate, A-53385. Diuretic activity in male mice, as shown in FIGURE 5, indicated that the (+)-enantiomer possesses all the diuretic activity and is approximately twice as potent as the racemate. This enantiomeric separation of diuretic activity was also confirmed in the dog and monkey assays (TABLE 1). In both the dog assay and in conscious Cebus monkeys, both enantiomers exhibited equivalent uricosuric activity as shown in TABLE 1.

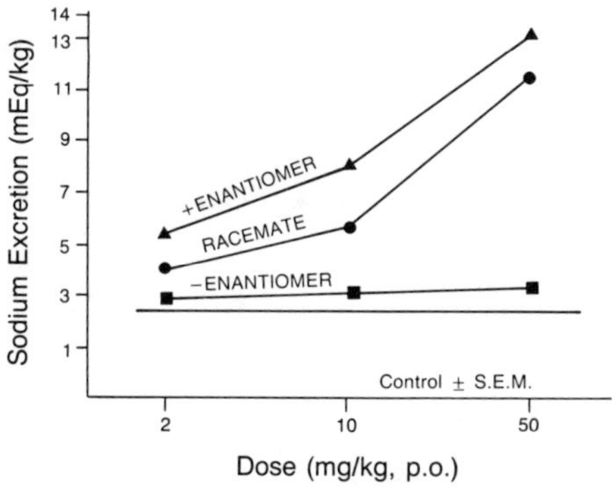

FIGURE 5: Sodium excretion during 4 hour period after p.o. administration of racemic A-53385 and resolved enantiomers to male saline-loaded mice. Each point is the mean of 4 cages of 5 mice/cage.

SUMMARY

A-53385 has been shown to be a potent salidiuretic uricosuric agent in four species. A-53385 has demonstrated minimal toxicity and is being scheduled for testing in man. The profile of a high ceiling salidiuretic with uricosuric activity will provide a unique therapeutic regimen when available.

REFERENCES

1. K.H. Beyer, Jr., J.E. Baer, J.K. Michaelson, and N.F. Russo, J. Pharmacol. Exp. Ther., 147, 1(1965).
2. R. Muschaweck and P. Hajdu, Arzneim-Forsch., 14, 44(1964).
3. Mullticenter Diuretic Cooperative Study Group, Arch. Intern. Med., 141, 482(1981).
4. E.D. Frohlich, New Engl. J. Med., 301, 25(1979).
5. F.D.A. Drug Bulletin, January, 1980.
6. A.G. Zacchei, T.I. Wishousky, B.H. Arison, and G.M. Fanelli, Jr., Drug Metab. Dispos., 4, 479(1976).
7. Z.E. Dziewanowska, K.F. Tempero, F. Perret, G. Hitzenberger, and G.H. Besselaar, Clin. Res., 24, 253A(1976).
8. P.H. Jones, D.S. Bariana, A.K.L. Fung, Y.C. Martin, J. Kyncl, and A. Lall, U.S. Patent 4,058,559 (1979).
9. C.M. Lee, J.J. Plattner, C.W. Ours, B.W. Horrom, J.R. Smital, Y.C. Martin, A.G. Pernet, P.R. Bunnell, S.E. ElMasry, and P.W. Dodge, J. Med. Chem., In Press.
10. J.J.Plattner, A.K.L. Fung, J.A. Parks, R.J. Pariza, S.R. Crowley, A.G. Pernet, P.R. Bunnell, and P.W. Dodge, J. Med. Chem., In Press.
11. G.M. Shutske, L.L. Setescak, R.C. Allen, L. Davis, R.C. Effland, K. Ranbom, J.M. Kitzen, J.C. Wilker, W.J. Novick, Jr., J. Med. Chem., 25, 36(1982).
12. O.W. Woltersdorf, Jr., S.J. deSolms, and E.J. Cragoe, J. Med. Chem., 24, 874 (1981).
13. G.M. Fanelli, Jr., L.S. Watson, D.L. Bohn, and H.F. Russo, Pharmacol. Exp. Ther., 212, 190(1980).
14. G. Stokker, J. Org. Chem., 48, 2613(1983).

VASO-ACTIVE INTESTINAL PEPTIDE (VIP): AN ENDOGENOUS DIURETIC AND ANTIDIURETIC SUBSTANCE.

G.E. PLANTE,* R. HEBERT,* A. FOURNIER,** N. FRANCO,* and S. ST-PIERRE,**
*Departments of Nephrology, and **Physiology-Pharmacology, University of Sherbrooke, Sherbrooke, Canada, J1H 5N4.

INTRODUCTION

The net transport of sodium and water across the tubular epithelium results from active baso-lateral pumping of sodium and/or chloride, and from passive (influx/outflux) movements of fluid and solutes across the tubular barrier (1). Passive movements are determined by both the peritubular physical forces (2) and the transepithelial permeability (3) predominantly operative along the proximal nephron. Most diuretics increase natriuresis by inhibition of active sodium and/or chloride transport in specific segments of the nephron. A limited number of substances are known to influence natriuresis through changes in the passive components of net fluid and solutes transport (4). The vaso-active intestinal peptide (VIP) influences the trans-epithelial permeability (5). The present study was designed to examine the effects of VIP on renal sodium excretion and hemodynamics.

METHODS

Anesthetized mongrel dogs were studied during acute extra-cellular expansion: in this model proximal tubular permeability is increased and maximal expression of peritubular physical forces on passive movements of fluid and solutes obtains (2, 3). In the first group of 5 dogs, successive bolus of VIP (100, 150 and 200 pM) were administered through the femoral vein. In the second group of 5 dogs, a single bolus of VIP (100 pM) was given in the left renal artery (right kidney as control). In the third group of 4 dogs, a single bolus of VIP (150 pM) was administered through the femoral vein during saralasine infusion. Three control periods (20 min. each) were obtained before each bolus of VIP (given in 2 min.). Four or 5 consecutive experimental periods of similar duration were obtained after each bolus of VIP. Synthetic VIP dissolved in isotonic saline was used in these experiments (purity 99.9%). Absolute and fractional excretion of sodium, phosphate and urea were measured, as well as inulin and para-amino-hippurate (PAH) clearances according to methods previously described (6, 7). Changes in exogenous creatinine/inulin clearance ratio were taken as index of changes in transepithelial permeability (8).

RESULTS

As shown in Fig. 1, the administration of VIP resulted in a biphasic effect on fractional excretion of sodium, phosphate and urea (FE_{Na}, PO^4, Urea, respectively): FE_{Na} rose from 16 to 24, 17 to 19, and 15 to 18% immediately after each bolus in Group 1. A rise of similar magnitude for and FE_{urea} was observed. Thereafter, FE decreased with time, to reach approximately initial control values for sodium and phosphate, but below control values for urea. When the peptide was administered in the left renal artery, a similar decrease of absolute and fractional sodium excretion obtained as shown in Table I: natriuresis decreased from 493 to 375 while inulin clearance remained almost unchanged. Angiotensin II receptor blockade with saralasine abolished the natriuretic and anti-natriuretic effect of VIP as shown also in Table I. This manoeuvre was associated with constant inulin clearance values. There was a close relationship between the changes in absolute sodium and urea excretion measured in Group I, as illustrated in Fig. 2. The increment over, as well as the decrease below control values were

Published 1984 by Elsevier Science Publishing Co., Inc.
Diuretics, Jules B. Puschett, Editor

both perfectly correlated. A similar relationship obtained between sodium and phosphate excretion (data not shown). In contrast, as depicted in Fig. 3, there was no relationship between the decrement in FE_{Na} and the calculated changes in filtration fraction (inulin/PAH clearances). It is of interest to note that the rise in urinary sodium excretion was associated with a significant increment in creatinine/inulin clearance ratio, as shown in Fig. 4. Similarly, the decrement of urinary sodium below control values was associated with "normalization" of this clearance ratio.

TABLE I: Urinary sodium and inulin clearance in Groups II and III (left kidney).

		$U_{Na}V$ µEq/min	C inulin ml/min
Group II	Control	493 ± 54	19 ± 3
	VIP	375 ± 48[a]	17 ± 2
Group III	SAR	438 ± 59	21 ± 2
	SAR VIP	470 ± 56	20 ± 2

a) significance: $p<0.01$

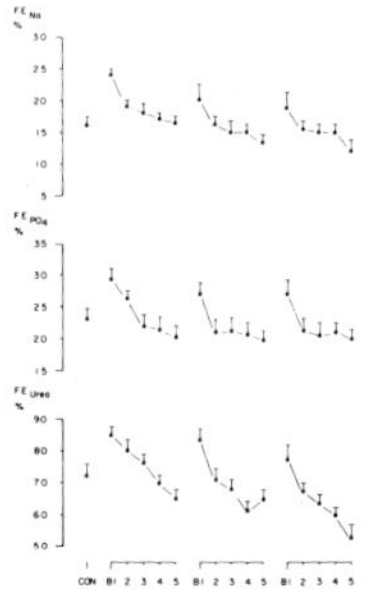

Fig. 1. FE_{Na}, PO^4, urea during and after VIP bolus.

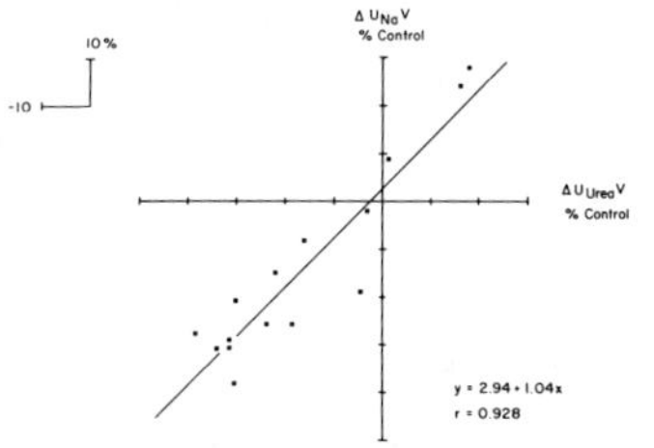

Fig. 2. Relation between changes in Na and Urea excretion.

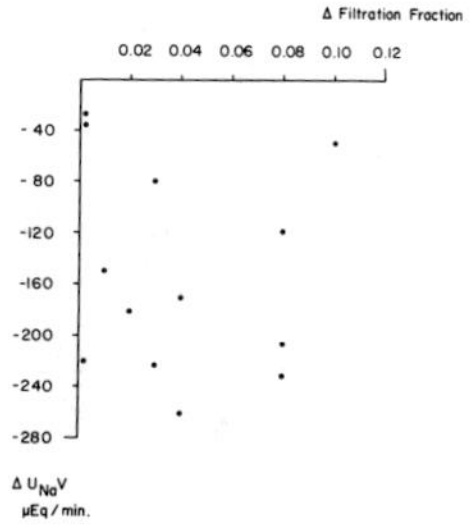

Fig. 3. Absence of relation between filtration fraction and urinary sodium.

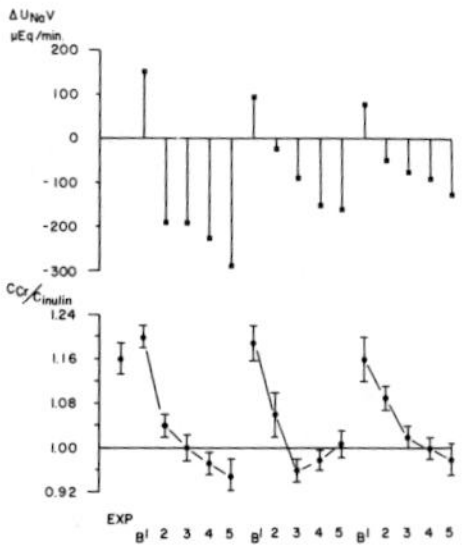

Fig. 4. Changes in creatinine/inulin clearances ratio.

DISCUSSION

Therefore, VIP injection resulted in a biphasic effect on sodium excretion: a brisk increment followed by a gradual decrease (over a period of 80 min.). VIP did not alter filtration rate but reduced renal plasma flow by less than 20%. The biphasic nature of VIP on urinary sodium almost excludes an effect of this peptide of the active component of net transport. Therefore, VIP is likely to affect the passive fluxes of fluid and solutes. Since there was no relationship between changes in natriuresis and filtration fraction, the role of peritubular physical forces on passive fluxes would also appear unlikely (2). By exclusion then, VIP has to influence the trans-epithelial permeability. The arguments in favor of such an effect are as follows. The changes in natriuresis were closely related to urinary excretion or urea, a compound known to be only passively transported (9). The increment and the decrease of natriuresis were also associated with the rise and "normalization" of the creatinine/inulin clearance ratio. Finally, the proposed mechanism of action of VIP on the nephron would appear similar to that documented on the intestinal epithelium (5). The localized effect of VIP on the left kidney (Group II) suggests that no systemic physical or humoral intervention is required for its expression on the tubular epithelium. However, the abolition of VIP action with saralasine (Group III) indicates that angiotensin II is required for the renal expression of VIP.

CONCLUSIONS

When administered in bolus (which may mimic the pattern of endogenous secretion), VIP results in a biphasic action on the net renal transport of sodium, phosphate and urea: an initial rise in excretion then a progressive abatement at or below control values. This phenomenon is not related to changes in renal hemodynamics nor alterations in peritubular physical forces. A direct effect of VIP on the active tubular transport of sodium appears improbable, but the eventual influence of this endogenous peptide on trans-epithelial permeability cannot be excluded.

REFERENCES

1. E.E. Windhager and G. Giebisch, Proximal sodium and fluid transport. Kidney Internat. 9: 121-133 (1976).
2. B.M. Brenner, K.H. Falchuk, and R.I. Keimowitz, The relationship between peritubular capillary protein concentration and fluid absorption by the proximal tubule. J. Clin. Invest. 48: 1519-1531 (1969).
3. W.B. Lorentz, Jr, The effect of cyclic AMP and dibutyryl cyclic AMP on the permeability characteristics of the renal tubule. J. Clin. Invest. 53: 1250-1257 (1974).
4. W.N. Suki, G. Eknoyan and M. Martinez-Maldonado, Tubular sites and mechanisms of diuretic action, A. Rev. Pharmac. 13: 91-106 (1973).
5. G.R. Davis, C.A. Santa Ana, S.G. Morawski and J.S. Fordtran, Effect of vasoactive intestinal polypeptide on active and passive transport in the human jejunum. J. Clin. Invest. 67: 1687-1694 (1981).
6. J. Jobin, T. Nawar, C. Caron and G.E. Plante, Effect of acetazolamide on renal bicarbonate reabsorption in volume-expanded dogs. Am. J. Physiol. 232: F484-F489 (1977).
7. G.E. Plante, R. Erian and C. Petitclerc, Renal excretion of levamisole. J. Pharmacol. Exp. Ther. 216: 617-623 (1981).
8. G.E. Plante and H. Hermkens, Endogenous creatinine: an inappropriate marker for glomerular filtration measurement. Proc. VIIth Internat. Congress Nephrol. C12 (1978).
9. J.A. Shannon, The renal reabsorption and excretion of urea under conditions of extreme diuresis. Am. J. Physiol. 123: 182-191 (1938).

RATE OF ADMINISTRATION AND RESPONSES TO INTRAVENOUS BUMETANIDE

G.T. McINNES, W.G. RAPEPORT,* A. COOK, A.M. THOMSON,** AND A. GOLDBERG
University Department of Medicine, Western Infirmary, Glasgow G11 6NT, Scotland; *MRC Clinical Pharmacology Unit, Radcliffe Infirmary, Oxford OX2 6HE, England; **University Department of Materia Medica, Stobhill General Hospital, Glasgow G21 3UW, Scotland

ABSTRACT

Urine electrolyte composition and bumetanide excretion in the eight hours after intravenous bumetanide (1mg) given as bolus injection and as constant rate infusion over four hours were compared in eight healthy subjects. Following infusion, sodium excretion, potassium excretion and urine volume were increased but the difference from bolus was significant ($p < 0.01$) only for natriuresis. However, bumetanide excretion was significantly greater after bolus injection ($p < 0.05$). Hourly urine excretion rates of sodium and bumetanide were correlated significantly after both bolus and infusion ($r = 0.95$ and $r = 0.73$ respectively, $p < 0.001$ in each case). These findings suggest that the diuretic response cannot be described simply by a concentration-effect relationship and support the proposition that the sodium response to loop diuretics also depends on the time during which drug is available at active sites. Consideration of rate of administration may result in more effective therapy.

INTRODUCTION

The primary action of loop diuretics is blockade of sodium/chloride transport at intraluminal sites in the ascending limb of the loop of Henle, necessitating adequate drug concentrations in renal tubular fluid [1]. Their influence on urine sodium excretion is characterised by a steep dose-response relationship but enhancement of natriuresis with high doses may be a function of prolonged diuretic availability at receptor sites rather than direct concentration dependent increased blockade of electrolyte transport [2,3]. If so, slow intravenous infusion of a loop diuretic might be expected to be more effective than the same dose administered by rapid bolus injection. The objective of this study was to examine this hypothesis using bumetanide as the test drug.

METHODS

Eight healthy male subjects (age 23-37 years; weight 52-78Kg) participated in the study after written explanation of its purposes and risks. The protocol was approved by the hospital ethical committee.

The study was a subject-blind, balanced, randomised, crossover comparison of the urine responses to intravenous bumetanide 1mg given by bolus or constant rate infusion. Intervals of at least one week separated each treatment.

Treatments were:

(a) Bumetanide 1mg (4ml active drug) as rapid intravenous bolus + 20ml normal saline by intravenous infusion (Sage pump) over four hours.

(b) Bumetanide 1mg (made up to 20ml in normal saline) by intravenous infusion over four hours + 4ml normal saline by rapid intravenous bolus.

Bolus injections were given simultaneously with the start of infusions.

Diuretics, Jules B. Puschett, Editor

On study days, drug administration commenced at 0900h and urine was collected hourly until 1700h. Water (200ml) was taken at 0900h and every hour until 1700h. An additional 300ml water was ingested at 1300h. Between 0900h and 1300h, subjects remained supine and threafter were ambulant. From 1700h on the evening prior to study days until urine collections were completed, diet was constant within subjects in both phases of the study. No alcohol or caffeinated drinks were allowed. Other medication was proscribed from one week before the study until its completion and strenuous exercise was prohibited from 24 hours before medication.

Urine was collected without preservative. After measurement of volume, aliquots were taken for assay of sodium and potassium concentration by flame photometry with lithium as the internal standard, and for analysis of bumetanide concentration by high performance liquid chromatography [4].

Statistical comparison of the urine electrolyte responses was by analysis of variance. Bumetanide excretion after bolus and infusion was compared by Student's t-test for paired observations. Correlations between hourly sodium excretion and hourly bumetanide excretion were by linear regression analysis.

RESULTS

Results for urine electrolyte and bumetanide excretion are presented in Table I.

TABLE I. Mean (SEM) urine electrolyte and drug excretion in eight hours following intravenous bumetanide 1mg given as bolus and infusion.

	Bolus	Infusion	Statistical significance of difference
Volume (ml)	2169(49)	2673(171)	N.S.
Sodium excretion (mmol)	179.2(13.5)	253.3(17.3)	$p < 0.01$
Potassium excretion (mmol)	48.7(4.8)	55.5(4.0)	N.S.
Bumetanide excretion (mcg)	500.1(24.0)	442.1(25.0)	$p < 0.05$

Natriuresis, kaliuresis and urine volume were greater following infusion but the difference was significant only for sodium excretion. Bumetanide excretion in the eight hours after bolus injection was significantly greater than that after infusion. Urine excretion rates for sodium and bumetanide are shown in Fig. 1. Hourly excretion rates of sodium and bumetanide correlated significantly after both bolus and infusion. Linear regression equation for infusion $y = 1.72 + 0.54x$; coefficient of correlation $r = 0.73$ ($p < 0.001$); for bolus, $y = 2.49 + 0.32x$; $r = 0.95$ ($p < 0.001$).

DISCUSSION

When compared to bolus injection, slow infusion of bumetanide enhanced natriuresis and diuresis at the expense of some increase in urine potassium loss. Although there was a close association between urine drug levels and natriuresis after both regimens, the pattern of drug excretion (greater after bolus than after infusion) suggests that the diuretic response cannot be described simply by a concentration-effect relationship. However, the findings support the proposition that the sodium response to bumetanide also depends on the time during which the drug is available at active sites. Similar conclusions can be drawn from the results of studies with frusemide in a number of experimental circumstances [1,5,6]. Thus, for the most efficient use of loop diuretics, maintenance of adequate drug levels in renal tubular fluid seems to be at least as important as achievement of high peak concentrations.

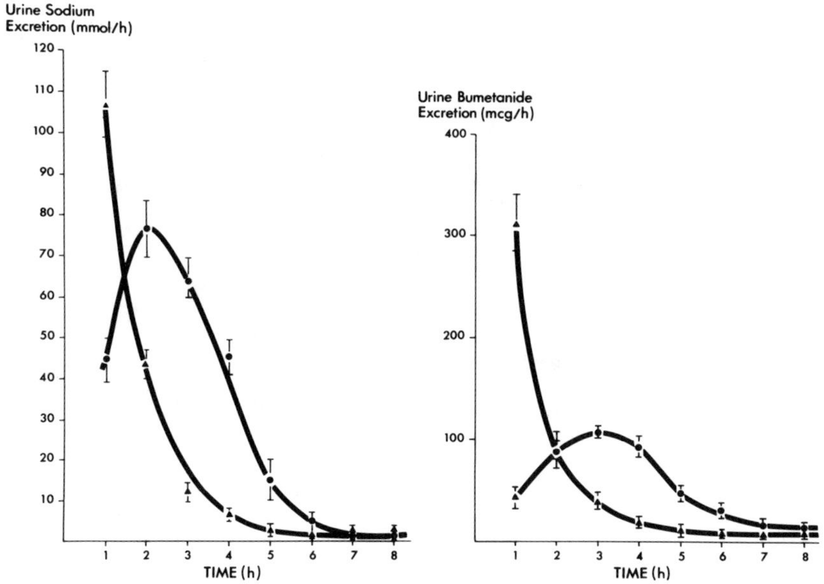

FIG. 1. Mean (vertical bars, SEM) excretion rates for sodium and bumetanide after bolus injection (▲) and infusion (●).

Consideration of the rate of administration of loop diuretics may result in more effective therapy and clinical benefit. An appreciable number of patients require intravenous doses of these drugs and often have prolonged hospital stays. In such cases, a controlled infusion provides a flexible approach allowing titration of dose according to response. Worthwhile natriuresis may be achieved at blood concentrations below those at which adverse extrarenal effects are seen, the risk of over rapid depletion of intravascular fluid volume may be avoided, and not least, the patient's time in hospital may be shortened substantially.

REFERENCES

1. L.Z. Benet, J. Pharmacokin. Biopharm. 7, 1-27 (1979).
2. R.E. Cutler, A.W. Forrey, T.S. Christopher, and B.M. Kimpel, Clin. Pharmacol. Ther. 15, 588-596 (1974).
3. D.L. Davies, A.F. Lant, N.R. Millard, A.J. Smith, J.W. Ward, and G.M. Wilson, Clin. Pharmacol. Ther. 15, 141-155 (1974).
4. L.A. Marcantonio, W.H.R. Auld, and G.G. Skellern, J. Chromatograph. 183, 118-123 (1980).
5. M. Homeida, C. Roberts, and R.A. Branch, Clin. Pharmacol. Ther. 16, 659-666 (1974).
6. C.D. Brater, Clin. Pharmacol Ther. 24, 548-554 (1978).

CROSS-OVER COMPARISON OF A FIXED COMBINATION OF HYDROCHLOROTHIAZIDE AND TRIAMTERENE (DYTENZIDE®, DYAZIDE®) AND A FREE COMBINATION OF FUROSEMIDE (LASIX®) AND TRIAMTERENE (DYTAC®, DYRENIUM®) IN THE MAINTENANCE TREATMENT OF PATIENTS WITH CARDIAC EDEMA.

F.A.TH. LUSTERMANS [1], H. FINTELMAN [2], M.C. HUIGE [3], J.J. KOOLEN [4], K.L. LIEM [5], A.J. FUNKE KÜPPER [6].

1. Dept. Int. Med., De Wever Ziekenhuis, Heerlen; Depts of Cardiol. of
2. Gemeente Ziekenhuis, Dordrecht; 3. St. Josef Ziekenhuis, Eindhoven;
4. Acad. Ziekenhuis W.G., Amsterdam; 5. Ziekenhuis Zonnestraal, Hilversum;
6. Acad. Ziekenhuis V.U., Amsterdam.

INTRODUCTION

The fixed combination of hydrochlorothiazide (25 mg) and triamterene (50 mg) was compared with the free combination of furosemide (40 mg) and triamterene (50 mg) in a randomized cross-over study of patients with chronic congestive heart failure (CHF), on salt restriction and treated with digitalis. Each treatment lasted 8 weeks. Other diuretics were not allowed.

PATIENTS

34 Outpatients (26 M, 8 F; age 31-82, mean 65 years) entered the study. MI was the cause of CHF in 23 patients. Functional Class was II in 25 and III in 9 of them.
Two-third was normotensive (diastolic BP < 95 mm Hg). All had normal liver and kidney function and serum potassium of 3,5-5,4 mmol/l. Excluded were patients with MI, coronary surgery or CVA in the last 3 months, and those with diabetes, gout and secondary or malignant hypertension.

RESULTS

4 Patients were withdrawn due to adverse signs and symptoms. In 3 of them this was not related to the trial drugs. Treatment failed in one patient with a cardiac aneurysm. Treatments could be compared in 30 patients (Table I):

Diuretics, Jules B. Puschett, Editor

TABLE I. Physical exam, symptoms and signs, lab. parameters and patients preference after 8 weeks treatment with the fixed and free combination

			Hydrochlorothiazide + 25 mg Triamterene 50 mg (Fixed comb.)	Furosemide 40 mg + Triamterene 50 mg (Free comb.)
Dose	1 Tablet	N	24	24
	2 Tablets		6	6
Physical exam	Bodyweight (kg)	$\bar{X}$	73,3	72,9
	BP syst/diast sitting		147,6/84,1	140,0*/80,6
	(mm Hg) supine		144,3/84,6	138,5*/80,0*
Symptoms/ signs	Rales	N	3	5
	Heartsound 3 or 4		7	7
	Dyspnoea		13	12
Lab	Serum creat. (µmol/l)	$\bar{X}$	104,5	106,3
	Serum K (mmol/l)		4,16	4,18
	Serum K < 3,5 mmol/l	N	2	2
Pat. preference (no difference in 2 pat.)		N	24	4

* $p < 0.05$

CONCLUSIONS

1. The fixed combination of hydrochlorothiazide with triamterene and the free combination of furosemide with triamterene maintain a "steady state" in patients with chronic CHF equally well.
2. The bloodpressure was lower after treatment with the free combination.
3. The fixed combination is more often preferred by the patient because of it's lower micturition frequency.

EFFECTS OF METOLAZONE COMBINED WITH BUMETANIDE IN NORMAL MEN

D. CRAIG BRATER, M.D., SHIRLEY A. ANDERSON, R.N.
The University of Texas Health Science Center at Dallas, Departments of Pharmacology and Internal Medicine, 5323 Harry Hines Blvd., Dallas, TX 75235

INTRODUCTION

Many clinicians have observed that the combination of metolazone and a loop diuretic can cause a profound diuresis in some patients who show a negligible response to either diuretic alone. The mechanism of this synergistic effect, or the supra-additive effect of other agents plus loop diuretics is unknown, but it seems to occur in patients with severe disease who have received chronic treatment with diuretics [1-6]. The presumed explanation is that patients who manifest a synergistic response are those with avid proximal tubular reabsorption of solute. Response to metolazone alone is minimal because solute rejected proximally is reclaimed at more distal nephron sites. Similarly, response to loop diuretics alone is minimal because most solute is reclaimed more proximal to their site of action [7]. In this setting, the combination allows effects of both drugs to become manifest whereas neither had before. Our aim is to explore mechanisms of this synergistic effect. Before studies in disease, studies in normal subjects are needed; hence, the motivation for this study. Our goal, then, was to assess response to bumetanide alone, metolazone alone and the combination in normal men receiving differing sodium intakes using clearance methodology so that mechanisms of interactions could be assessed.

METHODS

We performed 2 studies in each of two different phases. Phase 1 involved 7 normal men who had ingested an *ad libitum* diet for 4 days prior to study. These subjects were presumed to be sodium replete. A baseline 24 hr urine sample revealed excretion of 70 ± 10 mEq of sodium per day. In phase 2, we wished to employ a model of enhanced proximal reabsorption of sodium [8]. To effect this condition 5 normal men ingested a sodium deficient diet for 4 days prior to study. A baseline urine collection revealed 23 ± 4 mEq of sodium per day.

In each phase, subjects were studied twice in random order. All studies employed clearance methodology and were conducted during water diuresis with inulin and PAH infusions. In one study, after control collections, subjects received a bolus intravenous injection of 1.0 mg of bumetanide followed by six 20 min collections. In the other study, after control collections, subjects received 5.0 or 7.5 mg of oral metolazone followed by a 45 min equilibration period, followed by three 20 min collections to assess the effects of metolazone alone. Subjects then received 1.0 mg of bumetanide as before.

In this fashion, we assessed the effects of bumetanide alone, of metolazone alone and of the combination during both the sodium

Diuretics, Jules B. Puschett, Editor

replete and deplete state. To assess synergism, then, we compared the effects of coadministration of both diuretics to the sum of their individual effects.

RESULTS

Effects on urinary sodium, chloride, free water clearance (CH_2O) and delivery of solute to the diluting segment ($CCl + CH_2O$) are presented in Tables 1 and 2 for sodium replete and sodium deplete phases, respectively.

Since both diuretics can affect proximal tubular reabsorption of solute which will increase delivery of substrate to the diluting segment (which by itself will increase absolute CH_2O) and they can also affect the diluting segment (which by itself will decrease absolute CH_2O), the mechanism of the effects must be assessed as free water clearance relative to delivery of solute to the diluting segment [9,10] as shown in Table 3.

In the sodium deplete subjects, then, the combination of diuretic had a supra-additive effect compared to the sum of their individual effects.

DISCUSSION

This study provides preliminary evidence that normal subjects, particularly when sodium deplete, show a synergistic natriuretic and chloruretic response to metolazone plus bumetanide. The mechanism of this effect appears to be a supra-additive inhibition of the diluting segment as opposed to supra-additive increased delivery from proximal sites as evidenced by

1. The effect of bumetanide combined with metolazone on $CCl + CH_2O$ (ml/min) is no different from the effects of bumetanide alone plus metolazone alone on this same parameter:

	Sodium Replete		Sodium Deplete	
Bumetanide Alone	39.3	43.7	33.2	35.6
Metolazone Alone	4.4		2.4	
Bumetanide Plus Metolazone	42.3		35.6	

2. In contrast, in the sodium deplete subjects, free water clearance relative to delivery (Table 3) is increased by a greater degree with the combination of bumetanide plus metolazone (73%) compared to the effects of each diuretic alone (61%).

REFERENCES

1. K.H. Olesen. Acta Med. Scand. 190, 229 (1971).
2. K.H. Olesen, B. Dupont, E. Flensted-Jensen. Acta Med. Scand. 187, 33 (1970).
3. K.H. Olesen, B. Sigurd. Acta Med. Scand. 190, 223 (1971).

4. B. Sigurd, K.H. Olesen. Acta Med. Scand. 203, 113 (1978).
5. B. Sigurd, K.H. Olesen. Am. Heart J. 94, 168 (1977).
6. B Sigurd, K.H. Olesen, A. Wennevold. Am. Heart J. 89, 163 (1975).
7. D.C. Brater. Drugs 22, 477 (1981).
8. L.E. Earley, J.A. Martino. Circulation 42, 323 (1970).
9. D.W. Seldin, G. Eknoyan, W.N. Suki, F.C. Rector. Ann. N.Y. Acad. Sci. 139, 328 (1966).
10. D.W. Seldin, F.C. Rector. Excerpta Medica 268, 97 (1972).

TABLE I. Effects of bumetanide, metolazone and the combination in sodium replete subjects (n=7)*.

	Bumetanide Alone	Metolazone Alone	Bumetanide Plus Metolazone
Sodium Excretion Rate (mEq/min)	2.97 ± 0.15	0.16 ± 0.03	3.60 ± 0.22
Chloride Excretion Rate (mEq/min)	3.47 ± 0.17	0.20 ± 0.04	4.20 ± 0.24
CH_2O (ml/min)	5.8 ± 1.1	2.6 ± 1.2	2.0 ± 1.2
$CCl+CH_2O$ (ml/min)	39.3 ± 2.2	4.4 ± 1.2	42.3 ± 2.0

*Increase over control

TABLE II. Effects of bumetanide, metolazone and the combination in sodium deplete subjects (n=5)*.

	Bumetanide Alone	Metolazone Alone	Bumetanide Plus Metolazone
Sodium Excretion Rate (mEq/min)	2.19 ± 0.24	0.04 ± 0.03	2.80 ± 0.30
Chloride Excretion Rate (mEq/min)	2.80 ± 0.28	0.04 ± 0.03	3.33 ± 0.29
CH_2O (ml/min)	7.1 ± 1.0	2.0 ± 0.8	3.4 ± 1.2
$CCl+CH_2O$ (ml/min)	33.2 ± 5.0	2.4 ± 0.8	35.6 ± 2.1

*Increase over control

TABLE III. Effects of bumetanide, metolazone and the combination on the percent decrement in free water clearance relative to delivery of solute to the diluting segment: ($CH_2O/CCl + CH_2O$ X 100).

	Sodium Replete		Sodium Deplete	
Bumetanide Alone	60 ± 2	69	58 ± 5	61
Metolazone Alone	9 ± 3		3 ± 3	
Bumetanide Plus Metolazone	69 ± 2		73 ± 3	

ACUTE RENAL EFFECTS OF A NEW ANTIHYPERTENSIVE AGENT : BN 1270. COMPARISON WITH HYDROCHLOROTHIAZIDE AND FUROSEMIDE.

N. POZET, A. HADJ AISSA, M. LABEEUW, P. ZECH. Nephrology Department. Pr. J. TRAEGER. Hop. E. Herriot. INSERM U 80. 69374 LYON cédex 08. FRANCE

INTRODUCTION

The acute renal effects of a new antihypertensive agent : BN 1270 (Lab. BEAUFOUR - IPSEN) (1, 3-dihydro p-chlorophenyl-3 hydroxy-7 methyl-6 furo [3, 4-C] pyridine chlorhydrate) were studied in 10 normotensive subjects with normal glomerular filtration rate (GFR = 120,1 ± 18,7 ml/min/1,73 m2), after a single oral dose of 300 mg. Results were compared to the effects of hydrochlorothiazide (HCT) in 6 subjects (GFR = 116,2 ± 26,9 ml/min/1,73 m2) and Furosemide (F) in 6 other subjects (GFR = 105,5 ± 20 ml/min/1,73 m2), given respectively 50 mg and 40 mg per os.

METHOD

The same protocol was used in each treatment group. Both protocol and analytical methods were similar to those previously used and described in details elsewhere [1] : the studies were performed after a 12 h fast. Prior to the beginning of the study, subjects ingested a 10 ml/kg water load. After a 20 min equilibrium period, urine was collected for 2 control periods. Then, BN 300 mg, HCT 50 mg or F 40 mg, was administered orally with 100 ml water. Thereafter urine was collected for 7 hours : every 30 min for the first 2 h and every hour for the following 5 h. Urinary fluid losses were replaced orally (100 ml water every hour) and intravenously (isotonic glucose + saline infusion). Blood samples were drawn in the midpoint of each urine collection period. Continuous infusion of inulin and PAH allowed the measurement of glomerular filtration rate (GFR) and renal plasma flow throughout the study. Blood pressure and heart rate were measured every 30 min.

RESULTS

1 - Effects on renal function

. BN, like HCT, induced a slight (- 18 % mean maximal decrease) but not significant decrease in GFR. After F, the decline in GFR was more pronounced and significantly lower than after BN ($p<0.001$), while there was no significant difference between changes following HCT and F administration.

. No significant change in PAH clearance occured in either treatment group.

2 - Effects on Na and K excretion

Diuretics, Jules B. Puschett, Editor

Fig 1

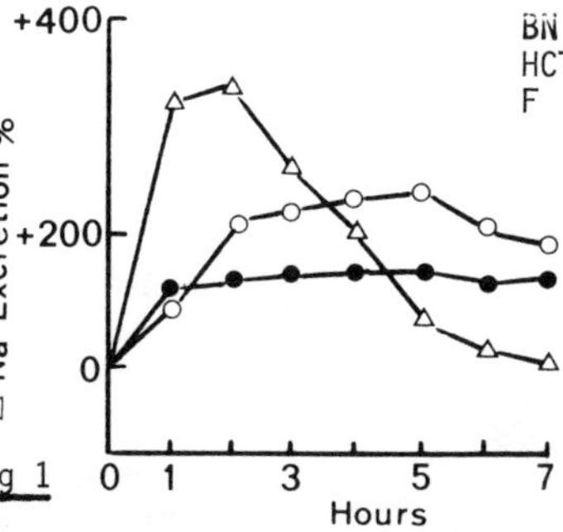

Fig 2

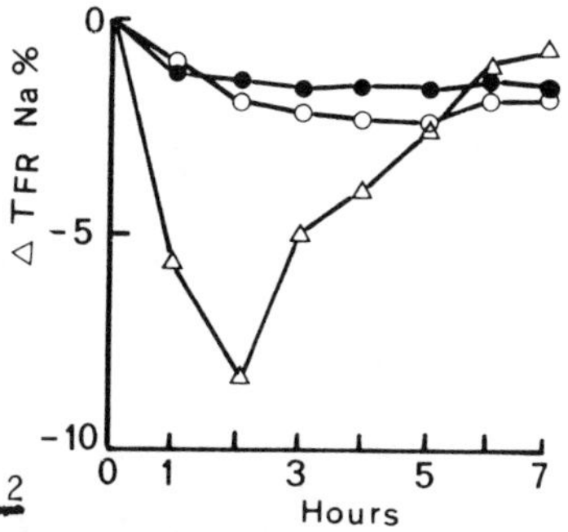

Percent changes in mean Na excretion rate over the 7 hours period (fig 1) and in mean Na tubular fractional reabsorption (fig 2) compared to control value.

- As shown in figures 1 and 2, BN induced a slight increase in Na excretion and decrease in Na tubular fractional reabsorption (TFR), being detectable within the first hour after its administration. The natriuresis was sustained up to the following 6 hours observation, averaging a two fold increase compared to control value. The pattern of natriuresis after BN was similar to that of HCT, while when compared to F, the increment of Na excretion after BN and HCT was lower but of longer duration. However, in spite of the highest efficiency of F, the cumulative increase in Na excretion over a 7 hours period was identical for all treatment group (table I)

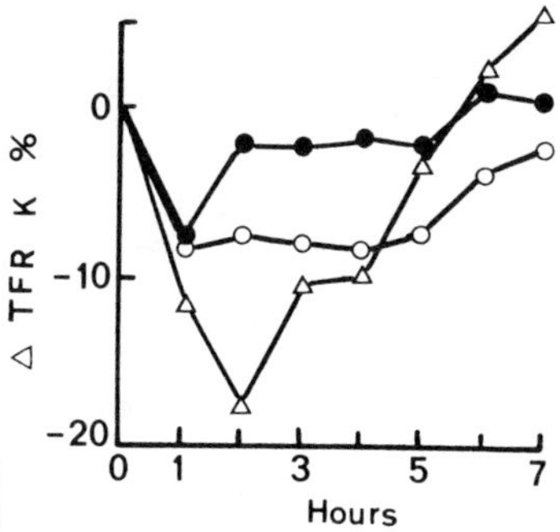

Fig 3

Changes in mean K tubular fractional reabsorption compared to control value.

BN induced a slight decrease in K TFR between the first and the fifth hour after its administration (figure 3). HCT caused a greater inhibition of net K TFR, and of longer duration. While after F, a deeply impaired K reabsorption occured : K TFR was minimal at the 2nd hour, and returned quite above control level after the 5th hour.

So that, over the 7 hours observation, cumulative K excretion was the lowest after BN (table I), but the differences between the 3 treatment groups were not significant. Urinary Na/K ratio rose similarly after BN and HCT, being higher after BN. Urinary Na/K ratio exhibited a larger increase after F, reaching a maximal value at the 2nd hour and then decreased sharply, remaining still above baseline at the 7th hour.

	Δ Na %	Δ K %	Δ Ca %
BN	+ 95	- 10	- 12
HCT	+ 150	+ 20	- 3
F	+ 140	- 3	+ 80

Table I : Percent changes in excretion rates over the 7 hours period compared to control values.

3 - Effects on urine volume (V) and free water excretion (CH_2O) (table I)

	V ml/min		C osm ml/min		CH_2O ml/min	
	T o	T m	T o	T m	T o	T m
BN	6,99	7,20	5,19	6,90	1,80	0,30
HCT	7,30	7,80	4,33	7,10	2,97	0,70
F	7,33	15,90	5,46	13,30	1,87	2,60

Table II : mean values of V, C osm and CH_2O at T o = control
and T m = C osm maximum

In water loaded subjects, BN nor HCT, did not induce any significant change in urine flow rate, while F caused a further increase in urine volume. Changes in osmolar clearance (C osm) paralleled that of Na excretion in each treatment group, and the maximal C osm was the highest after F. The free water excretion remained positive after F but decreased significantly following BN and HCT.

4 - Other results

. As expected from the well known effects of F and HCT, only F induced an increase in calcium excretion. Similarly to HCT, there was no detectable change in net calcium excretion following BN at least over a 7 h period (table I).

. Uric acid excretion remained unchanged following BN, while HCT and F induced a parallel significant decrease in uric acid clearance.

. Finally no significant change occured in the other measured urinary parameters nor in blood pressure or heart rate throughout the study in all treatment groups.

CONCLUSIONS

Thus BN whose antihypertensive effect has been demonstrated previously, exhibits a natriuretic effect comparable to that of HCT and F within 7 hours observation. The pattern of its diuretic activity appears to be similar to that of thiazide group. However more information should be gathered about its effectiveness in long term therapy.

REFERENCES

1. N. POZET, A. HADJ AISSA, M. PELLET and J. TRAEGER, Br. J. Clin. Pharmac. 9, 577 - 583 (1980)

DIFFERENT THERAPEUTIC STRATEGIES IN TREATING ASCITES WITH ALDACTONE.

FAEDDA R., SATTA A., BRANCA G.F., SANNA M., BARTOLI E.
Institute of Patologia Medica, University,Viale S.Pietro 12,Sassari (Italy).

ABSTRACT

We treated ascites in 41 patients with Liver Cirrhosis with different doses of Aldactone averaging 200, 300,400, and 600 mg daily respectively.The different amounts chosen were based on previous response to treatment, degree of renal failure, estimated volume of ascites and tubular avidity for Na.The effectiveness of diuretic response rose significantly with the daily dosage, the change in BW rising from 0.1±0.04 with 200 mg to 0.53±0.1 Kg/day with 600 mg of Aldactone.This indicates that the clinical judgement on the anticipated response can effectively guide to choice of an appropriate regimen based on the administration of Aldactone.

INTRODUCTION

The diuretic therapy of ascites creates conflicting problems for the physician:the use of drugs causing Na and volume depletion,can cause prerenal azotemia,a common consequence of effective circulating volume depletion (1). The extracellular volume contraction should be kept at a minimum,continuously counterbalanced by ascites reabsorption from the peritoneal capillaries,which acts by replenishing the circulating volume.Excessive diuresis has significant side effects.Both their incidence and the effectiveness of treatment can be optimalized through therapeutic strategies designed to keep the benefit/risk ratio high (2).We report herein the results obtained with Aldactone alone when used in different doses tailored to produce a response predicted on the grounds of clinical data and simple laboratory measurements. The results show that Aldactone alone may represent a flexible option within effective therapeutic strategies.

MATERIAL AND METHODS

The studies were performed on 41 patients with Liver Cirrhosis,diagnosed by standard clinical and histologic criteria (3).Different amounts of Aldactone were used for treating ascites,chosen on the grounds of the anticipated clinical response.The initial dose was 200 mg daily when ascites was estimated to be 3L,Plasma Creatinine was normal,renal avidity for Na slightly increased because of a slow weight gain(over weeks)in the face of unrestricted Na intake.The next dose of 300 mg was chosen when only the volume of ascites exceeded 3 liters, all other considerations being equal.
When 1 or 2 of the other conditions were not met, 400 mg were given, and 600 mg when more than two were not met,or when a previous trial with a lower

Diuretics, Jules B. Puschett, Editor

dosage of Aldactone had been unsatisfactory.All patients were studied during a recommended water restriction of 0.5 L per day and a Na restriction of 50 mEq per day.Compliance with these restrictions was checked by extensive questioning of the patients and their relatives.For inhospital patients, compliance was controlled directly by us and by the hospital staff.Urine output,Na excretion and laboratory values were obtained at the beginning,approximately at the middle and again at the end of treatment.Body weight,clinical conditions,encephalopathy,dehydration,blood pressure were checked daily.The response was considered a success when ascites either disappeared or decreased to the extent of representing a minor cosmetic problem in the absence of major side effects.These were hyponatremia(PNa<130 mEq/L),renal failure(PCr> 1.5 mg% or a rise>0.7 mg%),dehydration,hypotension encephalopathy,GI bleeding and death.A non success was scored when at least one of these complications supervened or when the weight loss was clinically unsatisfactory.We used a clinical rather than a numerical end-point since it is known that many of these patients are better off with some residual ascites and their clinical response is what the doctor and the patient want, rather than complete loss of ascites in the face of unacceptable encephalopathy or severe hyponatremia. The data were analized statistically,means and standard errors of the mean were calculated,and differences tested by either paired or unpaired "t" test.

RESULTS

Table I shows the average weight loss,change in PNa,PK,PCr for all patients treated with the different dose of Aldactone guided by a rational strategy.

Table I. M and SE before (B) and after (A) Aldactone at the indicated doses. ΔBW indicates the change in body weight ,N the number of patients (pts) studied.

PTS N.	Daily dose mg	ΔBW Kg	Treat/ days	Pcreat B	Pcreat A	PNa B	PNa A	PK B	PK A	Success Rate %
10	200	-1.8± 0.5	18.2± 2.5	1.2± 0.2	1.4 0.3	133.8± 2.1	134.8± 1.6	4.4± 0.4	4.4± 0.4	80.0%
16	300	-4.2± 0.8	16.2± 1.9	1.1± 0.2	1.3± 0.4	135.6± 1.8	136.0± 0.9	4.3± 0.2	4.6± 0.1	87.5%
8	400	-4.5± 1.2	13.3± 2.8	0.9± 0.1	0.9± 0.1	136.5± 1.1	133.7± 1.3	4.0± 0.2	4.5± 0.1	62.5%
7	600	-7.3± 0.1	19.3± 6.8	1.0± 0.1	1.0± 0.1	133.3± 2.9	132.0± 5.0	4.3± 0.6	4.8± 0.1	95.0%

It is apparent that the effectiveness increases with increasing dosage in average values,though not in the percentage of success rate.The side effects,mainly hyperkalemia and hyponatremia,do not increase.The data also show that the success rate remains independent of the dose.Figure 1 shows the average daily weight loss plotted against the corresponding dose schedule employed.The higher doses were more effective in inducing weight loss and did not result in any significant difference in PCr,while producing an improved success rate.

DISCUSSION

The treatment of ascites requires a careful clinical evaluation of the patient and of the factors that can influence the response,rather than the use of different diuretic agents either alone or in association. The diuresis must be even,continuous and less than the rate of ascites reabsorption, with

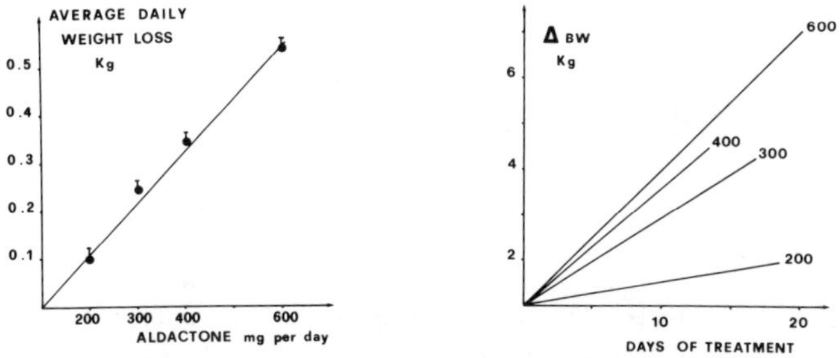

Fig.1.The average daily weight loss is plotted against Aldactone dose on the left.The absolute weight loss against time of treatment is on the right:separate regression lines are reported for each dose.

a desirable weight loss of <0.5 Kg/day.Thus,powerful diuretics are required only in the presence of a marked enhancement of the tubular avidity for Na (4,5,6).However, a successful diuresis could be induced by appropriately increasing the daily Aldactone dosage,which causes a slow and even diuresis by directly antagonizing the aldosterone hypersecretion.In Liver Cirrhosis, because of almost complete reabsorption at more proximal sites,the Na reaching the aldo-sensitive segment of the distal tubule is so low,that higher doses could hardly be expected to restore its effectiveness.However,loop diuretics may deliver Na to the aldo-sensitive segment at rates larger than before therapy, though still lower than the aldo-enhanced distal capacity (7).Since Na-free urines are produced along this segment,complete aldo inhibition would always result in natriuresis.This hypothesis is verified by our data demonstrating that there is an unmistakable dose response curve for aldactone and that most patients unresponsive to conventional dosages can be safely freed of their ascites by higher doses.In addition,our data demonstrate that clinical judgement is a sensitive tool that can guide the dose necessary to obtain the desired response,as it can effectively predict the refractoriness to the diuretic therapy and lack of response to low or conventional amounts.When even the larger dosage of aldactone prove ineffective,it seems reasonable to associate other powerful agents like Muzolimine.

REFERENCES

1. Soggia G. et al. in:Liver and Kidney,F.Fiaccadori Ed.(Piccin 1980) 97-108
2. Satta A. et al. Postgraduate Medical Journal 59,64-72 (1983).
3. Satta A. et al. Ital.J.Gastroenterol.15,10-13 (1983).
4. Chiandussi L. et al. Gut 19,497-516 (1978).
5. Bartoli E. et al. J.Clin.Pharmacol. 23, 56-64 (1983).
6. Satta A. et al. in:Recent advances in diuretic therapy (Excerpta Medica 1983) pp 235-241.
7. Bartoli E. et al. Ital.J.Gastroenterol. In press.

AKNOWLEDGEMENTS . This paper was supported by grants from the Consiglio Nazionale delle Ricerche (CNR) and the Ministero della Pubblica Istruzione (MPI), Rome, Italy.

MUZOLIMINE:A NEW LOOP DIURETIC IN VARIOUS FORMS OF HYPERTENSION.

SATTA A., FAEDDA R., BRANCA G.F., MANCA A., BARTOLI E.
University Institute of Patologia Medica,Viale San Pietro 12,Sassari(Italy).

ABSTRACT

We tested the effectiveness of Muzolimine,a long acting diuretic that inhibits Henle's Loop transport,in 7 patients with essential hypertension(EH)and 10 subjects with Chronic Renal Failure(CRF):Blood pressure(BP)fell from 138±11 to 106.5 in EH,and from 129±5 to 113±3 mmHg in CRF($P<0.05$ for both).Body weight(BW)fell only by 1.3±0.2 Kg in CRF,to remain stable when the patients had reached their dry weight and/or normal BP.PCr rose from 1.1±0.1 to 1.2±0.1 in HE, from 3.9±0.6 to 4.3±0.7 $mg \cdot dL^{-1}$ in CRF($P>0.05$ for both). When compared to 14 patients treated with Furosemide for CRF,Muzolimine,at the average dose of 23.0±1.5 mg daily, was equally effective in achieving the clinical end-points, and was more effective on a weight basis in reducing BP and BW.

INTRODUCTION

Of the powerful diuretics acting on Henle's Loop,Furosemide 40 mg iv completely inhibits transport for 30 minutes (1),while the effect of Muzolimine is dose dependent with a T/2 of 4 hours (2).Muzolimine should be useful at low doses when a continuous,mild inhibition of Na transport is important,as in EH,at high doses in CRF when a steady,maximal inhibition of reabsorption is required.We assessed their effectiveness by evaluating Na excretion,loss of body fluids and changes in GFR together with clinical end points,cost/benefit ratios,BP control and patient well being.

MATERIALS AND METHODS

The study was performed on 31 patients,7 affected by EH and 24 by CRF, diagnosed by standard criteria (5,6).All patients with EH were treated with Muzolimine.Of the patients with CRF, 10 were treated with Muzolimine,14 with Furosemide.The dose was chosen on clinical end points aimed at the optimum for the patient and for the therapeutic goals.These were normalization of BP, increased tolerance for salt and water,disappearance of edema,achievement of dry BW,control of hyperkalemia,absence of a rise in PCr,of orthostatic hypotension,of dehydration and of uremic symptoms.One side effect plus one benefit missing was the cut-off between success and failure.All patients with CRF were on a 0.5 gr/Kg protein,low Na diet,tailored to the patients' excretory ability and its modification by diuretic treatment.Additional drugs included β-blockers and peripheral vasodilators.All patients with EH underwent a wash-out period of 7 days.All data were analyzed statistically,Means

Diuretics, Jules B. Puschett, Editor

and Standard errors calculated and the significance of differences were tested by the paired and unpaired "t" test.

RESULTS

The data are reported in Table I. In 7 patients with EH, Muzolimine was given at the average dose of 30 mg qd: BP fell from 138±11 to 106±5 mmHg, BW, PNa, PK, and PCr remained unchanged. Thus, Muzolimine contributes to control hypertension by producing a fall in renal Na reabsorption without side effects, such as hypokalemia and renal failure. In 10 patients with CRF Muzolimine was given at the average dose of 23 mg qd: BP fell from 129±5 mmHg to 113±3 mmHg,

TABLE I. Means and SE of change in body weight (A) and of mean arterial pressure (MAP), Plasma Na, and Creatinine before (left) and after (right) treatment.
M = Muzolimine, F = Furosemide

PTS N	CONDITION	DRUG	ΔKg	PCreat. mg%		PNa $mEq \cdot L^{-1}$		PK $mEq \cdot L^{-1}$		M.A.P. mmHg	
7	EH	M	-0.7± 0.3	1.1± 0.1	1.2± 0.1	140.8± 1.0	138.0± 1.2	3.9± 0.1	3.9± 0.1	137.9± 11.5	105.8± 4.6
10	CRF	M	-1.3± 0.2	3.9± 0.6	4.3± 0.7	140.5± 1.5	137.8± 1.6	4.6± 0.2	4.8± 0.2	128.8± 5.3	112.8± 2.9
14	CRF	F	-0.7± 0.2	5.7± 1.3	5.8± 1.4	140.1± 1.1	141.1± 0.8	4.4± 0.6	4.4± 0.7	121.5± 0.2	104.9± 0.4

BW by -1.3±0.2 Kg, while PNa and PCr remained constant. The data obtained with an average dose of 45 mg qd of Furosemide were very similar, and are also in Table I.

DISCUSSION

EH is attributed to excessive circulating volume (7) due to a genetically determined rise in Na reabsorption (8). Thus, an effective diuretic should depress Na resorption to the normal value, thereby normalizing the circulating volume required to achieve a renal salt loss equal to the daily intake. Therefore, the ideal diuretic should exhibit a mild continuous effect, not suppressed by Na retaining mechanisms. The weight loss should be limited to that necessary to restore a normal circulating volume, and should not be progressive. Muzolimine appears to be a good candidate, because of the wide range of effectiveness allowed by the large dose flexibility. Our data show that Muzolimine is at the same time effective and safe in treating EH, and that a very low dose is required in the presence of normal renal function. The agent results in neither excessive nor progressive weight loss: therefore, the defect in reabsorption that it induces can be tailored by an appropriate dosage to match the alledged increase in reabsorption which is considered by some causative of hypertension. In CRF it is established that the defect in excreting the normal salt load stems from the reduced number of functioning nephrons, although each surviving unit exhibits an increased Na rejection fraction (9). The mainstay of diuretic therapy is to increase the resorptive defect to a maximum, thus allowing Na excretion to match the intake. This requires a progressive rise in diuretic effectiveness, as disease progresses, to be continuously kept at peak values in advanced stages.With Furosemide this is achieved by 250 mg q.6 hours.Although the T/2 of Furosemide is normally of a few minutes (10),it is markedly prolonged in CRF,where its effectiveness can be rendered more uniform.Muzolimine already exhibits a prolonged action,and complete inhibition of Henle's Loop transport can be reached by high dosage(11). Diuretic therapy in CRF improves the control of circulating volume and increases tolerance to the conservative management,particularly Na-K intake, because of its action on the kidney.Also it contributes significantly to controlling hypertension,mainly through the volume effect.This,in turn,ameliorates or relieves congestive heart failure (CHF).BP control is essential in CRF,as it prolongs survival (12),slows down the speed of disease progression, relieves CHF while preventing late cardiovascular complications(13).Our data demonstrate that Muzolimine is highly effective in controlling hypertension. The patients had an excess BW that was reduced on average by 1.3 Kg,with improvement in symptoms of CHF and in quality of life.The weight loss was not progressive,indicating that the dosage could be successfully tailored to the degree of residual renal function and to match an Na intake acceptable to the patients after the obtainment of dry weight and BP control.Again,the large flexibility of the Muzolimine dose makes these therapeutic goals possible by monitoring their clinical response and simple laboratory data without sophisticated or costly measurements.With the improved tolerance to less rigid dietary restrictions,the quality of life improves.These same goals were reached with Furosemide,because of a favorable prolongation of its T/2 in CRF,where it becomes a long acting diuretic.The paired comparison of the two agents indicates equal effectiveness,although the average amounts necessary were significantly less for Muzolimine.The danger of Furosemide toxicity at high doses,though remote,remains the only possible draw back for its indefinite use.

REFERENCES

1. Bartoli E. et al. J.Clin.Pharmacol. 20, 452-458 (1980).
2. Loew D. et al. E.J.Clin.Pharmacol. 12,341-344 (1977)
3. Rose H.J. et al.Clin.Pharmacol.Therap. 24,199-207 (1978)
4. Kaojarern S. et al. Kidney International 22,69-74 (1982)
5. Branca G.F. et al. Panminerva Medica (In press).
6. Branca G.F. et al. Panminerva Medica 25,13-18 (1983).
7. Beretta-Piccoli C. et al. Am.J.Med. 61,739-747 (1976).
8. Bianchi G. et al. Kidney International 13,452-466 (1978).
9. Schreiner G.E. et al.in:The Kidney,B.Brenner and F.Rector Eds (Saunders Company 1976) 1423-1447.
10. Brater C.D. et al. Kidney International 22,171-176 (1982)
11. Dal Canton A. et al.in:Recent advances in diuretic therapy.V.E Andreucci Ed.(Excerpta Medica 1983) 156-164.
12. Feld L.G. et al. Kidney International 20,606-614 (1981).
13. Ikkan H. et al. Kidney International 24,371-376 (1983)

AKNOWLEDGEMENTS . This paper was supported by grants from the Consiglio Nazionale delle ricerche (CNR) and the Ministero della Pubblica Istruzione (MPI), Rome, Italy.

DIURETIC POTENCY OF LOOP, THIAZIDE AND POTASSIUM SPARING AGENTS: A REAPPRAISAL OF RELATIVE ACTIVITY.

Hamdy R.C.,* Vinson M,* Robbins A.D.,** Struthers L.P.L.,** Chapman S.F.** Norris R.J.,** Shaw H.L.,**
* St. John's Hospital, London SW11, U.K. **Berk Pharmaceuticals Ltd., Eastbourne, U.K.

INTRODUCTION

Diuretics are traditionally classified into high, medium and low potency/ceiling groups. Frusemide is the prototype of the high potency/ ceiling group, the thiazides and their derivatives are regarded as medium potency, and the potassium sparing diuretics as low potency preparations. We feel that although this is correct for the first few hours following administration, a different picture may be seen if the action of the various preparations is followed for a longer period. In this study we undertook to assess over a 24 hour period the effects of administering various diuretic preparations.

PATIENTS AND METHODS

Five diuretics were selected for the study, frusemide, 40mg, hydrochlorothiazide, 25 and 50mg, triamterene, 50mg and amiloride 5mg. The effects of each diuretic on the urine volume, specific gravity and sodium, potassium, calcium and magnesium excretion were followed and compared with a control day, the day immediately preceding administration. The study, therefore, consisted of five legs, each separated from the next by five days during which the patients were not administered any diuretic preparation.

Patients were only included in the study if they had an indwelling catheter. The diagnosis was mild congestive cardiac failure and patients with severe orthopnoea or paroxysmal nocturnal dyspnoea recent myocardial infarction, chest infection or pulmonary embolism, and patients who required additional diuresis, were excluded. Other exclusion criteria included high output failure, anaemia, malabsorption, impaired renal function and impaired hepatic function. In the majority of patients included heart failure was secondary to ischaemic heart disease or valvular lesions. The nature and aims of the study were explained to the patients who then gave their consent. The study was approved by the appropriate ethical committee.

On the first day of each leg of the study the indwelling catheter bag was emptied at 6 am and the urine discarded. Urine was then collected 3, 6, 9, 12 and 24 hours later. The diuretic preparation was administered after 24 hours and the urine collections were continued at identical times for the next 24 hour period. At each urine collection the volume and specific gravity were carefully recorded and a sample taken and frozen to be later assayed for sodium, potassium, calcium and magnesium content. Urinary sodium and potassium were assessed using flame photometry with atomic absorption spectroscopy for calcium and magnesium.

RESULTS

12 patients completed the study. The urine volume, specific gravity and hourly urinary excretion rates, as well as cumulative excretion of sodium, potassium, calcium and magnesium, are shown in the accompanying tables.

Published 1984 by Elsevier Science Publishing Co., Inc.
Diuretics, Jules B. Puschett, Editor

URINARY VOLUME (ml)

COLLECTION PERIOD (hours)		FRUSEMIDE 40mg		HC-THIAZIDE 25mg		HC-THIAZIDE 50mg		TRIAMTERENE 50mg		AMILORIDE 5mg	
		CONTROL	TEST	CONTROL	TEST	CONTROL	TEST	CONTROL	TEST	CONTROL	TEST
0-3	Mean	120.00	624.17	130.42	196.25	129.09	205.46	130.00	172.50	119.75	184.58
	S.D.	94.48	437.81	76.47	129.81	81.39	110.22	71.26	65.52	82.84	113.37
3-6	Mean	65.83	281.25	60.58	79.83	66.73	117.27	68.08	76.25	76.83	92.75
	S.D.	40.83	180.61	40.94	79.22	38.59	102.16	55.22	38.21	89.17	50.65
6-9	Mean	74.17	152.50	78.75	121.67	89.09	145.46	91.25	106.67	83.75	115.83
	S.D.	39.42	72.38	44.32	91.64	48.05	93.18	71.55	41.41	45.58	71.41
9-12	Mean	91.25	100.83	105.00	235.00	106.82	213.46	120.83	132.08	99.58	128.33
	S.D.	56.89	49.08	77.37	197.14	47.55	122.49	59.19	65.97	42.13	84.08
12-24	Mean	645.83	512.08	663.75	822.92	573.18	1054.55	573.33	660.83	474.17	794.17
	S.D.	430.89	216.96	348.48	456.70	314.42	445.65	332.19	262.59	307.05	275.27
0-24	Mean	997.08	1670.83	1038.5	1455.67	964.91	1736.18	983.50	1148.33	854.08	1315.67
	S.D.	514.77	661.43	495.20	795.08	369.56	573.65	446.63	365.91	448.50	427.96

EXCRETION RATE OF SODIUM (mmol/hr)

COLLECTION PERIOD (hours)		FRUSEMIDE 40mg		HC-THIAZIDE 25mg		HC-THIAZIDE 50mg		TRIAMTERENE 50mg		AMILORIDE 5mg	
		CONTROL	TEST	CONTROL	TEST	CONTROL	TEST	CONTROL	TEST	CONTROL	TEST
0-3	Mean	3.33	18.71	4.55	7.43	4.19	7.19	3.05	4.71	3.72	5.75
	S.D.	2.69	18.42	3.17	5.94	3.49	4.77	2.58	3.43	3.27	4.55
3-6	Mean	1.58	7.38	1.50	3.40	1.73	3.33	1.68	2.68	2.10	3.56
	S.D.	1.17	5.34	0.93	3.47	1.32	2.10	1.78	2.14	2.66	2.38
6-9	Mean	1.71	2.80	1.52	4.23	1.91	5.18	1.68	3.40	1.68	3.39
	S.D.	1.21	1.74	1.41	3.54	1.22	4.19	1.98	3.18	1.32	1.91
9-12	Mean	1.70	2.11	1.71	8.12	2.16	7.80	2.03	3.91	1.82	3.11
	S.D.	1.49	2.28	1.11	7.19	2.24	4.53	2.29	3.85	1.37	1.67
12-24	Mean	3.24	1.90	3.60	5.12	2.81	7.33	2.75	4.31	2.21	3.73
	S.D.	2.44	1.32	2.09	2.84	1.35	3.80	2.19	2.82	2.41	1.77
0-24	Mean	2.66	4.82	2.96	5.46	2.65	6.60	2.43	3.99	2.27	3.84
	S.D.	1.65	3.05	1.43	2.94	1.19	2.37	1.79	2.47	1.24	1.72

EXCRETION RATE OF POTASSIUM (mmol/hr)

COLLECTION PERIOD (hours)		FRUSEMIDE 40mg		HC-THIAZIDE 25mg		HC-THIAZIDE 50mg		TRIAMTERENE 50mg		AMILORIDE 5mg	
		CONTROL	TEST	CONTROL	TEST	CONTROL	TEST	CONTROL	TEST	CONTROL	TEST
0-3	Mean	1.28	2.97	1.56	2.20	1.27	1.86	1.29	1.46	0.95	1.08
	S.D.	1.00	1.98	1.15	2.07	0.75	0.93	0.76	0.87	0.60	0.47
3-6	Mean	0.86	1.67	0.82	1.08	0.88	1.07	1.06	0.55	0.96	0.49
	S.D.	0.54	0.86	0.48	0.85	0.46	0.41	1.01	0.30	1.16	0.40
6-9	Mean	1.30	1.36	1.21	1.75	1.28	1.63	1.21	1.06	1.25	0.46
	S.D.	0.78	0.88	0.71	1.00	0.66	0.89	0.84	0.68	0.77	0.23
9-12	Mean	1.25	1.23	1.21	3.32	1.56	2.30	1.56	1.12	1.58	0.46
	S.D.	0.83	0.64	0.71	3.10	0.82	1.55	0.73	0.60	0.83	0.24
12-24	Mean	1.08	0.84	1.24	1.12	1.15	1.63	1.14	1.15	0.95	0.65
	S.D.	0.46	0.37	0.44	0.47	0.57	0.75	0.38	0.59	0.50	0.66
0-24	Mean	1.13	1.33	1.22	1.60	1.20	1.67	1.21	1.10	1.07	0.63
	S.D.	0.35	0.57	0.34	0.66	0.30	0.45	0.41	0.35	0.49	0.40

DISCUSSION

Both amiloride and triamterene induced a small increase in urine volume in the first three hours after administration. The increase was more pronounced in the case of amiloride and was followed by a period of only marginal polyuria for the following 9 hours. Nevertheless, from 12 to 24 hours after administration, there was a significant increase in the volume of urine, again more pronounced with amiloride than triamterene. Over 24 hours the urine volume increased from an average of 854ml (±448) and 984.5ml (±447) during the control day to 1316ml (±428) and 1148ml (±366) with amiloride and triamterene respectively.

Similar changes were observed in the urinary specific gravity and sodium excretion. Both amiloride and triamterene are therefore, slow acting, but amiloride is more potent than triamterene. Similarly, although both preparations tended to retain potassium, this was more pronounced with amiloride than triamterene. Amiloride reduced the 24 hour potassium excretion from 25.7mmol (±11.6) to 15.2mmol (±9.5), but triamterene only from 29.1mmol (±9.9) to 26.3mmol (±8.4). In both instances, the potassium conservation was most pronounced 3 to 12 hours post dose. Amiloride and triamterene also appear to have different actions on calcium and magnesium excretion: amiloride tends to retain calcium and magnesium, whereas triamterene tends to increase their excretion.

Hydrochlorothiazide 25 and 50mg demonstrated peak activity from 9 to 12 hours following administration. Their effect nevertheless started within three hours and lasted for 24 hours. Over a 24 hour period the urine volume was increased from 1039ml (±495) to 1456ml (±795) and from 965ml (±370) to 1736 (±574) ml for the 25 and 50mg prepraration respectively. Similar changes occurred in the urine specific gravity and sodium excretion, and it is clear that for hydrochlorothiazide, the diuretic potency increases from 25 to 50mg. Both doses moderately increased the urinary calcium and magnesium excretion.

As expected, frusemide 40mg induced the highest increase in urine volume (about 5 fold) in the shortest time (0-3 hours). This, however, was followed by a gradual reduction in diuresis, and 9-12 hours after administration, the diuresis was not significantly different from that during the control day. Furthermore, during the period 12 to 24 hours post dose, the volume of urine produced after frusemide was actually less than during the equivalent control day. Sodium excretion followed a similar pattern, indicating that during this period there is actual salt and fluid retention. This "relative reactive oliguric and sodium conserving state" is not seen when other types of diuretic are studied. It could be due to an acute hypovolaemia developing during the 3 to 6 hours following frusemide administration which is of sufficient magnitude to stimulate the renin-angiotensin-aldosterone axis and/or the production of anti-diuretic hormone. This was particularly likely in the patients investigated, who had no gross salt and water retention prior to the study. More work is presently being undertaken to elucidate the underlying cause of this finding. Frusemide, 40mg also increased the urinary calcium and magnesium excretion.

The cumulative 24 hours urine volume and sodium excretion induced by the various diuretic preparations studied indicate that frusemide, 40mg is not more potent than hydrochlorothiazide 50mg and that amiloride 5mg has a potency not too different from hydrochlorothiazide, 25mg. We therefore believe that the classification of diuretics into high, medium and low potency preparations is inappropriate and misleading and we suggest that they should be classified as rapid, intermediate and slow acting agents. Frusemide would be included in the "rapid-acting group", the thiazides in the "intermediate-acting group" and amiloride and triamterene in the "slow-acting group".

RENAL EFFECTS OF ALTERING RATIOS OF ENANTIOMERS OF INDACRINONE AND THE INFLUENCE OF AMILORIDE

F.H. NOORMOHAMED, W.R. McNABB and A.F. LANT.
Department of Therapeutics, Westminster Hospital, London SW1. ENGLAND.

INTRODUCTION

Racemic indacrinone (IND), (Figure 1) is a novel uricouric diuretic which has been shown to have its principal site of action in the thick ascending limb of Henle's loop [1,2]. Considerable difference exists in the renal sites of action as well as the natriuretic potencies of the resolved enantiomers of IND. The (-) enantiomer has been shown to act in the TAL whilst the (+) enantiomer acts in the cortical diluting segment of the early distal tubule [3]. In the present study we have studied the renal effects of altering the enantiomeric ratios of IND and the influence of amiloride on these responses.

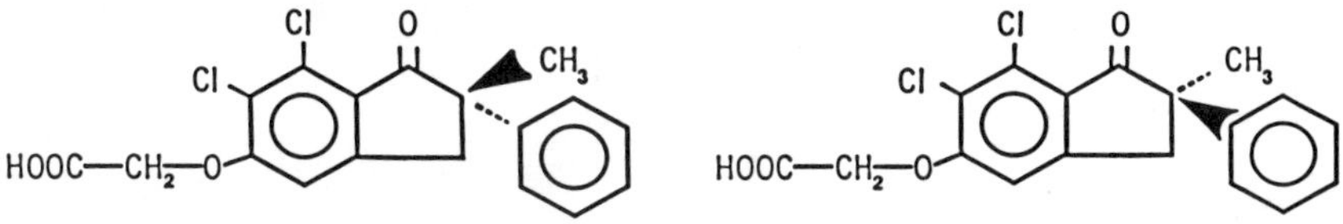

FIG 1. Enantiomers of Indacrinone.

METHOD

20 normal subjects received IND at various dose levels, alone and in combination with 5mg amiloride, in a double blind, placebo controlled study. A group of 12 subjects received 5/5 (-/+) IND and 10/10 (-/+) IND, whilst a second group of 8 subjects received 5/45 (-/+) IND with and without amiloride. Changes in plasma concentrations and renal excretion of electrolytes, urate, creatinine and pH were followed over 8 hours post dosing. All results are expressed as mean changes over matched control periods. Results were analysed using analysis of variance and students t-test with significance level $p<0.05$.

RESULTS

All doses of IND produced significant diuresis, saluresis and kaliuresis over 0-8 h period. The saluretic response was x 2.8 (5/5 IND); x3.3 (5/45 IND) and x 4.0 (10/10 IND) over control. The mean changes(0-8h) post-dosage over matched control are shown in Figure 2. A significant increase in excretion of magnesium was also seen with all three doses, (mmol/period) (+0.67±0.17, 5/5 IND; +1.30±0.21, 10/10 IND and +0.78±0.20, 5/45 IND) with an accompanying increase in calcium excretion seen only with 5/45 IND (+1.22±0.43 mmol/period). Excretion of urate increased by +30.6% (5/5 IND, $p<0.05$), +52.3%, 10/10 IND, $p<0.01$) and +47.6% (5/45 IND, $p<0.01$)

Published 1984 by Elsevier Science Publishing Co., Inc.
Diuretics, Jules B. Puschett, Editor

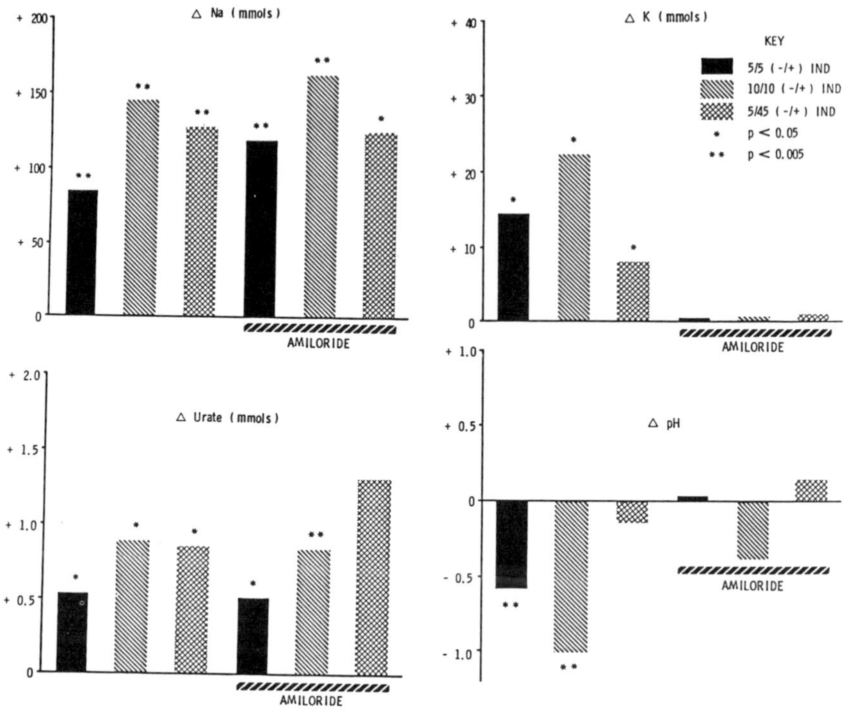

FIG 2 Changes in urinary parameters over matched controls (0-8 h)

over 0-8h. Addition of amiloride blunted the decrease in urinary pH ($p<0.05$) and kaliuresis seen with IND. A small additive natriuretic effect was seen with racemic IND whilst the excretion of magnesium was generally reduced by the addition of amiloride.

Plasma parameters remained largely unchanged with the exception of plasma urate. A fall in plasma urate concentration was seen only with 5/45 IND 4h post-dosage. (0.29 ± 0.02 compared to 0.38 ± 0.03 mmol/l on placebo).

DISCUSSION

All three doses of IND produced an effective diuresis. The saluresis produced by 5/45 IND was intermediate to that produced by the other two doses studied. Changes in urinary excretion of sodium, potassium, magnesium, urate and pH occurred in a dose-related fashion and were comparable to those reported previously [2]. In the absence of amiloride, the fractional excretion of sodium C_{Na} / C_{Cr} x 100%) increased from a control value of 0.62 ± 0.12% to 1.56 ± 0.15% with 5/5 IND and to 2.16 ± 0.13% with 10/10 IND in the group of 12 subjects, whilst in the second group of 8 subjects, fractional excretion of sodium increased from 0.54 ± 0.08% (control) to 1.63 ± 0.14% after 5/45 IND. The magnitudes of these changes in fractional excretion are similar to those reported for benzothiadiazines [4] and the uricosuric diuretic, tienilic acid [5].

Two of the most commonly encountered side effects associated with diuretic therapy are hypokalaemia and hyperuricaemia. Hypokalaemia can be alleviated by concurrent potassium supplements or by the addition of potassium sparing diuretics such as amiloride or triamterene. In the present study 5mg amiloride was very effective in producing an isokaliuretic response. Hyperuricaemia on the other hand has proved to be a more difficult problem to avoid on diuretic therapy. Introduction of a uricosuric diuretic such as indacrinone could therefore be a useful alternative. The uricosuric response of 5/45 IND equalled that of 10/10 IND in the presence of a lower natriuretic response indicating, that the (+) enantiomer can be an effective uric acid mobilizing agent. Changes in enantiomer ratios of IND can be effectively used to promote uric acid loss in absence of overt changes in extracellular fluid volume by diminishing the contribution of the saluretic potential of the (-) enantiomer of IND. In the present study a decrease in plasma urate was seen at 4h post dosage with 5/45 IND only. Long-term studies are currently in progress to see whether such a decrease can be seen on continued therapy.

REFERENCES

1. Brooks, B.A. Blair, E.M., Finch, R. and Lant, A.F. Br. J. clin. Pharmac., 10, 249-258. (1980)
2. Brooks, B.A., Lant, A.F., McNabb, W.R. and Noormohamed, F.H. Br. J. clin. Pharmac. 17, In press (1984)
3. Brooks, B.A., Lant, A.F., McNabb, W.R. and Noormohamed, F.H. Renal Physiol. 7, In press (1984)
4. Steinmuller, S.R., and Puschett, J.B. Kidney Internat. 11, 169-181 (1972)
5. Maas, A.R. and Snow, I.B. Postgrad. med. J. 55, (Suppl 3) 37-46 (1979).

THE DIURESIS IN CAPD PATIENTS (pts). THE EFFICACY OF A LOOP DIURETIC.

M. Querques, M. Ktena, P. delli Carri and A. Tappi.
Division of Nephrology and Dialysis, OO.RR. Foggia (Italy).

INTRODUCTION

Continuous Ambulatory Peritoneal Dialysis was introduced for the treatment of Uremia in 1976 (1). It has become an alternative treatment to Hemodialysis (2) (3). The role played by a loop diuretic (furosemide) in sustaining a strong diuresis during CAPD treatment, has been examined in a retrospective analysis.

Patients and Methods

31 pts. (17 males, 14 females) with a mean age of 56 ± 9,7 years (yrs) entered into the study as they began CAPD and have been followed for a cumulative period of 488 months (mts) (mean 15,7 ± 9,2) (range 3 - 34) tab. I.

The primary renal diseases included diabetic nephropathy (8), hypertensive nephropathy (6), interstitial nephritis (4), polycystic renal disease (4), chronic glomerulonephritis (5), SLE (1), gouty nephropathy (1) and unknown end-stage renal disease (2).

CAPD was carried out using standard techniques with 2 liter Viaflex (R) bags, and 3-4 exchanges/day.

The raccomanded diet contained 28 - 30 KCal and g. 1,2 of protein per Kg/body weight/day.

In the first 18 mts. the 24/hrs urine collection was performed twice a month in each patient. In the last 12 mts. all the patients were instructed to-perform the 24/hrs urine collection daily.

The values reported from patients didn't differ significantly from those observed during hospitalization (peritonitis, peritoneal clearances).

For statistical processing of the results it was used paired and unpaired t tests as well as linear regression analysis. Statistical significance was accepted at $p < 0{,}05$ levels. In the description of the results all values are expressed as means ± (SD).

Results

The patients were divided into two groups:
Group T: treated (18 pts; 3 diabetics)
Group NT: not treated (13 pts; 5diabetics).

Tab. I patients investigated

group	N°	age (yrs)	CAPD (mts)	GFR (ml/m')
T	18	56,4 ± 8,4	15,8 ± 9,4	4,5 ± 2,1
NT	13	55,1 ± 11,5	15,5 ± 9,2	° 2,6 ± 2,1

Diuretics, Jules B. Puschett, Editor

Tab. II 24/hrs diuresis (ml) and mean diuretic dosage (N°pts)

group	To	1-10(mts)	11-20	21-30
	(18)	(18)	(9)	(3)
T	1394 ± 589	1261 ± 640	1122 ± 591	1300 ± 781
NT	° 611 ± 545	° 273 ± 301	270 ± 421	150 ± 120
	(13)	(13)	(5)	(2)
furosemide mg/day	55 ± 31	66 ± 29	80 ± 17	93 ± 23

Tab. III biochemical parameters and body weght

glycemia mg%				
T	79 ± 20	82 ± 7	91 ± 22	91 ± 2
NT	105 ± 50	106 ± 43	102 ± 38	74 ± 21
triglyceridemia mg%				
T	152 ± 177	213 ± 189	217 ± 114	183 ± 96
NT	214 ± 170	263 ± 269	° 367 ± 154	295 ± 120
body weight Kg				
T	61 ± 9	64 ± 12	65 ± 14	70 ± 20
NT	61 ± 8	65 ± 14	71 ± 12	72 ± 8

Tab. IV hypertonic/isotonic solutions ratio

T	-----	1 / 5,8	1 / 4,7	1 / 3,7
NT	-----	1 / 4,1	1 / 3,7	1 / 3,2

° p 0,05

Discussion

Mean age and body weight were not significantly different at the beginning of CAPD treatment, whereas GFR (endogenous creatinine clearance) and 24/hrs diuresis were significantly different

($p < 0{,}05$) in the two groups (tab. I). In the treated group (T) the daily diuresis was uniform in the long run, whereas in the other group (NT) it was observed a significantly decrease in the first 10 mts of CAPD treatment (ml 611 vs 273; $p < 0{,}05$)

There was a direct relationship between 24/hrs diuresis and loop diuretic dosage ($r = 0{,}39$; $p < 0{,}05$). This relationship was closer during bouts of peritonitis (characterized by fluid retention). The higher glycemic levels in the NT group may be due both to the higher number of hypertonic solutions employed (tab. IV) and to the higher number of diabetic pts (five).

A correlation was found between weight gain, use of high dextrose solutions and change in plasma triglycerides (tab. III tab. IV).

Conclusions

The early use of loop diuretic (furosemide) in CAPD pts, plays a role in sustaining a strong diuresis in the long run and contributes to-reduce the use of hypertonic solutions, responsable of hyperglicemia, hypertriglyceridemia and increase in body weight. The hypertonic solutions may deteriorate the peritoneal membrane. Moreover the manteinance of diuresis exerts a benefical effect from a psichological viewpoint.

REFERENCES

1. Popovich RP, Moncrief JW, Decherd JB et al: Abstract Am. Soc. Artif. Intern. Organs. 5 , 64 (1976).
2. Popovich RP, Moncrief JW, Nolph KD et al: Ann. Intern. Med. 88 , 449-456 (1978).
3. Oreopoulos DG, Robson M, Izatt S et al: Trans. Am. Soc. Artif. Intern. Organs 24 , 484-487 (1978).

SECTION X

EXTRA-RENAL EFFECTS OF DIURETICS

Extrarenal effects of diuretics - Are prostanoids involved?

J.C. Frölich J. Filep H. Kroemer G. Fejes-Toth
Institute of Clinical Pharmacology Auerbachstr. 112 7000 Stuttgart 50 FRG

A highly desirable property of diuretics is their capability to lower peripheral resistance after chronic administration. Numerous suggestions have been made to explain this effect including changes in the kallikrein-kinin system, vascular electrolyte concentrations and, more recently, the prostaglandin system. However, while changes in all of these systems have been observed none have been proven conclusively to be causally responsible for the antihypertensive effect of diuretics. The lack of an antihypertensive effect of diuretics in dialysis patients could cast doubts on the significance of any extrarenal antihypertensive effects. However, there are many reasons why diuretics might not reduce blood pressure in these patients not the least of which is an expanded extracellular fluid volume.

There is clear evidence that some diuretics, in particular furosemide and bumetanide can cause an immediate reduction of renal vascular resistance (1, 2). Interestingly, this vascular effect seems to depend on prostanoids as it can be blocked by indomethacin (3). We reported already in 1976 that the diuretic action of furosemide can be blunted by indomethacin (4). An extensive discussion of the interaction has appeared elsewhere (5,6) and in contributions to this symposium. It has become apparent, that part of the interaction between furosemide and indomethacin may be due to pharmacokinetic interference. Thus, we found that the amount of furosemide excreted into the urine was lowered by indomethacin administration (4). The blunting of the diuretic effect of furosemide may, therefore, be in part the consequence of an interference with its intrarenal transport rather than an effect on prostaglandin synthesis as furosemide has to reach the tubular lumen to exert its diuretic effect.

Interpretation of biological effects following administration of indomethacin to block endogenous synthesis of prostanoids is hampered as indomethacin in addition to inhibiting cyclooxygenase has numerous other effects (15).

An alternate way to study the involvement of prostanoids in the action of diuretics is to study their effect on prostanoid synthesis. Indeed, administration of furosemide not only causes an acute rise

Published 1984 by Elsevier Science Publishing Co., Inc.
Diuretics, Jules B. Puschett, Editor

which in plasma renin activity is blocked by indomethacin (4, 6) but also increases urinary output of PGE_2 in man. As we have shown that urinary PGE_2 may reflect renal PGE_2 synthesis (7, 8) this action of furosemide might be thought to indicate enhanced renal PGE_2 synthesis. However, as we indicated earlier, such data need to be interpreted with greatest caution as PGE_2 is a weak acid and thus would be expected to be excreted flow and pH dependently (9). Indeed, studies from various laboratories have shown, that PGE_2 and PGF_{2a} excretion in dog and man is enhanced when urine flow increases (10, 11, 12). Recent studies from our laboratory indicate, that this may be true for prostanoid metabolites as well (unpublished).

There are, however, important species differences with respect to flow dependency of prostanoid excretion. A recent study carried out in our laboratory showed that in the rat in contrast to man, enhancement of urine flow by induction of an osmotic diuresis or hyposmolar volume expansion or administration of furosemide did not increase the urinary excretion of prostanoids (13). Thus, the rat would appear to be a useful model to study the effect of a diuretic on prostanoid synthesis.

When considering the type of prostanoid to study with respect to vascular resistance one has to realize that the most abundant prostanoid released from isolated perfused or incubated resistance vessels is PGI_2. Its major metabolite in the circulation and appearing in urine after intravenous administration is 6-keto-PGF_{1a} (14). Thus, we decided to measure this substance in the urine of awake rats previously prepared with chronic bladder canulae (13). After a 120 min control period (period 1) 1 mg/kg of piretanide was given i.p. and urine collected for 30 min (period 2), a first post-drug control period of 60 min (period 3) and a second post drug control period of 120 min (period 4). Piretanide caused a prompt increase of sodium excretion from $0.55 \pm 0,65$ u m/min to 14.5 ± 2.0 u m/min ($p < 0.05$). 6-keto-PGF_{1a} excretion determined by radioimmunoassay also showed a significant 200 % increase (Fig. 1). These data strongly suggest that piretanide causes an increase in the synthesis of the vasodilator prostacyclin. Whether stimulated prostacyclin synthesis contributes to the known antihypertensive and after-load reducing effect of piretanide remains to be elucidated.

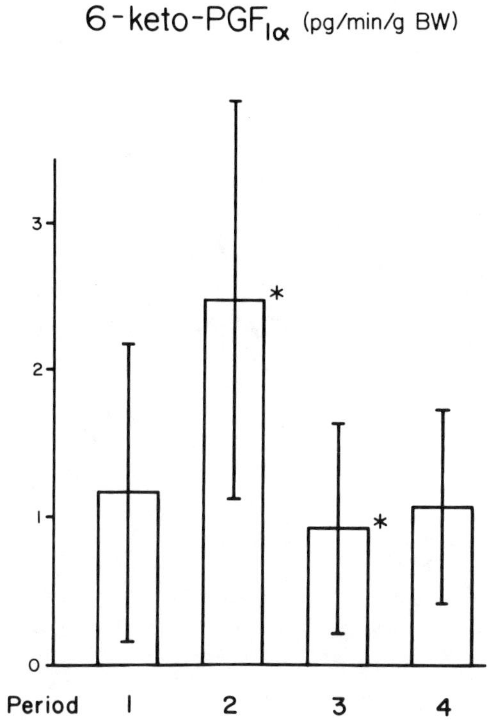

Legend Fig.1 Effect of piretanide (1 mg/kg i.p.) on urinary 6-keto-PGF_{1a}. 1:Control period 1 of 120 min duration, 2: 30 min period following piretanide, 3: first post-piretanide control period of 60 min duration, 4: second post-piretanide control period of 120 min. duration.

References

1. Vorburger, C., A.M. Harvey and R.L. Malvin: Direkter Nachweis der renalen Hyperämie nach intravenöser Injektion von Furosemid beim Hund.
Arch. Pharmak. exp. Path. 261: 346-352 (1968)

2. Olsen, U.B. and Ahnfelt-Ronne, I.: Bumetanide induced increase of renal blood flow in conscious dogs and its relation to local renal hormones.
Acta pharmacol. toxicol.38:219-228 (1976)

3. Olsen, U.B.: Indomethacin inhibition of bumetanide diuresis in dogs.
Acta pharmacol. toxicol. (Kbh) 37: 65-78 (1975)

4. Frölich, J.C., Hollifield, J.W., Dormois, J.C., Seyberth, H.J., Michelakis A.M., Oates, J.A.: Suppression of plasma renin activity by indomethacin in man.
Circ. Res. 39:447-452 (1976)

5. Nies, A.S., S. Fadul, J. Gal and J.G. Gerber: Indomethacin - furosemide interaction: The importance of renal blood flow.
J. Pharmacol. Exptl. Therap. 226: 27-32, 1983

6. Oliw, E., Köver, G., Larsson, C., and Änggard, E.: Reduction by indomethacin of furosemide effects in the rabbit.
Eur. J. Pharmacol. 38: 95 (1976)

7. Frölich, J.C., Wilson, T.W., Sweetman, B.J., Smigel, M., Nies, A.S., Carr, K., Watson, J.T. and Oates, J.A.: Urinary prostaglandins: Identification and origin.
J. Clin. Invest. 55:763-770 (1975)

8. Williams, W.M., Frölich, J.C., Nies, A.S. and Oates, J.A.: Urinary prostaglandins: Site of entry into renal tubular fluid.
Kidney International 11:256-260 (1977)

9. Frölich, J.C., Gill, J.R.,McGiff, J.C., Needleman, P. and Nies, A.S.: Prostaglandins. Subgroup Report of the Hypertension Task Force. DHEW Publication No(NIH) 79-1629, US Government Printing Office, Washington p. 1-98 (1979)

10. Kaye, J., R. Zipser, J. Hahn, P. Zia and R. Horton. Water Diuresis is a major regulator of prostaglandin E excretion in man. Advances in Prostaglandin and Thromboxane Research. 7, ed. by B. Samuelsson, P.W. Ramwell and R. Paoletti. Raven Press, New York, 1980, p. 1017

11. Kirschenbaum, M., E. Serros. Effects of alterations in urine flow rate on prostaglandin E excretion in conscious dogs.
Am. J. Physiol. 238: F107-F111 (1980)

12. Wright, L.F., S.G. Rosenblatt and M.D. Lifschitz. High urine flow rate increases prostaglandin E excretion in the conscious dog.
Prostaglandins 22: 21-34 (1981)

13. Fejes-Tóth, G., A. Náray-Fejes-Toth, B. Rigter and Jürgen C. Frölich: Urinary prostaglandin and kallikrein excretion are not flow dependent in the rat.
Prostaglandins 25, 99-103 (1983)

14. Rosenkranz, B., Fischer, C., Weimer, K.E., and Frölich, J.C.: Metabolism of prostacyclin and 6- keto- prostaglandin F_{1a} in man.
J.Biol. Chem. 255:10194-10198 (1980)

15. Flower,R.J.: Drugs which inhibit prostaglandin biosynthesis.
Pharmacol. Reviews. 26: 33-67 (1974)

CARDIOVASCULAR EFFECTS OF DIURETICS IN MAN

Jochen Schaefer, M.D.
Kurklinik Kueppelsmuehle, 6482 Bad Orb and
Christian-Albrechts-Universitaet Kiel, 2300 Kiel, FRG

ABSTRACT

The application of diuretics of various chemical structure and differing biological sites of action and time-courses leads to profound changes in the cardiovascular system. The effects on left ventricular performance of diuretics alone in patients with chronic ischemic heart failure also clearly demonstrate the impact of these drugs in reducing left heart filling pressure both at rest and during exercise. Due to the complicated pathophysiological situation in various disease states the extent and the grade of these changes cannot be quantitatively assessed in a reliable fashion. Therefore, it seems to be mandatory to use diuretics with caution being aware of their profound actions on the water and electrolyte content of the normal and diseased person and the resulting changes and alterations of the cardiovascular system.

CARDIOVASCULAR EFFECTS OF DIURETICS IN MAN

Diuretics are increasingly used in the therapy of cardiac patients and have gained considerable importance in the treatment of acute and chronic cardiac failure. To a certain extent they seem to be able to replace cardiac glycosides.

Before reviewing our knowledge on the cardiovascular effects of diuretics in man, I want to introduce a few terminological aspects of the subject which I shall cover in my talk.

a) The term cardiovascular effects of course is widely chosen and may incorporate many different parameters and variables of the cardiovascular system such as cardiac output, peripheral and pulmonary pressure, pulmonary and total blood volume, venous and arterial impedance, heart rate, ventricular chamber sizes and filling pressures. - The role of these parameters is evident in the complicated regulatory system of various cardiovascular determinants. A change in any one may influence alterations in the others.

b) Diuretics are those substances which act on the total body's composition of water and electrolyte content. They by this very action interfere with the complex chains of reflexes which are responsible for the homoiostatic regulation of the cardiovascular system. Diuretics which are used today in the clincal setting consist of a very heterogeneous group of substances. They have

Diuretics, Jules B. Puschett, Editor

quite different sites of actions in the kidney. And besides this they have extrarenal effects, which may influence the cardiovascular system. In addition, they differ in their short, fast and long acting efficacies, thus introducing an important time variable, which according to the changes induced by them in the water and electrolyte content of the body, may gain considerable impact on the dynamical interactions of the various cardiovascular subsystems. In addition, the nature of these interactions may differ with the severity of disease in its various stages.

c) When I chose the term man instead of patient in the title of this lecture, I wanted to have the liberty to discuss various aspects of the cardiovascular effects of diuretics as well in the non-diseased normovolumic subject as in the diseased with the signs of acute or chronic cardiac failure of various origins.

Having introduced these aspects of my talk I want to mainly concentrate on the following points:

1. Cardiovascular effects of fast and short-acting diuretics in the normovolumic subject.

2. Cardiovascular effects of fast-acting diuretics in the patient with acute myocardial infarction (and patients with coronary artery disease).

3. Cardiovascular effects of diuretics in the patients with chronic cardiac insufficiency and coronary artery disease.

4. Finally I want to mention the limitations in measuring and assessing the changes in cardiovascular parameters in patients who are sick (1).

With regard to the first point, in normovolumic patients the short-acting diuretics Furosemid and Piretanid reduce cardiac output and pressures in the pulmonary circulation, whereas systemic vascular resistance increases significantly. Both drugs slightly increase pulmonary blood volume but not significantly. Total blood volume decreases less rapidly than cardiac output, so that the ratio of cardiac output to total blood volume decreases with time. Both drugs seem to enhance venous compliance in normovolumic subjects and probably increase the compliance of the pulmonary vasculature (2). In addition a lowering of the left ventricular end diastolic pressure was observed. These changes are probably not only due to the fall in total blood volume but also to the marked water and salt diuresis caused by both substances.

It has been long known however (3) that an acute fall in left ventricular filling pressure occurs within a few minutes after the intravenous administration of the drug, before a diuretic response is apparent. This effect was thought to be due to a direct action of Furosemid on venous capacitance, thus reducing venous return dramatically. Recently it could be shown, however, that the early effect of Furosemid to increase venous capacitance in man requires functioning kidneys, a salt retaining state, and prostaglandin synthesis. Individuals without renal function or who are receiving indomethacin, do not show increased venous capacitance in the lower extremity which is the early effect of Furosemid (4).

Thus the early non-diuretic vascular effect of Furosemid on venous capacitance in humans is dependent on salt balance, prostaglandin synthesis, and renal function. A high salt intake, indomethacin and the lack of renal function will abolish the ability of Furosemid to produce effects on venous capacitance in man, whereas these factors do not influence the venodilatory response to nitroglycerin as Johnston et al. (4) recently described.

With regard to the point number two, in acute heart failure during acute myocardial infarction Furosemid has profound effects on left ventricular filling pressure and to a certain extent also on cardiac output (5). Sometimes however cardiac output may drop drastically, maybe because the left ventricular filling pressure declined too much. Kiely et al., (6) therefore cautioned the use of Furosemid or similarly fast acting saluretic drugs as the treatment of first choice in patients with acute left heart failure. To my knowledge no comparable data is available as to the effect of other diuretics in acute heart failure such as thiazides and similar substances. In spite of the often drastic improvement of the clinical condition after the injection of short and fast acting diuretics it is open to question up until now, if survival rate is really improved (7).

Also in the less dramatic phases of coronary arterial disease or some time after the survival of an acute myocardial infarction the application of short-acting diuretics leads to a lessened increase of pulmonary arterial pressure during exercise (8). Comparable findings were obtained by Nechwatal et al. (9) with Furosemid. Similar results were reported after the application of 12 mg Piretanid showing that mean as well as diastolic pulmonary arterial pressures declined (10).

With regard to the third point, it is a common clinical experience that marked subjective and objective improvement may follow diuresis in patients with chronic heart failure, but this accepted clinical fact appears to have attracted little investigative interest (7). In 18 patients with chronic heart failure due to a variety of causes Rader et al. (11) found large reductions in the right atrial, right ventricular and pulmonary artery pressures without substantial decrease in cardiac output after diuresis induced by mercurial diuretics at that time. Stampfer et al (12) observed also the short term effects of the addition of thiazide diuretics to digitalis in 15 patients with valvular heart disease. The resulting diuresis was accompanied by significant reductions, both in the pulmonary vascular pressures and cardiac output at rest and during treadmill exercise. Also, the duration of exercise was found to increase. Similar effects could be observed in patients with mitral valvular disease who received either Furosemid or ethacrynic acid (13).

The effects on left ventricular performance of diuretics alone in patients with chronic ischemic heart failure have also clearly demonstrated the impact of these drugs on various hemodynamic parameters and variables. Wilson et al (14) showed an improved performance of the failing left ventricle though left ventricular diastolic dimension was not altered as assessed by tm mode echocardiography.

In patients without overt signs of hydropic cardiac insufficiency Schaefer and Sievert (15) and Valette et al. (16) found a significant decrease in left ventricular filling pressure, measured by pulmonary capillary pressure, and in total and pulmonary vascular resistance as well as an increase in cardiac output after three weeks of treatment with 30 mg of Hydrochlorothiazide and Triamteren 60 mg per day. Similar observations were reported by Bauer et al (17) after chronic treatment with low dose Piretanid (6 mg per day).

The exact mechanisms by which diuretics achieve their action in heart failure is not entirely clear. There seems to be some evidence that their hemodynamic results are related to their site of action in the renal tubule (7). - Thiazide diuretics largely induce their circulatory effects by reduction in the blood volume whereas the loop diuretics may also incorporate an element of venodilation, under the conditions as outlined above, in their overall circulatory effects.

With regard to the final point, in spite of rather long-standing clinical experience with using diuretics in patients with various cardiovascular afflictions it has remained difficult to exactly measure and assess the effects of these quite different pharmacological agents on the cardiovascular system. Mainly three reasons may be responsible for this dilemma:

a) The patient with acute or chronic heart failure is never in a stage of a so-called stable equilibrium. The disease process itself as well as the effects of the drugs applied cause non--steady-state conditions which do not allow to obtain a really stable situation in which measurements can be made which are pertinent to the clinical and to the pathophysiological situation in which the patient is at this very moment.

b) The quality and the kind of measurements that can be reliably performed under the conditions of severe sickness and illness differ very much. In a rather critical review on this subject

Taylor et al (1) put together various notes of cautions which show that only very few clinically applicable measurements fulfill the criteria of being acceptable to evaluate cardiovascular effects or changes during or under the treatment with diuretics.

c) In spite of the widespread use of diuretics in the treatment of cardiac diseases there is no clear cut proof that survival is improved by the sole or the combined therapy with diuretics. This may seem disappointing to most of us since the subjective improvement which usually can be seen after the introduction of a therapy with diuretics and which in many cases seems to be supplemented by objective improvement as to various clinical parameters is sometimes impressive but does not show up in an improved prognosis (7). The reason for this may be that the chronic nature of the underlying cause of the disease cannot be changed. In so far only prophylactic improvement, which in itself is an important therapeutic goal, can be achieved.

In summary then it can be stated that the application of diuretics of various chemical structure and very differing biological sites of action and time-courses leads to profound changes in the cardiovascular system. The effects on left ventricular performance of diuretics alone in patients with chronic ischemic heart failure have also clearly demonstrated the impact of these drugs in reducing left heart filling pressure both at rest and during exercise. Due to the complicated pathophysiological situation in various disease states the extent and the grade of these changes cannot be quantitatively assessed in a reliable fashion. Therefore, it seems to be mandatory to use these substances with caution being aware of their profound actions on the water and electrolyte content of the normal and diseased person and the consecutively resulting changes and alterations of the cardiovascular system.

References

1. Taylor, S.H., Proceedings of the European Prazosin Symposium. Excerpta Medica. Amsterdam Oxford (1978) pp.101-132
2. Valette, H., Hebert, J.L., Raffestin, B., Lockhart, H., Apoil, E., J. Cardiovasc Pharmacol (1980) 2:103-111
3. Dikshit, K., Vyden, J.K., Forrester, J.S., Chatterjee, K., Prakash, R., Swan, H.J.C., New Engl. J. Med. (1973) 288: 1087-1090
4. Johnston, J.D., Hiatt, W.R., Nies, A.S., Payne, N.A., Murphy, R.C., Gerber, J.G., Circ. Research (1983) 53:630-635
5. Taylor, S.H., Silke, B., Nelson., G.I.C., European Heart Journal (1982) 3:Suppl. D, 19-43
6. Kiely, J., Kelly, D.T., Taylor, D.R., Pitt, B., Circulation (1973) 48:581-587
7. Taylor, S.H., Storstein, L., European Heart Journal (1983) 4:Suppl. A, 153-159

8. Schroeder, R., Arzneimittelforschung. (1977) 27:722-728
9. Nechwatal, W., Z. f. Kardiologie (1978) 67:116-12177
10. Nechwatal, W. Stange, A., Sigel, H., Kress, P., Resch, A., Stauch, M., Herz/Kreislauf (1982) 14:91-96
11. Rader, B., Smith, W.W., Barger, A.R., Eichna, L.W., Circulation (1964) 29:328-345
12. Stampfer, M., Epstein, St.E., Beiser, G.D., Braunwald, E., Circulation (1968) 37:900-911
13. Austin, St.M., Schreiner, B.F., Kramer, D.H., Shah, P.M., Yu, P.N., Circulation (1976) 53:364-369
14. Wilson, J.R., Reichek, N., Dunkman, W.B., Goldberg, Sh., Am. J. Med. (1981) 70:234-239
15. Schaefer, G.E., Sievert, H., Deutsche Med. Wsch. (1983) 108:764-766
16. Valette, H., Hebert, J.L., Apoil, E., Eur. J. Clin. Pharmacol (1983) 24:163-167
17. Bauer, U., Frick, G., Mouselimis, N., Cernoch, K., Fehske, K.J., Herz/Kreislauf (1983) 15:493-500

DIURETIC ANTIHYPERTENSIVE TREATMENT: EVIDENCE FOR ALTERATION OF INTRACELLULAR Ca^{++} BY HORMONAL SUPPRESSION

Vetter, H., Losse, H., Heckmann, U., Zidek, W.
Med. Univ.-Poliklinik, Albert-Schweitzer-Str. 33, D-4400 Münster, F. R. Germany (phone 0251 838001)

INTRODUCTION

As to the pathogenesis of essential hypertension several partly contradictory theories have been proposed in the last years. From these suggestions two seem to be of major concern:

1. The " electrolyte theory": In essential hypertensives as well as in spontaneously hypertensive rats a generalized disturbance of cellular electrolyte metabolism has been found. In red blood cells [1-3], lymphocytes [4] and in arterial smooth muscle cells [5] elevated free Na^+ and Ca^{++} concentrations have been demonstrated. These results correspond with earlier findings that intracellular Na^+ concentration in red blood cells is elevated in essential hypertension [6-10]. From studies on intracellular electrolyte content and transmembraneous electrolyte fluxes in normotensive relatives of essential hypertensives an inborn defect of transmembraneous ion transport has been suggested [1, 11].
2. The "humoral theory": Indications for the role of humoral factors in the pathogenesis of essential hypertension have mainly been drawn from the observations that in plasma and urine of essential hypertensives a substance with natriuretic properties inhibiting active cellular Na^+ extrusion was demonstrated [12]. However, the existence as well as the nature of such substances remained speculative up to now.

In the present study we tried to reconcile the "electrolyte theory" with the "humoral theory" by demonstrating some important links between the humoral pathogenesis of hypertension and electrolyte metabolism. As will be shown, these interconnections give important insights into the mechanisms, by which antihypertensive treatment, e.g. with diuretics, may be effective. The studies were performed in spontaneously hypertensive rats and in essential hypertensives.

METHODS

The animal studies were performed in spontaneously hypertensive rats from the Münster strain aged 3-5 months. Systolic blood pressure was 170-200 mm Hg as measured by tail plethysmography. In a first series of experiments parabiotic rats were made by connecting two animals. In the flank the skin was removed over an area of about 3 x 4 cm. Then the lateral abdominal muscles and the skin were sewed together. The parabiotic animals were then observed for 3 weeks. In these experiments 14 spontaneously hypertensive rats were connected to normotensive Wistar rats, and 20 normotensive rats were coupled as controls.

In another series of experiments the circulations of two rats were connected by a peristaltic pump, which pumped blood from the carotid artery of one rat into the external jugular vein of the other, and vice versa. By this cross-perfusion no changes of blood volume in a single rat occurred. The pump shifted 5 ml blood/min in each direction. Blood pressure was measured manometrically by a plastic catheter inserted into the common carotid artery.

The human studies were performed in 14 essential hypertensives who had previously been untreated, aged 21 to 68. Blood pressure and intracellular Na^+ and Ca^{++} activities in red blood cells were measured before as well as 2 and 6 weeks after starting a treatment with the loop diuretic, piretanide, in a dosis of 12 mg daily. Measurements of intracellular Na^+ and Ca^{++} ac-

Diuretics, Jules B. Puschett, Editor

tivities in red blood cells were performed with ion-selective electrodes [1] after washing the red blood cells in an isotonic solution containing choline hydrogen tartrate with 5 mmol/l NaCl. With this washing procedure lower and more constant values of intracellular Ca^{++} activities could be achieved than using an isotonic $MgCl_2$ solution.

RESULTS

Tab. 1 shows the changes in blood pressure occurring in parabiotic rats. In normotensive rats connected with spontaneously hypertensive animals blood pressure increased during three weeks continuously. On the other hand, there was no significant change in blood pressure in the spontaneously hypertensive animals connected with normotensive rats, and in the couples with normotensive rats.

TABLE 1. Mean values and standard deviations of changes in systolic blood pressure during 3 weeks of parabiosis (NT = normotensive, SH = spontaneously hypertensive).

rats	Systolic blood pressure (mm Hg) 1 week	2 weeks	3 weeks
SH rats connected to NT rats	$-1,3 \pm 8,1$	$-4,5 \pm 9,8$	$1,7 \pm 12,6$
NT rats connected to SH rats	$21,9 \pm 9,5$ §	$25,5 \pm 9,9$ §	$36,3 \pm 11,1$ §
normotensive couples	$0,8 \pm 6,3$	$0,5 \pm 7,6$	$-1,25 \pm 7,44$

§ = $p < 0,01$

Fig. 1 shows the changes in blood pressure when parabiosis is made by connecting the circulations through the great vessels, using a peristaltic pump for perfusion. When cross-perfusion is performed for 30 min with a spontaneously hypertensive and a normotensive rat, mean blood pressure increased in the normotensive and decreased in the spontaneously hypertensive rat. When a spontaneously hypertensive rat was used after removal of 3-5 ml bloof from the circulation, no increase in blood pressure could be elicited in the normotensive rat during cross-perfusion (Fig. 1).

In Fig. 2 the course of mean blood pressure and of intracellular Na^+ and Ca^{++} activity in red blood cells from essential hypertensives during treatment with piretanide is displayed. Blood pressure decreased from $156,4 \pm 13,9/104,6 \pm 6,0$ to $148,2 \pm 15,0/94,6 \pm 8,9$ and $135,7 \pm 10,7/90,0 \pm 6,2$ mm Hg after 2 and 6 weeks. Intracellular Ca^{++} activity decreased from $6,01 \pm 2,04$ to $3,10 \pm 1,06$ ($p < 0,01$) and $4,01 \pm 2,07$ µmol/l cell water after 2 and 6 weeks. Intracellular Na^+ activity showed a tendency to increase during treatment. Intracellular Na^+ activity was $8,61 \pm 1,87$ mmol/l cell water before treatment and was $9,78 \pm 2,23$ and $10,68 \pm 2,19$ mmol/l cell water after 2 and 6 weeks.

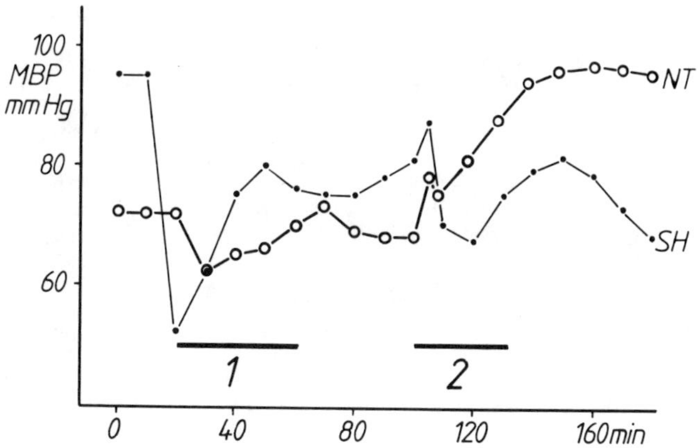

FIG. 1. Changes of mean blood pressure in a normotensive (open circles) and a spontaneously hypertensive rat (filled circles) during cross-perfusion. 1: cross-perfusion after removal of 3 ml blood in the spontaneously hypertensive rat. 2: cross-perfusion after injection of 5 ml 1,8 % NaCl solution in the spontaneously hypertensive rat.

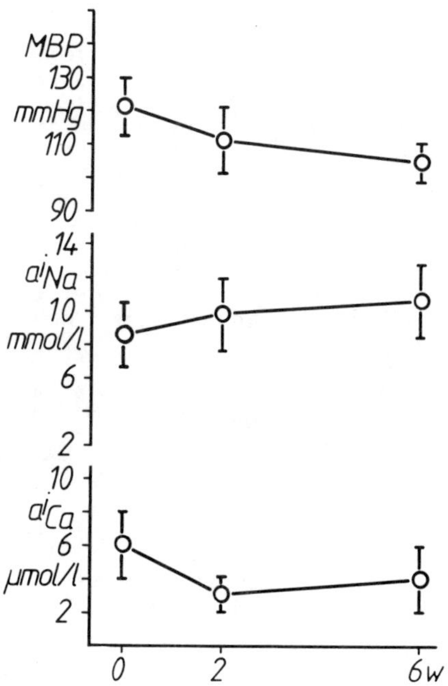

FIG. 2. Mean values and standard deviations of mean arterial blood pressure, intracellular Na^+ and Ca^{++} activities (a^i_{Na}, a^i_{Ca}) before as well as 2 and 6 weeks after starting treatment with 12 mg piretanide daily in 14 previously untreated essential hypertensives.

DISCUSSION

The analysis of relationships between the results in spontaneously hypertensive rats and in essential hypertensives appears to give important insights into the mechanisms of action of diuretics in the treatment of hypertension. As to the mode of action of diuretics in hypertension several theories have been proposed. On the one hand, diuretics were felt to induce hypovolemia, thus influencing blood pressure by a reduced stroke volume [13]. On the other hand it was shown that the blood pressure lowering effect of diuretics is not correlated with the hypovolemia. An additional important effect of diuretic antihypertensive treatment appeared to be the decrease of total peripheral resistance [14]. However, it has not been clarified conclusively up to now, by which mechanisms diuretics lower total peripheral resistance [15]. This problem may be further elucidated analyzing the alterations in the pathomechanisms of essential hypertension during diuretic treatment.

As to the pathomechanisms of essential hypertension, it is now possible to reconcile the aforementioned "electrolyte theory" and the "humoral theory". It has been demonstrated in several studies that in essential hypertension intracellular Na^{+} and Ca^{++} activities are elevated in red blood cells [1-3]. Some years ago these alterations in cellular electrolyte metabolism appeared to represent an "inborn error of metabolism" of cell membranes, i.e. an inherited defect of ion transport. In the aforementioned experiments it emerged then that primary hypertension can be transmitted by humoral factors, as was shown for salt-dependent hypertension in Dahl rats [16]. Therefore the described electrolyte abnormalities can rather be regarded as an effect of an unknown humoral factor than as an intrinsic membrane defect.

From this conception as well as from the cross-perfusion experiments described above the following mode of action can be suggested for the diuretics: Diuretics lower intracellular Ca^{++} but not intracellular Na^{+}. From the role of Ca^{++} ions in the activation processes of actomyosin filaments, resulting in an enhanced contractility of vascular smooth muscle with increasing Ca^{++} concentrations, the direct relationship between total peripheral resistance and intracellular free Ca^{++} is apparent. On the other hand the failure of diuretics to lower intracellular Na^{+} is in accordance with the view that intracellular free Na^{+} is not correlated with actual blood pressure, but rather represents a marker for the genetic disposition to hypertension [1]. The slight increase in intracellular Na^{+} activity in red blood cells during diuretic treatment can be expected from the ionic mechanisms in tubular cells leading to natriuresis, as an increased intracellular Na^{+} in renal tubular cells impairs Na^{+} diffusion from the tubular lumen into the tubular cells and then the peritubular space.

The cause, why diuretics lower intracellular free Ca^{++} and, as a corollary, blood pressure, lies in a suppression of the humoral factors associated with primary hypertension. This can be concluded from the cross-perfusion experiments shown above, since a hypovolemia suppresses the humoral factor. It is generally accepted that during diuretic treatment in the essential hypertensive patient similarly a state of slight hypovolemia is produced. If we assume that the same mechanisms are acting as in the spontaneously hypertensive rat, the hypertensive humoral factor is suppressed during diuretic treatment, which in turn leads to lower intracellular free Ca^{++}. The suppression of the factor by hypovolemia, which can be shown in the spontaneouslY hypertensive rat, is in accordance with the hypothesis, that this substance may act as a natriuretic factor [12], since a suppression of a natriuretic factor in hypovolemia is physiologically highly appropriate.

The nature of the hypothetical humoral factor is not clarified up to now. The cross-perfusion experiments show that the regulation of this factor is a very fast process acting within minutes. This can be concluded (1) from the rapid increase in blood pressure in the normotensive animal connected to a spontaneously hypertensive rat occurring within 10 min and (2) from the immediate effetc of hypovolemia on the level of the humoral factor in the spontaneously hypertensive rat, which is demonstrated by the failure to induce an increase in blood pressure in the normotensive rat.

In summary from the results demonstrated it can be concluded (1) that in primary hypertension the elevation of intracellular Ca^{++}, which is associated with vasoconstriction, is mediated by humoral factors and (2) that these factors can be suppressed by hypovolemia. By this mechanism hypovolemia, including diuretic-induced hypovolemia, can lower intracellular free Ca^{++} and thus normalize blood pressure.

REFERENCES

1. W. Zidek, H. Losse, K.G. Dorst, H. Zumkley and H. Vetter, Klin. Wschr. 60, 859-862 (1982).

2. W. Zidek, H. Vetter, K.G. Dorst, H. Zumkley and H. Losse, Clin. Sci. 63, 41s-43s (1982).

3. P.Baumgart, W. Zidek, H. Losse, Ch. Karoff, M. Wehling, W. Vetter and H. Vetter, Klin. Wschr. 61, 803-805 (1983).

4. W. Zidek, M. Knorr, H. Losse, P. Baumgart and H. Vetter, J. Hypertension, in press (1984).

5. W. Zidek, T. Kerenyi, H. Losse and H. Vetter, Res. Exp. Med. 183, 129-132 (1983).

6. E. Ambrosioni, F. Tartagni, L. Montebugnoli and B. Magnani, Clin. Sci. 57, 325s-327s (1979).

7. A. Fadeke-Aderounmu and A. Salako, Eur. J. Clin. Invest. 9, 369-375 (1979).

8. J.M. Hamlyn, R. Ringel, J. Schaeffer, P.D. Levinson, B.P. Hamilton, A.A. Kovarski and M.P. Blaustein, Nature 300, 650-652 (1982).

9. N.C. Henningsen, S. Mattson, B. Nosslin, D. Nelson and O. Ohlsson, Clin. Sci. 57, 321s-323s (1979).

10. A. Montanari, L. Borghi, M. Canali, A. Curti, P. Perinotti, A. Novarini and A. Borghetti in: Intracellular electrolytes and arterial hypertension, H. Zumkley and H. Losse, eds. (Thieme, Stuttgart 1980) pp. 135-143.

11. F. Wessels, G. Junge-Hülsing and H. Losse, Z. Kreislaufforsch. 56, 374-380 (1967).

12. D.A. MacGregor and H.E. De Wardener, Clin. Exp. Hypertension 3, 815-830 (1981).

13. I.M. Wilson and E.D. Freis, Circulation 20, 1028-1032 (1959).

14. J. Conway and P. Lauwers, Circulation 21, 21-27 (1960).

15. E.D. Freis in: Systemic effects of antihypertensive agents, M.P. Sambhi, ed. (Symposia Specialists, New York 1976) pp. 41-49.

16. L.K. Dahl, K.D. Knutsen and J. Iwai, Circ. Res. 24/25, 21-33 (1969).

CHLORIDE IONS IN VASCULAR SMOOTH MUSCLE

V.A.W. KREYE, F. GERSTHEIMER, M. MÜHLEISEN, D. NEHRING, AND K. WALTER
IInd Department of Physiology, University of Heidelberg,
Im Neuenheimer Feld 326, D-6900 Heidelberg, Fed. Rep. of Germany

INTRODUCTION

Little is known of the functional role of chloride ions in vascular smooth muscle (vsm), but their involvement in noradrenaline-induced vasoconstriction, and in vasodilatation induced by nitro-compounds such as sodium nitroprusside, nitroglycerin, and isosorbide dinitrate has been suggested (1,2). Using different methods of determination in various laboratories, the cellular chloride content of vsm has been found to be very large; values ranging from 30 to 90 mM were measured, and correspondingly, the calculated Nernst equilibrium potentials ranged from -40 to -11 mV which is considerably lower than the measured membrane potential of vsm (for review see (3,4)). Although these data suggest that chloride ions are not passively distributed across the cell membrane of vsm, intracellular binding and compartmentalization was assumed to underlie the high chloride content of vsm (5). No such mechanisms could be demonstrated however, by the use of the electron probe technique; instead, a high cytosolic chloride content in vsm was found, and a plea for the existence of an active chloride transport in vsm was made (6).

Here, we present evidence for a "furosemide-sensitive chloride transport" in vsm, and some very recent data on the possible mechanisms involved in this process. The effect of diuretic drugs, of chloride substitution by large non-permeant anions, and of bicarbonate withdrawal on transmembrane ion movements in the isolated rabbit aorta, and on the membrane potential of the isolated rabbit main pulmonary artery were investigated. Some of the material presented here has been published in detail (7) or abstract form (8,9,10).

METHODS

Ion flux studies

Steady-state ion exchanges (SSE) and unidirectional ion effluxes were studied by the dipping method (3, for references) on pieces (8 to 20 mg) of rabbit aorta from which the adventitia had been removed. After equilibration for 1 h in physiological salt solution (PSS), they were loaded for 2 h in PSS containing the radioactive nuclide (36-Cl or 86-Rb). Subsequently, by the use of a circular fraction collector and an electropneumatic hoisting device, the tissues were transported at fixed intervals of 1 or 2 min, and under permanent rotation, through a series of liquid scintillation vessels containing 5 ml of unlabelled washing solution (i.e. normal PSS, or salt solution with altered ion contents, or PSS containing drugs). - Determination of intracellular chloride concentration was based on the same type of study, i.e. SSE of 36-Cl in normal or furosemide-containing PSS. Subsequently, the method of residuals ("curve peeling") on curves relating time with the tissue content of 36-Cl was applied. The parameters of the resulting tri-exponential equation were used for the calculation of cellular compartments assuming a mixed mammillary-catenary multi-compartment system (for details see (7)). - For influx studies, equilibrated tissues were loaded for periods ranging from 1 to 10 min, and then washed in ice-cold PSS for 60 min in order to trap cytosolic nuclide inside the cell, and to remove extracellularly bound nuclide.

Microelectrode and contraction studies

Electric membrane potentials were measured with glass microelectrodes in

Diuretics, Jules B. Puschett, Editor

rabbit main pulmonary arteries, because this tissues permits better penetrations than the rabbit aorta. Microelectrodes (resistance 50-100 megohms) were made from Omega Dot capillary tubing HR-30-30-1, F.Haer and Co., Brunswick, ME/USA.- Isometric contraction studies were performed on helical strips of rabbit aorta by standard organ bath technique using Grass FT .03 force transducers.

Solutions and drugs

All experiments were done at 37 centigrade. Normal PSS was of the following composition (in mM): NaCl 128, KCl 4.7, NaH2PO4 1.2, NaHCO3 11.9, CaCl2 2.5, MgCl2 1.2, Ca-Na-EDTA 0.1, glucose 10, gassed with 95 % oxygen/ 5 % carbon dioxide mixture (pH=7.2). The salts used were of reagent grade (E. Merck, Darmstadt). - DIDS (4,4'-diisothiocyano-2,2'-disulfonic acid) was purchased from Sigma-Chemie GmbH, Taufkirchen. Diuretics (furosemide, piretanide, ethacrynic acid, hydrochlorothiazide,and amiloride) were kindly provided by Hoechst AG., Frankfurt; Merck and Dohme GmbH., München; and CIBA-GEIGY GmbH., Wehr).

RESULTS

Evidence for a "furosemide-sensitive" chloride transport in vsm

Furosemide, at a concentration of 1 mM, was found to interfere promptly and potently with the 36-Cl/Cl SSE in rabbit aorta (fig.1); the rate of SSE, i.e. the fractional loss of the nuclide from the tissue, fell from 0.083 +/- 0.004 1/min before addition of the drug to 0.049 +/- 0.004 1/min after addition of the drug to the washing solution (means +/- SE, n=8), i.e. by more than 40 %.

Based on the compartmental analysis of 36-Cl exchange curves, the intracellular chloride content of untreated rabbit aortic tissue was found to be 5.77 mmoles/kg wet weight. Preparations that had been incubated with 1 mM furosemide for 3 h, contained only 2.8 mmoles of chloride /kg wet weight. Taking into account an extracellular space (based on 14-C-sucrose labelling of aortic tissue) of 52 %, and an amount of dry matter of 24 % of the tissue's wet weight, the concentration of chloride in the intracellular water amounted to 24 mmoles/litre in the untreated preparations, and to only 11.7 mmoles/litre in the preparations that had been incubated with furosemide for a prolonged period. Substituting these data in the Nernst equation for (Cli), at a (Cle) of 140.1 mM, resulted in chloride equilibrium potentials of -47.7 +/- 2.3 mV (means +/- SE) in the untreated preparations, and of -66.1 +/- 1.3 mV in the furosemide-treated preparations.

In influx studies, furosemide, and the related loop diuretic, piretanide, were found to reduce the cellular uptake of 36-Cl. This became particularly obvious when the tissues had been preincubated for 90 min in a chloride-free PSS (chloride replaced by isethionate); after 10 min of incubation in 36-Cl-PSS, control preparations had taken up 132.4 +/- 14.8 cpm/mg wet weight (mean +/-SE, n=10), whereas in the presence of 2 mM of furosemide or piretanide, the strips took up only 59.5 +/- 10.2 or 71.0 +/- 4.6 cpm/mg w.w. (n=10), respectively. (These studies were performed in the presence of 1 mM ouabain in order to exclude an indirect contribution of the Na-K-ATPase.)

The 36-Cl/Cl-SSE proved to be highly temperature-dependent; decreasing the temperature of the washing solution from 37 to 17 centigrade reduced the fractional loss of 36-Cl from rabbit aorta from 0.0735 to 0.0146 1/min (means, n=6), i.e. to 20 % of the control value.

Incubation with 1 mM furosemide induced hyperpolarization of the rabbit main pulmonary artery (fig. 2). In a series of single penetrations, a membrane potential of -61.6 +/- 0.6 mV (mean +/- SE, no. of preparations: 11; no. of penetrations: 44) was measured under control conditions, whereas one of -67.1 +/- 0.8 mV (no. of preparations: 9; no. of penetrations: 23) was recorded on incubation with furosemide for 40 - 90 min. From the long-term penetration

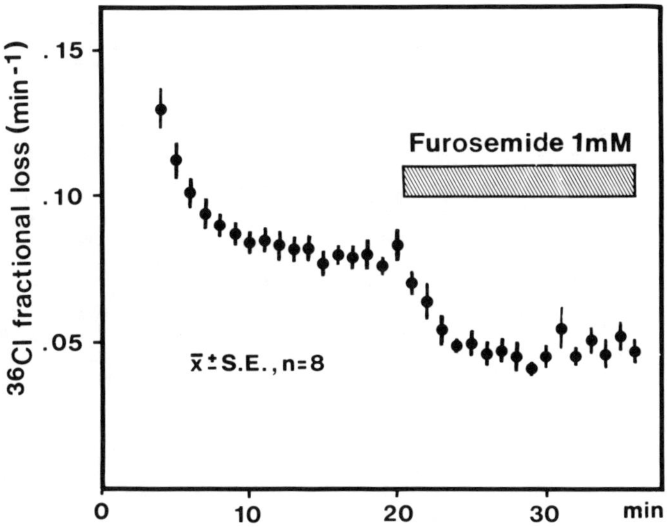

FIG. 1. Effect of furosemide on 36-Cl/Cl steady-state exchange in isolated rabbit aorta. Ordinate: 36-Cl fractional loss; i.e. rate of exchange = cpm in effluent/ 1 min/ cpm in tissue at time indicated. (Reproduced from (7).)

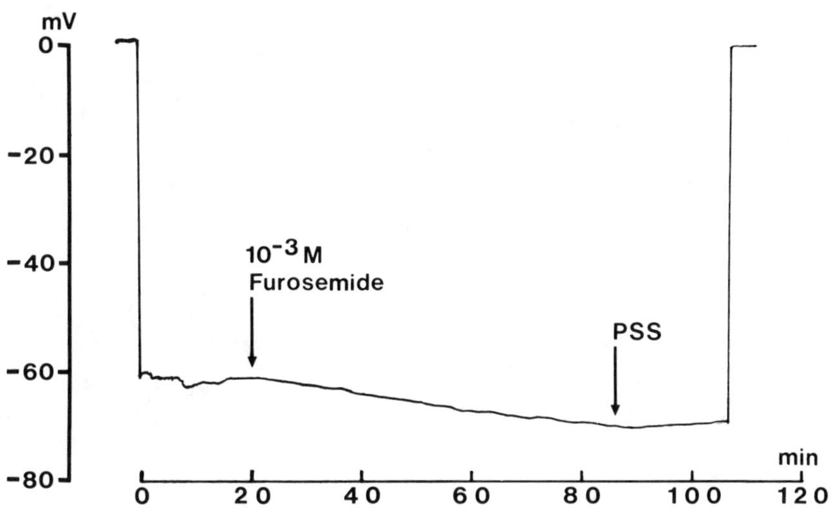

FIG. 2. Hyperpolarization of the membrane potential of rabbit main pulmonary artery by furosemide. Original recording of a long-term penetration with the glass microelectrode. PSS: washout of drug with physiological salt solution. At 110 min, the cell was lost.

shown in fig. 2 it is obvious that furosemide-induced hyperpolarization developed only slowly. Likewise, the suppressant effect of 1 mM furosemide on the contractile responses of helical strips made from rabbit aortae to 0.1 uM noradrenaline developed very slowly, too (fig.3).

Studies on the possible mechanisms involved in chloride transport in vascular smooth muscle

When during a washout of 36-Cl-labelled rabbit aorta, the standard-PSS buffered by bicarbonate/carbon dioxide was replaced by PSS buffered with 11.9 mM HEPES (gassed with pure oxygene), the rate of 36-Cl/Cl-SSE rose by a factor of 2.3, i.e. from 0.052 +/- 0.006 1/min (mean +/- SE, n=8) to 0.117 +/- 0.033 1/min (fig. 4). - This augmenting effect of bicarbonate withdrawal on the 36-Cl/Cl-SSE was partially inhibited when the washout of the preparations was performed in the presence of 4,4'-diisothiocyano-2,2'-disulfonic acid (DIDS), a known inhibitor of the anion carrier in erythrocytes (15). At 0.1 mM of DIDS, bicarbonate withdrawal only increased the fractional loss of 36-Cl by a factor of 1.4, i.e. from a control value of 0.060 +/- 0.006 1/min to 0.084 +/- 0.007 1/min (n=6). - A total suppression of the effect of bicarbonate withdrawal was achieved when the washout of the nuclide from the vascular preparations was performed in a PSS which instead of chloride ions contained large organic anions such as isethionate, benzenesulfonate, or proprionate.

All loop diuretics investigated (furosemide, piretanide, and ethacrynic acid) at concentrations ranging from 10 uM to 1 mM were found to interfere with the 36-Cl/Cl-SSE in rabbit aorta, and to suppress partially the contractile responses of helical strips of rabbit aortae. Whereas the latter effect was also demonstrated to occur with hydrochlorothiazide, this diuretic drug did not affect the 36-Cl/Cl-SSE even at 1 mM. - When aortic preparations were loaded with 86-Rb which is often used as a substitute for potassium ions in flux studies, the loop diuretic piretanide was found to interfere with 86-Rb/K-SSE. Similarly, loop diuretics were found to partially inhibit the influx of 86-Rb into potassium-depleted preparations (experiments performed in the presence of 1 mM ouabain); whereas the control tissues took up 857 +/- 38.2 nmoles/g wet weight (mean +/- SE, n=5) during 10 min of exposure to the 86-Rb-PSS, the uptake was considerably smaller in the presence of 2 mM furosemide (243 +/- 28.1 nmoles/g w.w., n=5) or 2 mM piretanide (128 +/- 6.8 nmoles/g w.w., n=5). - 0.1 mM of the sodium channel blocker, amiloride, was shown to interfere with 36-Cl/Cl-SSE. - Subtotal replacement of Na ions by choline in the PSS (128 mM choline, 13.2 mM Na) enhanced the fractional loss of 36-Cl from preparations loaded with 36-Cl.

DISCUSSION

The findings presented here provide strong evidence for the existence of a chloride transport system within the cell membrane of vsm. Loop diuretics have been found to interfere with ion transport systems in a variety of tissues such as erythrocytes, epithelia, the thick ascending limb of Henle, the rectal gland of the shark, and the toad cornea. In the presence of furosemide, we found the intracellular chloride content of the rabbit aorta considerably reduced, and a similar finding, although less in extent, was made in the dog carotid artery (11).

It is of particular interest that after prolonged incubation with furosemide, the calculated equilibrium potential for chloride became almost identical to the measured membrane potential. Previously, we had proposed this congruence to be a strong indication of an active nature of the chloride distribution in vsm; such a finding would have to be expected if active chloride transport were inhibited, and passive electro-chemical forces were left to account for a Donnan-like distribution of chloride ions (7). Recently however, on the basis of electrophysiological studies, it was suggested that

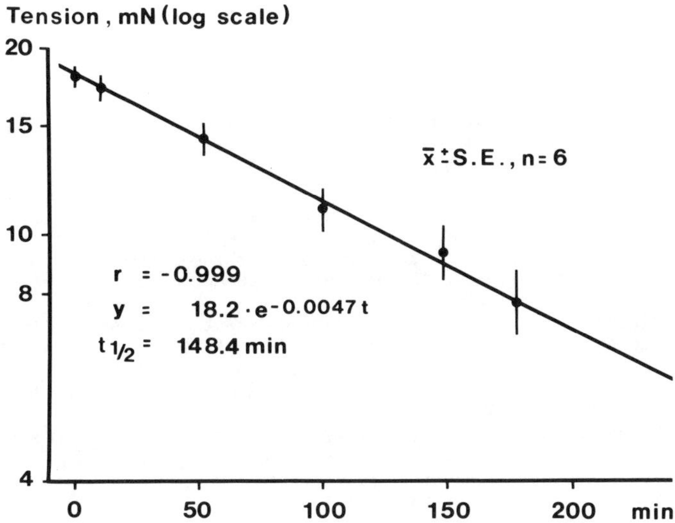

FIG. 3. Effect of 1 mM furosemide on contractile responses of helical strips from rabbit aorta to repeated additions of 0.1 uM noradrenaline to the organ bath. Immediately after the preparations had reached their peak response, the organ bath was rinsed with physiological salt solution containing furosemide. Note the roughly mono-exponential course, and the slow development of the decay of the contractile action of noradrenaline in the presence of furosemide.

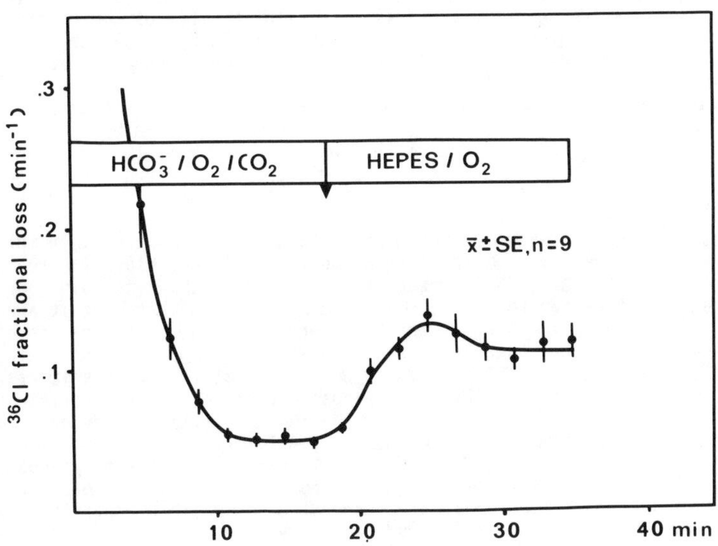

FIG. 4. Effect of bicarbonate withdrawal on 36-Cl/Cl steady-state exchange in isolated rabbit aorta. Ordinate: as in FIG. 1.

in the resting vsm, chloride permeability may be negligible (12); if this hypothesis can be validated, one has to face the possibility that in contrast to former belief (13), the chloride ion gradient across the cell membrane of vsm does not contribute to the resting membrane potential. With regard to our own results, it might come out that the described congruence of membrane potential and calculated equilibrium potential in the presence of furosemide may have been circumstantial rather causually related. Also, our finding that the cell membrane of the rabbit main pulmonary artery hyperpolarized on incubation with furosemide would require an explanation other than by a role of the chloride gradient. In spite of the so far missing explanation for the furosemide-induced hyperpolarization of vsm, we like to suggest that this effect may underlie the vasorelaxant property of furosemide (and other loop diuretics), since the time course for the development of hyperpolarization and vasorelaxation were similar.

Regardless of the shortcomings mentioned, another strong evidence for an active principle being involved in chloride distribution across the cell membrane of vsm is its high dependence on temperature; using the data presented, a Q10-value of 2.24 was calculated which is much greater than the maximum Q10-value of passive ion movements (i.e. 1.3 (3)).

What is the nature of chloride transport in vascular smooth muscle ? Two presumed types of transport may play their role, i.e. anion countertransport, and Na-K-Cl-cotransport. Recently, by applying the technique of ion-sensitive microelectrodes, Aicken and Brading (14) provided evidence for the existence of an anion transport system exchanging bicarbonate for chloride in the guinea-pig vas deferens. Our own data based on ion flux techniques suggest that anion countertransport takes place in vsm, too; removal of bicarbonate from the PSS used for the washout of 36-Cl-labelled rabbit aorta led to an increase of the rate of 36-Cl/Cl-SSE, and this effect was completely blocked on removal of extracellular chloride. These findings are in keeping with the notion that the mobility of the anion membrane carrier is enhanced when it is freed of bicarbonate ions thus permitting improved chloride self-exchange (15), and that chloride self-exchange is suppressed when extracellular chloride ions are not available at the extracellular binding sites of the carrier protein. The partial inhibition of the stimulation of 36-Cl/Cl-SSE on withdrawal of bicarbonate by DIDS, a known inhibitor of anion countertransport, conforms with the hypothesis of an anion carrier in vsm.

In contrast, the evidence for the existence of Na-K-Cl-cotransport in vsm is faint so far. The discovery of such a mechanism would be of great pathophysiological interest, since it has been claimed that ion cotransport being sensitive to loop diuretics may be disturbed in erythrocytes of patients suffering from hypertension (16); the demonstration of a related mechanism in vsm might add to a better understanding of this desease. Above, we have presented several examples which point to apparent links between chloride and cation movements in vsm. The fact alone that all loop diuretics tested, interfered with 36-Cl/Cl-SSE in rabbit aorta whereas thiazides did not, may be taken as a hint for the existence of Na-K-Cl-cotransport, but it should not be ignored that much larger concentrations of these drugs were necessary for measurable effects than in other tissues, e.g. the thick ascending limb of Henle (17); hence, we cannot exclude so far that in our experiments, the loop diuretics exhibited unspecific high-dose effects on anion countertransport or other, so far unknown mechanisms. Based on a related study of Geck (18) in Ehrlich ascites tumor cells, we have recently studied the furosemide-sensitive influx of 22-Na, 86-Rb, and 36-Cl into potassium-depleted pieces of rabbit aorta (in the presence of a high concentration of ouabain to suppress contributions of Na-K-ATPase) in order to establish a 1:1:2 relationship of the uptake of these ions; this study was a failure since total ion uptake (with the exeption of 86-Rb) exceeded furosemide-sensitive uptake manifold. Hence, the statistical variations of total uptake had a great impact on the measurement of the furosemide-sensitive portion of uptake, but on the basis of that study we feel that Na-K-Cl-cotransport is probably of minor importance for the distribution of monovalent ions, if existing at all, in vsm. -

REFERENCES

1. B.A. Wahlström, Acta physiol. scand. 92, 404-411 (1974).
2. V.A.W. Kreye, R. Kern, and I. Schleich in: Excitation-Contraction Coupling in Smooth Muscle, R. Casteels, T. Godfraind, and J.C. Rüegg, eds. (Elsevier/North Holland, Amsterdam 1977) pp. 145-150.
3. A.W. Jones in: Handbook of Physiology, Section 2, vol.II: Vascular Smooth Muscle, D.F. Bohr, A.P. Somlyo, and H.V. Sparks, eds. (The Williams and Wilkins Comp., Baltimore 1980) pp. 253-299.
4. V.A.W. Kreye and F.W. Ziegler, Adv. Microcirc. 11, 114-133 (1982).
5. M. Villamil, N. Yeyati, L. Barajas, and C.R. Kleemann, Am. J. Physiol. 215, 833-839 (1968).
6. A.P. Somlyo, A.V. Somlyo, H. Shuman, J. Cell Biol. 81, 316-335 (1979).
7. V.A.W. Kreye, P.K. Bauer, and I. Villhauer, Europ. J. Pharmacol. 73, 91-95 (1981).
8. V.A.W. Kreye, P.K. Bauer, and I. Villhauer, Blood Vessels 18, 217 (1981).
9. V.A.W. Kreye and F. Gerstheimer, Pflüger's Arch. 394, R89 (1982).
10. V.A.W. Kreye, F. Gerstheimer, M. Mühleisen, D. Nehring, and K. Walter, Naunyn-Schmiedeberg's Arch. Pharmacol. 325, R38 (1984).
11. M.F. Villamil, J. Ponce, C. Amorena, and A. Müller, T.-I.-T. J. Life Sci. 9, 9-14 (1979).
12. G.D.S. Hirst and D.F. van Helden. J. Physiol. 333, 53-67 (1982).
13. V.A.W. Kreye in: Vasodilatation, P.M. Vanhoutte and I. Leusen, eds. (Raven Press, New York 1981) pp.299-305.
14. C.C. Aicken and A.F. Brading, J.Physiol. (1984), in press.
15. A.G. Lowe and A. Lambert, Biochim. Biophys. Acta 694, 353-374 (1983).
16. R. Garay, G. Dagher, M.-G. Pernollet, M.-A. Devynck, and P. Meyer; Nature 284, 281-283 (1980).
17. E. Schlatter, R. Greger, and C. Weidtke, Pflüger's Arch. 396, 210-217 (1983).
18. P. Geck, C. Pietrzyk, B.-C. Burckhardt, B. Pfeiffer, and E. Heinz, Biochim. Biophys. Acta 600, 432-447 (1980).

DIRECT CARDIOVASCULAR EFFECTS OF DIURETICS

G. Dennis Johnston, M.D., M.R.C.P., D.C.H., Consultant Physician,
Belfast City Hospital and Royal Victoria Hospital, Belfast and
Senior Lecturer, Department of Therapeutics and Pharmacology,
Queen's University of Belfast, Belfast, Northern Ireland

INTRODUCTION

Frusemide is a potent diuretic which is frequently used for the treatment of acute left ventricular failure and pulmonary oedema. Although frusemide decreases cardiac preload by producing a natriuresis with a resultant reduction in extracellular fluid volume, an acute fall in the left ventricular filling pressure has been observed within a few minutes of intravenous drug administration, before a diuretic response is apparent (Dikshit et al, 1973). Plethysmographic studies in man have demonstrated that frusemide causes an increase in venous capacitance which probably accounts for the early decrease in venous return to the heart.

In addition to the peripheral venous effects, frusemide is known to increase renal blood flow acutely (Ludens et al, 1968), an effect which has been postulated as being of benefit in the early management of acute tubular necrosis (Cantarovich et al, 1971). There is increasing evidence in animals that both the renal and extra renal vascular effects are related to renal function and are not due to direct effects of the drug. To investigate the role of the kidney in producing these vasodilator effects, a series of experiments were carried out in man and in the unconscious dog.

In the first study, we examined the effects of salt balance, prostaglandin synthetase inhibition with indomethacin and angiotensin converting enzyme inhibition with captopril on the acute changes in wedge pressure and renal blood flow in the dog. In addition we examined the responses in a group of anephric dogs to determine whether functioning kidneys were essential for venodilatation. Since PGE_2 and PGI_2 are known vasodilators, evidence was sought for increased concentrations in the urine and since PGI_2 is the only vasodilator prostaglandin which produces systemic effects plasma concentrations of its main metabolite 6 keto $PGF_{1\alpha}$ were estimated.

EXPERIMENT I

FACTORS MODIFYING THE EARLY NON-DIURETIC VASCULAR EFFECTS OF FRUSEMIDE IN THE UNCONSCIOUS DOG: the possible role of prostaglandins and angiotensin II

Methods

Four groups of 6 salt depleted dogs and one group of salt overloaded dogs were studied.

1. SALT DEPLETED

   Four groups of 6 dogs weighing 15-20 kg received salt free diets for 5 days before each experiment.

   (a) Control.

   (b) Indomethacin pretreated: In addition, each dog received indomethacin 8 mg/kg intravenously 45 mins before receiving frusemide.

   (c) Captopril pretreated: Salt depleted dogs received captopril 1 mg/kg intravenously 45 mins before frusemide.

   (d) Anephric: Kidneys were removed one hour before starting the experiment.

2. SALT OVERLOADED

   A final group of 6 dogs received a normal diet with added salt in

Published 1984 by Elsevier Science Publishing Co., Inc.
Diuretics, Jules B. Puschett, Editor

the drinking water and 10 mg of intramuscular deoxycortisone acetate for a period of 5 days.

Dogs were anaesthetised with 30 mg/kg of sodium pentobarbitone and ventilated with room air. Through a retroperitoneal flank incision, an electromagnetic flow transducer was placed around the exposed renal artery to measure renal blood flow and the renal artery and vein cannulated for blood sampling except in the anephric and captopril pretreated groups. A Swan Gauz flow catheter was then introduced into the pulmonary artery via the jugular vein to record pulmonary wedge pressure and the femoral vein cannulated for drug administration and sampling.

Measurements of wedge pressure and renal blood flow were made for 30 mins before frusemide administration to ensure a stable baseline. In all but the anephric and captopril pretreated groups baseline urine samples were obtained for sodium and prostaglandin estimation (PGE_2 and PGI_2) and blood samples from the renal artery, renal vein and femoral vein were obtained for estimation of plasma renin activity and 6 keto $PGF_{1\alpha}$, a metabolite of PGI_2.

Frusemide (5 mg/kg) was then infused intravenously and measurements of renal blood flow and wedge pressure made over the next 15 mins at 3-min intervals. After 10 mins, blood samples were taken from the renal artery, renal vein and femoral vein for plasma renin activity and 6 keto $PGF_{1\alpha}$ in the salt depleted, salt overloaded, and indomethacin pretreated groups. At the end of 15 mins, urine samples were taken in these three groups for sodium and prostaglandin (PGE_2 and 6 keto $PGF_{1\alpha}$) estimation.

Mean comparisons of paired data were made by analysis of variance and Duncan's multiple range test for multiple comparisons or Student's paired t-test for single comparisons. Unpaired t-test was used to compare the means of unpaired data. The level of significance was chosen at the 5% level and the results expressed as mean ± standard error of the mean.

Fig. 1

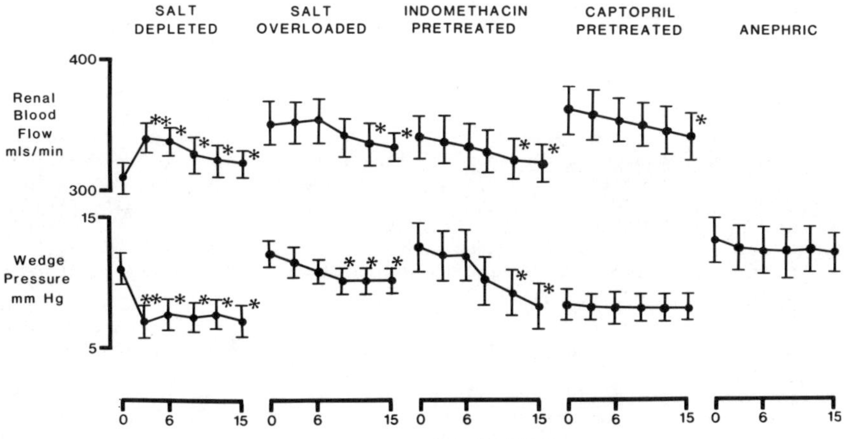

A significant increase in renal blood flow was observed within 3 mins of frusemide administration (312 ± 12 to 342 ± 14 ml/min, $p<0.01$) in the group of dogs who had received a low salt diet only and persisted during the 15 min period. No acute increase in renal blood flow was observed in the high salt, indomethacin or captopril pretreated groups (Fig. 1). In all 3 groups baseline blood flow was higher but these increases were not statistically greater than the low salt group. In the salt overloaded and indomethacin pretreated groups, renal blood flow was significantly reduced at 12 and 15 mins and at 15 mins in the captopril pretreated group (Fig. 1).

Wedge pressure decreased from 11.1 ± 1.3 to 7.0 ± 1.2 mm Hg ($p<0.01$) at 3 mins and remained reduced during the 15 min period ($p<0.05$) in the salt depleted groups. No acute decreases were observed in the other groups (Fig. 1) although in the high salt and indomethacin pretreated groups 15 min pressures were significantly less than baseline and comparable to the 15 min values in the low salt group.

Plasma renin output from the kidney was increased in the salt depleted group before ($p<0.05$) and increased significantly after frusemide administration (210 ± 24 to 512 ± 36 ng AI/hr/min, $p<0.01$) but no increases occurred in the indomethacin, salt overloaded or anephric groups. Urinary PGE_2 increased ($p<0.05$) in the salt depleted group but we were unable to detect increased plasma concentrations of the 6 keto $PGF_{1\alpha}$.

This study provides evidence that the non-diuretic effects of frusemide on renal blood flow and preload depend on intact kidneys, prostaglandin formation and activation of the renin angiotensin at least in the unconscious dog. No evidence was provided that the venodilator effects were due to the systemic effects of prostacyclin.

EXPERIMENT II

FACTORS MODIFYING THE NON-DIURETIC VASCULAR EFFECTS OF FRUSEMIDE IN MAN: the possible role of renal PROSTAGLANDINS (Johnston et al, 1983a)

This study was undertaken to determine whether the early extra renal vascular effect of frusemide on venous capacitance was influenced by the subject's salt balance or prior administration of the prostaglandin synthetase inhibitor, indomethacin. In addition, we studied a group of uraemic patients to determine whether a functional kidney was essential for the extra renal vascular responses to occur. Again evidence for increased levels of prostacyclin were sought.

Methods

The study was divided into two parts. Ten healthy female volunteers (23-32 years) participated in the first part of the experiment and five uraemic patients in the second part. The group of 10 volunteers was studied on 3 separate occasions with a period of at least one month between each study. Subjects received a low salt diet (10 mg/kg) on the first occasion, a high salt diet (250 meq/day) on the second and a 10 meq/day salt diet followed by oral indomethacin on the last occasion (50 mg qid for 2 days). In the second part, five uraemic patients - 2 surgically anephric and 3 functionally anephric were studied following dialysis when the patients were considered to be 'dry weight'.

Subjects rested in the supine position for a period of one hour before the experiment at the end of which a timed urine sample was obtained for estimation of urinary sodium. Three baseline measurements of venous capacitance were made at 5 min intervals over the next 15 mins. Blood was then withdrawn for determination of plasma renin activity (PRA) and 6 keto $PGF_{1\alpha}$ concentrations. Frusemide (80 mg) was then administered as an intravenous bolus, and measurement of venous capacitance repeated at 5 min intervals for 15 mins. Ten mins after frusemide blood was obtained for PRA and 6 keto $PGF_{1\alpha}$ concentrations. A second urine collection was obtained for sodium estimation at the end of the 15 min period. The study design in the five uraemic patients was similar except that no urine was produced and therefore no urinary sodium estimations were obtained. Statistical analyses were the same as in the first study and again the level of significance was chosen as $p<0.05$ and the results expressed as the mean ± SEM.

Fig. 2

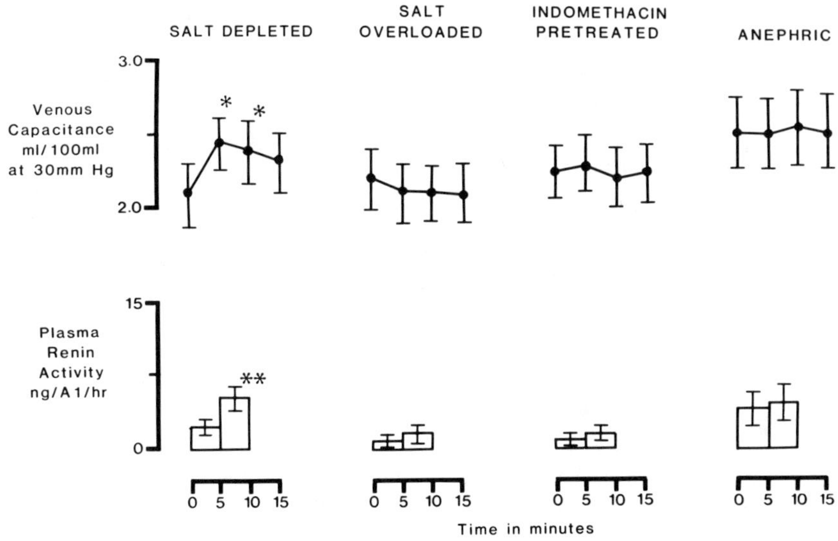

Results

In the salt depleted group venous capacitance increased following frusemide (2.11 ± 2.15 to 2.42 ± 2.40, $p<0.05$) and remained elevated during the 15 min period (Fig. 2). Indomethacin abolished the increase in venous capacitance produced by frusemide in the salt depleted subjects. In the salt overloaded group there was no increase in venous capacitance and small decreases were apparent (Fig. 2) following frusemide administration. The uraemic individuals had no change in venous capacitance with frusemide whether or not the kidneys had been surgically removed.

The sodium excretion rate for the 15 min period after frusemide was significantly higher than for the salt depleted groups but the response in the two salt depleted groups did not differ from each other. Frusemide induced increases in supline plasma renin activity (2.2 ± 0.3 to 4.8 ± 0.7 ng AI/ml/hr, $p<0.05$) were observed in the low salt group but not in any of the other groups (Fig. 2). The baseline supine plasma renin activities were significantly higher ($p<0.05$) when volunteers were salt depleted than when they were salt overloaded. Indomethacin treatment failed to reduce baseline plasma renin activity significantly. The high plasma renin activity in the uraemic group is accounted for by one patient with a value of 16 and 18.9 ng AI/ml/hr before and after frusemide respectively. No 6 keto $PGF_{1\alpha}$ was detected (<30 pg/ml) before or after frusemide administration.

This experiment confirmed most of the findings in the dog study and again no evidence that the venous effects were due to prostacyclin was obtained.

EXPERIMENT III

VENOUS DOSE-RESPONSE CHARACTERISTICS (Johnston et al, 1984)

In the previous two experiments, large doses of frusemide were used to demonstrate these non-diuretic effects. Since at these doses there was always a slight possibility that a small diuresis had occurred at the same time as the acute vascular effects, we decided to determine the dose response characteristics of the venodilator effects to determine the dose which would produce the greatest vascular effect with the least diuretic effect.

Methods

Nine healthy salt depleted volunteers were studied. The study was carried out on six separate occasions at the same time of day with a period of at least one week between studies. On each study day subjects were maintained in the supine position for a period of one hour following which 3 baseline measurements of venous capacitance were made at 5 min intervals. Subjects then received 0, 5, 10, 20, 40 or 80 mg frusemide according to a randomised, double-blind design. Venous capacitance was then measured at 5, 10 and 15 mins after intravenous frusemide administration.

Fig. 3

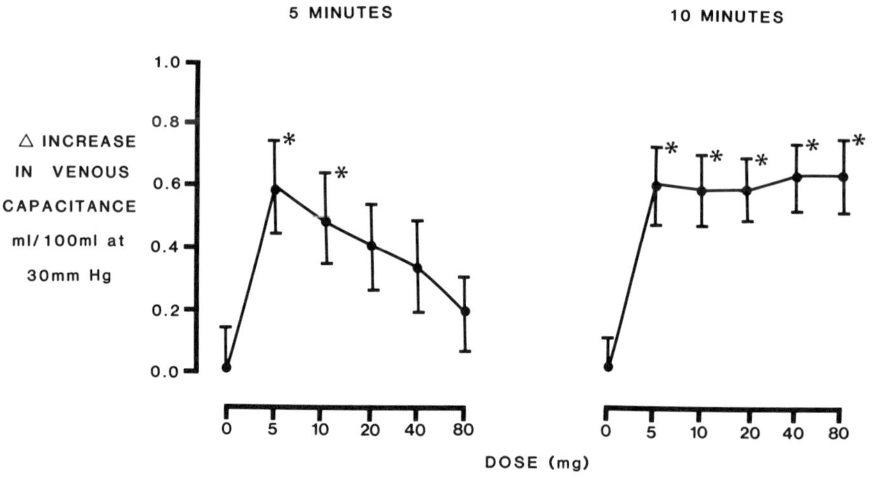

Results

The increases in venous capacitance 5 mins after 5 and 10 mg of intravenous frusemide were significantly greater than the corresponding placebo values (0.58 ± 0.12 and 0.47 ± 0.11 ml/100 ml respectively, $p<0.05$) (Fig.3). With increasing doses, a progressive decline in the venous responses at 5 mins was observed so that over the dose range 20-80 mg, no significant increase was apparent (Fig. 3). On the other hand, 10 min venous responses showed a flat dose response relationship (Fig. 3), the increases being statistically greater than placebo at all the doses studied ($p<0.05$).

In view of these findings it was decided to use 5 mg frusemide in subsequent experiments and so strengthen the argument that the vascular responses were truly unrelated to diuresis.

EXPERIMENT 4

THE EFFECTS OF CAPTOPRIL ON THE ACUTE VASCULAR RESPONSES TO FRUSEMIDE IN MAN (Johnston et al, 1984a)

In the previous experiments it has been shown that the acute vascular effects of frusemide only occur when frusemide stimulated renin release is abolished or when angiotensin II formation is attenuated. One explanation which would fit with these observations is that the drug causes renin release from the kidney, resulting in angiotensin II formation, which in turn causes release of vasodilator substances from the kidney or vein wall. In keeping with this theory is the observation that angiotensin II stimulates the production of vasodilatory prostaglandins PGE_2 and PGI_2 in several vascular beds (Messina et al, 1976; Gryglewski et al, 1980) and prostaglandins modulate the arteriolar constriction produced by angiotensin II. The formation of prostacyclin from the kidney or vasodilatory prostaglandins from the vein wall could result in a net increase in venous capacitance since angiotensin appears to have little or no direct venoconstrictor effect (De Pasquale, 1963). This study was undertaken to test this hypothesis by looking at the effect of pretreatment with captopril, an angiotensin converting enzyme inhibitor, on the acute peripheral venous effects of frusemide in man.

Methods

Ten healthy volunteers aged 18-22 years were studied. The study was carried out at the same time of day with at least one week between studies. Salt depletion was achieved in all subjects as previously described. After rest for one hour in the supine position, 3 baseline measurements of venous capacitance were made at 5 min intervals and a blood sample was taken for measurements of plasma renin and plasma aldosterone concentrations. Subjects then received 50 mg of captopril or identical placebo, according to a double-blind, randomised, cross-over design. Three further measurements of venous capacitance were taken over a 15 min period 2 hours after the first series of baseline measurements and a blood sample was obtained for plasma renin activity and aldosterone concentration. Immediately afterwards, 5 mg of frusemide was injected as an intravenous bolus over 10 seconds and further measurements of venous capacitance made over the next 30 mins at 5 min intervals. Ten mins after frusemide a further blood sample for plasma renin activity and plasma aldosterone was obtained.

Results

In the placebo treated group, increases in venous capacitance were observed in the 15 min period following 5 mg frusemide intravenously. In the captopril pretreated group, no changes were observed in the 15 min period following frusemide administration (Fig. 4). Increases in plasma renin activity (Fig. 4) and decreases in plasma aldosterone confirmed the effects of captopril on the renin-angiotensin-aldosterone system.

This study therefore confirms the findings of the dog study that pretreatment with captopril abolishes the acute vascular effects of frusemide and provides further evidence that angiotensin II is important in producing these vascular responses.

EXPERIMENT V

THE ACUTE VENODILATOR EFFECTS OF FRUSEMIDE IN MAN: The importance of frusemide stimulated renin release (Johnston et al, 1984b)

We have previously seen that acute increases in venous capacitance and renal blood flow are accompanied by acute renin release from the kidney. If frusemide stimulated renin release is inhibited by salt overloading or indomethacin, these acute vascular effects do not occur. Digoxin and propranolol, which are commonly used with frusemide in the treatment of heart disease have been shown to inhibit frusemide stimulated renin release (Ferrari et al, 1979; Bravo et al, 1979). In this study the effect of pre-treatment with each of these drugs was examined to determine if frusemide-induced renin release was inhibited and whether this was accompanied by an attenuation of frusemide's venodilator response.

Methods

Twelve salt depleted healthy volunteers aged 18-22 years were studied. After a one hour period in the supine position, 3 baseline measurements of venous capacitance were made at 5 min intervals. Subjects then received 750 μg digoxin, 10 mg propranolol (dissolved in 20 ml normal saline) or 20 ml normal saline delivered at a rate of 1 ml/min according to a double blind, randomised cross over design. One hour after the start of each infusion, a further 3 sets of readings were taken and 5 mg frusemide administered as an intravenous bolus over 10 seconds. Venous capacitance was again measured at 5 min intervals over the next 15 mins. Plasma renin activity and plasma aldosterone concentrations were measured immediately before digoxin, propranolol or placebo, before frusemide and 10 mins after frusemide administration.

Fig. 4

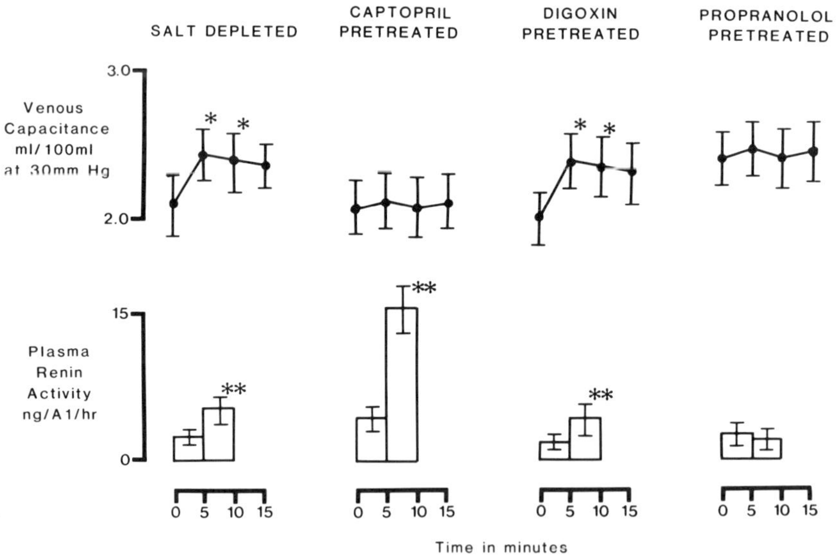

Results

Venous capacitance following frusemide increased from 2.85 ± 0.27 to 3.31 ± 0.33 ml/100 ml at 30 mm Hg ($p<0.05$) 10 mins after administration in the placebo treated group and from 2.05 ± 0.21 to 2.38 ± 0.21 ml/100 ml ($p<0.05$) in the digoxin treated group (Fig. 4). No venodilator response was observed following frusemide in the group pretreated with propranolol. (Fig.4)

An increase in plasma renin activity following frusemide was observed in the presence of placebo (1.41 ± 0.16 to 2.27 ± 0.17 AI/ml/hr, $p<0.01$) and digoxin (1.41 ± 0.29 to 1.86 ± 0.4, $p<0.01$) but not in the group pre-treated with propranolol (Fig. 4). Similarly, plasma aldosterone increased following frusemide in the placebo (109 ± 16 to 143 ± 21 pg/ml, $p<0.01$) and digoxin (105 ± 13 to 132 ± 10 pg/ml, $p<0.01$) treated groups but remained unchanged in the propranolol treated group.

This study provided further evidence of a relationship between acute renin release and the acute venodilator effects of frusemide in man.

CONCLUSION

These studies demonstrate that the acute non-diuretic vascular effects of frusemide on renal blood flow and venous tone are not due to direct effects of the drug but depend on the presence of functioning kidneys. They occur independent of diuretic activity and the venodilator responses do not increase with increasing dosage. Vasodilator prostaglandin formation (PGE_2 and possibly PGI_2) are probably involved in renal artery vasodilatation but we found no evidence that the venous effects were due to increased levels of circulating prostacyclin (PGI_2).

Acute frusemide induced renin release occurs in association with the non-diuretic effects and inhibition of renin release and angiotensin II formation prevents these effects occurring. The most satisfactory explanation of the acute venodilator effects is that frusemide gives rise to acute renin release with secondary angiotensin formation which causes release of vasodilator materials (probably prostaglandins) from the vein wall.

REFERENCES

1. Bravo, E.L., Tarazi, R.C. and Dustan, H.P. (1974). On the mechanism of suppressed plasma-renin activity during beta-adrenergic blockade with propranolol. J. Lab. Clin. Med. 83, 119-128.
2. Cantarovich, F., Locatelli, A., Fernandez, J.C., Perez Loredo, J. and Christhot (1971). Furosemide in high doses in the treatment of acute renal failure. Postgrad. Med. J. 47 (suppl), 13-17.
3. De Pasquale, N.P. and Burch, G.E. (1963). Effect of angiotensin II on the intact forearm veins of man. Circ. Res. 13, 239-245.
4. Dikshit, K., Vyden, J.K., Forrester, J.S., Chatterjee, K., Prakash, R. and Swan, H.J.C. (1973). Renal and extra renal haemodynamic effects of furosemide in congestive heart failure after acute myocardial infarction. N. Engl. J. Med. 288, 1087-1090.
5. Ferrari, M. (1979). Effects of digoxin and digoxin plus furosemide on plasma renin activity of hypertensive patients. Circ. Res. 44, 295.
6. Gryglewski, R.J., Splawinsk, J. and Korbut, R. (1980). Endogenous mechanisms that regulate prostacyclin release. In: Advances in Prostaglandin and Thromboxane Research, vol. 7, edited by B.Samuelson, P. Ramwell, R. Paoletti. New York, Raven Press, pp.177-287.
7. Johnston, G.D., Hiatt, W.R., Nies, A.S., Payne, N.A., Murphy, R.C. and Gerber, J.G. (1983a). Factors modifying the early non-diuretic vascular effects of furosemide in man: the possible role of renal prostaglandins. Circ. Res. 53, 630-635.
8. Johnston, G.D., Nicholls, D.P., Leahey, W.J. and Finch, M.B. (1983b). The effects of captopril on the acute vascular responses to frusemide in man. Clinical Science 65, 359-363.
9. Johnston, G.D., Nicholls, D.P. and Leahey, W.J. (1984a). The dose response characteristics of the acute non-diuretic peripheral vascular effects of frusemide in normal subjects. Br. J. Clin. Pharmacol. (In press).

10. Johnston, G.D., Nicholls, D.P., Leahey, W.J., O'Connor, P.C. and Finch, M.B. (1984b). The acute venodilator effects of frusemide in man: the importance of frusemide stimulated renin release. Br. J. Clin. Pharmacol.17, 192P.

11. Ludens, J.H., Hook, J.B., Brody, M.J. and Williamson, H.E. (1968). Enhancement of renal blood flow by furosemide. J. Pharmacol. Exp. Ther. 163, 456-460.

12. Messina, E.J., Weiner, R. and Kaley, G. (1976). Prostaglandins and local circulatory control. Fed. Proc. 35, 2367-2375.

MODE OF ACTION OF LOOP DIURETICS IN CHLORIDE TRANSPORTING EPITHELIA

R. KINNE*, J. HANNAFIN**, B. KOENIG*, AND E. KINNE-SAFFRAN*
*Max-Planck-Institut fuer Systemphysiologie, Rheinlanddamm 201, 4600 Dortmund, FRG; **Albert Einstein College of Medicine, 1300 Morris Park Avenue, New York, NY 10461, USA

Recent physiological [1] and biochemical [2,3,4] studies have shown that active chloride absorption in the renal thick ascending limb of Henle's loop (TALH) and active chloride secretion in the rectal gland of the dogfish, Squalus acanthias, are comprised of a similar chain of events. Chloride entry into the cell occurs via a sodium-chloride-potassium cotransport system which is energized by the sodium gradient across the membrane. This sodium gradient is maintained by the Na-K-ATPase which, in turn, requires a continuous supply of ATP for its operation. Chloride leaves the cell via a sodium independent, probably electrogenic route.

In order to study the cellular action of loop diuretics TALH cells were isolated from rabbit kidney outer medulla [5] and the effect of furosemide and bumetanide on the activity of the cotransport system, the activity of the Na-K-ATPase, and the intracellular ATP content were investigated. As shown in Table 1 the activity of the cotransport system, measured as KCl dependent sodium flux into plasma membranes prepared from isolated TALH cells, is inhibited by both diuretics in a dose dependent manner. The Na-K-ATPase activity and the intracellular ATP content, as indicator for cellular metabolism are, however, not affected [6,7]. The inhibition of the cotransport system parallels the inhibition of the NaCl-dependent O_2 consumption of the cells. The latter can be regarded as equivalent for the active transcellular chloride transport.

TABLE I. Effect of "loop" diuretics on cellular parameters involved in active chloride transport in TALH cells.

	furosemide				bumetanide		
	10^{-6}	10^{-5}	10^{-4}	10^{-3} M	10^{-6}	10^{-5}	10^{-4} M
NaCl-dependent O_2 consumption	72	43	19	0	47	21	0
KCl dependent sodium transport	73	34	18	0	25	12	0
Na-K-ATPase activity	100	94	97	100	87	100	90
ATP-content	107	103	97	112	99	108	94

Most of the data have been compiled from [6] and [7], the ATP-content represents mean values of 3 determinations performed as described in [6]. All values are given as percent of the control without diuretic.

These results clearly indicate that the diuretics inhibit chloride transport by interacting directly with the sodium-chloride-potassium cotransport system and not by affecting the driving force for the system by inhibiting the Na-K-ATPase or the cellular metabolism.

Diuretics, Jules B. Puschett, Editor

To characterize further the interaction of the diuretics with the cotransport system, binding studies on plasma membranes isolated from rectal glands were performed, which contain a cotransport system similar to the one found in the TALH cells [4]. Using labeled N-methylfurosemide (NMF) and piretanide, high affinity binding sites for the diuretics were detected. Bumetanide and furosemide displaced NMF from the high affinity binding sites indicating that these sites interact with a variety of "loop" diuretics. The binding increased in the presence of sodium and potassium, but was inhibited by high concentrations of chloride (Fig. 1 and 2). These studies suggest that the diuretics interact with the sodium-potassium-chloride cotransport system and that chloride seems to compete with the binding of the diurectics to the cotransport system. This assumption is supported by the finding that in sodium flux studies an increase in chloride concentration decreases the affinity of the transport system for piretanide (Fig. 3).

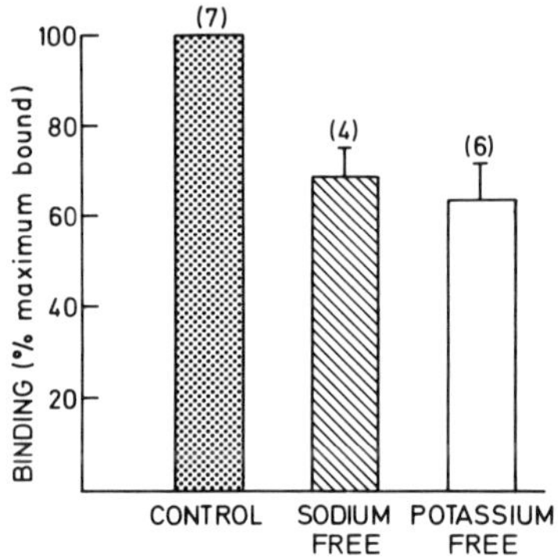

FIG. 1. Binding of piretanide to rectal gland plasma membrane vesicles: Effect of sodium and potassium.
Binding of 2 x 10^{-7} M ^{3}H-piretanide was studied as described previously [4]. In the sodium free medium potassium, and in the potassium free medium sodium were used as replacement. The results represent mean values $\pm$ SEM derived from at least 4 experiments and are expressed as % of binding observed in the presence of 200 mM NaCl and 10 mM KNO_3. Unspecific binding amounted to about 60% of maximum binding. Data are taken from Hannafin [8].

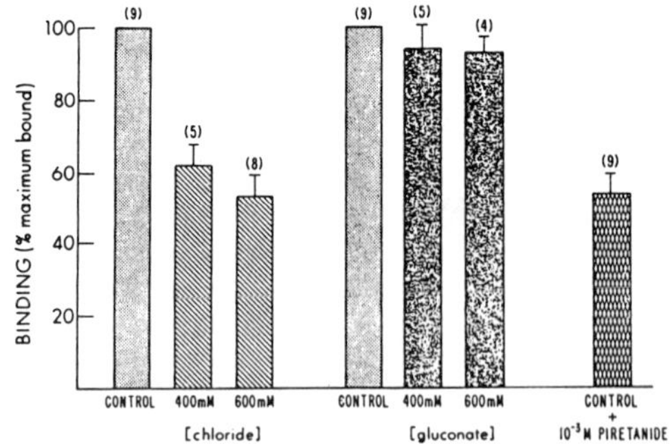

FIG. 2. Binding of piretanide to rectal gland plasma membrane vesicles: Effect of chloride and gluconate.
Binding of 2 x 10^{-7} M [^{3}H]-piretanide was studied as described previously [4]. Sodium salts of the anions were used. The results represent the mean values $\pm$ SEM derived from at least 4 experiments and are expressed as % binding observed in the presence of 200 mM NaCl and 10 mM KNO_3.
Data are taken from Hannafin [8].

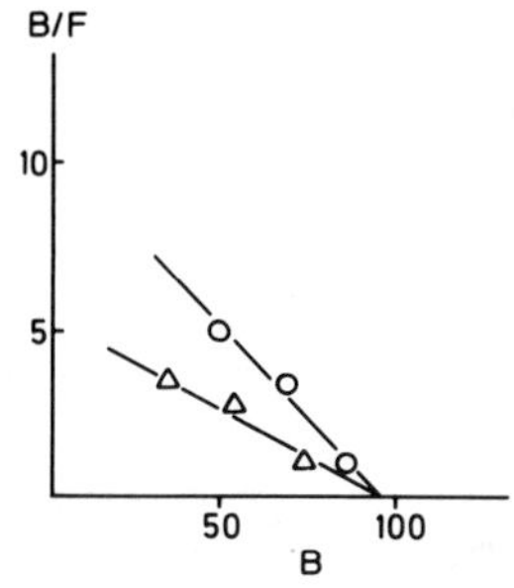

FIG. 3. The effect of chloride concentration on the inhibition by piretanide of chloride dependent sodium uptake into rectal gland plasma membrane vesicles.
Sodium uptake was measured as described previously [4] at different concentrations of piretanide (10^{-4} M, 2 x 10^{-4} M, 10^{-3} M) and in the presence of either 167 mM KCl (△-△) or 47 mM KCl, 120 mM K gluconate (o-o). The results are mean values obtained from 3 experiments and are expressed as % inhibition of sodium uptake in the absence of piretanide. B represents the % inhibition of sodium uptake and F the concentration of piretanide (x 10^5).

In summary, the major, if not exclusive action of "loop" diuretics on active chloride transport in epithelia is the inhibition of the sodium-chloride-potassium cotransport system. The binding of the diuretic to the transport system requires potassium and sodium, and the diuretic interacts with the transport system probably at the chloride site [9] as a pseudosubstrate with a very high affinity. A similar model has been proposed recently in studies on partially purified renal medullary membranes [9] and on erythrocytes [10].

REFERENCES

1. R. Greger, and E. Schlatter, Pfluegers Arch. 396, 325-334 (1983).
2. J. Eveloff, and R. Kinne, J. Membrane Biol. 72(3), 173-181 (1983).
3. B. Koenig, S. Ricapito, and R. Kinne, Pfluegers Arch. 399, 173-179 (1983).
4. J. Hannafin, E. Kinne-Saffran, D. Friedman, and R. Kinne, J. Membrane Biol. 75, 73-83 (1983).
5. J. Eveloff, W. Haase, and R. Kinne, J. Cell Biol. 87, 672-680 (1980).
6. J. Eveloff, E. Bayerdoerffer, P. Silva, and R. Kinne, Pfluegers Arch. 389, 263-270 (1981).
7. J. Eveloff, and R. Kinne in: Advances in Pharmacology 5: Cardio-Renal and Cell Pharmacology, H. Yoshida, Y. Harihara, and S. Ebashi, eds. (Pergamon Press, Oxford-New York 1982) pp. 301-308.
8. J. Hannafin, Ph.D. Thesis 1983, Albert Einstein College of Medicine, NY.
9. B. Forbush III, and H.C. Palfrey, J. Biol. Chem. 258, 11787-11792 (1983).
10. M. Haas, T.J. McManus, Am. J. Physiol. 245, C235-C240 (1983).

ACKNOWLEDGEMENT

Labeled piretanide and N-methylfurosemide were kindly provided by Hoechst A.G., F.R.G.

EXTRA-RENAL EFFECTS OF DIURETICS ON VASCULAR SMOOTH MUSCLE

NEIL L. BROWN, ANNE-MARIE MOURA and MANUEL WORCEL.
Centre de Recherches Roussel-Uclaf, BP. 9, F93230 Romainville, France.

The observation that long-term treatment with diuretics, especially thiazides, produces a reduced response to pressor stimuli, and lowered blood pressure despite normalized extracellular volumes [1] has lead to the hypothesis that these drugs may possess important extra-renal, or direct effects. Indeed, it has been suggested that part of the anti-hypertensive action of indapamide may be due to its direct myorelaxant effect on vascular smooth muscle [e.g. 2,3], and high concentrations of furosemide have been shown to directly inhibit ^{36}Cl efflux from rabbit aorta [4].

This paper will briefly summarize our recent findings on some possible extra-renal or direct effects of diuretics on vascular smooth muscle.

Following the results of Borkowski et al. [2] with indapamide, it appeared of interest to see if other diuretics had *in vitro* smooth muscle relaxing, or anti-spasmogenic properties. All the diuretics tested reduced the amplitude of rat portal vein spontaneous contractions and inhibited angiotensin II (Ag II)-induced contractions of the same preparations [5]. Similarly, they also inhibited contractions of rat aorta induced by $PGF_{2\alpha}$, showing the same order of potency as in the portal vein (Table I). Furthermore, the "low ceiling" type diuretics, indapamide and hydrochlorothiazide, gave dose-response curves which differed from those of the other compounds in both tissue preparations [5].

TABLE I. Concentrations (uM) of diuretics producing 50% inhibition of spontaneous activity and Ag II-induced contractions in portal vein and $PGF_{2\alpha}$-induced contractions of aorta.

	amplitude of* spontaneous contractions	Ag II* contractions	$PGF_{2\alpha}$* contractions
Amiloride	3.4 ± 1.2	6.8 ± 0.8	18.5 ± 1.9
Furosemide	4.5 ± 0.8	76.2 ± 15.0	68.3 ± 14.4
Piretanide	5.5 ± 0.9	83.8 ± 14.8	
Bumetanide	0.6 ± 0.2	82.6 ± 22.9	
Indapamide	53.7 ± 8.3	286.4 ± 20.6	131.3 ± 43.7
Hydrochlorothiazide	174.5 ± 34.9	840.7 ± 80.4	280.7 ± 82.3

* mean ± S.E.M. of 5-8 preparations.

Thus, the results demonstrate that a direct, anti-spasmogenic action *in vitro* is not unique to indapamide ; in fact, this compound was comparatively inactive when compared to amiloride and the loop diuretics.

Diuretics, Jules B. Puschett, Editor

A myorelaxant effect of some diuretics was also observed *in vivo*. Employing anesthetized, ganglion-blocked, intact rats with Ag II-supported blood pressure [see 6] (thus discounting reflex activity), an immediate and significant fall ($p < 0.05$, analysis of variance) in mean blood pressure was observed after i.v. injection of amiloride, furosemide and piretanide (10mg/kg) but not after hydrochlorothiazide and indapamide (10-30mg/kg). The falls in blood pressure preceded measurable diuresis (cannulated urinary bladder), which did not occur with amiloride. The hypotensive response to amiloride, furosemide and piretanide (10mg/kg) was also observed in rats which had been binephrectomized 24 hr beforehand (Fig. 1), suggesting that it was not dependent upon the kidney. It is not possible to conclude whether the hypotensive response was due to arterial or venous dilation. However, the fact that the hypotensive response to piretanide in binephretomized rats was partially blocked by indomethacin (10mg/kg per os) reveals some analogy with the observed effects of furosemide on venous capacitance [7,8] and may thus reflect a venodilating action.

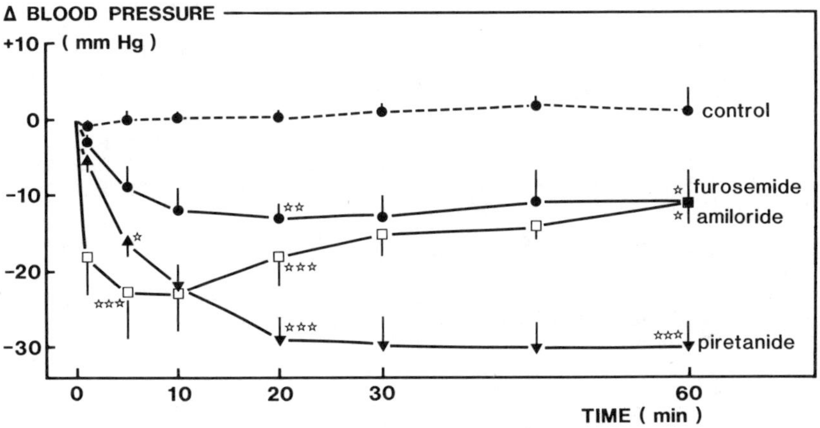

FIG. 1. Effects of furosemide (●), amiloride (□) and piretanide (▲) on changes in mean blood pressure in binephrectomized ganglion-blocked, Ag II-supported rats (*, **, *** ; $p < 0.05$, $p < 0.01$, $p < 0.001$ from control).

Another type of *in vivo* study revealed a direct, or extra-renal action of diuretics. It is well known that thiazides can produce hypokalemia, which can be prevented by concomitant treatment with "potassium-sparing" diuretics such as amiloride and triamterene. In rats treated *per os* with cyclothiazide (0.2-0.5mg/kg) [9] or hydrochlorothiazide (1.4mg/kg), the *ex vivo* rate of ^{86}Rb efflux (a marker of K^+ efflux) from the tail artery smooth muscle cells was significantly increased. The effect of cyclothiazide was inhibited by concomitant treatment of the rats with triamterene (10.0-25.0mg/kg) [9] which was by itself without action. Furthermore, these above effects on ^{86}Rb efflux were also observed in binephrectomized animals (Table II), suggesting an extra-renal effect. None of the diuretics directly affected Na efflux from the tail artery.

TABLE II. Effects of cyclothiazide (CT), triamterene (T) and their association on the ex vivo ^{86}Rb efflux rate from rat tail artery smooth muscle cells from binephrectomized rats.

Treatment	Dose (mg/kg)	^{86}Rb efflux rate (min^{-1})^{a}
Control	-	0.0100 ± 0.0004
Cyclothiazide	0.2	0.0128 ± 0.0001*
Triamterene	10.0	0.0102 ± 0.0002
CT + T	0.2 + 10.0	0.0103 ± 0.0002(**)
Cyclothiazide	0.5	0.0137 ± 0.0006*
Triamterene	25.0	0.0102 ± 0.0004
CT + T	0.5 + 25.0	0.0105 ± 0.0004(**)

[a] Mean±S.E.M. of 8 rats per group. * $p < 0.05$ from control, (**) $p < 0.01$ from cyclothiazide group (Dunnett).

In summary, the results demonstrate that some diuretics (amiloride, furosemide, piretanide, bumetanide) show a direct anti-spasmogenic activity *in vitro*, at concentrations compatible with therapeutic blood levels. Some of these diuretics can acutely lower blood pressure in binephrectomized, ganglion-blocked rats with Ag II-supported blood pressure, suggesting an extra-renal action. Finally, thiazides stimulate smooth muscle permeability to potassium. This membrane effect is blocked by triamterene. Thus the potassium sparing action of triamterene could be in part explained by a direct effect on potassium permeability of vascular smooth muscle.

ACKNOWLEDGEMENTS

The authors thank Mmes M. Badel,F. DaPonte and M.C. Hameau for the skilled technical assistance, and Mme M. Viallet for typing the manuscript.

REFERENCES

1. J. Conway in : Handb. Exp. Pharm. XXXIX Antihypertensive Agents. F. Gross, ed. (Springer-Verlag, Berlin 1977) pp. 477-494.
2. K.R. Borkowski, P.E. Hicks and R.A. Moore, Br. J. Pharmacol. 72, 172-173P (1981).
3. J. Kyncl, K. Oheim, T. Seki and A. Solles, Arzneim Forsch. 25, 1491-1495 (1975).
4. V.A.W. Kreye, P.K. Bauer and I. Villhauer, European J. Pharmacol. 73, 91-95 (1981).
5. N.L. Brown and M. Worcel, Br. J. Pharmac. 79, 332P (1983).
6. N.L. Brown and M. Worcel, European J. Pharmacol. 92, 285-289 (1983).
7. J.L. Data, A. Rane, J. Gerkens, G.R. Wilkinson, A.S. Nies and R.A. Branch, J. Pharmacol. Exp. Ther. 206, 431-438 (1978).
8. G.D. Johnston, W.R. Hiatt, A.S. Nies, N.A. Payne, R.C. Murphy and J.G. Gerber, Circ. Res. 53, 630-635 (1983).
9. A.M. Moura and M. Worcel, European J. Pharmacol. 86, 129-133 (1982).

RED CELL NA^+-K^+ COTRANSPORT: DOSE-RESPONSE EFFECTS OF FUROSEMIDE INHIBITION IN BLACK AND WHITE HYPERTENSIVES.

J.E. CROOK and P.J. MROCZKOWSKI
Department of Medicine and Pharmacology
Medical College of Wisconsin, Milwaukee, WI U.S.A.

INTRODUCTION

Hypertension is a major cardiovascular disease affecting a population which is heterogeneous with regard to race, sex and age. The size of the hypertensive population is variably estimated at 25 to 60 million, dependent on the criteria employed to define an elevated arterial pressure [1]. The scope and number of investigations directed toward a better understanding of the pathophysiology of the disease is matched only by the equally voluminous number of studies detailing treatment strategies. Despite this large body of data, it is quite clear that voids still remain in our knowledge of the genesis of the disease as well as what constitutes the best therapeutic modality.

What has evolved, with time, is that sequestered within the larger population of hypertensive persons is an important group composed of black individuals who are disproportionately affected in terms of number and severity. The prevalence of high blood pressure among blacks is 66 percent greater than that found among whites. An estimated 17 percent of the white population have definite high blood pressure (systolic blood pressure = 160 mm Hg or diastolic blood pressure = 95 mm Hg) compared to 28.2 percent for blacks. This same report also cites evidence that blacks continue to be over-represented in the higher blood pressure elevations (greater than 105 mm Hg diastolic) [2].

Renewed interest in the transport of sodium and potassium across red cell membranes has been generated by recent reports [3,4] demonstrating differences in translocation of these cations by hypertensive subjects.

The membrane surrounding the contents of the erythrocyte is a classic bilayer mixture of lipids and proteins that contains a sodium and potassium adenosine triphosphatase (ATPase) dependent mechanism responsible for the active transport of sodium and potassium across the membrane. The ubiquitous membrane bound sodium and potassium dependent ATPase is likely the most well-known and well-studied mechanism for transport of sodium and potassium. However, it is not the sole means by which red cells are able to exchange sodium and potassium ions.

There are other ATPase pump-independent transport systems for sodium and potassium. The inhibition of a simultaneous influx or efflux of both sodium and potassium by furosemide led to characterization of the cotransport system [5].

The collective results of a survey of international investigators who utilized the cotransport system to study hypertensive patients indicate that hypertensive individuals have cotransport systems with decreased activity [4].

Results in our laboratory show that the cotransport system is markedly less active in blacks compared to whites. As is illustrated in Table I, this system functions quite differently in white and black individuals. An all male population of 26 normotensive (14 white and 12 black) and 44 hypertensive (30 white and 14 black) individuals were studied. The hypertensive patients had been free of medications for at least three weeks and their blood pressures were greater than 140/95. As shown in Table I, the sodium effluxes for white and black hypertensives differed significantly ($p < 0.001$). Also, the red cell potassium effluxes of black hypertensives were significantly lower ($p < 0.001$) than those of the corresponding white hypertensives.

Diuretics, Jules B. Puschett, Editor

Interestingly, white normotensive males had significantly greater ($p < 0.001$) effluxes of sodium and potassium than black normotensives. In other words, black individuals transported out of their red cells sodium as well as potassium at a slower rate than white subjects irrespective of blood pressure. The reduction of potassium efflux in black hypertensives versus black normotensives achieved statistical significance ($p < 0.05$). The passive permeability rate constant, representing other mechanisms for translocating sodium and potassium after the ATPase pump and cotransport system have been inhibited, was significantly higher ($p < 0.05$) for sodium in white normotensive subjects when compared with the corresponding group of black individuals.

Table I. Kinetic Properties of Loaded Red Cells From Normotensives(NT) and Hypertensives(HT) Fluxed in a Magnesium Chloride-Sucrose-Ouabain Medium.

Group	N	Passive Permeability Na^+	K^+	Furosemide-Sensitive Effluxes Na^+	K^+	$\frac{Na^+}{K^+}$
		(rate constant, hr^{-1})*		(µmol/L cells/hr)*		Flux ratio
WHITE(W)						
Normotensive	14	0.031 ± 0.006^a	0.009 ± 0.001	629 ± 235^b	584 ± 172^b	1.07 ± 0.33^c
Hypertensive	30	0.030 ± 0.006	0.009 ± 0.001	608 ± 168^d	612 ± 154^d	1.00 ± 0.18
BLACK(B)						
Normotensive	12	0.025 ± 0.004	0.010 ± 0.002	264 ± 65	320 ± 49^e	0.83 ± 0.18
Hypertensive	14	0.026 ± 0.006	0.010 ± 0.002	256 ± 84	265 ± 65	1.00 ± 0.33

*Mean ± S.D. Unpaired t-test; WNT v. BNT: a= $p<0.01$; b= $p<0.001$; c= $p<0.05$. WHT v. BHT: d= $p<0.001$. BNT v. BHT: e= $p<0.05$

The purpose of this investigation was to further define the inhibition of erythrocyte cotransport of sodium and potassium in white and black hypertensives at subsaturating concentrations of furosemide by observing for differences in sensitivity to furosemide between hypertensive subjects.

METHODS

Erythrocytes from 22 male hypertensive subjects free of all drugs for two weeks were collected in pre-chilled heparinized tubes. Of the total group, 12 patients were white (mean age = 55 years, mean blood pressure = 146/99 mm Hg.)and 10 subjects were black (mean age = 50 years, mean blood pressure = 136/101 mm Hg.). The cotransport system was measured using the p-chloromecuribenzene sulfonate method described by Garay, et al. [6].

RESULTS

As shown in table 2, no significant differences in percent inhibition of cotransport were demonstrated at any of the inhibitor concentrations employed The relationship of log [F] to log (I/100-I) where [F] equals concentration of inhibitor and I equals percent inhibition was used to calculate concentrations at which 50 percent inhibition (IC_{50}) occurred. Although the IC_{50} values are similiar, the slopes of the lines are very dissimiliar. The data indicate that the two groups have similiar responses to and affinity for furosemide.

Table II. Dose-Response Effects of Furosemide on Red Cell Na^+-K^+ Cotransport Inhibition in White and Black Hypertensives.

[Furosemide] (μM)	Cotransport Inhibition (%) White Na^+	White K^+	Black Na^+	Black K^+
1	3	5	9	1
5	15	12	19	9
10	20	23	18	18
50	51	58	59	77
100	74	84	65	82
1,000	100	100	100	100
Hill Plot Data:				
IC_{50}(μM)	39	28	43	28
Correlation Coefficient(r)	0.996	0.984	0.969	0.996
Slope(m)	0.97	1.00	0.67	1.4

The lack of similiarity of the curves for the two groups is further emphasized in Figure 1. In this figure, the log concentration of inhibitor is plotted versus μMoles of cation inhibited.

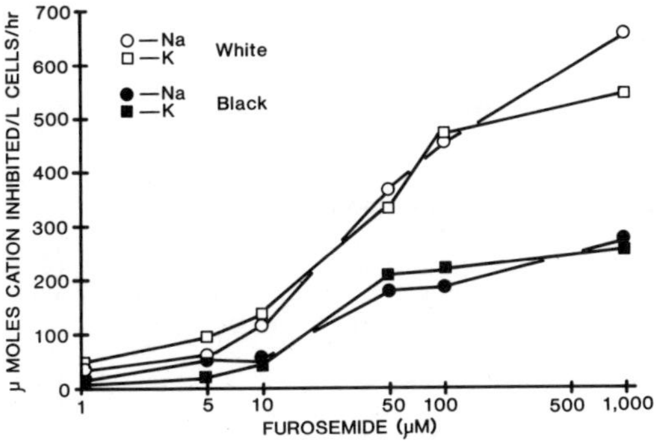

FIG. 1. Inhibition of sodium-potassium cotransport in hypertensives.

In summary, the data suggests that the lower cotransport values in black hypertensives are due to a reduced number of cotransport furosemide receptors.

REFERENCES

1. E.D. Freis, New Eng. J. Med. 307, 306-307 (1982).
2. Final Report on the National Black Health Providers Task Force on High Blood Pressure Education and Control. NIH Publication, No. 81-1474 (1981).
3. R.P. Garay, J.L. Elghozi, G. Dagher, P. Meyer, New Eng. J. Med. 302 769-771 (1980).
4. R.P. Garay, Lancet 1, 500-502 (1982).
5. J.S. Wiley and R.A. Cooper, J.Clin. Invest. 53, 745-755 (1974).
6. D. Cusi and R.P. Garay, Mol. Pharmacol. 19, 438-443 (1981).

Address correspondance to James E. Crook, M.D., Ph.D., Oak Ridge Associated Universities, Medical and Health Sciences Division, Oak Ridge, TN 37831. U.S.A.

STUDIES ON THE CARDIAC ACTION OF TRIAMTERENE IN HEALTHY VOLUNTEERS

R. DÜSING, B. WEISSER, K. GLÄNZER, E. MUTSCHLER*, and H.J. KRAMER

Medizinische Universitäts-Poliklinik Bonn and *Pharmakologisches Institut der Universität Frankfurt, Federal Republic of Germany

ABSTRACT

The present study investigates, whether triamterene (TA) interferes with the cardiac response to $ß_1$-receptor stimulation in vivo. In ten healthy volunteers the response of heart rate to increasing doses of isoproterenol and to graded exercise was recorded three times, during control, acutely following a single oral dose of 100 mg of TA, and after 12 days of TA administration (100 mg/day). Neither resting heart rate nor the chronotropic response to isoproterenol was altered after a single oral dose or following chronic administration of TA. Accordingly, no alterations could be observed in the heart rate response to graded treadmill exercise. Our results therefore suggest that TA does not interfere with the cardiac response to $ß_1$-stimulation in healthy volunteers.

INTRODUCTION

Triamterene (TA), a "potassium-sparing" diuretic has been widely used for about two decades in the therapy of edema and hypertension. Its predominant use is in combination with conventional diuretics such as hydrochlorothiazide to prevent potassium losses known to occur during diuretic therapy (1). In addition to its renal effects, TA has been suggested to possess antiarrhythmic properties and to exert an inotropic effect in isolated heart preparations (2-7). It has recently been suggested that TA may also interfere with the cardiac response to $ß_1$-receptor stimulation. Thus, in vitro-studies have suggested that TA may interfere with the signal transfer between the cardiac ß-adrenoceptor site and the adenylate cyclase system through the plasmalemma (6). Whether these effects can also be demonstrated in humans following acute or chronic TA administration is presently unknown. The present study therefore investigates the response of heart rate in response to isoproterenol administration and to graded treadmill exercise during control and after a single oral dose and chronic administration of TA.

METHODS

The cardiac response to increasing doses of the $ß_1$-receptor stimulator isoproterenol was investigated three times in ten healthy volunteers aged between 23 and 26 years. The first protocol served as control while the second and third protocol were performed following a single oral dose of 100 mg of TA and after 12 days of treatment with TA in a dose of 100 mg/day, respectively. In both the acute and chronic experiment, isoprenaline injections were performed 120 min after TA had been administered to the subjects. The experimental protocol was performed according to methods previously described (8). In brief, the procedure was carried out with the subjects supine in a quiet surrounding. An intravenous infusion of 5% glucose was started and baseline pulse readings were established. Isoproterenol sulfate was then injected as a bolus in amounts of 0.0025 to 0.02 µg/kg body weight. Heart rate

Diuretics, Jules B. Puschett, Editor

changes were measured using constant ECG monitoring with automatic recording of heart rate. Approximately one hour after the isoproterenol injections, all volunteers were exposed to graded treadmill exercise of 50, 100 and 150 watts, each for 2 min and heart rate was measured at the end of each exercise period.

Blood for measurements of serum concentrations of sodium, potassium and creatinine was drawn before each experimental procedure. In addition, blood for the measurement of serum concentrations of TA and the pharmacologically active phase II-metabolite p-hydroxytriamterene sulfuric acid ester (OH-TA-ester) was drawn on the day of the "chronic" experiment. Determinations of TA and OH-TA-ester were carried out according to methods previously described (9).

The results are given as means ± SEM. Statistical analysis of data was performed using the Wilcoxon matched pairs signed rank test (10).

RESULTS AND DISCUSSION

Serum concentrations of sodium, potassium and creatinine averaged 137 ± 1, 4.2 ± 0.1 mmol/l and 69 ± 3 µmol/l, respectively and were unchanged following 12 days of TA treatment (138 ± 1, 4.2 ± 0.1 mmol/l and 75 ± 4 µmol/l, respectively). After 12 days of treatment with 100 mg of TA per day, serum concentrations of TA and the OH-TA-ester averaged 103 ± 33 and 1234 ± 203 ng/ml, respectively.

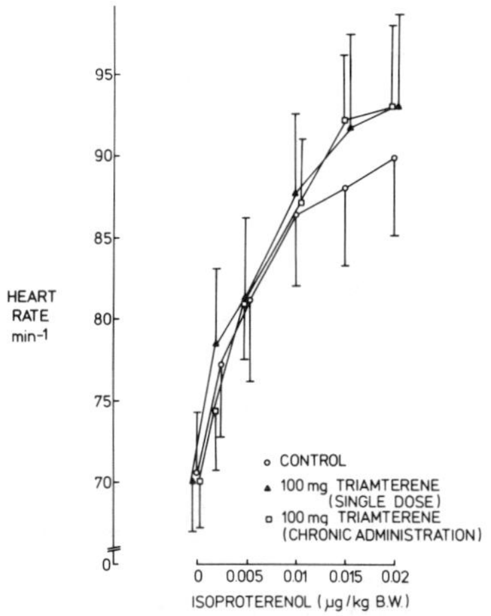

Fig. 1: Heart rate response to i.v. isoprenaline during control and following treatment with TA.

Mean heart rate responses to intravenous isoproterenol before and after a single oral dose and following chronic treatment with TA are shown in figure 1. Following injections of isotonic saline without isoproterenol, heart rate averaged 70.6 ± 3.4 beats/min and dose dependently increased to 89.8 ± 4.7 beats/min following isoprenaline in a dose of 0.02 µg/min. Following a single oral dose or after chronic treatment with TA, the respective values were 70.1 ± 4.1, 93.1 ± 5.3, 70.1 ± 2.8 and 93.1 ± 4.8 beats/min, respectively.

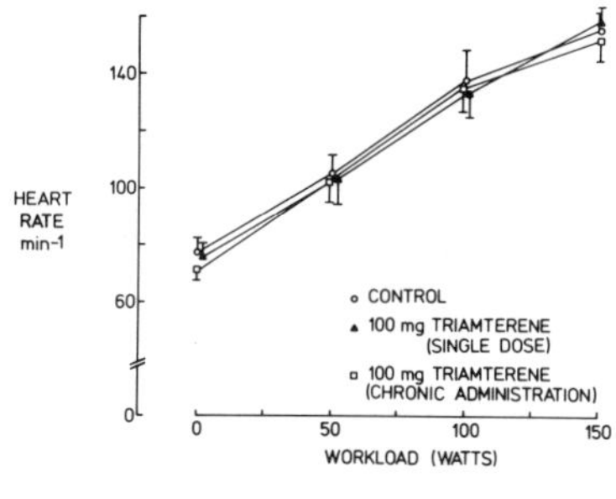

Fig. 2: Heart rate response to graded treadmill exercise during control and following treatment with TA.

Thus, no significant changes occurred in the heart rate response to intravenous doses of isoprenaline after a single oral dose or following chronic TA treatment. Accordingly, no changes occurred in the heart rate response to graded treadmill exercise both after a single dose of TA or following 12 days of TA treatment (Figure 2).

Previous in vitro-studies have suggested that TA may exert cardiac effects by acting as a phosphodiesterase-inhibitor and by inhibition of catecholamine-activated adenylate cyclase (6). The inhibitory effect on phosphodiesterase activity has been demonstrated for TA itself and for the OH-TA-ester (5,7). On the other hand, TA may also inhibit the positive inotropic action of ß-receptor agonists through a mechanism that involves the blockade of the signal transfer between the ß-adrenoreceptor and the adenylate cyclase complex (6).

In the present in vivo-study in healthy volunteers, TA did not interfere with ß-receptor stimulation either when an exogenous ß-receptor stimulator was administered or during graded physical exercise with activation of endogenous adrenergic activity. Determinations of serum TA and OH-TA-ester concentrations clearly demonstrate that therapeutic concentrations of both agents were present and therefore exclude subtherapeutic serum and tissue concentrations as a reason for the lack of an effect of TA treatment. Our data, therefore, suggest that TA treatment may not be associated with an altered cardiac ß-receptor responsiveness in humans.

REFERENCES

1. E.J. Cragoe, Diuretics, Chemistry, Pharmacology, and Medicine. John Wiley and Sons, Inc., 1983
2. B.K. Yeh, J.S. Francis, A.J. Gosselin, and R.A. Relias, Clin. Pharmacol. Ther. **17**, 141-145 (1975)
3. D.J. Weber, Clin. Pharmacol. Ther. **13**, 868-874 (1972)
4. K. Greef, E. Noack, Drug Res. **29**, 619-622 (1979)
5. K. Greef, P. Schuhmacher, Drug Res. **29**, 705-709, (1979)
6. E. Noack, P. Schuhmacher, J. Mol. Cell Cardiol. **15**, 319-324 (1983)
7. P. Schuhmacher, K. Greef, E.A. Noack, European J. Pharmacol. **95**, 71-77 (1983)
8. C.F. George, M.E. Conolly, T. Fenyvesi, R. Briant, and C.T. Dollery, Arch. Intern. Med. **130**, 361-364 (1972)
9. U. Gundert-Remy, D. von Kenne, E. Weber, H.E. Geißler, B. Grebian, and E. Mutschler, Eur. J. Clin. Pharmacol. **16**, 39-44 (1979)
10. R.C. Milton, J. Am. Statist. Ass. **59**, 925-934 (1964)

SECTION XI

USE OF DIURETICS IN ACUTE AND CHRONIC RENAL FAILURE

THE USE OF DIURETICS IN ACUTE RENAL FAILURE

Bernardo Rodríguez-Iturbe, M.D., Renal Service and Laboratory, Hospital Universitario de Maracaibo, Maracaibo, Zulia, Venezuela.

The purpose of this paper is to review the subject of the use of diuretics in patients with acute renal failure (ARF) attempting to give a balanced view of controversial issues and contributing with data from our own division. The task is made simpler by the recent publication of Levinsky et al. [1] that deals with the subject in a comprehensive and scholarly manner; from this work I have drawn extensively.

My remarks will be confined to the use of mannitol and loop diuretics in the prevention as well as in the treatment of oliguric acute renal failure. Promising as it presently seems, not enough data is available on the clinical use of dopamine to permit sensible conclusions of clinical relevance.

Acute renal failure may be the result of ischemia or nephrotoxins and, as shown in Table I, the pathophysiologic consequences of these insults are vasoconstriction, tubular cell damage with varying degrees of obstruction, backleak and further reflex vasoconstriction, and glomerular cell damage. The clinical result is a sudden impairment of renal function with azotemia and the urine flow rate may be normal or decreased.

TABLE I. Pathophysiology of acute renal failure.

INITIAL INSULT	PATHOPHYSIOLOGIC CONSEQUENCES	CLINICAL RESULT
Ischemia	Vasoconstriction → ↓GFR	Oliguria present or absent
Nephrotoxins	Tubular cell damage → (obstruction, backleak, vasoconstriction) Glomerular cell damage → (↓Kf, ↓GFR)	Azotemia

Kf = ultrafiltration coefficient.

In the experimental animal, the ischemic models of acute renal failure are the glycerol model, the norepinephrine infusion model and the renal artery clamping model. The classic nephrotoxic models are the ones induced by uranyl nitrate and mercuric chloride. These experimental models have been authoritatively reviewed by Stein et al. [2].

In all the different experimental models of ARF, with the possible exception of the uranyl nitrate model, there is an initial drop in renal blood flow and, in the ischemic models, the drop in renal blood flow is sustained past the initial insult throughout most of the maintenance phase of ARF. However, the role of influences other than ischemia is underscored by the fact that blood flow may be increased in the maintenance phase of ARF without restoration of glomerular filtration rate [2].

Tubular obstruction is evident in the mercuric chloride model [3] as well as in the renal clamping [4] and norepinephrine [5] models and backleak appears to be prominent in the nephrotoxic models [6-8] as well as in the ARF induced by renal artery clamping [9].

Published 1984 by Elsevier Science Publishing Co., Inc.
Diuretics, Jules B. Puschett, Editor

Decreased ultrafiltration coefficient (Kf) due to injury in the glomerular basement membrane induced by ischemia or toxic agents, appears to be a contributing factor in the norepinephrine and nephrotoxic models of ARF [7, 10, 11].

As indicated by Levinsky et al. [1], mannitol or furosemide may be beneficial by inducing vasodilation or reversal of the vasoconstriction. They may prevent or eliminate tubular obstruction by inducing a high urine flow. Furosemide may be useful by inhibiting the tubuloglomerular feedback mechanism that will induce vasoconstriction in the nephrons that present tubular obstruction, and finally, mannitol may prevent or decrease tubular cell swelling which may be a factor contributing to obstruction of urine flow. Alternatively, the effect of diuretics may be only to increase urine flow with no change in renal function or detectable effect in prognosis.

Diuretics in Prevention of Acute Renal Failure.

In most models of experimental renal failure, diuretic therapy appears to have a beneficial effect if administered prophylactically [2]. Mannitol and furosemide, when given before the insult, are useful in preventing or improving the ischemia-induced ARF (renal artery clamping and norepinephrine) [12-16] and methemoglobin [17] and cis-platinum-induced ARF [18]. Mannitol but not furosemide, may prevent glycerol-induced ARF [19] and furosemide may prevent ARF induced by cephaloridine (it worsens it if given later) [20-21] amphotericin [36], and folic-acid [48].

It appears, therefore, that diuretic therapy could be potentially useful if given prophylactically in clinical situations which are associated with a high incidence of ARF. Table II summarizes the patient groups in which prevention of ARF has been attempted with diuretic therapy.

TABLE II. Diuretics in the prevention of acute renal failure (ARF).

Patients	Renal Function	Incidence of ARF	Mortality	Ref
High Risk Surgery				
Cardiovascular	↑ Urine Volume	Unchanged	Unchanged	24-32
Obstructive Jaundice	Prevents GFR ↓, ↑ Urine Volume	Unchanged	Unchanged	33,34
Severe Trauma	↑ Urine Volume	Unchanged	Unchanged	35
Nephrotoxic Drugs				
Cis-Platinum DD	Renal function preserved with doses known to be nephrotoxic			36
Amphotericin B	Renal function preserved with doses known to be nephrotoxic			37
IV Radiocontrast in patients with RF		Improved		38-40
Acute Hyperuricemia, Severe Hemolysis		Improved		1

Several studies [24-32] have analyzed the use of Mannitol or furosemide in open-heart and cardiovascular surgery, and there is little question that urine volume may be increased. However, the mortality and incidence of ARF is not improved by diuretics.

Untura et al. [33] and Dawson et al. [34] reported that furosemide increased urine flow and prevents the decrease in glomerular filtration rate observed in patients with obstructive jaundice that undergo major surgery. Lucas et al. [35] observed increased urine flow in patients with severe trauma and emergency surgery. These series, nevertheless, failed to show a significant drop in the incidence of ARF in these patients with the use of diuretics.

Hayes et al. [36] reported that furosemide prevented renal failure in patients receiving cis-platinum DD in doses of 3.0 mg/kg, while nephrotoxicity occurs at doses higher than 1.0 mg/kg without the use of this diuretic. Olivero et al. [37] reported prevention of nephrotoxicity, but not of the acidosis, associated with amphotericin B. Several reports [38-40] indicate that the incidence of radiocontrast-induced ARF may be reduced by the prophylactic use of diuretics.

As noted by Levinsky et al. [1] acute hyperuricemia and severe hemolysis are clinical situations in which diuretic therapy should prevent the development of ARF.

Diuretics in the Treatment of Acute Renal Failure.

Acute renal failure may have two phases: one early or functional, and one late or organic [41-43]. The possibility exists that, if given in the first phase, the diuretics could revert the renal function to normal.

The problem is to establish objective criteria to define the early phase. There is no clear-cut dividing line in the functional tests to distinguish between the theoretical phases of evolution of ARF. Most cases of reversible ARF have less impaired U/P osmolar ratio, U/P urea ratio and renal failure index, but the overlap is so substantial [42] that it renders these tests useless to distinguish between functional and established ARF. In fact, the duration of ARF is as good as any indicator of "early" (less than 48 hrs) ARF susceptible to be rapidly reverted to normal. Because of these problems in definition it is difficult to evaluate the published reports [41-46]. From their review of the literature, Levinsky et al. [1] concluded that oliguria may be reversed by diuretics in two-thirds of the patients, and that those patients who respond with a diuresis will have a lower mortality than those who do not.

In established ARF, diuretics have been used extensively, but few authors report controlled trials [47-50]. Cantarovich et al. [47, 48] reported that high doses of furosemide induced a shorter course of oliguria and reduced the need for dialysis, whereas lower doses of furosemide (600 mg/day) were associated with minimal improvement. These authors found that the overall mortality of ARF was not significantly altered by diuretics, but diuretic therapy was recommended because of the lower dialysis requirements and shorter oliguria in the diuretic-treated patients. Karayannopoulos [51] also reported beneficial effects with loop diuretics.

Contrary to these investigations, Kleinknecht et al. [49] and Brown et al. [50] found no discernible effect of diuretics in established ARF. The conversion to non-oliguric ARF achieved with diuretics may be beneficial because it may shorten the course of the disease or because it may facilitate the medical management of the patient. Clearly, response to diuretics may identify a milder disease rather than reflect a change in natural history [1].

In the University Hospital we have seen 207 patients with oliguric renal failure between 1973 and 1983 (Table III). These patients failed to respond to volume expansion and had one or more of the following indices of parenchymal renal failure: urinary sodium > 30 mEq/L, U/P osm < 1.5:1, U/P urea < 5:1, fractional sodium excretion > 2.5%.

Table III. Mortality of oliguric acute renal failure. (Hospital Universitario de Maracaibo, 1973-1983).

ETIOLOGY		DEATHS/CASES	MORTALITY %
MEDICAL	Hemodynamic ("pure")	2/19	10.5
	Nephrotoxins	1/8	12.5
	All Others	19/35	54.2
	TOTAL	22/62	35.4
SURGICAL	Gastrointestinal	16/24	66.6
	Severe Trauma	11/18	61.1
	Peripheral Vascular	3/8	37.5
	Firearm Wounds	3/10	30.0
	Burns (less than 60%)	1/9	11.1
	Urologic	0/6	0.0
	TOTAL	34/75	45.3
OBSTETRICAL	1st Trimester	11/42	26.1
	3rd Trimester	7/28	25.0
	TOTAL	18/70	25.7
ALL CASES		74/207	35.7

Forty-seven of these patients were seen within 48 hours of the beginning of oliguric ARF and received, after volume expansion failed to induce a diuresis, furosemide 100-200 mg IV. If oliguria persisted no further diuretic treatment was given, but if the urine output increased to at least 20 ml/hr, additional doses of furosemide were administered by the urine flow rate, without exceeding 500 mg in 24 hours. As shown in Table IV, 16 patients had a transient response and 9 patients had a sustained increase in urine flow.

TABLE IV. Response to diuretics in established acute renal failure. Diuretics given only in cases with oliguria of less than 48 hours when first seen.

ETIOLOGY	PATIENTS RESPONDING (%)	TYPE OF RESPONSE	
		TRANSIENT	SUSTAINED
MEDICAL	4/12 (33.3)	3	1
SURGICAL	11/20 (55.0)	9	2
OBSTETRIC	10/15 (66.6)	4	6
TOTAL	25/47 (53.1)	16	9

We could detect no differences in mortality, hospital stay and number of patients requiring dialysis, between the group receiving and the group not receiving diuretics (Table V). The prognosis of patients showing a sustained diuretic response was essentially the same as that of patients that did not respond to diuretics (Table VI).

TABLE V. Diuretic treatment in established acute renal failure. Diuretic treatment only used in patients with less than 48 hrs of oliguric renal failure when first seen.
D = diuretics given, No-D = diuretics not given.

ETIOLOGY	MORTALITY		HOSPITAL STAY (days)		PATIENTS REQUIRING DIALYSIS	
	D	No-D	D	No-D	N	No-D
MEDICAL (n=62)	4/12 (33.3%)	18/50 (36.0%)	27.1 ± 3	21.6 ± 4	58.3%	60.0%
SURGICAL (n=75)	8/20 (40.0%)	26/55 (47.2%)	31.7 ± 4	23.0 ± 3	90.0%	72.7%
OBSTETRIC (n=70)	3/15 (20.0%)	15/55 (27.0%)	18.4 ± 2	23.1 ± 3	33.3%	36.3%
ALL CASES (n=207)	15/47 (31.9%)	59/160 (36.8%)				

TABLE VI. Mortality of acute renal failure responding to diuretics. Oliguric ARF includes patients who did not receive diuretics and those who did not have a sustained diuretic response with diuretics.

ETIOLOGY	SUSTAINED RESPONSE TO DIURETICS Cases resp.	Deaths	OLIGURIC ARF Deaths (%)	ALL CASES (%)
MEDICAL	1/12	0	22/61 (36.0%)	35.4%
SURGICAL	2/20	1	33/73 (45.2%)	45.3%
OBSTETRIC	6/15	2	16/64 (25.0%	25.7%
ALL CASES	9/47 (19.1%)	3/9 (33.3%)	71/198 (35.8%)	35.7%

In reviewing the literature (Table VII) it appears that non-oliguric ARF has a mortality ranging from 26-46%, while oliguric ARF has a mortality ranging from 35-71%. It is possible that ARF with non-oliguric natural history is milder than oliguric ARF.

Brown et al. [50], Minuth et al. [52] and our own data appear to indicate that response to diuretic therapy with sustained diuresis does not improve the prognosis.

In conclusion, the evidence indicates that loop diuretics will increase urine output in one-half to two-thirds of the patients with oliguric ARF and sustained diuresis may be expected in 19 to 20% of them. Yet, diuretics have not been proven to alter the prognosis of established ARF. Their use in medical practice is widespread among clinicians because there is evidence that they exert beneficial effects in some experimental models of the disease and because some studies indicate that non-oliguric ARF has a more favorable prognosis. It is reasonable to use them as long as they are not employed as a substitute of volume expansion in cases in whom prerenal factors need to be ruled out. The risks of mannitol (circulatory overload) and furosemide (chiefly ototoxicity and potentiation of gentamycin and cefaloridine toxicity) are comparatively minor if one keeps in mind that aggressive pursuit of a high urine volume does not appear justified in the light of available data.

TABLE VII. Prognosis of oliguric and non-oliguric acute renal failure.

STUDY	MORTALITY (%)*			Reference
	Oliguric ARF	Non-Olig ARF	Oliguric ARF Responsive to Diuretics	
Cantarovich et al, 1969-72	57		46 (NS)	48**
Lordon & Burton, 1972	62	46		54
Baek et al, 1975	71	39		53
Minuth et al, 1976	62	38		52
Anderson et al, 1977	50	26		55
Brown et al, 1981	57		64 (NS)	50
Present series	35		33 (NS)	

*Mortality expressed disregarding decimal points. NS = no significant differences.

**Mortality in this study is given for patients receiving and not receiving furosemide rather than for those who responded to treatment; however 71.7% of the patients responded.

REFERENCES

1. N.G. Levinsky, D.B. Bernard, P.A. Johnston. Mannitol and loop diuretics in acute renal failure. In Acute Renal Failure, edited by B.M. Brenner and M.J. Lazarus. W.B. Saunders Co., Philadelphia 1983, p. 712.
2. J.H. Stein, M.D. Lifschitz, L.D. Barnes. Current concepts on the pathophysiology of acute renal failure. Am. J. Physiol. 234:F171, 1978.
3. W.M. Flamenbaum, M.L. Huddleston, J.S. McNeal, R.J. Hamburger. Uranyl-nitrate induced acute renal failure in the rat: micropuncture and renal hemodynamic studies. Kidney Int. 6:408, 1974.
4. G.A. Tanner, M. Steinhausen. Tubular obstruction and ischemia-induced acute renal failure in the rat. Kidney Int. 10:565, 1976.
5. T.J. Burke, K.L. Duchin, R.E. Cronin, R.W. Schrier. Nephron and microcirculatory pressure changes in norepinephrine induced acute renal failure: modification by mannitol. Clin. Res. 25:96a, 1977.
6. N. Bank, B.F. Mutz, H.A. Aynedjian. The role of "leakage" of tubular fluid in anuria due to mercuric poisoning. J. Clin. Invest. 46:695-704, 1976.
7. R.C. Blantz. Mechanism of acute renal failure after uranyl nitrate. J. Clin. Invest. 57:419-439, 1976.
8. J.S. Stein, J. GottschalK, R.W. Osgood, T.F. Ferris. Pathophysiology of nephrotoxic model of acute renal failure. Kidney Int. 8:27, 1975.
9. W.J. Arendshorst, W.F. Finn, C.W. Gottschalk. Pathogenesis of acute renal failure following renal ischemia in the rat. J. Clin. Invest. 53:1497, 1974.

10. J.W. Cox, R.W. Baehler, H. Sharma, T. O'Dorisio, R.W. Osgood, J.H. Stein, T.F. Ferris. Studies on the mechanisms of oliguria in a model of unilateral acute renal failure. J. Clin. Invest. 53:1546, 1974.
11. R.W. Baehler, T.A. Kotchen, J.H. Burke, J.H. Galla, D. Bhathena. Considerations on the pathophysiology of mercuric chloride-induced acute renal failure. J. Lab. Clin. Med. 90:330, 1977.
12. M.J. Hanley, K. Davidson. Prior mannitol infusion in a model of ischemic acute renal failure. Am. J. Physiol. 241:F556, 1981.
13. C.R. Morris, E.A. Alexander, F.J. Bruns, N.G. Levinsky. Restoration and maintenance of glomerular filtration by mannitol during hypoperfusion of the kidney. J. Clin. Invest. 51:1555, 1972.
14. R.E. Cronin, A. deTorrente, P.D. Miller, et al. Pathogenic mechanisms in early norepinephrine-induced acute renal failure. Functional and histological correlates of protection. Kidney Int. 14:115, 1978.
15. R.V. Patak, S.Z. Fadem, M.D. Lifschitz, J.H. Stein. Study of factors which modify the development of norepinephrine-induced acute renal failure in the dog. Kidney Int. 15:227, 1979.
16. A. deTorrente, P.D. Miller, R.E. Cronin, et al. Effects of furosemide and acetylcholine in norepinephrine-induced acute renal failure. Am. J. Physiol. 4:F131, 1978.
17. W.L. Parry, J.A. Schaeffer, C.B. Mueller. Experimental studies of acute renal failure. I. The protective effect of mannitol. J. Urol. 89:1, 1963.
18. M.F. Pera, B.C. Zook, H.C. Harder. Effects of mannitol or furosemide diuresis on the nephrotoxicity and physiological disposition of cis-dichlorodiammine-platinum-(II) in rats. Cancer Res. 39:1269, 1979.
19. D.R. Wilson, G. Thiel, M.L. Arce, D.E. Oken. Glycerol induced hemoglobinuric acute renal failure in the rat. III. Micropuncture study of the effects of mannitol and isotonic saline on individual nephron function. Nephron 4:337, 1967.
20. R.R. Bailey, R. Natale, D.I. Turnbull, A.L. Linton. Protective effect of furosemide in acute tubular necrosis and acute renal failure. Clin. Sci. Mol. Med. 45:1, 1973.
21. M.G. Dodds, R.D. Foord. Enhancement by potent diuretics of renal tubular necrosis induced by cephaloridine. Brit. J. Pharmacol. 40:227, 1970.
22. A.A. Hellebusch, F. Salama, E. Eadie. The use of mannitol to reduce the nephrotoxicity of amphotericin B. Surg. Gynecol. Obstet. 134:241, 1973.
23. M.E. Huguenin, A. Birbaumer, F.P. Brunner, et al. An evaluation of the role of tubular obstruction in folic acid-induced renal failure in the rat. Nephron 22:41, 1978.
24. L.M. Berman, L.L. Smith, G.D. Chisholm, R.E. Weston. Mannitol and renal function in cardiovascular surgery. Arch. Surg. 88:239, 1964.
25. D.R. Kahn, J.C. Cerney, R.W.S. Lee, H. Sloan. The effect of dextran and mannitol on renal function during open heart surgery. Surg. 5: 676, 1965.
26. L.S. Nuutinen, M. Kairaluoma, S. Tuononen, T.K.I. Larmi. The effect of furosemide on renal function in open heart surgery. J. Cardiovas. Surg. 19:471, 1978.
27. K.G. Barry, A. Cohen, J.P. Knochell, et al. Mannitol infusion II. The prevention of acute functional renal failure during resection of an aneurysm of the abdominal aorta. New Engl. J. Med. 264:967, 1961.
28. R.J. Baird, W.B. Firor, H.W.K. Barr. Protection of renal function during surgery of the abdominal aorta. Canad. Med. Assoc. J. 89:705, 1963.
29. A.C. Beall, R.M. Holman, G.C. Morris, M.E. DeBakey. Mannitol-induced osmotic diuresis during vascular surgery. Arch. Surg. 86:34,1963.
30. L.L. Smith, L.B. Berman, G.D. Chisholm. Effect of mannitol on renal function during cardiovascular surgery. Forum 14:103, 1963.

31. S.R. Powers, A. Boba, W. Hostnik, A. Stein. Prevention of postoperative acute renal failure with mannitol in 100 cases. Surgery 55:15, 1964.
32. E.E. Etheredge, H. Levitan, K. Nakamura, W.W.L. Glenn. Effect of mannitol on renal function during open heart surgery. Ann. Surg. 161: 53, 1965.
33. A. Untura. Incidence and prophylaxis of acute postoperative renal failure in obstructive jaundice. Rev. Med. Chir. Soc. Med. Nat. IASI 83:247, 1979.
34. J.L. Dawson. Postoperative renal function in obstructive jaundice. Effect of a mannitol diuresis. Br. Med. J. 1:82,1965.
35. C.E. Lucas, J.G. Zito, K.M. Carter, et al. Questionable value of furosemide in preventing renal failure. Surgery 82:314,1977.
36. D.M. Hayes, E. Cvitkovic, R.B. Golbey, et al. High dose cis-platinum diammine dichloride. Amelioration of renal toxicity by mannitol diuresis. Cancer 39:1372, 1977.
37. J.J. Olivero, J. Lozano-Mendez, E.M. Ghafary, et al. Mitigation of amphotericin B nephrotoxicity by mannitol. Br. Med. J. 1:550, 1975.
38. H.R. Anto, S.Y. Chou, J.G. Porush, W.B. Shapiro. Mannitol prevention of acute renal failure associated with infusion intravenous pyelography. Clin. Res. 27:407A, 1979.
39. C.W. Old, L.M. Lehrner. Prevention of radiocontrast induced acute renal failure with mannitol. Lancet 2:885 (Letter), 1980.
40. C. Oguagha, J.G. Porush, S.Y. Chou, et al. Prevention of acute renal failure following infusion intravenous pyelography in patients with chronic renal insufficiency by furosemide. Proc. VIII Internat. Cong. Nephrology, p. 290, 1981.
41. H.E. Eliahou, A. Bata. The diagnosis of acute renal failure. Nephron 2:287, 1965.
42. R.G. Luke, J.D. Briggs, M.E.M. Allison, A.C. Kennedy. Factors determining response to mannitol in acute renal failure. Am. J. Med. Sci. 259:168, 1970.
43. R.G. Luke, A.L. Linton, J.D. Briggs, A.C. Kennedy. Mannitol therapy in acute renal failure. Lancet 1:980, 1965.
44. R.G. Muth. Furosemide in acute renal failure. Symposium on Acute Renal Failure. National Institutes of Health, 1973, p.245.
45. C.M. Kjellstrand. Ethancrynic acid in acute tubular necrosis. Indications and effect on the natural course. Nephron 9:337, 1972.
46. R.L. Scheer. The effect of hypertonic mannitol on oliguric patients. Am. J. Med. Sci. 250:483, 1965.
47. F. Cantarovich, A. Locatelli, J.C. Fernandez. Furosemide in high doses in the treatment of acute renal failure. Postgrad. Med. J. (April Suppl) 47:13, 1971.
48. F. Cantarovich, C. Galli, L. Benedetti, et al. High dose furosemide in established acute renal failure. Br. Med. J. 4:449, 1973.
49. D. Kleinknecht, D. Ganeval, L.A. Gonzalez-Duque, J. Fermanian. Furosemide in acute oliguric renal failure: A controlled trial. Nephron 17:51, 1976.
50. C.B. Brown, C.S. Ogg, J.S. Cameron. High dose furosemide in acute renal failure: a controlled trial. Clin. Nephrol. 15:90, 1981.
51. S. Karayannopoulos. High-dose furosemide in renal failure. Br. Med. J. 2:278, 1974.
52. A.N. Minuth, J.B. Terrell, W.N. Suki. Acute renal failure: A study of the course and prognosis of 104 patients and of the role of furosemide. Am. J. Med. Sci. 271:317, 1976.
53. S.M. Baek, G.G. Makabali, W.C. Shoemaker. Clinical determinants of survival from postoperative renal failure. Surg. Gynecol. Obstet. 140:685, 1975.

54. R.E. Lordon, J.R. Burton. Post-traumatic renal failure in military personnel in Southeast Asia: experience at Clark USAF Hospital, Republic of the Philippines. Am. J. Med. 53:137, 1972.
55. R.J. Anderson, S.L. Linas, A.S. Berns, W.L. Henrich, T.R. Miller, P.A. Gabow, R.W. Schrier. Nonoliguric acute renal failure. N. Engl. J. Med. 296:1134, 1977.

DIURETIC USAGE IN CHRONIC RENAL FAILURE

VITTORIO E. ANDREUCCI, ANTONIO DAL CANTON and GIUSEPPE CONTE
Department of Nephrology, Second Faculty of Medicine, University of Naples, Naples, Italy

SALT AND WATER METABOLISM IN CHRONIC RENAL FAILURE

A progressive loss of functioning nephrons is the typical feature of chronic renal failure. The impairment of renal function, however, is not followed by a fall in urine output until a glomerular fitration rate usually less than about 5 ml/min. The maintenance of urine output despite the severe reduction in functioning nephrons is attributed to an adaptation of residual nephrons to the uremic environment. This phenomenon occurs through the following mechanisms: (1) extracellular volume expansion which suppresses the fractional tubular reabsorption of filtrate; (2) increase in plasma concentration of filtrable, poorly reabsorbable solutes (e.g. urea, phosphate, sulphate) with a resulting osmotic diuresis in the survivng nephrons; (3) compensatory hypertrophy of residual nephrons; (4) a secondary hyperpathyroidism (parathyroid hormone is known to suppress the tubular reabsorption of phosphate and sodium); (5) a postulated natriuretic factor(s) (still to be identified) [1].

Thus, because of the uremic environment, the reduction in overall filtration of salt and water (due to the decrease in number of functioning nephrons) is compensated by a proportional reduction in the tubular reabsorption of surviving nephrons leading to a "spontaneous" intensive diuresis in each residual nephron. The external balance of sodium is maintained as in normal subjects; but the fractional excretion of filtered sodium is greatly increased [1].

Hypertension in Chronic Uremia

The price paid by the uremic patients for maintaining (despite a progressive reduction of functioning nephrons) the external balance of salt and a fairly constant urine output is a progressive expansion of extracellular fluid volume which will cause the uremic hypertension. Hypertension is, in fact, almost constant in chronic renal failure. The important role played extracellular fluid volume expansion in uremic hypertension becomes evident when the patients begin dialysis therapy;in a few dialisis sessions the loss of salt and water by dialysis ultrafiltration (a) will greatly reduce the body weight, (b) will significantly decrease urine output and (c) will normalize blood pressure.

Congestive Heart Failure in Chronic Uremia

In patients with chronic renal failure the long-standing hypertension may cause a congestive heart failure; in this condition renal function deteriorates further, urine output decreases and the patient becomes edematous [1].

Diuretics, Jules B. Puschett, Editor

Nephrotic Syndrome in Chronic Uremia

It is unusual for patients with advanced chronic renal failure to exhibit a nephrotic syndrome. As renal function deteriorates, in fact, any great urinary loss of protein subsides and the edema disappears. In some patients, however, a severe proteinuria persists despite the marked fall in glomerular filtration rate; these patients remain edematous and may excrete urine virtually free of sodium [1].

DIURETICS IN CHRONIC RENAL FAILURE

Hypertension, congestive heart failure and nephrotic syndrome represent the main indications for a diuretic therapy in patients with chronic renal failure. The efficacy of diuretics in chronic renal failure, however, is greatly reduced by at least two factors: (a) the decrease in number of functioning nephrons; this is the major limiting factor when the glomerular filtration rate is greater than 15 ml/min [2]; but undoubtedly it is an important cofactor also when the glomerular filtration rate is less than 15 ml/min; (b) the "spontaneous" inhibition of tubular reabsorption in residual nephrons due to the uremic environment. In patients with glomerular filtration rate of less than 15 ml/min, in fact, the saluretic effect of diuretics is reduced out of proportion to the reduction in nephron mass [2]. Thus, thiazide appeared to be of little value when glomerular filtration rate was less than 15-20 ml/min.

Loop Diuretics in Advanced Chronic Renal Failure

It was only two decades ago that very powerful (so-called high-ceiling) diuretics were made available for clinical use and proved to substantially increase salt and water excretion in advanced chronic renal failure. They were called "loop diuretics" for their site of action in the ascending limb of the loop of Henle. Ethacrynic acid and furosemide were the first loop diuretics utilized for treating salt retention in chronic renal failure. Furosemide in particular has been widely used for treating edematous and/or hypertensive uremic patients.

High dosage (up to 2 g/day per os) furosemide therapy has been shown to increase the fractional excretion of sodium up to 50% in edematous patients with creatinine clearance as low as 1.8 ml/min [3]. Treatment may start with an oral dose of 80 to 120 mg/day in a single morning dose and increase, if necessary, up to a 1,000 mg/day. I.v. infusion of the drug may be indicated in patients with incipient left ventricular failure (100 to 500 mg given i.v. very slowly).

It is important to note that furosemide does not reduce the glomerular filtration rate (unless severe volume depletion occurs) [3]. It has been demonstrated that it increases renal blood flow when given acutely[4]; this effect, however, is prevented by pretreatment with inhibitors of prostaglandin synthesis [5]. Even the saluretic effect of furosemide, on the other hand, has been attributed, at least in part, to an increased synthesis and release of prostaglandins [6]; it is, in fact, inhibited by indometacin [7, 8]. The main site of action of furosemide is the thick ascending limb of Henle's

Muzolimine: a New Loop Diuretic

In the last few years a new high ceiling diuretic has been introduced in clinical pharmacology: muzolimine. It is the 3-amino-1-(3,4 dichlormethyl benzyl)-2-pyrazolin-5-one, a loop diuretic with no structural similarity to currently available diuretics (FIG. 1).

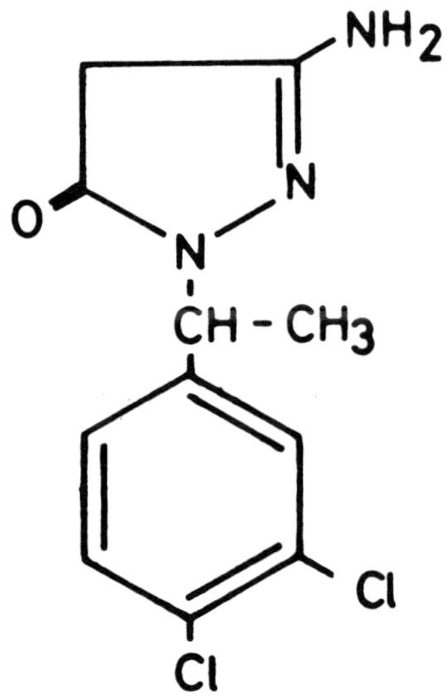

FIG. 1. Structural formula of muzolimine

Muzolimine has been shown to be at least as efficient as furosemide in advanced chronic renal failure, possibly with some advantages and apparently with no side effects [27]. Its pharmacodynamics is different from that of other high-ceiling diuretics. It has a slightly slower but a much longer duration of action than furosemide, so that no "rebound phenomenon" occurs after a single daily dose [27]. It is rapidly absorbed after oral intake and eliminated from the blood by biotransformation to inactive metabolites that then undergo biliary and urinary excretion [28]. Thus its elimination in chronic renal failure is not different from that in healthy subjects.

In 1981 we have demonstrated the efficacy of muzolimine in treating edema and/or hypertension in patients with advanced chronic renal failure. When given at high doses (1 to 5 mg/kg b.w./day) per os to twenty edematous and/

loop; it has been demonstrated that the fall in fractional excretion of sodium after indomethacin is due to overreabsorption of salt in the thick ascending limb of the loop of Henle [9]. Experimental studies in dogs, on the other hand, appear to support the view that only the vascular effect of furosemide (that is prostaglandin-mediated) is inhibited by indomethacin; hence, only that portion of overall natriuresis caused by furosemide is inhibited by indomethacin [10].

Despite the enormous advantages in using furosemide in chronic renal failure, some problems may arise even with this very powerful diuretic:
(1) Furosemide has a very short duration of action. Thus after an initial brisk diuresis with depletion of circulating blood volume, a "rebound phenomenon" may occur: as soon as the diuretic effect is exhausted, salt and water excretion falls below control values [11]. To face this problem repeated doses of the drug have to be given at short intervals.
(2) Furosemide has to reach the tubular lumen to inhibit salt reabsorption. Experimental studies have demonstrated that the drug enters the tubules primarily via active tubular secretion [12-14] and that probenecid blocks its natriuretic effect suggesting that the drug is secreted by the same transport system as for organic acids [15]. In advanced chronic renal failure (i.e. glomerular filtration rate less than 15 ml/min), tubular transport is inhibited by the uremic environment [16-18]. The accumulation of endogenous organic acids in chronic renal failure may further inhibit the secretory transport of furosemide into the tubular lumen [19, 20] in a condition of reduced filtration of the drug. To overcome this problem very high blood levels of furosemide are to be attained in chronic uremic patients. These high levels may increase the ototoxic effect of the drug [21].
(3) Occasionally uremic patients are resistant to furosemide even at high i.v. dosage [22]It is possible, however, that oral dosing could overcome such a "resistance" by increasing the time course of delivery of the drug into urine thereby allowing a longer maintenance of the furosemide excretion rate with maximum efficiency [23, 24].

More recently bumetanide has shown similar efficacy in chronic renal failure. We have used bumetanide in chronic uremic patients. Unfortunately our experience was disappointing when high doses (10 mg) were used in advanced chronic renal failure: muscular pain, tachicardia and general malaise were frequently observed [25]. Hence we had to stop the use of this diuretic in advanced chronic renal failure.

Loop Diuretics in Dialysis Patients

Loop diuretics have been also suggested in chronic uremic patients on regular dialysis therapy, with the purpose of alleviating the severe diet restrictions and obtaining an easier control of water and salt balance. Furosemide has been shown particularly efficient in this respect: when given at a daily dosage of 500 mg per os to patients on regular dialysis therapy, the body weight increment between dialyses was significantly reduced [26]. Our experience with bumetanide was negative also in patients on regular dialysis therapy: when given per os at a dosage of 10 mg to 4 patients, all of them complained of severe muscular pain, forcing us to stop any further attempt [25].

or hypertensive patients with glomerular filtration rate less than 30 ml/min (mean value of 16.8 ± 1.5 SEM ml/min) for a mean period of 9.3 days, sodium and chloride excretion was triplicated and urine output doubled. No changes occurred in calcium and hydrogen excretion, in serum concentration of sodium, potassium, calcium, bicarbonate, glucose and creatinine and in creatinine clearance [27]. Similar efficacy of muzolimine was then reported by others [29-32].

In terms of activity 1 mg of muzolimine corresponds to about 1.5-2.0 mg of furosemide. Table I shows the equally potent doses of muzolimine and furosemide in relation to different degrees of renal function impairment. When creatinine clearance is 20 to 30 ml/min, the suggested dose of muzolimine is 1.8 mg/kg b.w./ day, that corresponds to 2.5 mg/kg b.w./day of furosemide. When creatinine clearance is 10 to 20 ml/min, the dose of muzolimine may be 2.4 mg/kg b.w./day that corresponds to 4 mg/kg b.w./day of furosemide. Finally, when creatinine clearance is 5 to 10 ml/min, the suggested dose of muzolimine is 4.6 mg/kg b.w./day that corresponds to 8 mg/kg b.w./day of furosemide [22]. Obviously these doses may be increased if necessary.

TABLE I. Equally potent doses of muzolimine and furosemide in relation to different degrees of renal function impairment.

Creatinine Clearance ml/min	Muzolimine mg/kg b.w.	Furosemide mg/kg b.w.
20 - 30	1.8	2.5
10 - 20	2.4	4.0
5 - 10	4.6	8.0

It is interesting to note that muzolimine has occasionally shown a greater efficacy than furosemide in treating edematous patients with advanced chronic renal failure. Thus, in 1981 we reported four uremic patients with congestive heart failure and/or nephrotic syndrome (one with diabetic nephropathy) who resulted unrensponsive to 500 mg/day of furosemide intravenously, but increased significantly salt excretion and urine output after 120 to 480 mg/day of muzolimine per os [27]. Similar results have then be reported by others [33]. The efficacy of muzolimine when furosemide has failed may be due to an action of the two drugs on different sides of the tubular cells. Experimental studies in rats by micropuncture techniques (split oil-droplet) [34] have, in fact, demonstrated that muzolimine, unlike furosemide (and bumetanide), does not act from the luminal side but from the peritubular side only [35]. Should this interesting observation be confirmed, muzolimine would become the ideal diuretic for treating acute renal failure in the early stage [36].

EFFECTS OF LOOP DIURETICS ON PLASMA UREA

Long-term treatment of chronic uremic patients with loop diuretics is followed by a significant increase in plasma urea without further impairment in renal function [27, 37]. Our group has studied this effect in uremic patients treated with furosemide.

As reported elsewhere [38], we have demonstrated that the rise in azotemia after long-term treatment of uremic patients with furosemide is secondary to extracellular volume depletion; under such circumstances urea retention is not due to a decrease in glomerular filtration rate, but to a tubular overreabsorption of urea, presumably in the distal part of the nephron.

REFERENCES

1. V.E. Andreucci, in: The treatment of renal failure, J.E. Castro, ed. (MTP Press, Lancaster 1982) pp. 33-167.
2. W.D. Shelp and R.E. Rieselbach, Nephron 8, 427-439 (1971).
3. M.E.M. Allison and A.C. Kennedy, Clin. Sci. 41, 171-187 (1971).
4. J.B. Hook, A.H. Blatt, M.J. Brody and H.E. Williamson, J. Pharmacol. Exp. Ther. 154, 667-673 (1966).
5. M.D. Bailie, J.A. Barbour and J.B. Hook, Proc. Soc. Exp. Biol. Med. 148, 1173-1176 (1975).
6. A.A. Attallah, Prostaglandins 18, 369-375 (1979).
7. J.C. Frolich, W. Hollifield, J.C. Dormois, B.L. Frolich, H. Seyberth, A. M. Michelakis and J.A. Oates, Circ. Res. 39, 447-452 (1976).
8. G. Hover and Tost, Pflugers Arch. 273, 215-220 (1977).
9. S. Kaojarern, P. Chennavasin, S. Anderson and D.C. Brater, Am. J. Physiol. 244, F134-139 (1983).
10. J.G. Gerber, Federation Proc. 1707-1710 (1983).
11. K. Meng, Dtsch. Med. Wochenschr 95, 2089-2094 (1970).
12. P. Deetjen, Ann N. Y. Acad. Sci. 139, 408-415 (1966).
13. B. Odlind and B. Beermann, Clin Pharmacol. Ther. 27, 784-790 (1980).
14. B. Odlind, Federation Proc. 42, 1703-1706 (1983)
15. J.B. Hook and H.E. Williamson, J. Pharmacol. Exp. Ther. 149, 404-408 (1965).
16. T.H. Steele and R.E. Rieselbach, Am. J. Med. 43, 876-886 (1967).
17. N.S. Bricker, S. Klahr, M. Purkerson, R.G. Schultze, L.V. Avioli and S.J. Birge, Nature 219, 1058-1059 (1968).
18. R. Podevin, F. Paillard and G. Richet, Proc. 4th Int. Congr. Nephrol. (Stockholm 1969) vol. 2, pp. 278-282.
19. A. Rane, J.P. Villeneuve, W.J. Stone, A.S. Nies, G.R. Wilkinson and R.A. Branch, Clin. Pharmacol. Ther. 24, 199-207 (1978).
20. H.J. Rose, K. O'Malley and A.W. Pruitt, Ciln. Pharmacol. Ther. 24, 199-207 (1978).
21. K. Gallagher and J.K. Jones, Ann. Inter. Med. 91, 744-745 (1979).
22. A. Dal Canton, D. Russo, R. Gallo, G.F. Ardillo, S. Trevico, B. Cianciaciaruso and V.E. Andreucci, Proc. Fourth Capri Conference (1983) (in press).
23. S. Kaojarern, B. Day and D.C. Brater, Kidney Int. 22, 69-74 (1982).
24. D.C. Brater, Federation Proc. 42, 1711-1713 (1983)
25. V.E. Andreucci, A. Papa, V. Calderaro, P. Stanziale and M. Usberti, XIV th Congress of E.D.T.A., Helsinki (1977), p.272 (Abstract).
26. P.J.C. Vereerstraeten, F. Dupuis and C. Toussaint, Nephron 14, 333-338 (1975).
27. A. Dal Canton, D. Russo, R. Gallo, G. Conte and V.E. Andreucci, Brit. Med. J. 282, 595-598 (1981).

28. W. Ritter, Clin. Nephrol. 19, S26-S31 (1983).
29. P. Schimdt, D. Loew, J. Dycka, H. Kopsa, P. balcke, J. Zazgornik and E. Deutsch, Clin Nephrol. 19, S45-S49 (1983)
30. N. Sugino, A.Ando, T.Saruta, Clin. Nephrol. 19, S59-S61 (1983).
31. G. Orsoni, A Di Felice, P. Cucudis, A. Vangelista, S. Stefoni and V. Bonomini, in: Recent Advances in Diuretic Therapy, V.E.Andreucci, ed. (Excerpta Medica, Amsterdam 1983) pp. 246-258.
32. V.Mioli, M. Ragaiolo, E. Ohnmeiss and M. Carosi, in: Recent Advances in Diuretic Therapy, V.E. Andreucci, ed. (Excerpta medica, Amsterdam 1983) pp. 259-268.
33. N. Belovezhdov, A.Astrug, V.Vlahov, D. Tzekova, M. Vretenarska and N. Bakracheva, in: V.E. Andreucci, ed. (Excerpta Medica, Amsterdam 1983) pp. 292-298.
34. V.E. Andreucci, Manual of Renal Micropuncture (Idelson, Naples 1978).
35. D. Loew and K. Meng, Pharmaterapeutica 1, 333-340 (1977).
36. V.E. Andreucci, Acute Renal Failure, Pathophysiology, Prevention and Treatment (Martinus Nijhoff Publishing, Boston 1984).
37. A. Dal Canton, D. Russo, R. Gallo, G. Conte and V.E. Andreucci, Clin. Nephrol. 19, S54-S58 (1983)
38. A. Dal Canton, G. Fuiano, G. Conte, M. Terribile, M. Sabbatini, B. Cianciaruso and V.E. Andreucci, Proc E.D.T.A. 19, 744_ 748 (1982).

USEFULNESS OF HIGH DOSE DIURETICS IN CAPD PATIENTS WITH REDUCED ULTRAFILTRATION CAPACITY

G. BAZZATO, U. COLI, S. LANDINI, A. FRACASSO, F. RIGHETTO, F. SCANFERLA and P. MORACHIELLO
Nephrology Dept., Umberto I Hospital, Venice-Mestre, Italy.

ABSTRACT

Among 72 uremic pts who entered our CAPD program, 11 showed a reduction or loss of ultrafiltration capacity (UF) of peritoneal membrane (PM). They have been treated with high dose of Furosemide (F) to force residual urine volume (UV). Seven appeared "responders" to drug with a significant increase in UV, Na excretion and, within a week gained their dry body weight (BW). In the remaining 4 pts where drug therapy resulted uneffective, fluid removal was obtained by hemofiltration (HF). In both groups we noted an increase in the UF capacity of the PM when their dry BW was reached either by pharmacological or technical approach. These results support the assumption that overhydration status of PM plays a major role in maintaining its UF process.

INTRODUCTION

Increasing clinical experience has shown that CAPD is an effective modality of treatment for uremic pts on short and middle term period. Nevertheless long term CAPD pts even with normal peritoneal clearances, not infrequently, are not able to maintain a satisfactory water and electrolytes balance. The aim of this study was to assess the effectiveness of diuretic therapy with high dose of F to maintain water and electrolytes balance by forcing residual UV. In addition pts who appeared refractory to F, were evaluated after occasional HF, which similarly led to dry BW. This approach allowed us to screen the pure effect of pts dehydration from the direct action of diuretic compound on PM.

PATIENTS AND METHODS

The reduction or loss of the UF capacity of PM was observed in 11 (15%) pts (8 M and 3 F) of 72 pts who were admitted to our CAPD program using double bag system described elsewere (1). They have been on CAPD from 16 to 54 mos (mean 27.2 mos) showing a progressive water and salt retention with a mean Δ BW increase of 7.21 ± 0.6 kg. The investigation was carried out during hospitalization, by administering IV high dose of F (15 mg/kg/day) and daily UV UF, Na^+, BUN, creatinine, P, uric acid removal with dialysate and protein losses were evaluated. The pts refractory to diuretic therapy underwent HF by removing fluid overload and thus ruling out the diuretic action of F per se on PM. Routine lab data were performed at basal condition and every 2-3 days. Also CAPD pts "not responders" followed the same lab controls.

RESULTS

Among our 11 pts 7 resulted "responders" to F with a significant increase in UV from 380 ± 154 to 1270 ± 475 ml/24h ($P<0.001$) and in Na^+ excretion from 32 ± 10 to 110 ± 28 mEq/24h ($P<0.001$) in the meantime a decrease of BW with return to normal value was observed with an average of 1.2 ± 0.3 kg/day. After hav-

Published 1984 by Elsevier Science Publishing Co., Inc.
Diuretics, Jules B. Puschett, Editor

ing reached dry BW we observed a progressive increase in the UF capacity of PM already present in the 3rd day of therapy, from 288±123 to 1220±154 ml/24h ($P < 0.001$) leading to ideal BW within a week. Thus the pts were discharged and at home they were advised to follow an oral dose of 500 mg F, 2-3 times a week. No side effects were observed, and a satisfactory water and electrolytes balance was mainained (fig. 1).The 4 pts "not responders" whom residual UV remained unchanged after F administration, were treated by HF (Amicon 20) using a subclavian or jugular catheter. Mean BW decrease/HF session was 3.5 kg allowing these pts to gain their dry BW. (fig. 2). Thereafter we observed a progressive increase in the UF capacity of the PM from 460±192 to 1215±202 ml/24h ($P < 0.001$) associated with an increase in Na^+ removal with dialysate from 61±8 to 158±20 mEq/24h ($P < 0.001$). Only 2 pts needed additional HF every 40 days to maintain their dry BW. During F therapy or HF, we didn't observe any significant change in BUN, creatinine, P, Uric acid removal with dialysate, nor in protein loss (fig. 3). Similarly lab data remained stable indicating an unchanged effectiveness in the peritoneal diffusive capacity during altered UF.

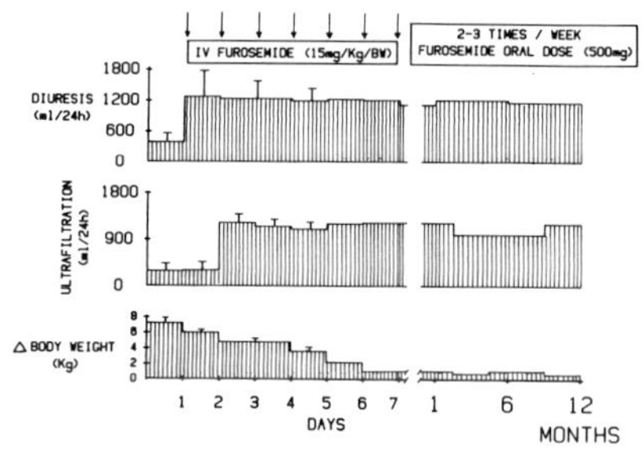

FIG. 1 Effect of high dose diuretics on 7 CAPD pts with reduction of peritoneal UF (mean values ± SD)

DISCUSSION

The reduction or loss of the UF capacity of PM is a not infrequent complication in long term CAPD pts. It has been reported a direct relationship between the reduction of the UF capacity and the duration of CAPD (2). Indeed the longer the pts have been treated, the higher is the total number of hypertonic bags exchanged in long-term treatment to maintain fluid balance. High glucose osmolality of dialysis solution has been claimed responsible for PM alteration and metabolic disorders, because of its large amount absorption. However the

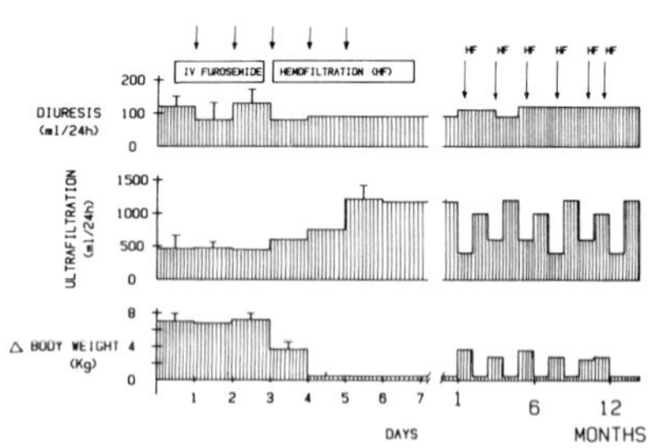

FIG. 2 Effect of high dose diuretics and hemofiltration on 4 CAPD pts with reduction of peritoneal UF.

loss or reduction of the UF capacity of PM may be related to the high incidence of peritonitis, unrespectively to the duration of CAPD(3). Among our 11 pts with reduced peritoneal UF, 7 demonstrated a significant increase in UV and Na excretion after high dose of F, while 4 didn't respond to diuretic therapy, even with an incidence of peritonitis and period of CAPD similar to those with normal peritoneal UF function. The restoration of UF capacity of PM which occured later than diuretic effect, suggest not a direct action on peritoneum of F. In fact it is well known that F doesn't affect peritoneal UF and Na removal since its peritoneal clearance is negligible(4).The recovery of UF may be due to the dehydration of the interstitial space of PM promoting a better action of the physic-hydraulic forces involved in UF process. Considering the 4 "not responders" pts, they showed an increase in UF capacity of PM after having gained dry BW by HF. These results support the assumption that the improvement of physic-chemical status of PM, is related to the normalization of its hydration obtained either with F or HF. In such a manner F therapy and/or HF achieve the same results, keeping dry BW stable in ourCAPD pts. This therapeutic approach besides, allowing to continue peritoneal treatment, also demonstrates that reduction of UF was functional and reversible rather than permanent structural alteration.

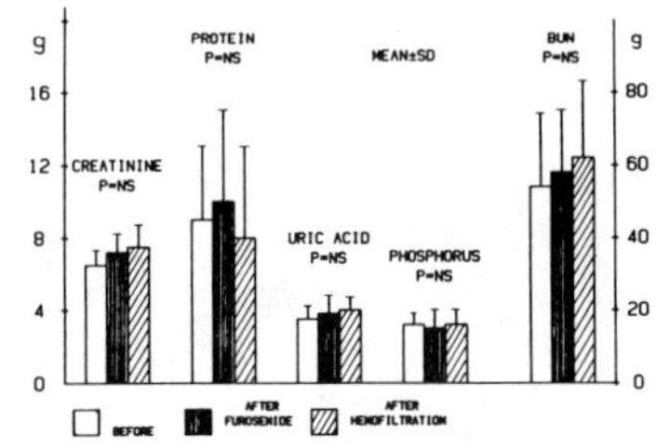

FIG. 3 Solutes removal with dialysate (g/week) and protein losses (g/day) before, after F and HF in 11 CAPD pts with reduced peritoneal UF

CONCLUSIONS

Our data suggest these considerations:-High dose of diuretics allows the "responders" pts a satisfactory water-electrolytes balance and BW control, leading to UF recovery of PM.-Occasional administrations of high-ceiling diuretics in pts with reduced UF may maintain an adequate PM function.-If diuretic therapy fails("not responders"pts) HF also leads to restore UF capacity by obtaining dry BW.-High dose of diuretics and/or HF, normalizing PM hydration and water-electrolytes balance, plays an important role for the recovery of UF in CAPD pts.-These therapeutic modalities consent to continue CAPD program.

REFERENCES

1. G. Bazzato, S. Landini, U. Coli, S. Lucatello, A. Fracasso, M. Morachiello A new technique of CAPD: double-bag system for freedom to a patient and significant reduction of peritonitis. Clin. Nephr. 13, 251 (1980).
2. B. Faller, J.F. Marichal, Loss of ultrafiltration in CAPD: clinical data. In: Advances in peritoneal dialysis. Exc. Medica, 227 (1981).
3. A. Slingeneyer, B. Canaud, C. Mion, Permanent loss of UF capacity of the peritoneum in long-term PD: an epidemiological study.Nephron,33,133(1983).
4. H.F. Boutron, J.F. Brocard, E. Singlas, D. Fries, Pharmacokinetics of furosemide in CAPD.In: Advances in peritoneal dialysis. Exc. Med. 90 (1981)

ACUTE RENAL FAILURE: INFLUENCE OF LOOP DIURETIC MUZOLIMINE AND CALCIUM ANTAGONIST NISOLDIPINE.

BERNWARD GARTHOFF* AND LOTHAR HERTLE**
*Institute of Pharmacology, Bayer AG, P.O.Box 101709, D 5600 Wuppertal 1, FRG; ** Deptm. of Urology, Ruhruniversität Bochum, Herne, FRG.

INTRODUCTION

A variety of agents have been claimed to prevent acute renal failure in different experimental models. The calcium antagonist verapamil has been found to exert such an effect in norepinephrine- or ischemia-induced models of acute renal failure (1, 2) both at least sharing one common pathogenic mechanism, i.e. tubular obstruction. Although the main mechanism underlying calcium antagonistic action is vasodilation, there are additional properties of these drugs, which designate them for usage in acute renal failure: preservation of tissue integrity by preventing cytosolic and mitochondrial calcium overload (3), and a certain yet undefined diuretic activity, also found in a dog model of acute renal failure more recently (4).

In order to further clarify the mechanism of calcium antagonists, we employed the potent calcium antagonist nisoldipine (IC_{50} in KCl-induced concentrations aortic strips: 2.4×10^{-9} mol/l, 5), structurally different from verapamil, and the loop diuretic muzolimine in a rat model of acute renal failure. Rats were treated with either calcium antagonist or loop diuretic or a combination of both.

METHODS

Acute renal failure was induced in male Wistar rats by clamping of the left renal pedicle for 60 minutes with a microsurgery clamp with a closing force of 0.4-0.5 Newton. The right kidney had been removed four days before ischemia. From that date on, the following diets were fed in the different ischemia groups:

I: standard diet (control ischemia)
II: standard diet plus muzolimine (800 ppm)
III: standard diet plus nisoldipine (300 ppm)
IV: standard diet plus combination (muzolimine 800 ppm/nisoldipine 300 ppm)

In addition to the pretreatment, rats were treated with either substance one hour before ischemia by gavage (10 mg/kg of each substance). Clearance data were obtained one the first and third day after ischemia by 24 h endogeneous creatinine clearance in the surviving animals according to standard procedures (2).

RESULTS

Results obtained in the different groups are demonstrated in fig. 1 and fig. 2. Whereas in the control group urine volume excretion and creatinine clearance fell to almost zero, renal function was significantly improved in the treated groups. On the third day after ischemia, creatinine clearance could be determined only in two out of the surviving four control animals, because the other two animals were anuric. Survival rate and values for serum creatinine and serum urea (tab. 1) in the different groups indicate that muzolimine was superior to nisoldipine in the dosage employed, as was the combination.

Diuretics, Jules B. Puschett, Editor

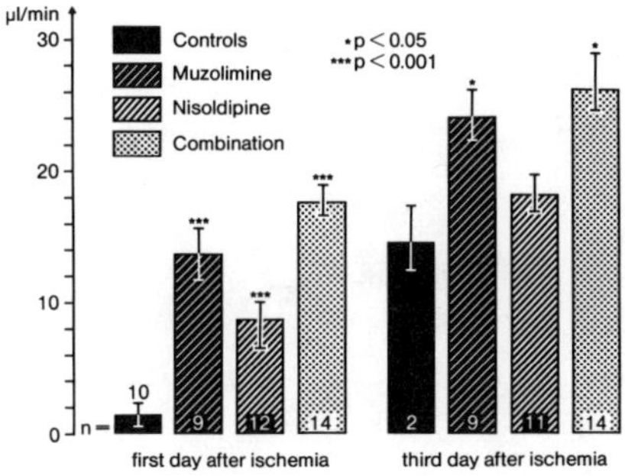

FIG. 1. Urine volume in uninephrectomized rats after 60 min. ischemia ($\bar{x} \pm$ SEM).

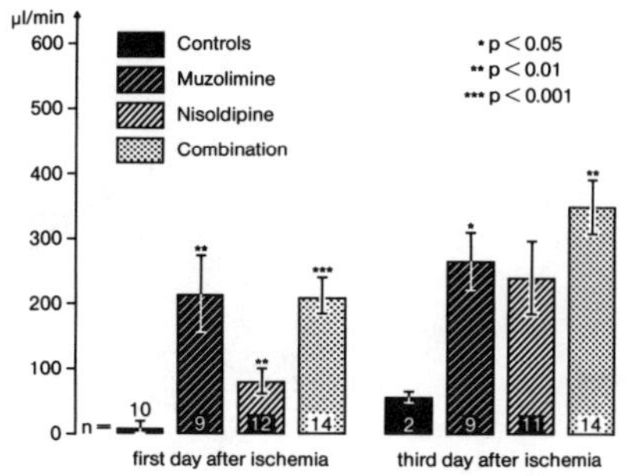

FIG. 2. Creatinine clearance in uninephrectomized rats after 60 min. ischemia ($\bar{x} \pm$ SEM)

TABLE I. Serum creatinine and serum urea in uninephrectomized rats after 60 min. ischemia ($\bar{x} \pm$ SEM).

Group	day	n[a]	serum creatinine µmol/l	serum urea mmol/l
I	0	(10)	68.2 ± 11.2	9.2 ± 0.2
	1	(10)	375.7 ± 13.6	58.4 ± 1.5
	3	(4)	460.5 ± 47.4	86.3 ± 2.4
II	0	(9)	73.0 ± 1.7	13.4 ± 0.4
	1	(9)	182.3 ± 32.5 b)	40.6 ± 5.3 b)
	3	(9)	169.1 ± 35.8 b)	41.8 ± 8.7 b)
III	0	(12)	61.4 ± 1.8	10.3 ± 0.2
	1	(12)	263.8 ± 23.9 b)	48.4 ± 3.6 b)
	3	(11)	211.4 ± 38.5 b)	56.3 ± 7.8 b)
IV	0	(14)	79.6 ± 2.1	14.7 ± 0.6
	1	(14)	149.1 ± 18.2 b)	35.4 ± 3.8 b)
	3	(14)	108.4 ± 13.6 b)	31.4 ± 4.3 b)

a) surviving animals in bracketts, b) $p < 0.05$ versus controls I

SUMMARY

Investigations in a rat model of ischemia-induced acute renal failure indicate that both calcium antagonist and loop diuretic muzolimine prevent postischemic acute renal failure. Although muzolimine treatment ensured an almost complete prevention, addition of nisoldipine led to better results.

This might indicate that the main mechanism underlying prevention of acute renal failure with calcium antagonist could be a diuretic effect leading to flushing of the obstructed tubule, as suggested by Wait et al. (4). But as addition of a calcium antagonist still optimizes the preventive effects of a loop diuretic, there is apparently a different mechanism at the cellular level. Addition of a calcium antagonist to a loop diuretic might therefore be a therapeutic advantage in the treatment of acute renal failure.

REFERENCES

1. H.L.Mc Crorey, A.de Torrente, T.J.Burke, T. Berl, and R.Schrier, Clin. Res. 27, 424 (1979).
2. D.Goldfarb, A.Iaina, I.Serban, S.Gavendo, S.Kapuler, and H.E.Eliahou, Proc. Soc. Biol. Med. 172, 389-392 (1983).
3. A.M.Katz and H.Reuter, Am. J. Cardiol. 44, 188-190 (1979).
4. R.B.Wait, G.White, and J.H.Davis, Surgery 94, 276-282 (1983).
5. S.Kazda, B.Garthoff, H.Meyer, K.Schloßmann, K.Stoepel, R.Towart, W. Vater, and E.Wehinger, Arzneim.-Forsch./Drug Res. 30, 2144-2162 (1980).

SECTION XII

DIURETICS: METABOLIC AND HORMONAL EFFECTS

CHANGES IN SERUM CALCIUM, PARATHYROID HORMONE AND ALKALINE PHOSPHATASE ISO-ENZYMES IN SHORT-TERM TREATMENT WITH ACETAZOLAMIDE IN END-STAGE RENAL DISEASE. EVIDENCE OF AN EXTRARENAL MECHANISM FOR ACETAZOLAMIDE-INDUCED ACIDOSIS.

S. De Marchi, E. Cecchin, D. Schinella, G. Calianno, S. Maganuco, F. Tesio.

Unit of Nephrology and Dialysis, Stabilimento Ospedaliero di Pordenone.
Unit of Dialysis, Stabilimento Ospedaliero di Maniago
Department Internal Medicine, Stabilimento Ospedaliero di Codroipo, Italy.

INTRODUCTION

Evidence from previous studies suggest that acetazolamide (AZ) produces a mild self-limiting acidosis by inhibition of carbonic anhydrase in the proximal tubular epithelium which results in a bicarbonate diuresis (1). A serious acidosis frequently develops in patients with chronic renal failure submitted to AZ therapy (2). Muldowney (3) suggested that in uremic patients excessive bicarbonate may be lost by the tubule and AZ would be expected to inhibit the partial reabsorption of this bicarbonate.
We report that a short-term therapy with AZ causes a severe metabolic acidosis in patients with end-stage renal disease receiving long-term haemodialysis. A complex extrarenal mechanism, probably involving at least in part the parathyroid hormone effects on bone resorption and calcium metabolism, has a major role in the pathogenesis of this metabolic derangement induced by AZ in such patients.

MATERIALS AND METHODS

We investigated 25 patients with end-stage renal disease receiving long-term haemodialysis (12 women and 13 men, mean age 45 years, range 25-63 years, mean dialytic age 4.5 years).Only patients without a significant residual diuresis have been included in the study. AZ was administered orally in a dose of 500 mg daily for a period of 6 days. Arterial blood pH, PCO_2, serum levels of calcium, parathyroid hormone (iPTH), alkaline phosphatase and its bone and liver isoenzymes were measured before, during AZ treatment (3rd and 6th day), 10 and 20 days after its cessation. Arterial blood pH and PCO_2 were measured on a blood gas analyzer (Radiometer, Copenhagen). Bicarbonate was calculated from the pH and PCO_2 relations using the Henderson-Hasselback equation. Serum calcium was determined by atomic absorption. Serum iPTH was measured by radioimmuneassay using an antiserum for C-terminal fragments. Alkaline phosphatase was evaluated by Autoanalyzer. The liver and bone isoenzymes of alkaline phosphatase were separated by electrophoresis.

RESULTS

The modifications of arterial blood pH and bicarbonate, serum calcium, iPTH, alkaline phosphatase and its bone isoenzyme are shown in Table I. A six days course of AZ therapy resulted in a significant decrease of arterial blood pH (7.39 ± 0.02 vs 7.24 ± 0.02), bicarbonate (21.2 ± 2 vs 12.5 ± 2 mmol/l) and serum calcium (9.2 ± 0.9 vs 8.4 ± 0.7 mg/dl). On the contrary there was a significant increase in iPTH (230 ± 100 vs 300 ± 50 pmol/l), alkaline phosphatase (105 ± 14 vs

Diuretics, Jules B. Puschett, Editor

136+22 U/l) and its bone isoenzyme (72.45±13.65 vs 103.36±14.96 U/l). All these investigated parameters returned to the pre-therapy levels in a period of 10-20 days after AZ cessation.

TABLE I. Modifications of arterial blood pH (pH) and bicarbonate (HCO_3^-), serum calcium (Ca), parathyroid hormone (iPTH), alkaline phosphatase (AP) and its bone isoenzyme (bAP) caused by a 6 day course of acetazolamide therapy.

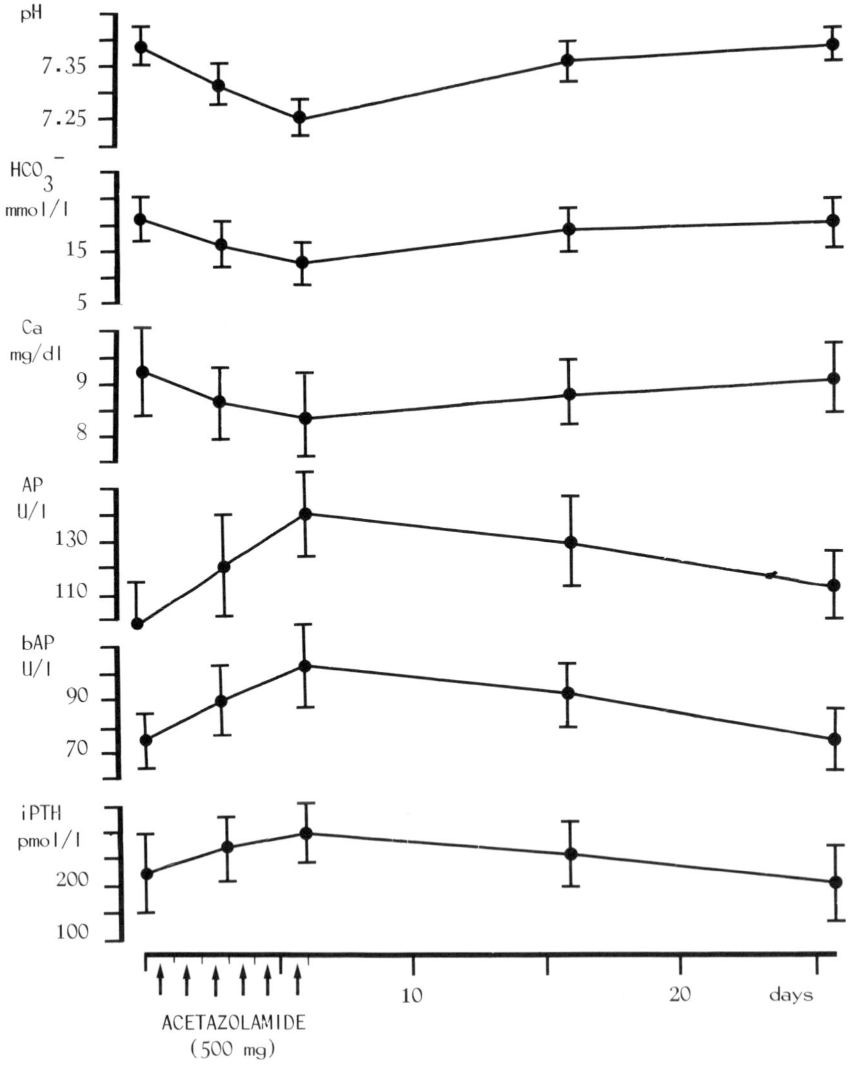

DISCUSSION

We observed that AZ produces a serious metabolic acidosis in patients with end-stage renal disease receiving long-term haemodialysis. It is not clear how the acidosis develops in these patients. It has been suggested that in chronic renal failure excessive bicarbonate may be lost by the tubules and AZ would be expected to inhibit the partial reabsorption of this bicarbonate (3). None of our patients had a significant residual diuresis so that an extrarenal mechanism must be involved in the pathogenesis of the severe acidosis. The increase of serum levels of iPTH, total alkaline phosphatase and its bone isoenzyme as well as the decrease of serum calcium suggest a complex mechanism probably involving, at least in part, PTH action on bone resorption and calcium metabolism. Whereas Siegmund et al (4) have concluded that carbonic anhydrase is important in PTH-induced bone resorption in the chicken, the role of this enzyme in mammalian bone metabolism is more controversial (5). Our data confirm the hypocalcemic effect of AZ in uremia previously described in nephrectomized rats (6). AZ seems to block the hypercalcemic response to PTH but is not capable of inhibiting the final resorption of bone as indicated by the increase of serum levels of alkaline phosphatase and its bone isoenzyme. The importance of the bone buffers, such as phosphates and carbonates, in maintaining the hydrogen balance has been emphasized for many years (7). The availability of these bone buffers depends on the action of PTH mediated by carbonic anhydrase and by vitamin D (8). It is conceivable that AZ by inhibiting the enzyme may impair the PTH action on the bone reducing the availability of these bone buffers.
In conclusion these data suggest that in patients with end-stage renal disease receiving long-term haemodialysis AZ produces a serious metabolic acidosis by an extrarenal mechanism, probably involving at least in part the PTH action on bone metabolism.

REFERENCES

1. Goodman and Gilman's. The pharmacological basis of therapeutics. MacMillan ed (New York 1980) pp 896-899.
2. D.N. Maisey, R.D. Brown, Br. Med. J. 283, 1527-1529 (1981).
3. F.F. Muldowney in: Renal disease, D.A.K. Black, N.F. Jones, eds (Blackwell Scientific Publications 1979) pp 588-614.
4. P. Siegmund, H.J. Dulce, Hoppe Seyler Z Physiol Chem. 320, 149-160 (1960).
5. L.C. Waite, W.A. Volkert, A.D. Kenny, Endocrinology 87, 1129-1139 (1970).
6. D.T. Baran, S. Klahr, E. Slatopolsky, L.V. Avioli, J Clin. Endocrinol. Metab. 48, 766-770 (1979).
7. G. Mioni, M. Gropuzzo, A. Favazza, P. Messa, D. Montanaro, M. Adorati, G. Paviotti, F. Antonucci, P. Lo Greco, Physiopathology of acid base balance in chronic renal failure, in: Uremic Acidosis, E. Petrella, ed (Wichtig Editore 1983) pp 19-39.
8. J.A. Arruda, V. Alla, H. Rubinstein, M. Cruz-Soto, S. Sabatini, C.D. Battle, N.A. Kurtzmann, Am. J. Physiol. 239, 533 (1980).

S. T. Kau, Ph.D., W. J. Pritchard, M.S. and C. L. Yochim, B.S., Biomedical Research Dept., Stuart Pharmaceuticals, Division of ICI Americas Inc., Wilmington, DE 19897

ABSTRACT: Following a 14 to 21 day maintenance on low Mg (70 ppm) or normal Mg (426 ppm) diet, the rats were used for studying diuretic effects of amiloride and hydrochlorothiazide (HCTZ). In both dietary regimens, amiloride demonstrated the sparing effect on Mg and K excretion after saline loading while HCTZ promoted both electrolyte outputs. Contrary to HCTZ, amiloride in the low Mg group caused less excretion of Mg and K than in the normal Mg group. The low Mg intake led to a two-fold increase in natriuresis and in the excretion ratio of U_{Na}/U_K of amiloride compared to the normal Mg diet. This unique finding was not obtained with HCTZ. The possible mechanisms through which Mg deficiency enhances amiloride-induced natriuresis are discussed.

INTRODUCTION: Magnesium (Mg) is the second most abundant cation in the intracellular fluids. Magnesium deficiency per se can cause potassium depletion and Mg is required for both the maintenance and the restoration of cellular potassium (1,2). Urinary excretion of Mg is enhanced by loop diuretics and thiazides, leading to hypomagnesemia after continuous administration. There is increasing evidence indicating that potassium sparing diuretics can reduce urinary Mg excretion (3). To our knowledge, the role of Mg homeostasis in the renal effect of diuretics has not been well defined. Hence, the purpose of the present study is to evaluate the influence of the dietary Mg intake on the diuretic effect of amiloride and HCTZ in conscious rats.

Materials and Methods: Male Wistar rats weighing 200-250 g were used. Rats were chosen and paired according to the method described previously (4). The selected pairs of rats were fed with standard diet containing low Mg (70 ppm, 6.5 μEq/g) or normal Mg (426 ppm, 35.4 μEq/g) (Bioserv Inc., Frenchtown, N.J.). Low Mg diet contained Na, 1700 ppm and K, 4400 ppm, while normal Mg diet contained Na, 1600 ppm and K, 4900 ppm. Following a 14-to 21-day maintenance on either dietary regimen, the pairs of rats were divided into the placebo and the treated groups, and were fasted overnight with water *ad lib*. On the next day, each pair of rats was given an oral load of normal saline (4% body weight) containing the test agent and placed in a metabolism cage. Urine was collected over a 6-hour period and its volume (UV), sodium (Na) and potassium (K) were measured. Placebo animals were only given saline. At the end of the 6-hour experimental period, the rats were cervically dislocated and blood samples were taken via the puncture of vena cava. Hematocrit and plasma electrolytes were analyzed. In addition, similar blood biochemistry were monitored during the period of the dietary adaptation.

Saline suspension of the test substance (amiloride, 10 mg/kg or HCTZ, 5 mg/kg) were prepared with the aid of 0.25% hydroxymethylcellulose. Sodium and K were determined by flame photometry (Instrumentation Laboratory, Model 914) in urine and plasma. Magnesium levels were analyzed by atomic absorption photometry (Instrumentation Laboratory). Hematocrit was measured with a microhematocrit centrifuge (Autocrit II). Data were presented as mean ± S.E.M. The Student's t-test was used to compare the results with the 0.05 level of probability as the criterion of significance.

Results: Figure 1 demonstrates that following a 10-day maintenance on

Diuretics, Jules B. Puschett, Editor

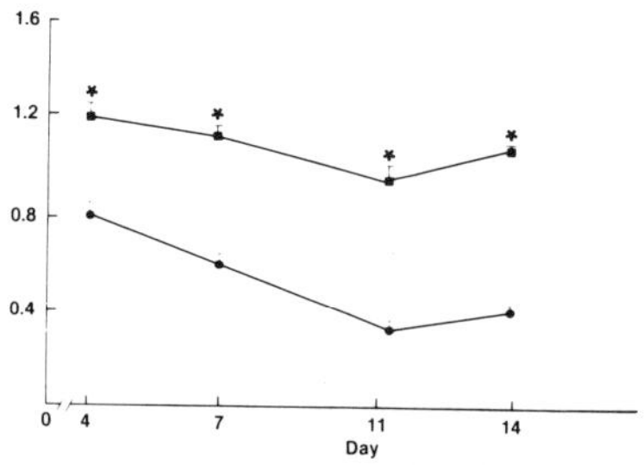

FIGURE 1

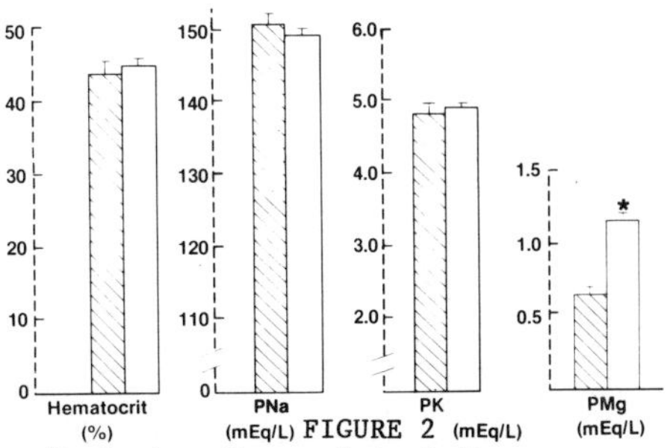

FIGURE 2

FIG. 1. Change in the level of plasma Mg during the period of dietary adaptation. *$p<0.05$ significantly different from the low Mg diet.

FIG. 2: Hematocrit, plasma Na, K and Mg levels 6 hours after saline loading (4% body weight) in placebo rats on low and normal mg diets. *$p<0.05$ significantly different from the low Mg diet.

low Mg, plasma Mg in the rat reached a steady state, being significantly less than that obtained with the normal diet. However, between these two dietary regimens, the placebo values of body weight, hematocrit, and plasma Na and K were not significantly different throughout the period of the dietary adaptation. After saline loading, hematocrit, plasma Na and K of the placebo rats were not different between these two dietary groups, while plasma Mg was consistently lower in the low Mg intake group (Figure 2). However, the placebo rats which received low Mg diet excreted less Mg and more K than those treated with the normal diet over 6 hours (Table 1).

TABLE I. Comparison of urine flow and electrolyte excretions in rats treated with low and normal Mg diet.

	UV	$U_{Na}V$	U_KV	$U_{Mg}V$	U_{Na}/U_K
	mg/6 hrs/100 g		μEq/6 hrs/100g		
Low Mg (n=8)	1.42±0.13	238+25	82±6	2.8±0.8	2.97 ±0.32
Normal Mg (n=8)	1.34±0.19	270±29	59±4*	10±1.7*	5.00* ±0.56

*$P<0.05$, significantly different from the low Mg diet.

Also, the excretion ratio of U_{Na}/U_K was significantly lower in the low Mg group. In both dietary regimens, amiloride demonstrated the sparing effect on Mg and K excretion while HCTZ promoted both electrolyte outputs (Table 2).

TABLE II. Diuretic effects of amiloride and HCTZ in rats treated with low and normal Mg diet.

		ΔUV	$\Delta U_{Na}V$	ΔU_KV	$\Delta U_{Mg}V$	$\Delta U_{Na}/U_K$
		ml/100 g/6 hrs		μEq/100 g/6 hrs.		
Amiloride	Low Mg (n=5)	0.67 ±0.20	341 ±10	-86 ±1	-2.0 ±0.4	122.2 ±12.6
	Normal Mg (n=4)	0.41 ±0.19	141* ±37	-51* ±2	-12* ±1	67.7* ±14.5
HCTZ	Low Mg (n=4)	1.63 ±0.13	300 ±21	60 ±29	0.9 ±0.3	1.55 ±1.27
	Normal Mg (n=4)	±1.48 ±0.15	253 ±33	32 ±2	1.6 ±0.8	2.02 ±0.47

Each value indicates the net change from the placebo rats fed with low or normal Mg diet. *$P<0.05$, significantly different from the low Mg diet.

Contrary to HCTZ, amiloride caused less K excretion in the low Mg diet group than in the normal diet group. The low Mg intake led to a two-fold increase in natriuresis and in the ratio of U_{Na}/U_K of amiloride compared to the normal Mg intake, which was not noted with HCTZ. Table 3 shows that hematocrit, plasma Na, K and Mg were not altered with both drugs.

TABLE III. Effects of amiloride and HCTZ on hematocrit and plasma electrolytes in rats treated with normal or low Mg diet.

		Hematocrit (%)	P_{Na}	P_K (mEq/L)	P_{Mg}
Amiloride	Low Mg (n=11)	-0.5±0.8	-1.6±0.5	0.25±.18	0.07±.03
	Normal Mg (n=11)	-0.4±0.6	-1.1±0.6	-0.02±0.10	0.02±.06
HCTZ	Low Mg (n=7)	2.0±1.1	-3.1±0.8	-0.4±0.2	-0.03±.05
	Normal Mg (n=5)	1.2±0.7	0.1±1.2	0.0±0.1	0.14±.06

Each value represents the net change from the placebo animals fed with normal or low Mg diet.

Discussion: The results of the present studies confirm the previous observation (1) that the plasma and urinary Mg decreased in the low Mg intake rat, but the excretion of K increased as compared to those obtained with the normal Mg diet. The consistent lack of difference in the level of Na or K in the plasma between these dietary regimens suggests the enhancement of K excretion which accompanied Mg deficiency in the present studies is less likely associated with alteration of the level of plasma aldosterone concentration (PAC). Our preliminary observation confirms that the PAC levels between both dietary groups were not significantly different throughout the entire period of the Mg dietary adaptation. There is an abundance of evidence (2,5) that Mg is an essential cofactor for the activity of Na-K-ATPase and the enzyme is necessary to release energy for the Na-K pump. In view of this premise, the present information is in agreement with the hypothesis (1) that Mg deficiency may have impaired the ability of the cell to maintain an appropriate K concentration in the extracellular fluid at a normal level.

The data show that dietary Mg deficiency augmented the natriuretic effect of amiloride in rats after saline loading, while the potentiation of the natriuresis produced by HCTZ, if any, was minimal. It is also these findings alluded to above concerning the possibility that Mg deficiency may have decreased energy supply by means of the reduction of Na-K-ATPase activity. The minimal energy requirement of the net Na transport per mEq for the cortical collecting tubule (i.e., amiloride-action-site) has been estimated to be 1.7 times that for the distal convoluted tubule (i.e., HCTZ-action-site) (5,6). It is conceivable that Mg deficiency would cause a greater inhibitory response on Na transport in the cortical collecting tubule, which, in turn, may have predominantly potentiated the natriuretic response of amiloride.

In summary, we have demonstrated that Mg deficiency enhances K excretion and amiloride-induced natriuresis in the rat after saline loading. The hypothesis that Mg deficiency decreases the activity of Na-K-ATPase and potentiates the natriuresis produced by amiloride remains to be verified.

References

1. R. Whang and L. Welt, J. Clin, Invest. 42, 305-313 (1963).
2. W. P. Leary and A. J. Reyes, SA Med. J. 20, 279-280 (1982).
3. J. Devane and M. P. Ryan, Br. J. Pharmac. 72, 285-289 (1981).
4. S. T. Kau, J. R. Keddie, and D. Andrews, J. Pharmacol. Methods 11, 67-75, 1984.
5. H. J. Rodriguez and S. Klahr in: Textbook of Nephrology, S. G. Massary and R. J. Glassock, eds. (Williams and Wilkins, Baltimore 1983) pp. 1.65-1.78.
6. W. N. Suki and R. C. K. Ng in: Textbook of Nephrology, S. G. Massary and R. J. Glassock, eds. (Williams and Wilkins, Baltimore 1983) pp. 3.158-3.173.

ACETAZOLAMIDE AND INTESTINAL CALCIUM ABSORPTION IN NEPHROTIC SYNDROME.

Messa P.,Mioni G.,Favazza A.,Montanaro D.,Antonucci F.,Adorati M.,Paviotti G.,Messa M.,Paduano R.-Department of Nephrology - O.C. Udine - ITALY.

ABSTRACT

In order to better clarify the role of TmPi/GFR in affecting the levels of Intestinal Ca absorption(I.A.)in Nephrotic Syndrome(NS),the effect of a phosphaturic drug(Acetazolamide,ACZ)on Ca I.A. in 14 nephrotic patients was studied.The results demonstrate a stimulating effect of ACZ on I.A. of Ca,mainly mediated by a reduction in TmPi/GFR.

INTRODUCTION

The reduced levels of Ca I.A. found in NS is commonly thought to be due to Vit D depletion secondary to urinary losses of Vit D binding globulin (VDBG) (1,2,3).However,though increased excretion of VDBG and reduced serum concentration of 25(OH)D_3 are common findings in NS, Ca I.A. has not been invariably found reduced by some Authors(4,5).Recently a role for TmPi/GFR in affecting Ca I.A. in NS has been proposed(6,7).The aim of the present study was to further investigate on this aspect.

PATIENTS AND METHODS

Twentyfour patients(12 M,12 F;aged 14-74 years)with NS(u-prot.>3.5 g/day s-Alb<0.6-2.8 g/dl)were studied.Their renal function ranged from 60 to 138 ml/min(Cr.Cl.).No patient received any drug affecting Ca metabolism in the 2 months preceding the study.The study was performed in autumn-winter period in 12 patients and in spring-summer period in the others.All the patients had a comparable dietary intake of Vit D.After a stabilization period of at least a week with a diet of 800 mg of Ca and 1000 mg of Phosphorus per day,Ca I.A., TmPi/GFR,s-VDBG,seric and urinary electrolytes,acid-base balance in blood and urine and s-PTH-COOH were evaluated.Fourteen of these patients received ACZ(5 mg/kg b.w./day)over 15 days period;at the end of the treatment all the above mentioned parameters were again evaluated.The Ca I.A. was calculated using Sr^{85} 3 µCi i.v. and Ca^{47} 10 µCi p.os,according to Wooton and Reeve(8);TmPi/GFR was assessed by infusional methodology;s-VDBG by radial immunodiffusion (Behring Institut kit);Ca in serum and urine by atomic absorption spectrophotometry(Perkin Elmer 403);phosphate by green malachite micromethod;s-PTH by radioimmunoassay using bovine antiserum direct against COOH terminal fragment pH,pCO_2 in blood and urine and T.A. and ammonium in urine were evaluated by current methodology;serum and urinary bicarbonate were calculated by Henderson-Hasselbalch equation.Statistics were performed using variance analysis, simple and multiple correlation and stepwise analysis.

Diuretics, Jules B. Puschett, Editor

RESULTS

The basal parameters of the 24 nephrotic patients are reported in the table :

TABLE I.

	Ca I.A. %	TmPi/GFR mg/dl	s-VDBG mg/dl	s-PTH ng/ml
M	36.5	4.38	26.6	2.87
SE	± 3.9	± 0.22	± 3.5	± 0.26
n.v.	(35-60)	(2.2-4.4)	(20-60)	(1.8-3.3)

The values of Ca I.A. resulted extremely scattered throughout a wide range (11.4-76%).The TmPi/GFR also showed considerably dispersed values,though a trend toward the upper limit of the normal range was evident.The values of Ca I.A. were negatively correlated with TmPi/GFR at a high significant level on a log-log scale:

$$\ln \text{Ca I.A.} = 5.4 - 1.33 \ln \text{TmPi/GFR} \quad (r=0.66; p<0.01)$$

The possible effect of various factor was considered which may theoretically affect Ca I.A.(i.e.:patient age,illness duration,kidney function,proteinuria degree,s-Alb concentration and s-VDBG)with a multiple correlation where Ca I.A. was the dependent variable and the above mentioned parameters,plus TmPi /GFR,the independent ones.The table illustrates the results:

TABLE II. Multiple correlation(the standardized coeff. are used in the eq.)

Ca I.A.= 84.9 - 0.07 age + 0.39 duration(months) + 0.18 Cr.Cl. + 0.04 s-Alb. -0.13 u-prot. -0.3 s-VDBG - 0.65 TmPi/GFR.

F= 4.34; $p=0.0072$ total explained variance= 65.5%

Stepwise: TmPi/GFR= 44%; s-Alb.= 10%; Others= 11%

As one can see the TmPi/GFR seems to be the major factor in affecting the levels of Ca I.A.(44/65.5% of the explained variance);a minor but significant influence was wielded by serum albumin concentration(10/65.5% of the explained variance);no significant role was played by the other independent variables.The effect of ACZ are summarized in the followinf table/

TABLE III. Effect of ACZ (n=14, M ± SE).

	Ca I.A.%	TmPi/GFR mg/dl	s-pH	s-HCO_3 mEq/l	NAE mEq/day
B	39.9	3.91	7.39	26.3	37.4
	± 2.6	±0.08	±0.01	±0.39	± 5.5
ACZ	49.0	3.28	7.35	21.0	39.0
	± 3.7	± 0.05	±0.01	± 0.9	± 2.3
p	< 0.01	< 0.01	< 0.05	< 0.01	n.s.

ACZ resulted in a significant decrease of TmPi/GFR and a significant increase of Ca I.A.The extent of the increase of the Ca I.A. was correlated with the degree of the reduction of TmPi/GFR/

$$\text{Ca I.A.} = 5.9 - 6.78 \ \text{TmPi/GFR} \quad (r=0.57,\ p<0.05).$$

DISCUSSION

The cause of the derangement of calcium homeostasis in NS is still a matter of controversy.Alon and Chan(9)recently pointed out that factors other than vit D deficiency may explain the fact that some authors have reported changes in Ca metabolism whereas others failed to substantiate these findings.These factors may include the age of the patient,illness duration,kidney function,degree of proteinuria and serum albumin concentration.Our recent reports stressed a role for TmPi/GFR in affecting Ca I.A. in NS.Actually little weight has been given to the possible role of phosphate in the alterations of Ca metabolism of NS.It is probably due to 2 factors:first,s-iP levels are not frequently elevated in NS and,second,TmPi/GFR is currently assessed by Bjivoet nomogram.It has indeed been postulated that the phosphate content of the renal tubular cells rather than the s-iP could provide the signal for $1,25(OH)_2D_3$ synthesis(10).Furthermore Sutton et al.(11)have recenly pointed out that TmPi/GFR in NS need to be obtained by direct measurement using phosphate infusion,because of falsely low values when TmPi/GFR is calculated by Bjivoet nomogram.If we further consider that the diet of nephrotic patients is often abounding in iP and that the Int. iP Abs.has been found normal also when Ca I.A. was reduced(12),it is not difficult to immaginate that in the presence of an enhanced TmPi/GFR,phosphate pool may be increased.This fact may also explain the resistance to the calcemic action of PTH found in NS(5).By our data patient age,illness duration,kidney function,degree of proteinuria and s-VDBG,factors postulated as probably influencing the variable findings of Ca metabolism in NS,did not seem to play any role. Serum Alb.concentration resulted to have a significant,but minor,weight on the levels of Ca I.A..ACZ,a well known phosphaturic drug(13),when given to 14 nephrotic patients,resulted in a significant increase of Ca I.A. proportional to its phosphaturic effect.These data seem to confirm a key role for TmPi/GFR in affecting Calcium homeostasis in NS.

REFERENCES

1 .Barragry J.M.,France M.W.,Carter N.D. et al.,Lancet,ii,629,1977.
2 .Schmidt-Gayk,Schmitt W.,Grawunder C.,Ritz E.,Tschope W.,Pietsch V.,Andrassy K.,Bouillon R.,Lancet,ii,105,1977.
3 .Goldstein D.A.,Yoshitaka O.,Kurokawa K.,Massry S.G.,Ann.Int.Med.87,664,77
4 .Mountokalakis Th.,Virvidakis C.,Shingellakis P.,Alevizaki C.,Ykkos D., Ann.Int.Med.86,746,1977.
5 .Goldstein D.A.,Haldiman B.,Sherman D.,Norman A.W.,Massry S.G;J.Clin.Endocrinol.Metab.52,116,1981.
6 .Messa P.,Mioni G.,Favazza A.,et al.Min.Metab.Res.in Italy,2,97,1981.
7 .Messa P.,Mioni G.,Adorati M, et al. Kidney Internat. A659,23,1983.
8 .Wootton R. and Reeve J.Clin. Sci. 58,287,1980.
9 .Alon U.,Chan J.C.M.Nephron ,36,1,1984.
10.Bikle D.D.,Rasmussen H. J.Clin.Invest. 55,292,1973.
11.Sutton J.V.,Brown C.,Adler A.J.,Feinroth M. et al.Nephron,32,108,1982.
12.Farrington K.,Newman S.P.,Varghese Z.,Moorhead J.F. Clin.Sci.65,437,1983.
13.Fulop M.,Brazeau P. J.Clin.Invest. 47,983,1968.

EFFECTS OF SEVERAL DIURETIC FORMULATIONS ON URINARY MAGNESIUM OUTPUT IN HEALTHY ADULTS

W. P. LEARY,* AND A. J. REYES**
*Department of Clinical Pharmacology, University of Natal, Durban, South Africa; **Departamento de Investigación Cardiovascular, Fundación Procardias, Montevideo, Uruguay

ABSTRACT

The effects of monodoses of placebo and a number of diuretic formulations on 24 h urinary excretions of several electrolytes, including Mg, were studied in healthy volunteers. All common (loop and thiazide-like) diuretics, except indapamide 2.5 mg, induced hypermagnesiuresis. Amiloride did not affect 24 h urinary Mg output significantly.

INTRODUCTION

Magnesium depletion caused by diuretics contributes to the pathogenesis of cardiac arrhythmias, sudden death, myocardial infarction, vasospasm in the coronary and cerebral vessels and partially underlies alterations in lipid and carbohydrate metabolism induced by diuretics. The objective of this study was to evaluate the acute effects of several diuretics on the urinary eliminations of Mg and K.

SUBJECTS AND METHODS

Healthy student volunteers aged 18-25 were studied. Monodoses of diuretics or placebo were given double-blind and in random order, at 08h00 and urine was collected at intervals for 24 h thereafter. Seven days elapsed between experiments and a standard diet was prescribed throughout.

RESULTS

The 24 h percentage changes in urinary outputs after medication, in comparison with placebo, are shown in Table I; statistical results refer to mean values.

FIGS. 1, 2 and 3 show the urinary Na and Mg flows after placebo, furosemide 40 mg or hydrochlorothiazide 50 mg respectively. While flows of both cations were almost parallel after placebo, Mg flow was delayed with respect to Na after furosemide or hydrochlorothiazide.

DISCUSSION

All formulations which cause acute hypermagnesiuresis may induce Mg depletion upon prolonged administration. Since urinary Mg flows were delayed with respect to Cl, Na and volume flows after administration of the diuretics concerned, the hypothesis was advanced that slow-acting endocrine-type mechanisms might account, at least partially, for the hypermagnesiuresis. A system analysis of pertinent data reveal loop diuretics

Diuretics, Jules B. Puschett, Editor

TABLE I. Percentage changes in mean 24-h urinary excretions after monodosing with several diuretic formulations with respect to corresponding outputs after placebo.

N° of cases	Drug and dose (mg)	% change in 24-h renal output Cl	Na	Volume	K	Mg
13	amiloride 5	10^{ns}	39^{b}	19^{a}	-27^{c}	-4^{ns}
13	amiloride 10	32^{d}	65^{e}	43^{e}	-32^{d}	-7^{ns}
9	chlorthalidone 100	152^{e}	165^{e}	69^{d}	69^{d}	87^{d}
9	furosemide 40	49^{b}	48^{d}	49^{d}	21^{a}	52^{a}
19	hydrochlorothiazide 50	63^{e}	61^{e}	38^{e}	31^{a}	24^{a}
9	hydrochlorothiazide 50	59^{a}	63^{d}	35^{a}	22^{a}	44^{a}
7	indapamide 2.5	87^{c}	139^{e}	26^{c}	23^{e}	-8^{ns}
10	muzolimine 30	38^{e}	34^{c}	14^{c}	20^{ns}	8^{ns}
13	xipamide 5	39^{e}	46^{c}	20^{e}	40^{a}	27^{c}
13	xipamide 10	106^{e}	120^{e}	63^{e}	55^{a}	50^{e}
13	xipamide 20	101^{e}	111^{e}	63^{e}	79^{e}	40^{e}

Significances of the differences between mean excretions after drug and after placebo: $^{a}P < 0.05$; $^{b}P < 0.02$; $^{c}P < 0.01$; $^{d}P < 0.005$; $^{e}P < 0.001$; ns: non-significant.

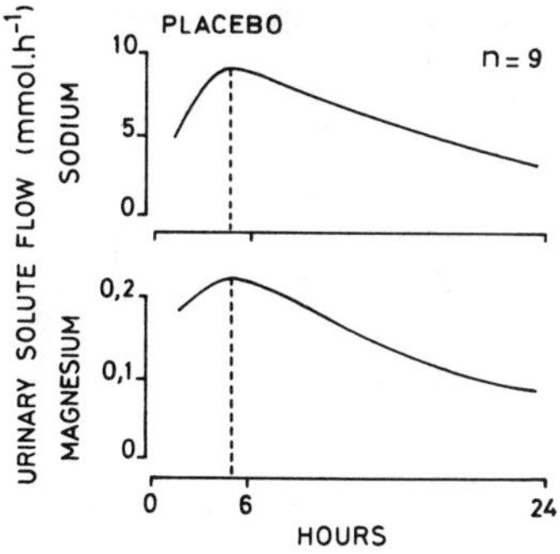

FIG. 1. Urinary Na and Mg flows after placebo administration to healthy volunteers. Adapted from Reyes and Leary [1], by courtesy of Current Therapeutic Research.

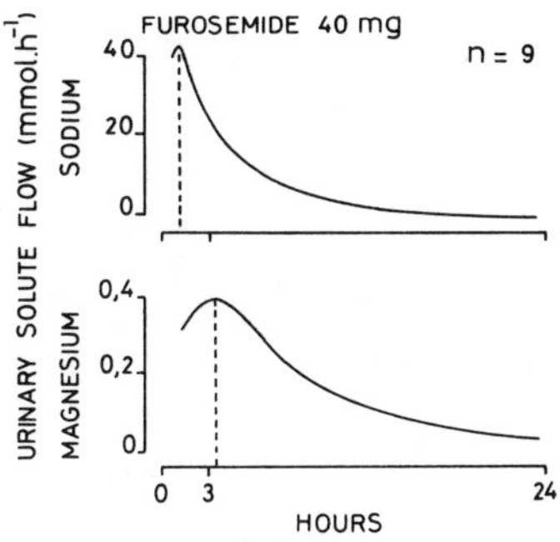

FIG. 2. Urinary Na and Mg flows after administration of furosemide 40 mg to healthy volunteers. Adapted from Reyes and Leary [2], by courtesy of Current Therapeutic Research.

cause hypermagnesiuria by direct blockade of Mg reabsorption which is aggravated by a further increase in Mg filtration at the glomerulus which follows Mg mobilisation from bone secondary to an increase in plasma parathyroid hormone (PTH) level which occurs in response to hypercalciuria provoked by loop diuretics. Thiazide-type diuretics block Mg reabsorption in the early portion of the distal tubule but the principal mechanism whereby they provoke hypermagnesiuresis is a decrease in

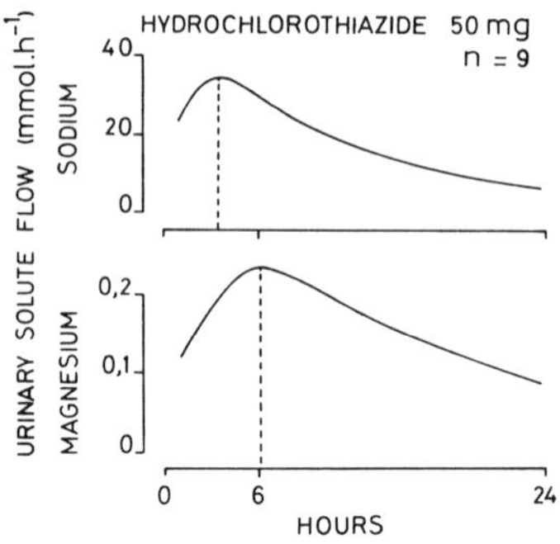

FIG. 3. Urinary Na and Mg flows after administration of hydrochlorothiazide 50 mg to healthy volunteers. Adapted from Leary and Reyes [3], by courtesy of Current Therapeutic Research.

reabsorption of Mg at the loop of Henle. This occurs because decreased Ca excretion induced by these substances reduces plasma PTH and thus diminishes PTH-dependent Mg reabsorption in the loop [4] (FIG. 4).

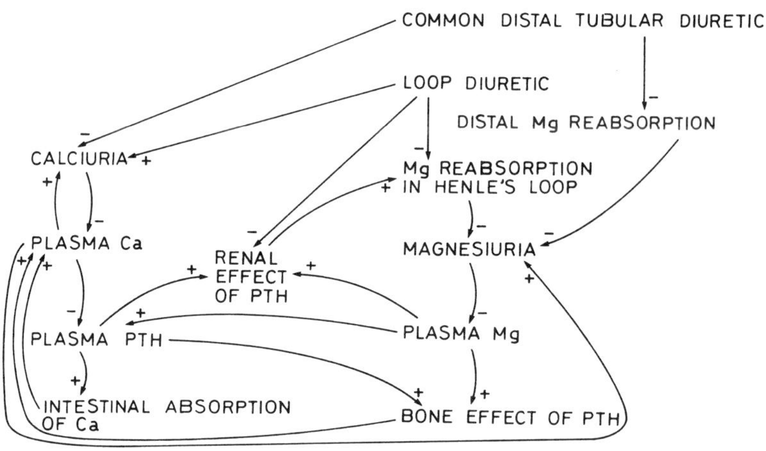

FIG. 4. Causal diagram of the determination of Mg deficiency provoked by loop and distal tubular diuretics. The diagram depicts changes (+: augmentation; -: diminution) resulting from increases in the variables at which arrows start (system dynamics notation). PTH: parathyroid hormone. Adapted from Reyes [4], by courtesy of La Prensa Médica Argentina.

REFERENCES

1. A.J. Reyes, and W.P. Leary, Curr. Ther. Res. 32, 128-137 (1982).
2. A.J. Reyes, and W.P. Leary, Curr. Ther. Res. 32, 406-416 (1982).
3. W.P. Leary, and A.J. Reyes, Curr. Ther. Res. 32, 425-431 (1982).
4. A.J. Reyes, Pren. Méd. Argent. 70, 448-456 (1983).

AN ANALYSIS OF THE STIMULATORY EFFECT ON RENIN RELEASE OF FUROSEMIDE AND ACETAZOLAMIDE

KATSUNORI HONDA, KENZO MATSUZAKI, AND MASAHITO NAGASAKA
First Department of Medicine, Faculty of Medicine, University of Tokyo, 7-3-1, Hongo, Bunkyo-ku, Tokyo, 113, Japan.

ABSTRACT

Clearance studies were performed to analyze the stimulatory effect of furosemide(F) and acetazolamide(A) on the plasma renin activity(PRA) under 3 different Na balance conditions(+, 0, -). PRA increased in both groups in Na (-) balance condition. It is demonstrated that PRA increased with F and A only when ECF volume contracted, and it is suggested that macula densa mechanism may not be operative without volume depletion. By factor analysis, stimulation of renin release by 2 diuretics appears to have different mechanisms.

INTRODUCTION

In the kidney, renin secretion is held to be controlled by at least 2 different mechanisms; renal baroreceptors and macula densa. Until now among the controversial views on the macula densa theory(1, 2), there is a rough agreement in that, under many experimental and clinical situations, the decrease of Na load to the distal tubule coincides with the increase of renin secretion. It is shown that procedures to decrease body Na content, such as giving low Na diet or forcing Na loss, stimulate the renin secretion, and conversely its increase results in the renin suppression(3). In clinical practice, intravenous F administration is a routine to check the renin responsiveness. However, there exists a problem what is the direct signal to the JG cells; the decrease of Na transport or load, body Na depletion or volume depletion. We studied, first, the stimulatory effect on PRA by the injection of F and also of A under 3 different Na balance conditions(+, 0, -) to elucidate this problem with clearance technic. Secondly, we investigated the difference in the effect of F and A for renin stimulation with factor analysis technic.

METHODS

Female mongrel dogs, average body weight 15kg, were anesthetized with pentobarbital and catheter was placed in the urinary bladder. After the control period of about 1 hour, F 20mg was injected intravenously followed by (1) saline infusion 1500ml/90min(Na (+) balance), (2) only replacement of urinary volume with saline (Na (0) balance), and (3) no replacement(Na (-) balance). Blood and urine samples were collected begining from the control period before the injection, and at each 30min interval during all experimental periods of 120-210min. Blood and urine samples were analyzed for Na, K, Cl and creatinine. Blood samples were, in addition, determined for PRA and plasma aldosterone concentration(PAC). In another group, A 500mg and isotonic sodium bicarbonate solution were given in place of F and saline.

RESULTS

Among the time course of the changes in plasma Na, K, Cl concentration (P_{Na}, P_K, and P_{Cl}, respectively), urinary Na, K and Cl excretion rate(E_{Na}, E_K and E_{Cl}), PRA and PAC, average and SD values of PRA, PAC and E_{Na} for 3 experimen-

Diuretics, Jules B. Puschett, Editor

tal conditions in F group were shown in Fig. 1(Na (+) balance is shown in the left, (0) in the middle and (-) in the right column). Natriuresis caused by F was found the largest in the Na (+) balance group, and became smaller in the (0) and (-) balance groups in this order. PRA elevation was found only in the Na (-) balance groups and was not found in others. PAC values were almost unchanged in all cases. In case of A, PRA, PAC, E_{Na} and P_{Cl} were shown in Fig. 2. Natriuresis was found largest in the Na (+) balance groups, but in other groups, in difference from F experiments, E_{Na} was found to be similarly small. PRA elevation was found only in the Na (-) balance groups, and it was unchanged in Na (0) and (+) balance groups as in F experiments. However, although PRA was low during isotonic bicarbonate infusion, it was followed by a slight increase after the end of infusion that was distinctly different from F experiments. PAC was unchanged in all groups. PRA increment along with P_{Cl} decrease was not found throughout, and this is different from Kotchen's theory. PRA and PAC were correlated only in F experiments. Table 1 shows that PRA and PAC have different correlation patterns with serum electrolyte concentrations and urinary electrolyte excretion rates which implies that there seems to be different mechanisms between the stimulatory effect of renin release by the 2 diuretics.

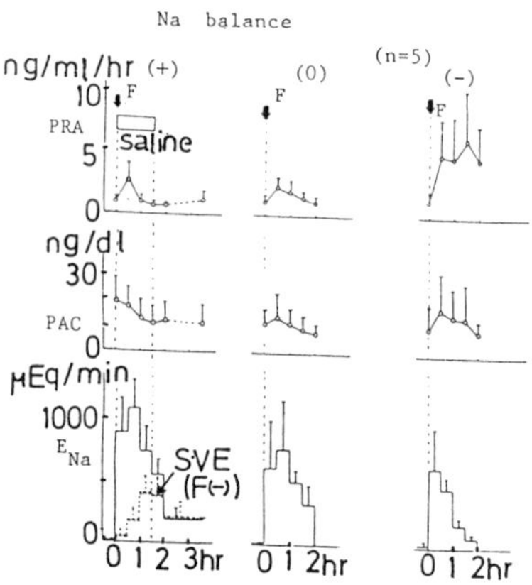

FIG. 1. Furosemide effect in 3 Na balance(+, 0, -) conditions.
In the low left panel E_{Na} for saline expansion without F is shown, as S-VE.

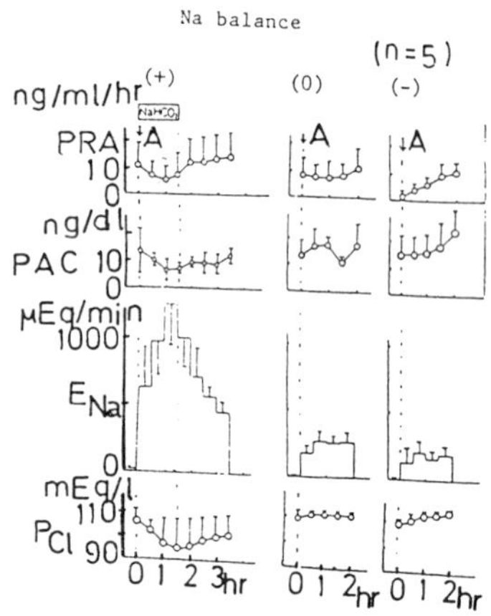

FIG. 2. Acetazolamide effect in 3 Na balance.

DISCUSSION

In F experiments, PRA was increased only in Na (-) balance groups which was in accordance with routine clinical practice. Under Na (+) balance condition PRA was suppressed during the whole period of saline infusion which represents the inhibitory effect of volume expansion(4). NaCl transport is considered to be an important signal to the macula densa(1, 5) and Kotchen et al. suggested that the inhibition of renin release by increased NaCl delivery is specifically related to the increased Cl transport in the ascending limb of the loop of Henle (6, 7). Our results did not confirm this in A experiments as mentioned above. It was demonstrated that such diuretics that inhibit NaCl transport in the ascending limb (e. g. F and ethacrynic acid) stimulated renin release, even if volume contraction was prevented (8, 9). But our results showed that PRA was not elevated, rather suppressed under the Na (0) balance condition. This result implies that renin stimulatory action of F may not operate without volume depletion in our experimental settings.

In A experiments, PRA increased under Na (-) balance condition that is the same as in F experiments. A was known to act mainly in the proximal tubules, but our result shows this diuretic may also act in the ascending limb of Henle similarly to F. Friedman et al. has demonstrated that this was indeed the case(10). However, our correlation table could not confirm that E_{Na} would influence PRA neither in F nor in A experiments. The difference in the correlation between PRA and PAC between F and A experiments is an unexpected finding. This may show that the stimulatory effect on the renin-aldosterone system of the 2 diuretics are dissimilar.

TABLE 1. Analysis of correlations

Acetazolamide

		PAC	P_{Cl}	P_K	P_{Na}	pH	P_{HCO_3}	E_{Cl}	E_K	E_{Na}	E_{HCO_3}
PRA	r		0.19	0.21	0.21		0.18				
	p		0.049	0.029	0.026		0.053				
PAC	r	/	0.38	0.36		0.49	0.42	0.28		0.432	0.35
	p	/	1×10^{-4}	2.9×10^{-4}		1.4×10^{-6}	4×10^{-5}	0.0062		1.3×10^{-5}	0.0014

Furosemide

		PAC	P_{Cl}	P_K	P_{Na}	pH	P_{HCO_3}	E_{Cl}	E_K	E_{Na}	E_{HCO_3}
PRA	r	0.33			0.25	/	/		0.24		/
	p	<0.05			<0.05	/	/		<0.05		/
PAC	r	/				/	/		0.30		/
	p	/				/	/		<0.05		/

r: significant correlation coefficient

p: p values for significance

REFERENCES

1. A. J. Vander, Physiol. Rev. 47, 359-382 (1967).
2. K. Thurau, Am. J. Med. 36, 698-719 (1964).
3. J. H. Laragh and J. E. Sealey in: Handbook of Physiology, Vol. 8, Renal Physiology, Am. Physiol. Soc., Washington, 831 (1973).
4. M. L. Tuck, R. G. Dluhy and G. H. Williams, J. Clin. Invest. 53, 988-995 (1974).
5. J. O. Davis and R. H. Freeman, Physiol. Rev. 56, 2-56 (1976).
6. T. A. Kotchen, J. H. Galla and R. G. Luke, Kidney Int. 13, 201-207 (1978).
7. K. A. Kirchner, T. A. Kotchen, J. H. Galla and R. G. Luke, Am. J. Physiol. 235, 444-450 (1978).
8. A. J. Vander, J. Carlson, Cir. Res. 25, 145-152 (1969).
9. P. Meyer, J. Menard, N. Papanicolaou, J. M. Alexandre, C. Devaux and P. Milliez, Am. J. Physiol. 215, 908-915 (1968).
10. P. E. Friedman and T. E. Andreoli, J. Gen. Physiol. 80, 683-711 (1982).

INTERACTION OF CONVENTIONAL AND K-SPARING DIURETICS WITH THE RENAL PROSTAGLANDIN (PG)-SYSTEM. STUDIES IN HEALTHY SUBJECTS AND IN PATIENTS WITH ESSENTIAL HYPERTENSION

J. KIPNOWSKI, R. DÜSING, and H.J. KRAMER

Medizinische Universitäts-Poliklinik Bonn, Bonn, W-Germany

INTRODUCTION

To date, conflicting results have been presented concerning the role of the renal PG-system in the regulation of renal sodium excretion and its possible participation in the tubular actions of diuretics (1). The present study was therefore performed to investigate the effects of acute inhibition of PG synthesis with indomethacin on renal excretion of sodium and potassium, respectively, in the presence of the conventional diuretics furosemide (F) and hydrochlorothiazide (HCT), and of the K-sparing diuretics amiloride (A), triamterene (TA), and K-canrenoate (K-C) in healthy subjects and in patients with essential hypertension.

EXPERIMENTAL PROTOCOL AND METHODS

All subjects who participated in this study were maintained on their regular intake of food and fluid which contained 100 to 200 mmol sodium and 50 to 80 mmol potassium per day. Twenty-four h urines were collected daily from 8.00 A.M. to 8.00 A.M. throughout the entire study. After a control period of two days each diuretic was given on two occasions for one day in random order without and with oral indomethacin, 50 mg t.i.d., at intervals of six days for subjects to regain normal sodium and fluid balance. In a first series of experiments which was performed in six (2 female and 4 male) healthy subjects and in seven male patients with essential hypertension, F, 40 mg t.i.d., and HCT, 25 mg t.i.d, were given orally. In a second series of experiments the K-sparing diuretics A, 5 mg t.i.d., and TA, 50 mg t.i.d., were given orally to seven female healthy subjects. In a last series K-C, 200 mg i.v. at 8.00 A.M., was administered to six (2 female and 4 male) healthy volunteers. Aliquots of urine samples were stored frozen at $-18^{\circ}C$ for determination of PGE_2 concentrations by radioimmunoassay (2) and of sodium and potassium by flame photometry. For statistical analysis of results Wilcoxon's signed-rank test was used. Results are expressed as means $\pm$ S.E.M.

RESULTS

Effects of conventional diuretics on urinary excretion of sodium and PGE_2 in the absence and presence of indomethacin in control subjects and in patients with essential hypertension.

Administration of F resulted in a significant rise in urinary excretion of sodium which was accompanied by a similar increase in urinary excretion of PGE_2 in control subjects and in hypertensive patients. Indomethacin significantly suppressed the F-induced increases in urinary excretion of sodium and PGE_2 in both groups (Table I). Treatment with HCT was accompanied by a significant increase in urinary excretion of sodium in control subjects and in hypertensive patients. Whereas the HCT-induced rise in urinary PGE_2 excretion was variable and not statistically significant in normotensive subjects, PGE_2 excretion significantly increased in hypertensive patients during HCT administration. The HCT-induced rise in urinary sodium and PGE_2 excretion was markedly suppressed by indomethacin in both groups (Table I).

Diuretics, Jules B. Puschett, Editor

Table I. Effects of orally administered furosemide (4O mg t.i.d.) and hydrochlorothiazide (25 mg t.i.d.) on urinary excretion of sodium and PGE_2 in normotensive controls (n = 6) and hypertensive patients (n = 7) without and with simultanoeous inhibition of PG synthesis with indomethacin (I) (5O mg t.i.d.).

	Normotensives		Hypertensives	
	$U_{Na}V$ (mEq/24h)	$U_{PGE_2}V$ (ng/24h)	$U_{Na}V$ (mEq/24h)	$U_{PGE_2}V$ (ng/24h)
Control	155±24	434±111	194±26	3O7±1O8
Furosemide	326±42*	915±228*	369±29*	1O89±312*
Furosemide + I	2O9±27*	367±125*	29O±21*	538±129*
Control	145±19	453±117	162±22	263±33
Hydrochlorothiazide	389±48*	1O32±269	375±2O*	757±135*
Hydrochlorothiazide + I	279±45*	248±85*	2O7±39*	433±39*

* Diuretic vs. control and without vs. with I, resp.: $p < 0.05$

Table II. Effects of amiloride (5 mg t.i.d.), triamterene (5O mg t.i.d.), and K-canrenoate (2OO mg i.v.) on urinary excretion of sodium, potassium, and PGE_2 without and with simultaneous inhibition of PG synthesis with indomethacin (I) (5O mg t.i.d.) in healthy volunteers.

	$U_{Na}V$ (mEq/24h)	U_KV (mEq/24h)	$U_{PGE_2}V$ (ng/24h)
Control	11O±16	53± 7	278± 44
Amiloride	195±24*	3O± 7*	739± 74*
Amiloride + I	149±12*	43±16	33O±138*
Control	11O±16	53± 7	278± 44
Triamterene	198±32*	52± 4	39O± 48
Triamterene + I	147±12	37± 9	117± 15*
Control	154±22	8O± 8	435± 65
K-canreonate	214±25*	55± 9*	15OO±37O*
K-canreonate + I	181±38	91± 9*	155± 5O*

* Diuretic vs. control and without vs. with I, resp.: $p < 0.05$

Effects of K-sparing diuretics on urinary excretion of sodium and potassium, urinary Na/K-ratio, and on urinary PGE_2 excretion.

Urinary sodium excretion increased significantly with the administration of A, TA, and K-C. While urinary potassium excretion was significantly reduced in the presence of A and K-C, potassium excretion remained unaltered during administration of TA (Table II). These changes in urinary electrolyte excretion were accompanied by a significant increase in urinary PGE_2 excretion following administration of A and K-C, whereas TA only slightly and variably stimulated urinary PGE_2 excretion (Table II). The diuretic-induced rise in PGE_2 excretion was suppressed by indomethacin in most instances to below control levels. This was paralleled by a suppression of diuretic-induced natriuresis which, however, was significant only during administration of A (Table II).

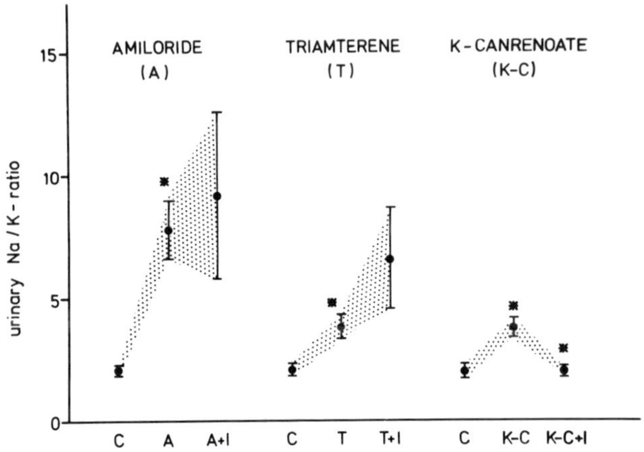

Figure 1: Urinary Na/K-ratio during administration of anti-kaliuretic diuretics without and with concomitant administration of indomethacin (I). (C = control; * p O.O5).

The urinary Na/K-ratio increased significantly with A and T from 2.1 $\pm$ O.2 to 7.8 $\pm$ 1.2 and to 3.7 $\pm$ O.5, respectively, and with K-C from 2.O $\pm$ O.3 to 3.8 $\pm$ O.4. Urinary potassium excretion in the presence of A and TA was variably affected by indomethacin, whereas the K-sparing effect of K-C was completely abolished by inhibition of PG synthesis. Thus, the urinary Na/K-ratio of 3.8 in the presence of K-C fell to 2.O $\pm$ O.2 ($p < O.O5$) when indomethacin was administered simultaneously (Figure 1).

DISCUSSION

Non-steroidal antiinflammatory drugs, such as indomethacin, have been shown to inhibit PG synthesis at the level of the cyclooxygenase enzyme system (3). In the present study we have shown that urinary excretion of PGE_2 increases with administration of conventional and K-sparing diuretics. These diuretic-induced effects on the renal PG system accompanied the rise in urinary sodium excretion, while inhibition of PG synthesis by concomitant administration of indomethacin with the diuretics markedly diminished their natriuretic effects. In the case of conventional diuretics this effect is probably related to hemodynamic (4) and tubular functional alterations in the presence of indomethacin (5,6).

The variable effects of indomethacin on the urinary Na/K-ratio in the presence of A and TA may be due to unspecific mechanisms such as competitive inhibition of proximal tubular secretion of these diuretics through interference at the level of the organic anion pump and/or increased NaCl-absorption in the ascending limb of Henle's loop (5). In contrast, the effects of indomethacin which completely abolished the K-sparing effect of K-C (7), may be related to more specific mechanisms such as interference with the renin-angiotensin and aldosterone system or with tubular aldosterone receptors. Whatever the mechanisms of this interaction are, inhibition of renal PG synthesis by non-steroidal antiinflammatory drugs during treatment with conventional and K-sparing diuretics at least partially abolishes the tubular effects of these diuretics. Thus, especially in patients with hypertension and/or edema non--steroidal antiinflammatory drugs should be given with caution.

ACKNOWLEDGMENTS

This study was supported in part by grants No. FA-76O4 and FA-8476, Ministerium für Wissenschaft und Forschung, Nordrhein-Westfalen, W-Germany. The authors gratefully acknowledge the skillful technical assistance of Mrs. A. Bäcker, Mrs. H. Stelkens, Mrs. S. Krämer, and Mrs. J. Eden.

REFERENCES

1. Düsing, R., Kramer, H.J., In: Annual Research Reviews - The renal prostaglandins, J.B. Lee, ed. (Eden Press, Montreal 1978) pp. 92-1O7

2. Kramer, H.J., Moch, T., Düsing, R., Renal Physiol. (Basel) 2: 3O2-31O (1979/8O)

3. Flower, R.J., Pharmacological Reviews 26: 33-67 (1974)

4. Williamson, H.E., Bourland, W.A., Marchand, G.R., Farley, D.B., van Orden, D.E., Proc. Soc. exp. Biol. Med. 15O: 1O4-1O6 (1975)

5. Düsing, R., Nicolas, V., Glänzer, K., Kipnowski, J., Kramer, H.J., Renal Physiol.(Basel) 5: 115-123 (1982)

6. Düsing, R., Nicolas, V., Glatte, B., Glänzer, K., Kipnowski, J., Kramer, H.J., Br. J. Pharmac. 16: 377-384 (1983)

7. Kramer, H.J., Düsing, R., Stinnesbeck, B., Prior, W., Bäcker, A., Eden, J., Kipnowski, J., Glänzer, K., Krück, F., Clin. Sci. 59: 67-7O (198O)

EFFECT OF TRIPAMIDE ON RENAL HEMODYNAMICS AND KALLIKREIN-KININ SYSTEM

Yoshito Fujiki, Satoru Fujishima, Susumu Uneda, Shoji Sesoko, Osamu Tochikubo and Yoshihiro Kaneko.
Yokohama City University School of Medicine,Yokohama, Japan

ABSTRACT

Twenty essential hypertensives were given 30 mg of tripamide orally for 10 weeks to investigate its effect on renal hemodynamics and the kallikrein-kinin system. Tripamide lowered arterial pressure significantly and also reduced serum Na and K. Plasma renin activity, urinary aldosterone excretion and kallikrein excretion (Ukal) increased significantly after tripamide. Renal blood flow and glomerular filtration rate revealed no significant change. However, renal vascular resistance (RVR) was diminished significantly by tripamide. Moreover, a significant negative correlation was seen between changes in RVR and Ukal as well as pretreatment RVR. In conclusion, our findings suggest that the increase in kallikrein activity participates in the reduction in RVR as one of the factors in antihypertensive action of tripamide.

INTRODUCTION

Tripamide (aminobenzen-sulphonamide derivative) has been reported to produce a hypotensive effect partly by saliuresis and partly by a reduction in peripheral vascular resistance, but the effect of this agent on renal hemodynamics and the kallikrein-kinin system in essential hypertension (EH) has not yet been investigated. This study was designed to evaluate the chronic effect of tripamide on the renal kallikrein-kinin system as a possible mediator of changes in renal hemodynamics.

METHODS

Twenty patients with EH (10 men and 10 women aged 38 to 60 years) were included in this investigation after a full survey to rule out secondary forms of hypertension. None had proteinuria or serum creatinine levels higher than 1.4 mg/dl. We classified 6 patients as stage I in accordance with WHO criteria, 12 as stage II and 2 as stage III with hemorrhagic retinopathy. All antihypertensive therapies were discontinued 4 weeks or more prior to the study. Then a daily dose of 30 mg tripamide was administered orally for 7 to 17 weeks with no dietary restriction imposed.

On the day before the termination of the placebo or tripamide treatment, patients were asked to come to the hospital in a fasting condition, and their arterial pressures (AP) were measured after a 30 minute period of supine rest. Blood was drawn to determine serum electrolytes (SNa, SK, SCa), serum creatinine (SCr), hematocrit (Hct) and plasma renin activity (PRA). Urine was collected after an hour period of supine rest to test for glomerular filtration rate (GFR, Ccr). Patients were also asked to collect urine for a 24-hour period prior to the examinations using a new device ("MEMORETTE" [1]) to determine the urine volume (UV), sodium (UNa), potassium (UK), aldosterone (Uald) and kallikrein activity (Ukal).

Kallikrein was determined by the method of Hitomi, et al. [2]. Results are expressed as Naphthol units per day (NU/day), and recovery was within 6%. Aldosterone was determined by direct radioimunoassay and renin activity by

Diuretics, Jules B. Puschett, Editor

radioimunoassay.

Renal plasma flow (RPF) was measured using the method of constant infusion of para-amino-hippurate after GFR measurement. Renal blood flow (RBF) was calculated from effective RPF by using the peripheral venous hematocrit value. Renal vascular resistance (RVR) was calculated in dyne·sec·cm-^{5}/1.73 m^{2} = MAP [mm Hg]/RPF (ml/min/ 1.73 m^{2}) X 80000. The GFR, RBF and RVR were corrected to 1.73 m^{2} of body surface.

RESULTS

Arterial pressure, Chemical and Biochemical Determinations

After long-term tripamide treatment, AP, SNa and SK were significantly reduced concomitantly with the significant increase in SCr, SCa, PRA, Uald and Ukal, whereas no significant changes occurred in UNa, UK, UV, body weight or Hct (Table 1).

TABLE 1. Arterial Pressure, Clinical and Biochemical Data and Renal Function After Long-Term Treatment with Tripamide.

Arterial Pressure (mmHg)		before treatment	after treatment	P
	Systolic	172 ± 4	151 ± 5	<0.001
	Diastolic	106 ± 2	96 ± 3	<0.001
	Mean	128 ± 2	114 ± 3	<0.001
Hct	(%)	41.7 ± 1.0	41.3 ± 1.1	ns
Serum Na	(mEq/L)	140.3 ± 0.4	139.1 ± 0.5	<0.02
Serum K	(mEq/L)	3.7 ± 0.1	3.3 ± 0.1	<0.001
Serum Ca	(mg/dl)	8.9 ± 0.1	9.1 ± 0.1	<0.05
Serum Cr	(mg/dl)	0.97 ± 0.04	1.04 ± 0.04	<0.01
PRA	(ng/ml/hr)	0.83 ± 0.12	1.41 ± 0.18	<0.01
Weight	(Kg)	59.4 ± 1.7	58.4 ± 1.7	ns
UV	(ml/day)	1668 ± 137	1775 ± 123	ns
UNa	(mEq/day)	222 ± 20	220 ± 20	ns
UK	(mEq/day)	56 ± 4	53 ± 4	ns
Uald	(μg/day)	10.3 ± 1.1	13.5 ± 1.6	<0.01
Ukal	(NU/day)	8.15 ± 0.94	11.08 ± 1.22	<0.05
RVR	(dyme·sec·cm^{-5}/1.73 m^{2})	14523 ± 1113	12144 ± 858	<0.01
RBF	(ml/min/1.73 m^{2})	784 ± 59	809 ± 49	ns
GFR	(ml/min/1.73 m^{2})	109 ± 6	102 ± 8	ns

Renal Function

After long-term tripamide therapy, the PRA, Uald and Ukal increased significantly (Table 1). Changes in Ukal did not correlate with the changes in the mean AP (Figure 1).

The GFR tended to be lower as compared with the placebo period, but the difference was not significant (Table 1). As compared with the placebo period, the RBF tended to be higher, but the difference was also not significant (Table 1). Changes in RBF correlated with changes in Ukal (r=0.47, P<0.05), and inversely with the changes in RVR (r=0.86, P<0.001). The RVR was significantly reduced (Table 1). The pretreated RVR correlated inversely with changes in RVR (r=0.62, P<0.01) and moreover the changes in RVR with changes in Ukal (r=-0.53, P<0.02) (Figure 2).

DISCUSSION

In hypertensives, thiazides elevate kallikrein and decrease RVR [3].

However, the site of action of tripamide differs from that of the thiazides. Our findings that the increase in Ukal after tripamide correlated with the decrease in RVR could mean that renal kallikrein may be one of the factors which diminish RVR. However, the absence of a correlation between changes in Ukal and MAP supports the concept that the action of kallikrein is a factor affecting RVR. From our findings, we cannot be completely certain that tripamide caused the changes in RVR and therefore in MAP by increasing Ukal. In another study from this laboratory, RVR decreased with no increase in Ukal after the administration of captopril in man.

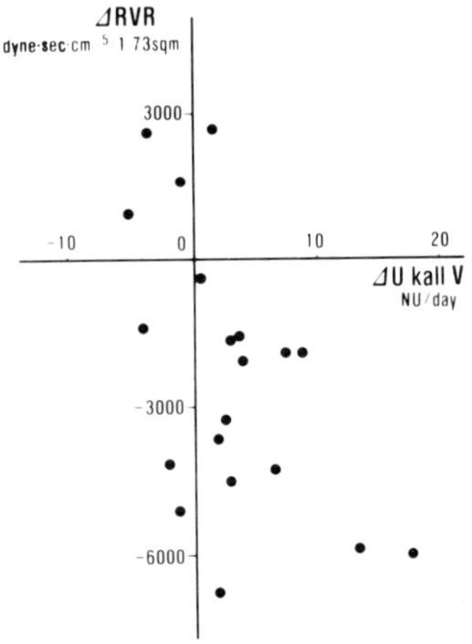

FIGURE 1. A significant inverse correlation between changes in RVR and Ukal occurred with tripamide administration ($r=-0.53$, $P<0.02$, $n=20$).

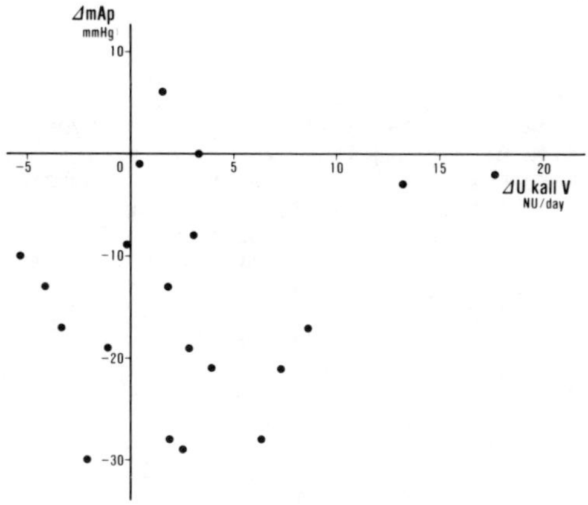

FIGURE 2. There was no correlation between changes in AP and Ukal (r=0.19, P>0.25, ns)

One of the mechanisms whereby tripamide decreased RVR was probably the activation of the kallikrein-kinin system. This hypothesis is supported by the facts that: 1) There was a significant correlation between RBF and kinins in the urine in dogs after the administration of an ACE inhibitor, and 2) RBF, GFR and urinary PGE2 were decreased in rats after aprotinin administration [4]. The kallikrein-kinin system may also be important in preventing the excessive vasoconstriction caused by the renin-angiotensin system that was enhanced by tripamide [5].

REFERENCES

1. O. Tochikubo, S. Uneda and Y. Kaneko, Hypertension 5, 270 (1983).
2. Y. Hitomi, M. Niinobe and S. Fujii, Clinica Chimica Acta 100 275-283, (1980).
3. D.T. O'Connor, R.A. Preston, J.A. Mitas, R.P. Frigon and R.A. Stone, Hypertension 3, 139-147, (1981).
4. H.J. Kramer, T. Moch, L. Von Sicherer and R. Dusing, Clin. Sci. 56, 547-553 (1979).
5. P.A. Johnston, D.B. Bernard, N.S. Perrin, L. Arbeit, W. Lieberthal and N.G. Levinski, Circ. Res. 48, 728-733 (1981).

Effects of tripamide on aortas and blood levels of lipids and prostaglandin (6-keto-PGF and TXB) in SHR

Y. Matsuda*, R. Sato*, T. Suzuki*, K. Unno*, K. Kawamura**, and T. Shozawa**
*Department of Pharmacy, Akita University Hospital, **Second Department of Pathology, Akita University School of Medicine, Akita 010, Japan

INTRODUCTION

Both Hypertension and hypercholesterolemia are risk factors of arteriosclerosis. It has been reported that some kinds of hypertensive agents, especially hypotensive diuretics, lower the blood pressure in hypertensive patients, but on the other hand they aggravate a disturbance in cholesterol metabolism, and that their practical utility is thus reduced to naught.

A disturbance in the synthesis of prostacyclin (PGI) in the vascular system is believed not only to promote a rise in blood pressure and arteriosclerosis but to facilitate the progress of atherosclerosis. In 1981 Gryglowski et al. reported that hyperlipemia itself was not only a risk factor of arteriosclerosis, but also it facilitated the deposition of lipids on the blood vessel wall, and that the resulting lipoperoxide diminished PGI formation in the blood vessel wall.

Diminished PGI formation has important implications relative to the persistence of hypertension and progress of arteriosclerosis. The present study was therefore undertaken to determine the effects of the hypotensive diuretic tripamide on lipometabolism and blood levels of PGI and TXA in spontaneously hypertensive rats (SHR).

MATERIALS AND METHODS

Experimental Animals

Spontaneous Hypertensive Rats (SHR) Wistar Kyoto Strain(Charles River Japan Inc.)

Sex and Age : Male , 12 weeks of age

Drug : Tripamide (Eisai Co Ltd.)

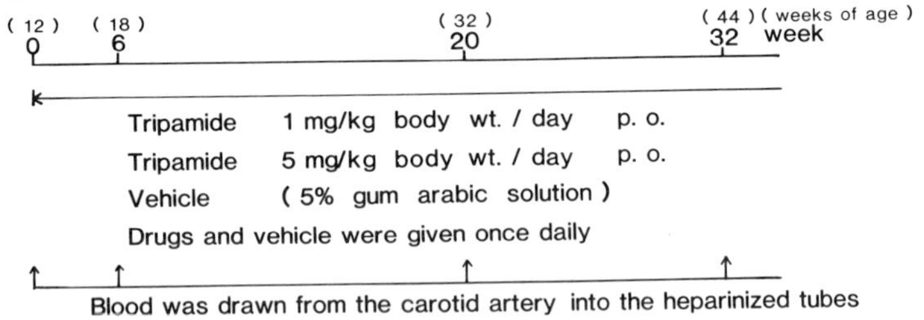

Determination methods

Blood pressure (Tail cuff)

Total cholesterol (Enzyme method)

HDL-cholesterol (Phospho tungstic method)

6-keto-$PGF_{1\alpha}$ and TXB_2 (Radioimmumoassay method)

Diuretics, Jules B. Puschett, Editor

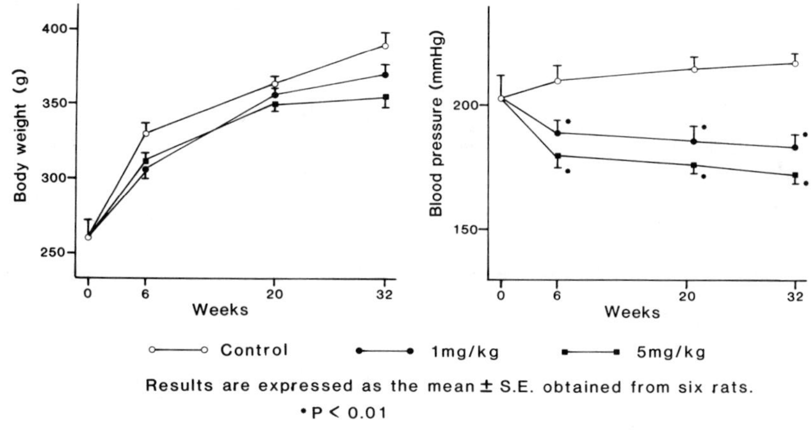

Fig. 1. Effect of tripamide on body weight and blood pressure in SHR.

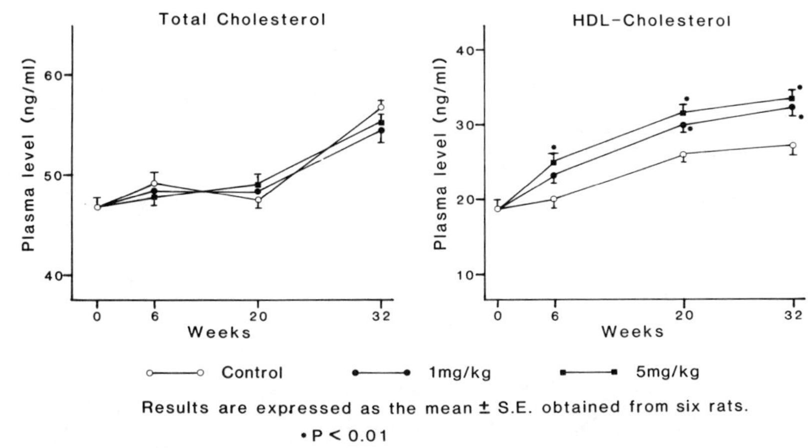

Fig. 2. Effect of tripamide on serum lipids in SHR.

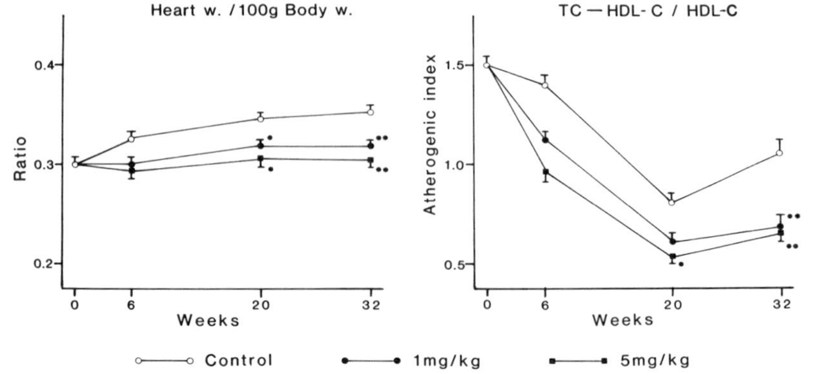

Results are expressed as the mean ± S.E. obtained from six rats.
•P < 0.05 ••P < 0.01

Fig. 3. Effect of tripamide on atherogenic index and heart weight in SHR.

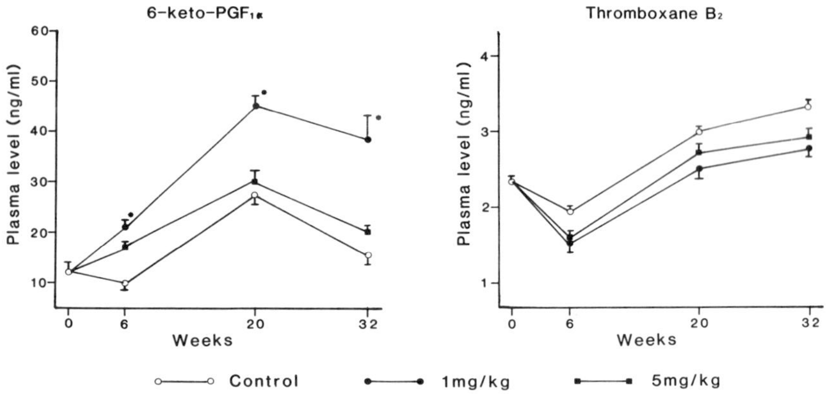

Results are expressed as the mean ± S.E. obtained from six rats.
•P < 0.01

Fig. 4. Effect of tripamide on serum content of prostaglandins in SHR.

RESULTS

Tripamide induced a drop in blood pressure, an increase in PGI and a slight decrease in TXA . It was also shown that tripamide hardly affected the blood levels of total cholesterol, but produced a significant increase only in blood level of HDL cholesterol. These results suggest that tripamide not only benefits hypertension which is an important risk factor of arteriosclerosis, but produces a favorable effect on the PG system and cholesterol metabolism.

LONG-TERM METABOLIC CHANGES AFTER CONVERTING DIURETIC TREATMENT OF HYPERTENSION TO TREATMENT WITH VERAPAMIL

A. LEHTONEN, AND A. GORDIN
Department of Medicine, Turku University Central Hospital, Turku, and Clinical Research Department, Orion Pharmaceutical Company, Espoo, Finland

ABSTRACT

We have studied the effect of verapamil on different metabolic parameters after converting the treatment of hypertension with hydrochlorothiazide monotherapy to treatment with verapamil monotherapy. Verapamil therapy was continued for 6 months in doses of 80 to 160 mg b.i.d. The antihypertensive efficacy of verapamil was comparable with that of hydrochlorothiazide. None of the patients reported side-effects on verapamil. Plasma total cholesterol, LDL-cholesterol, HDL-cholesterol, triglycerides and free fatty acids did not change significantly after converting diuretic treatment to verapamil. Neither were marked changes observed in fasting blood glucose, insulin or C-peptide values. Serum uric acid concentration decreased significantly and serum potassium levels increased significantly on verapamil compared to the diuretic period. Serum concentration of calcium decreased and calcium excretion increased significantly during verapamil from the levels on diuretic.

INTRODUCTION

It is well known that unfavourable changes occur in risk factors for coronary heart disease during diuretic treatment: Increase in total cholesterol and triglycerides and decrease in HDL-cholesterol to total cholesterol ratio (1, 2), glucose intolerance (2, 3), insulin resistence (2) and other well known adverse effects in serum potassium and uric acid concentrations. These changes probably even increase the risk of developing coronary heart disease (4).

Calcium channel blockers are increasingly used in the treatment of hypertension and angina pectoris (5). However, there is sparce information on their long-term metabolic effects, especially on lipid metabolism.

The present study was thus performed to evaluate the long term effect of a calcium channel blocker, verapamil, on different metabolic parameters in hypertensive patients treated earlier with hydrochlorothiazide monotherapy.

Diuretics, Jules B. Puschett, Editor

PATIENTS AND METHODS

Fifteen patients with essential hypertension (mean age 53.5 years, range 36-70) were included in the study. All patients had had antihypertensive therapy for mild - to - moderate hypertension with either 25 mg or 50 mg of hydrocloro-thiazide once daily for at least 6 months as monotherapy. Thereafter the hydrocholorothiazide treatment was discontinued and verapamil 80 mg twice daily was started. The dose of vera-pamil was increased to 160 mg twice daily if the diastolic pressure was over 90 mmHg after one months treatment. Blood pressure, heart rate and weight measurements as well as bio-chemical determinations were performed at the end of the diuretic treatment and after 1, 3 and 6 months´ treatment with verapamil.

RESULTS

Systolic blood pressure was slightly, but not signifi-cantly, higher in both the supine and standing position after one month of treatment with verapamil than during diuretic therapy. Otherwise there were no differences. The weights of the patients increased significantly during the first month on vera-pamil, and was about constant during the following months.

The concentrations of plasma free fatty acids and lipids did not change significantly after converting diuretic treatment to verapamil. The levels of plasma triglycerides, cholesterol and LDL-, VLDL-, HDL-cholesterol and the ratio of HDL-choles-terol to total cholesterol were rather similar during the 6 months on verapamil as compared to the hydrochlorothiazide period.

There were no significant differences in fasting blood glucose or serum insulin levels between the two treatment periods. The fasting C-peptide level was significantly lower ($p < 0.01$) at 6 months on verapamil than at the end of the diuretic period. There were, however, no differences in the C-peptide levels at other points of time.

Serum uric acid concentration was significantly lower during the whole verapamil period compared to the situation at the end of the hydrochlorothiazide treatment.

The concentration of serum potassium increased signifi-cantly after converting the diuretic therapy to verapamil. Serum calcium level was significantly lower at 6 months on verapamil than on diuretics, but the concentration of serum magnesium did not change significantly. The 24 h urinary calcium excretion increased significantly during the verapamil treatment period.

DISCUSSION

In the present study, hydrochlorothiazide monotherapy was converted to verapamil monotherapy, and the antihypertensive effects of these drugs were comparable when verapamil was used in doses from 160 to 320 mg daily.

According to the present study, there was no change in the lipid profile after converting diuretic therapy to verapamil. None of the parameters measured were markedly elevated either on the diuretic or verapamil period.

In the present study, no marked changes were observed in the basal glucose, insulin or C-peptide levels. Again, the material did not include patients with overt diabetes.

In contrast to diuretics, calcium channel blockers offer the prospective of a specific cardioprotective action by antagonizing the increase in myocardial calcium influx induced by sympathetic stimulation or electrolyte imbalance (6, 7). Verapamil also appears preferable to diuretic agents as the latter induce depletion of potassium as well as increase in serum uric acid levels. Verapamil is very well tolerated, and it has an antihypertensive efficacy comparable with diuretics.

REFERENCES

1. R.P. Ames, P. Hill, Improvement of glucose tolerance and lowering of glycohemoglobin and serum lipid concentrations after discontinuation of antihypertensive drug therapy. Circulation 65, 899-904 (1982).
2. R.P. Ames, Negative effects of diuretic drug on metabolic risk factors for coronary heart disease. Possibly alternative drug therapies. Am J Cardiol 51, 632-638 (1983).
3. O.O. Andersen, I. Persson, Carbohydrate metabolism during treatment with chlorthalidone and ethacrynic acid. Br Med J 2, 798-801 (1968).
4. Editorial, Antihypertensive drugs, plasma lipids, and coronary disease. Lancet 2, 19-20 (1980).
5. Editorial, Calcium antagonists in hypertension. Lancet 2, 307-308 (1982).
6. A.M. Katz, H. Reuter, Cellular calcium and cardiac cell death. Am J Cardiol 44, 188-190 (1979).
7. W.G. Nayler, The heart cell: some metabolic aspects of cardiac arrhythmias. Acta Med Scand (Suppl) 647, 17-31 (1981).

ENZYMURIA IN RATS UNDER TREATMENT WITH DIURETICS.

H. GROETSCH, M. HROPOT, H. KIEF AND E. KLAUS
Hoechst AG, Postfach 80 03 20, D-6230 Frankfurt am Main 80, FRG

ABSTRACT

The effect of daily treatment with high- and low-ceiling diuretics on enzymuria in rats during a four week experiment was studied. The following enzymes were measured daily in 24-hour urine samples: alanine-aminopeptidase (AAP), gamma-glutamyl-transferase (GGT), N-acetyl-β-glucosaminidase (NAG) and lactate-dehydrogenase (LDH). The excretion of electrolytes and the histology were also evaluated. As early as 24-hours after administration of furosemide (32 mg/kg) and piretanide (8 mg/kg), the measured enzymes AAP, GGT and NAG showed a clear increase in excretion. In addition, indapamide caused an increase in LDH. Furosemide and piretanide did not cause any histological alterations in the kidneys.

INTRODUCTION

The excretion of renal enzymes may be interpreted as a normal activity of kidney cells. Particularly proximal tubular cells reveal a high level of enzymes in the microvilli of the brush border and cytosol. These enzymes pass over in the urine by regular protein turnover and permeation. Among other drugs, diuretics cause also an increase in enzymuria in man and animal, respectively. However the increased enzymuria must not indicate a permanent damage of renal tubules. The effect of increased enzymuria has already been shown in rats after treatment with a high single dose of furosemide as far as furosemide induced diuresis was concerned. The postulated circadian rhythms could not be established (1).

The aim of this study was to examine the effect of daily treatment with high oral doses of loop- and low-ceiling diuretics over a prolonged period of time on enzymuria and nephrotoxic effects. The diuretics used were administered in equipotent doses, i.e. in doses which caused equal increased urine excretion within 24 hours.

METHODS

35 male Wistar rats with an initial body weight of 161±6 g were kept in single metabolism cages with free access to food and water. The rats were randomized in five groups as followed: control (vehicle 5 ml water/kg b.wt.), 32 mg/kg p.o. furosemide, 8 mg/kg p.o. piretanide, 4 mg/kg p.o. hydrochlorothiazide and 2 mg/kg p.o. indapamide.

24-hour urine samples were collected by addition of sodium acide as preservative. After centrifugation of an aliquot for

Diuretics, Jules B. Puschett, Editor

10 minutes at 1000 g, 2.5 ml of the supernatant were gelfiltered by a Sephadex G25M column. The following enzymes were determined in the filtrate:

1. Alanine-aminopeptidase (AAP),
2. Gamma-glutamyltranspeptidase (GGT) and
3. Lactate-dehydrogenase (LDH)
   by kinetic reaction at 25° C.
4. N-Acetylglucosaminidase (NAG)
   by an endpoint reaction at 37° C.

In addition the electrolytes sodium,potassium, calcium, magnesium, chloride as well as creatinine were measured. At the end of the experiment histological examinations were performed.

RESULTS AND DISCUSSION

The results have shown that high- and low-ceiling diuretics could not be dissociated with respect to an increased excretion of urinary enzymes in 24-hour urine samples. As shown

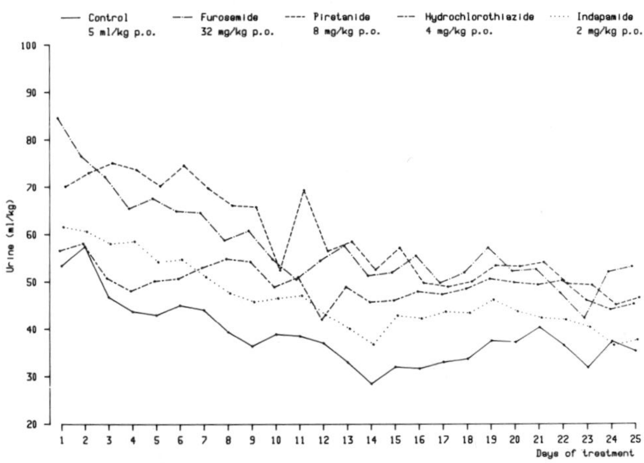

FIG. 1. 24-hour urine volumes during the treatment period of 25 days ($\bar{x}$, n = 7).

in figures 2 - 5 high doses of all diuretics produced a pronounced increase in the enzymes AAP, GGT and NAG in the urine compared to the control group. The total excreted enzyme activities over the period of treatment are shown in table 1. In addition LDH only rose in the indapamide group within the first decade of treatment. Throughout the whole treatment period the diuretic effect has been observed with the diuretics, whereas natriuresis was not consistent. Histological examinations did not show any damage after furosemide and piretanide, whereas indapamide caused changes in the distal tubular cells of the kidney.

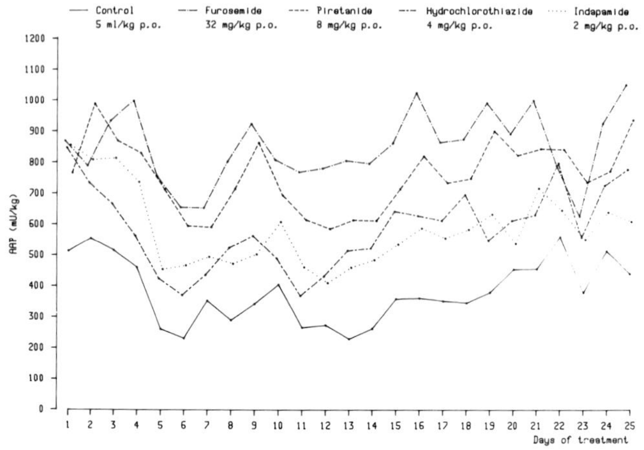

FIG. 2. Urinary excretion of AAP during the treatment period of 25 days ($\bar{x}$, n = 7).

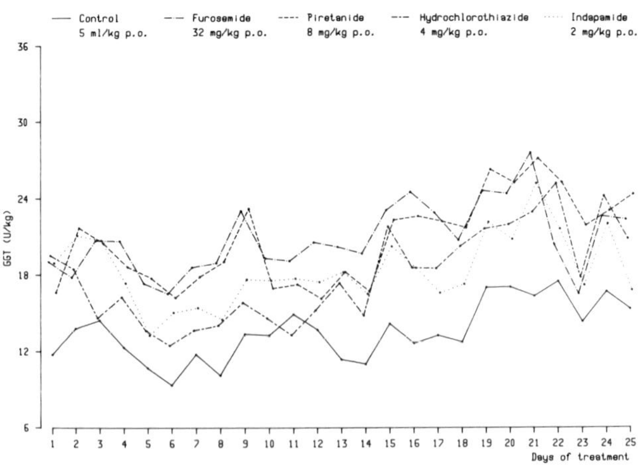

FIG. 3. Urinary excretion of GGT during the treatment period of 25 days ($\bar{x}$, n = 7).

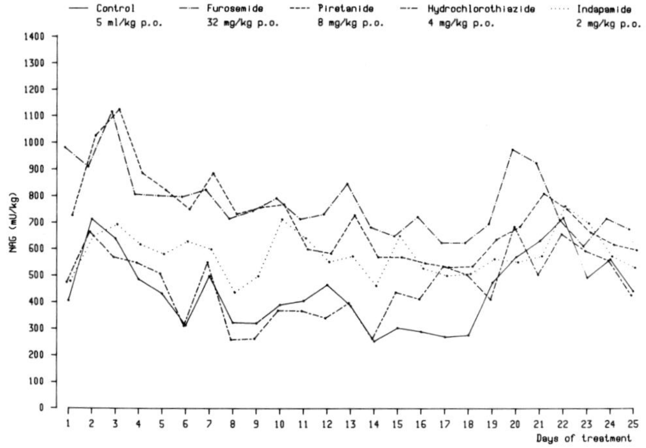

FIG. 4. Urinary excretion of NAG during the treatment period of 25 days ($\bar{x}$, n = 7).

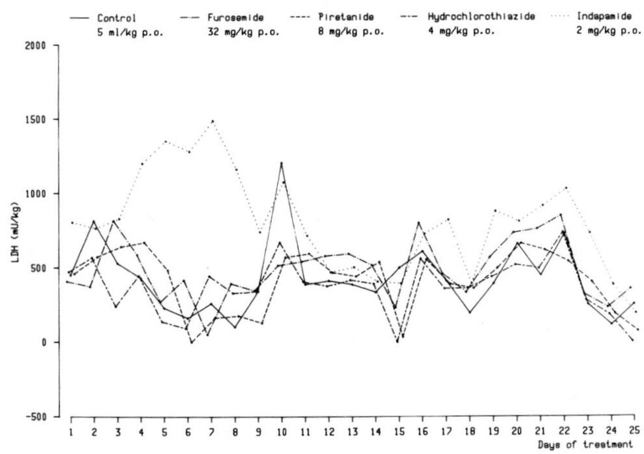

FIG. 5. Urinary excretion of LDH during the treatment period of 25 days ($\bar{x}$, n = 7).

TABLE 1 : TOTAL EXCRETED ENZYME ACTIVITIES OVER 25 DAYS-TREATMENT WITH DIURETICS
VALUES ARE MEAN ± S.D. (N = 7). ASTERISKS DENOTE P 0.05 (•) AND P 0.01 (••) [U-TEST]

	AAP (mU/kg)	GGT (U/kg)	NAG (mU/kg)	LDH (mU/kg)
CONTROL	9535 ± 4256	339 ± 106	11035 ± 4530	10567 ± 7120
FUROSEMIDE	21167 •• ± 6195	521 ± 157	19318 ± 3032	12030 ± 2675
PIRETANIDE	18858 •• ± 3475	518 • ± 126	17829 • ± 3326	10214 ± 2257
HYDROCHLORO - THIAZIDE	14637 ± 4723	447 ± 86	11569 ± 2251	9237 ± 3099
INDAPAMIDE	14579 • ± 2268	460 ± 102	14498 ± 6483	20560 • ± 5027

In summary it can be said that oral administration of high doses of diuretics for a prolonged period of time induced an increased enzymuria. In combination with the histological findings the increased enzymuria after furosemide and piretanide can be interpreted as a result of an elevated metabolic activity of renal tubular cells.

REFERENCE

1. M. Hohenegger and W. Raab, Clin. chim. Acta 28, 61-65 (1970).

EFFECT OF TRIPAMIDE, A NEW ANTIHYPERTENSIVE DIURETICS, ON THIAZIDE INDUCED HYPERGLYCEMIA

TORU YAMAGAMI, M.D., YASUHARU MAEDA, M.D., HIROSHIGE KUBO, M.D., HIROTAKA AKAGAMI, M.D., KAZUO SAWAMI, M.D. AND SEIICHI TOYAMA, M.D.
Department of Cardiology, The Center for Adult Diseases, Osaka
3-1 Nakamichi Higashinari, Osaka 537, Japan

SUMMARY

Effect of Tripamide on blood pressure and fasting blood sugar was studied in 43 cases with essential hypertension. Antihypertensive activity of Tripamide was as same as that of thiazide. 15 mg tripamide may have equal antihypertensive activity to 4 mg Trichlormethiazide.

Diabetogenetic activity of Tripamide was less than that of Thiazide. Hyperglycemia induced by Trichlormethiazide was improved by replacement with Tripamide.

INTRODUCTION

Tripamide (TPM), a new antihypertensive diuretics, was synthesized by Hamano et al [1]. A pharmacological action of TPM was investigated by several investigators and reported that antihypertensive activity was almost equal to thiazide [2], while it has little effect on potassium excretion [3] and no diabetogenetic activity on animal model of diabetes in rats [4].

To confirm these phenomena in clinical medicine, effect of TPM on blood pressure and fasting blood sugar (FBS) was studied in the patients with essential hypertension and the results were compared with that of Trichlormethiazide (TCMT).

MATERIALS AND METHODS

43 patients with essential hypertension were selected from out patient clinic of our hospital. These patients were divided into two groups. The first group, untreated group, was consisted of 23 hypertensives who had never received diuretics before trial. They were 12 males, aged 61.6, and 11 females, aged 53.6. The second group, TCMT group, was consisted of 20 hypertensives with thiazide induced hyperglycemia. They were treated with TCMT, mean dose of 3.8 mg and mean period of 23 months, and their initial FBS were less than 108 mg/dl and increased to more than 112 mg/dl during TCMT administration. They were 13 males, aged 60.4, and 7 females, aged 56.3.

15-45 mg of TPM, mean dosage of 19 mg, was administered orally to the patients in untreated group and same dose of TPM was also administered to TCMT group instead of TCMT. The other drugs, including non-diuretic anti-hypertensive agents, were continued without any change during experimental period.

Each value was expressed as mean ± s.e. and student t test was employed for statistical analysis.

RESULTS

Effects of TPM on blood pressure was summarized in Table 1. In the untreated group, initial systolic pressure was 179.5 ± 5.3 mmHg and reduced to 147.1 ± 2.9 mmHg after treatment ($p<0.001$). Initial diastolic pressure was 102.3 ± 3.0 mmHg and reduced to 85.1 ± 2.1 mmHg after treatment ($p<0.05$). In the TCMT group, initial systolic pressure was 190.2 ± 5.1 mmHg

Diuretics, Jules B. Puschett, Editor

Table 1. Effect of TPM on blood pressure.

	Untreated Group		TCMT Group	
No. of cases	23		20	
	Systolic	Diastolic	Systolic	Diastolic
Initial	179.5 ± 5.3	102.3 ± 3.0	190.2 ± 5.1	105.9 ± 3.5
TCMT			162.7 ± 4.2	91.7 ± 2.3
TPM	147.1 ± 2.9	85.1 ± 2.1	152.5 ± 3.6	87.9 ± 2.0

and reduced to 162.4 ± 4.2 mmHg during TCMT administration ($p<0.005$). After replacement of TCMT with TPM, it was 152.5 ± 3.6 mmHg and showed no difference compared with that of TCMT treatment. Initial diastolic pressure was 105.9 ± 3.5 mmHg and reduced to 91.7 ± 4.2 mmHg during TCMT administration ($p<0.005$). After replacement of TCMT with TPM, it was 87.9 ± 2.0 mmHg and showed no significant difference.

To compare the hypotensive effect of TPM with TCMT, changes in mean blood pressure was studied. A reduction of 19.1 ± 3.3 mmHg was observed during TCMT administration compared with initial value and a reduction of 24.6 ± 3.5 mmHg was observed during TPM administration. Therefore, it seems that hypotensive effect of TPM was stronger ($p<0.05$) than that of TCMT on the dosage of 20 mg and 4 mg respectively.

Fasting blood sugar during TPM administration was summarized in Table 2 and 3. In the untreated group, it was 121.8 ± 7.9 mg/dl at initial and 123.1 ± 7.4 mg/dl after treatment and showed no difference between them. This group was divided into two subgroups according to initial FBS. The first subgroup was the patients with normal blood sugar, whose FBS was less than 110 mg/dl, and the second subgroup was the patients with high FBS, whose FBS was larger than 112 mg/dl. In the first subgroup, initial FBS was 95.4 ± 1.2 mg/dl and increased to 102.9 ± 2.1 mg/dl after administration of TPM and showed significant difference ($p<0.005$). On the other hand, in the second group, it was 146.6 ± 11.5 mg/dl and 141.6 ± 12.0 mg/dl respectively and showed no difference.

Table 2. Effect of TPM on FBS, untreated group.

	No. of cases	Initial	TPM
Normal FBS	11	95.4 ± 1.2	102.9 ± 2.1
High FBS	12	146.1 ± 11.5	141.6 ± 12.0
Total	23	121.8 ± 7.9	123.1 ± 7.4

Table 3. Effect of TPM on FBS, TCMT group.

No. of cases	Initial	TCMT	TPM
20	98.1 ± 1.7	124.6 ± 2.3	111.8 ± 3.2

In the TCMT group, initial FBS was 98.1 ± 1.7 mg/dl and significantly increased to 124.6 ± 2.3 mg/dl during TCMT administration ($p<0.005$). when TCMT was replaced with TPM, it decreased to 111.8 ± 3.2 mg/dl. This value was higher than initial value ($p<0.005$) but lower than that of TCMT treatment ($p<0.005$). FBS during TPM administration was higher in the TCMT group than that in the patients with normal FBS in the untreated group, although initial FBS level was almost same in both groups.

DISCUSSION

Since many investigators were studied on antihypertensive effect of TPM, TPM was accepted as a new antihypertensive diuretics in Japan.

Comparative study of TPM on essential hypertension was studied with

Me iclothiazide in the manner of double blind procedure [5] and showed almost same potency of antihypertensive activity.

In this study, antihypertensive activity of TPM was compared with that of TCMT and showed almost same activity, however, mean blood pressure reduced more during TPM administration than TCMT. In this study, dosage of TCMT was 3.8 mg and that of TPM was 19.6 mg. Consequently, antihypertensive activity of 4 mg TCMT may meet that of 15 mg TPM.

Patients with essential hypertension should be controlled by antihypertensive drugs for long period, sometimes their life long. Therefore, side effects of the drugs should be considered by physicians. Antihypertensive diuretics are recognized in many country as a first choice of antihypertensive drugs. Main side effects of thiazide derivatives are hypokalemia, hyperuricemia, azotemia and diabetogenetic activity. In the previous report on double blind trial with Methiclothiazide [5], it was suggested that these side effects were observed as same possibility in TPM as in thiazide. On the other hand, animal experiment suggested that diabetogenetic activity of TPM was less than that of thiazide [4], moreover in clinical open study, it was reported that TPM administration did not increase FBS [6].

McMahon [7] reviewed that an incidence of hyperglycemia due to thiazide was 0.1 - 5 %. In Japan, it seems a little higher than that report. Ebihara [8] reported hypokalemiz in 5.2 %, hyperuricemia in 4.2 % and hyperglycemia in 5.2 % of 213 cases with thiazide treated hypertensives. In our out patient clinic, hypokalemia was 11.2 %, hyperuricemia was 1.0 % and hyperglycemia was 4.9 % of 493 cases [9].

In 20 cases with thiazide induced hyperglycemia, thiazide was replaced with TPM in this study. FBS showed significant decrease by the replacement of thiazide. In the individual case, 13 cases showed 120 mg/dl or more FBS by thiazide administration. In these cases, replacement of TCMT decreased FBS under 120 mg/dl in 8 cases. These results suggested that TPM may have less diabetogenetic activity than thiazide and thiazide induced hyperglycemia may improved by replacement of thiazide with TPM.

On the other hand, initial FBS in untreated group was 95 mg/dl and in TCMT group was 98 mg/dl. However, during TPM administration, it was 103 mg/dl in the former and 112 mg/dl in the latter and significantly higher in the latter ($p<0.05$). These results suggest that cases with thiazide induced hyperglycemia may also be sensitive to TPM.

It is assumed that mechanism of diabetogenetic activity in TCMT may be same in TPM but an activity may be less in TPM than TCMT.

REFERENCES

1. Hamano, H. et al: Chem. Abst., 78:364 (1973).
2. Igarashi, T. et al: Shinryo to Shinyaku, 16:1253 (1979).
3. Noguchi, M. et al: Yakubutsu Ryoho, 12:539 (1979).
4. Noguchi, M. et al: ibid., 12:549 (1979).
5. Masuyama, Z. et al: Igaku no Ayumi, 113:928 (1980).
6. Kubo, H. et al: Prog. in Med., 2:585 (1982).
7. McMahon, F.C.: Management of Essential Hypertension (Futura, New York, 1978), p. 47.
8. Ebihara, T. et al: Rinshoyakuri, 9:45 (1978).
9. Yamagami, T. et al: Rinsho to Kenkyu, 49:771 (1972).

EFFECTS OF SULFAMOYLBENZAMIDE (TRIPAMIDE, NORMONAL^R) ON PLASMA LIPOPROTEIN LIPIDS

H. NAKAMURA*, T. ISHIKAWA, N. TADA, N. SUZUKI, K. KONDO AND E. MIYAZIMA*
* National Defense Medical College*, Tokorozawa.
Jikei University, Aoto Hospital, Tokyo.

ABSTRACT

It has been recognized that certain types of diuretics may alter plasma lipids which might decrease the beneficial effects of diuretics to hypertensive subjects. Elevated LDL cholesterol and triglyceride and decreased HDL-cholesterol could be an risk factor in developing coronary heart diseases.

The aim of the present study is to evaluate whether Tripamide may alter plasma lipoprotein lipids during the treatment of hypertension. Twenty hypertensive subjects (9 male, 11 female) with ages ranging from 32 to 73 were subjected to receive Tripamide 30 mg per day for 3 to 6 months. Systolic blood pressure decreased significantly from 153.5±11.9 mmHg to 139±4.6 mmHg in 3 months, and from 153.5± 11.9 mmHg to 130.5±5.1 mmHg in 6 months. Diastolic blood pressure also decreased significantly from 92.2±4.3 mmHg to 86.8±3.2 mmHg in 3 months, and from 92.2±4.2 to 86.4±1.7 mmHg in 6 months. During this treatment, total cholesterol did not change significantly. Triglyceride tended to increase but this change was not significant. HDL-cholesterol remained unchanged.

Phospholipids increased significantly during the treatment, from 215.5±26.1 mg/dl to 240.4±39.9 mg/dl (P 0.01). Uric acid also remained unchanged.

Compared with the alterations frequently induced by chorthalidone or thiazids, Tripamide seemed to have no consistent adverse effects on plasma lipids.

INTRODUCTION

Hypertension is probably one of the most dreadful, but the most readily treatable risk factors for coronary heart disease either by dietary or by drug therapy.

In the past decade or two, antihypertensive agents such as diuretics have been increasingly used as a first-choice in controlling moderate to severe hypetension. Yet a number of large intervention trials have failed to show any substantial benefit of blood pressure-lowering on coronary heart disease mortality. This fact has raised the question of whether the anti-hypertensive diuretics commonly used may be offsetting the potential benefits of blood pressure reduction [1].

Some alterations of plasma lipids have been cited as probable causes.

The aim of the present study is to examine whether tripamide would impair the blood lipid levels during the course of the treatment of hypertensive patients.

METERIALS AND METHODS

Twenty mild hypertensive subjects with the age ranging from 32 to 73 years old were advised to take dietary instruction not to change any particular habits of foods to minimize the dietary effects on plasma lipids. Blood Pressure was measured every two weeks in the sitting position and fasting blood specimens were obtained every four weeks. Plasma total cholesterol, triglyceride and phospholipids were determined by the enzymatic method. Free fatty acids (FFA) were also measured by Duncombe's method. HDL-cholesterol was determined after the precipitation of the plasma by heparin-Ca and LDL-cholesterol was calculated by the equation of Friedewald.

RESULTS

The changes of total cholesterol, triglyceride and phospholipids were shown in Table 1 according to the length of the administration periods. Total cholesterol remained essentially unchanged during the both periods. Triglyceride tended to increase slightly but this change was not statistically significant. Phospholipids increased significantly in both experimental periods. Changes of HDL and LDL cholesterol were not significantly different. FFA levels were also shown in Table 1 which were again essentially the same before and during therapy. The percentage of beta, pre-beta, alpha lipoprotein remained unchanged during the therapy.

For the comparison of the effects by different diuretics, trichlormethiazide (4 mg/day) was administered to 17 mild hypertensive subjects for 2 months. Changes of plasma lipids are shown in Table 2, indicating the significant decrease in HDL-cholesterol after 2 month administration. Triglyceride tended to increase, but this change was not statistically significant.

In order to ascertain further the effect of these two agents, trichlormethiazide and tripamide were administered alternatively to the same subjects (Table 3). After 6 week administration of each drug, total cholesterol remained almost at the same level. Triglyceride, however, increased and HDL-cholesterol decreased on trichlormethiazide.

Fifty gram of glucose was ingested in each therapeutic period. Blood glucose curve appeared to be impaired and FFA tended to respond more sharply to the glucose in later part of the test on trichlormethiazide (Fig. 1).

Table 1. Effects of Tripamide on plasma lipoprotein lipids

	3 Month Administration		6 Month Administration	
	(1)	(2)	(1)	(2)
Total cholesterol	226.9±39.5	236.5±40.0	227.9±36.0	240.8±172.8
Triglyceride	157.0±71.7	182.3±82.1	172.7±83.0	196.7± 74.7
Phospholipid	215.5±26.1	225.9±36.3*	215.9±26.3	240.4± 39.9**
HDL-cholesterol	46.6±47.6	47.6±10.4	41.7± 7.3	39.6± 5.9
LDL-cholesterol (mg/dl)	148.9±33.5	152.4±28.9	151.7±30.1	161.9± 34.6
Free Fatty Acid (mEq/L)	0.41±0.31	0.31±0.21	0.33±0.19	0.33± 0.21
Beta lipoprotein	54.7± 9.6	51.2± 9.8	57.1±10.6	54.2± 11.4
Pre beta lipoprotein	29.6±13.7	33.7±13.8	28.8±14.6	32.8± 15.0
Alpha lipoprotein (%)	15.1± 6.6	15.1± 6.0	14.0± 5.5	13.9± 4.1

(1) : before therapy (2) : during therapy (mg/dl)
* $P < 0.05$ ** $P < 0.01$

Table II. Effects of Trichlormethiazide on plasma lipids (4 mg/day, N=17)

	before therapy	after 2 monthe administration
Total cholesterol (mg/dl)	238.6± 52.2	221.5± 54.4
Triglyceride (mg/dl)	135.0± 60.4	179.2±114.0
HDL-cholesterol (mg/dl)	53.4± 11.1	42.2± 13.0* ($P < 0.05$)
TC-(HDL-C) (mg/dl)	174.8± 49.4	167.5± 51.3

Table III. Plasma lipids of the same subject by different therapies

N.W. Female 61 years old

	Total cholesterol	Triglyceride	HDL-cholesterol
Off	268	145	38.2
Fluitran (4 mg/day)	260	186	34.6
Normonal (45 mg/day)	250	160	38.5

Fluitran : Trichlormethiazide (6 weeks) (mg/dl)
Normonal : Tripamide (6 weeks)

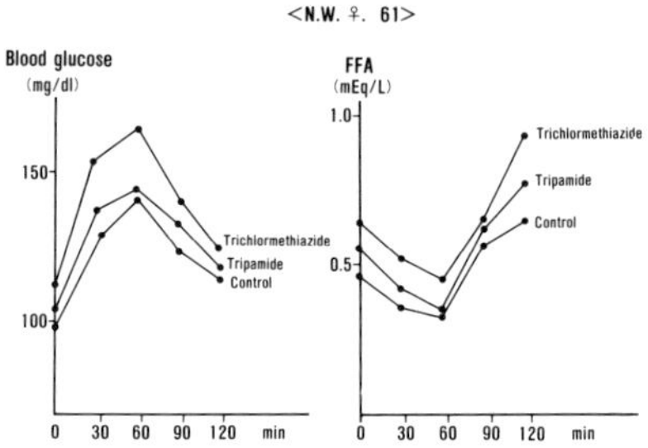

Fig. 1. Changes of blood glucose and free fatty acid on different therapies during 50g GTT.

DISCUSSION

Several studies have examined the effects of diuretics in the treatment of hypertension on the plasma lipids.

Hydrochlorothiazide and chlorthalidone were shown to increase plasma triglyceride. Chlorthalidone increased LDL cholesterol. These particular agents produced very little change in HDL-cholesterol levels [2]. However, various types of diuretics appear to differ significantly in this respect.

The present study revealed that tripamide did not change the distribution of cholesterol in various lipoproteins, compared with the results obtained by trichlormethiazide. Increase of phospholipid was noticed after the administration of tripamide, the significance of this change need to be evaluated by further experiment. High FFA level and increased glucose level on trihlormethiazide might imply that certain diuretic agent may increase plasma triglyceride and decrease HDL-cholesterol by altering the link of glucose and lipids.

In conclusion, tripamide that does not have an adverse effect on plasma lipids, may be a preferable choice for initial therapy in hypertension.

REFERENCES

1. R. Cutler, Am. J. Cardiol. 51, 628-631 (1983).
2. R.P. Ames, AM. J. Cardiol. 51, 632-638 (1983).

TRANSMEMBRANE POTASSIUM MOVEMENTS, DIURETIC DRUGS, AND THE ARACHIDONATE CASCADE: ICOSANOIDS AND K^+ TRANSPORT — AN IN VIVO MODEL

C. DEBY*, G. DEBY-DUPONT*, R. GARAY**, R.H. BOURGAIN***, F.V. DEFEUDIS**** AND P. BRAQUET****
*Lab. de Biochimie Appliquée, University of Liège, Sart-Tilman, 4000 Liège 1, Belgium; **INSERM U7, CNRS LA 318, Hôpital Necker, 161 rue de Sèvres, 75015 Paris, France; ***Laboratorium voor Fysiologie en Fysiopathologie, Free University of Brussels, Laarbeecklaan 103, 1090 Brussels, Belgium; ****Institut de Recherches Henri Beaufour, 17 Avenue Descartes, 92350 Le Plessis Robinson, France

INTRODUCTION

Certain diuretics, such as furosemide (1), bumetanide (2,3) and cicletanide, stimulate prostacyclin (PGI_2) synthesis *in vivo* and *in vitro* (4), and enhance the release of PGI_2 into plasma that is produced by intravascular injection of arachidonic acid (AA) in the rabbit (5). These drugs might act directly on cyclooxygenase, or they might alter the availability of AA, the precursor of prostanoids. This latter effect might involve either an increased phospholipase activity or a modification of cell membrane permeability, thus facilitating the penetration of AA into endothelial cells. The membrane-modifying properties of diuretics and the stimulation of PGI_2 release could be inter-related (4,5), and furosemide and bumetanide have been shown to inhibit Na^+, K^+, Cl^- co-transport in various *in vitro* systems (8-14). Also, it appears evident now that cicletanide stimulates a K^+ transport system (15).

The present report describes the *in vivo* and *in vitro* effects of ion transport modifiers, such as cicletanide, bumetanide, furosemide, verapamil, diethylmaleate (DEM), and N-ethylmaleimide (NEM), on the release of PGI_2 and thromboxane A_2 that is induced by exogenous AA.

MATERIALS AND METHODS

In vivo model

Anaesthetized male rabbits, 2.5 to 3.0 kg, with a low plasma haptoglobin level (40 mg/ml) were used (16,17). Arterial (carotid) and venous (right atrium) pressures and the ECG were recorded. In these animals, intravascular injections of AA produce arterial hypotension which is mediated by the conversion of AA to active derivatives such as PGI_2. Rabbits were sensitized in one hour to AA by heparinization, followed by i.v. administration of autologous hemolyzed blood (18). The AA_{50} (dose of i.v.-injected AA, which induces a 50% decrease in mean arterial blood pressure) decreased from about 400 µg/kg to about 60 µg/kg and even lower, and remained relatively constant for several hours. The following protocol was then applied: AA_{50} was determined; 12 minutes later, the first blood sample was taken, followed by injection of AA and by taking a second blood sample (2 minutes after AA injection). Prostanoid determinations for the first and second samples permitted calculation of the newly-formed prostanoids. The agent under investigation was then administered and, at different time intervals, the formation of AA metabolites was measured as described above. Modifications in AA_{50} produced by the drug were expressed as *sensitization coefficients*: the number by which the AA_{50} observed after the administration of a drug must be multiplied to obtain the initial AA_{50} value.

In vitro biosynthesis of PGs

Biosynthesis of PGs was studied in bull seminal vesicle microsomes, as

Published 1984 by Elsevier Science Publishing Co., Inc.
Diuretics, Jules B. Puschett, Editor

previously described (19).

Radioimmunoassays

Radioimmunoassays of samples of crude plasma were performed according to Granström and Kindahl (20).

Solubility of test substances

Furosemide (F), bumetanide (B) and verapamil (V) were readily soluble in aqueous solutions. Cicletanide (C), insoluble in water, was solubilized in dimethylsulfoxide (DMSO), and then the DMSO solution was mixed with saline or buffer to make an emulsion.

RESULTS AND DISCUSSION

F, B, V and C produced increases in the sensitization coefficient when administered in a single dose. F, V and B induced a rapid and transient (30 min) sensitization to AA in rabbits that were heparinized and injected with homologous blood. Cicletanide acted more slowly than the other drugs, but its action increased progressively for more than 2 hours; a potent sensitization was evident after 40 min. B was the weakest agent tested. The effects of all drugs on AA_{50}, and thus on the sensitization coefficient, were dose-dependent.

The enhancement of AA-induced hypotension by these four agents was well correlated with an increased release of 6-oxo-$PGF_{1}\alpha$, corresponding to a stimulation of PGI_2 synthesis. V released the greatest amounts of PGI_2 during the 30 minutes following drug injection; the same phenomenon, though less pronounced, was observed with F and B. On the contrary, C administration initiated a progressive enhancement of 6-oxo-$PGF_{1}\alpha$ release which was maintained for more than 2 hours.

A significant dose/effect relationship was produced by NEM, which sensitized rabbits to the hypotensive effects of AA at doses of 10^{-6} and 10^{-5} mole/kg. However, the decrease in AA_{50} was of short duration, the sensitization coefficient returning to unity after 50 minutes. The other thiol-blocker, DEM, used in the same dose range, was more effective than NEM in sensitizing rabbits to AA-induced hypotension.

As shown in Table I, major disparities existed among the *in vitro* actions of the agents tested. B had slight stimulant activity at high molarity. F and V were not significantly active. In the case of C, which is not water soluble, the experiments were more difficult to perform, since this drug had to be solubilized in DMSO which, itself, is a cyclooxygenase activator (Table I). After correction for the cyclooxygenase-activating activity of DMSO, C appeared to be an effective cyclooxygenase inhibitor, with an $IC_{50} = 2.10^{-5}M$ (Table I).

An enhancement of prostanoid production by various agents has been demonstrated in a rabbit model. Diuretics such as F, B and C, a Ca^{2+}-channel blocker such as V, and thiol-blockers such as NEM and DEM, all acted on the cell membrane, possibly through ion displacement effects. A major discrepancy is evident when the *in vivo* and *in vitro* effects of the diuretics are compared. On the one hand, all of the drugs tested increased *in vivo* PGI_2 production (results shown herein) and PGI_2 synthesis by cultured smooth muscle cells (4). On the other hand, while B, F and V are weak or inefficient stimulators of *in vitro* cyclooxygenase activity, cicletanide appears to be an efficient inhibitor of this enzyme. These observations imply that these

TABLE I. Effects of several ion transport modifiers on *in vitro* cyclooxygenase activity, measured as percentage of control activity

Drug	Molarity of drug			
	10^{-6}	10^{-5}	10^{-4}	10^{-3}
	Effects of hydrosoluble drugs on cyclooxygenase activity			
Furosemide	97.5% ± 11*	104% ± 8**	113% ± 11*	124% ± 8**
Bumetanide	98 % ± 7*	100% ± 10**	106% ± 12*	127% ± 9**
Verapamil	97 % ± 6**	98% ± 7**	96% ± 8**	93% ± 9**
	Effects of DMSO and of a DMSO-soluble drug (cicletanide)			
	Molarity of drug			
	5.10^{-4}	5.10^{-3}	5.10^{-2}	5.10^{-1}
DMSO	114% ± 10**	150% ± 12**	201% ± 22**	249% ± 32*
	Molarity of drug			
DMSO	5.10^{-4}	5.10^{-3}	5.10^{-2}	5.10^{-1}
+ Cicletanide	10^{-6}	10^{-5}	10^{-4}	10^{-3}
A	96% ± 8**	67% ± 9*	18.3% ± 2.5	9.1% ± 0.7**
B	110% ± 9**	100% ± 13*	36.9% ± 5	22.4% ± 1.8**

*p < 0.05; **p < 0.01; A: in % of DMSO control; B: in % of control in absence of DMSO.

drugs (particularly cicletanide) enhance PGI_2 production indirectly *in vivo* and in cultured cells. Therefore, no correlations exist between the direct action of the drugs studied on cyclooxygenase activity and on *in vivo* PGI_2 synthesis. These compounds seem to control other phenomena, such as ion transport and membrane potential, by modifying the influx of AA into cells.

REFERENCES

1. J.G. Gerber, Fed. Proc. 42, 1707 (1983).
2. U.B. Olsen, Acta Pharmacol. Toxicol. 37, 65 (1975).
3. J. Kaufman, R. Hamburger, J. Matheson and W. Flamenbaum, J. Clin. Pharmacol. 21, 11 (1981).
4. P. Braquet, B. Dorian, J. Larrue, C. Deby, H. Salari, R. Bourgain and P. Borgeat, Biochem. Pharmacol. (submitted) (1984).
5. P. Braquet, J. Larrue, B. Dorian, C. Deby, G. Deby-Dupont, J. Maclouf, P. Sirois and P. Borgeat, Rev. Portug. Bioqui. Aplic. 5, 161 (1982).
6. P.C. Weber, B. Scherer and C. Larsson, Eur. J. Pharmacol. 41, 329 (1977).
7. J.G. Gerber and A.S. Nies, Adv. Prostaglandin Thromboxane Res. 7, 1079 (1980).
8. M. Tuck, R.P. Garay, F. Russo-Marie and P. Meyer, Amer. Fed. Clin. Res. Meeting, Washington (USA) (1982).
9. P. Geck, C. Pietrzyk, B.C. Burckhardt, B. Pfeiffer and E. Heinz, Biochim. Biophys. Acta, 600, 432 (1980).
10. R.P. Garay, N. Adragna, M. Canessa and D.C. Tosteson, J. Membr. Biol. 62, 169 (1981).
11. M. De Mendoça, A. Knorr, M.L. Grichois, D. Ben-Ishay, R.P. Garay and P. Meyer, Kidney Int. 21 (suppl. 11), S69 (1982).
12. M.B. Burg, Kidney Int. 22, 454 (1982).
13. H.C. Palfrey, P. Feit and P. Greengard, Amer. J. Physiol. 238, C139 (1980).

14. R.P. Garay, C. Nazaret and J. Diez, Biochem. Pharmacol. (submitted) (1984).
15. P.K. Lauf, J. Comp. Physiol. 146, 9 (1982).
16. C. Deby, P. Van Caneghem and Z.M. Bacq, Biochem. Pharmacol. 27, 613 (1978).
17. S.A. Saaed, W.S. Mc Donald-Gibson, J. Cuthbert, J.L. Copas, C. Schneider, P.J. Gardiner, N.M. Buut and H.O.J. Collier, Nature 270, 32 (1977).
18. C. Deby, Biochem. Pharmacol. 30, 2243 (1981).
19. C. Deby, M. Descamps, F. Binon and Z.M. Bacq, Biochem. Pharmacol. 24, 1089 (1975).
20. E. Granström and H. Kindahl, Adv. Prostaglandin and Thromboxane Research, vol. 5, ed. by J.C. Frölich, Raven Press, New York, p.119 (1978).

STIMULATION OF K FLUXES BY NATRIURETIC FUROPYRIDINES IN HUMAN ERYTHROCYTES

PIERRE BRAQUET AND RICARDO GARAY
I.H.B.17,av.Descartes,Le Plessis-Robinson and INSERM U7/CNRS LA 318. Hôpital Necker. Paris 75015 . France.

ABSTRACT

Two different families of diuretic drugs: (i) (Aryloxy)acetic acid diuretics: ethacrynic acid, tienilic acid and (-)indacrinone and (ii) natriuretic furopyridines: cicletanide and BN 50157 stimulate K movements across human red cell membranes. The kinetic properties of this effect (K-specificity saturability,optical isomerism,antagonism by structural analogues,etc...) strongly suggest that it is mediated by a K transport system with a specific binding site for some diuretic drugs. The stimulated K fluxes are resistant to ouabain,bumetanide and quinine,thus suggesting that they are not mediated by the Na,K-pump,Na,K-cotransport system or by the Ca-dependent,K-permeability ("Gardos effect").

The study of structural analogues showed that the intensity of stimulation of K fluxes is strongly correlated with the magnitude of the natriuretic effect.

INTRODUCTION

Several observations suggest that diuretic drugs may decrease renal Na reabsorption by a direct inhibition of a Na transport carrier in different segments of the nephron(Fig.1 and ref.1). The injection of ouabain directly into the renal artery inhibits basolateral Na reabsorption which is catalyzed by the Na,K-pump,inducing a profound natriuresis. Furosemide and bumetanide provoke natriuresis by inhibition of another Na transport carrier: the

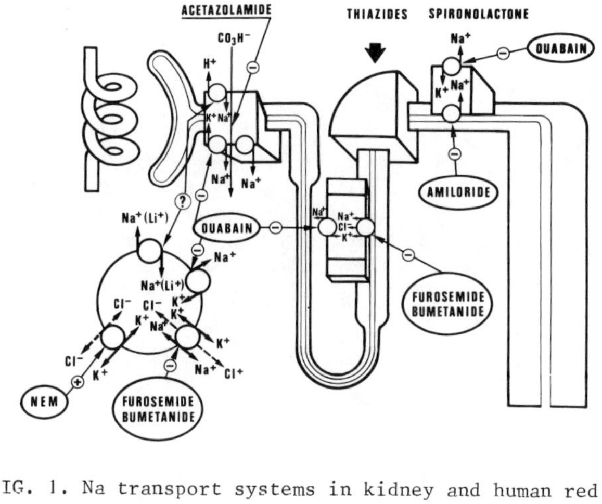

FIG. 1. Na transport systems in kidney and human red cells.

Diuretics, Jules B. Puschett, Editor

Na,K,Cl-cotransport system which is located in the luminal side of Henle's loop cells. Amiloride inhibits a Na carrier located apically in distal tubular cells. Spironolactone antagonizes the aldosterone-induced synthesis of a Na transport protein in distal and collecting tubules. Acetazolamide abolishes proximal tubular acidification thus inhibiting the net reabsorption of $NaHCO_3$. The mechanism of action of thiazide drugs is unclear.

In contrast to the mode of inhibition by the drugs mentioned above, tienilic acid, an (aryloxy)acetic acid diuretic, modifies K rather than Na fluxes in human red cells (2). This effect did not stem from the Na,K-pump, Na,K cotransport system or from a "Gardos effect" (Ca-dependent,K-permeability). A similar stimulation could not be obtained with hydrochlorotiazide, amiloride or furosemide. We report here that a new family of diuretic drugs: natriuretic furopyridines are also able to stimulate K fluxes in human red cells. This effect appears to be correlated with the natriuretic activity of these compounds.

METHODS

K fluxes were measured in fresh human red cells following a previously published method (1,2). Briefly, fresh cells were washed with cold isosmotic $MgCl_2$ and resuspended in Mg,sucrose medium containing ouabain and bumetanide External K concentrations were measured at 0 time and after 0.5 and 1h incubation at 37°C. K efflux was obtained by the difference in K concentration divided by the final hematocrit and the incubation time.

RESULTS

Table 1 shows that <u>(aryloxy)acetic acid diuretics</u>: ethacrynic acid, tienilic acid and (-) indacrinone and <u>natriuretic furopyridines</u> (see chemical structures in ref.1): cicletanide and BN 50157 are able to stimulate K movements across red cell membranes.

TABLE I. The effect of diuretic drugs on K fluxes in human red cells

Compound	concentration (mM)	ouabain and bumetanide-resistant K efflux. (μmol(l.cells x h)$^{-1}$)
Ethacrynic acid	0.4	3590±500 (5)
Tienilic acid	1.0	1445±110 (5)
(-) Indacrinone	0.7	1820±100 (4)
(+) Indacrinone	0.7	1010± 65 (4)
Cicletanide	0.85	1215± 85 (4)
BN 50157	0.6	5070±560 (5)
Control	-	895± 80 (7)

Values are given as mean±SD. The number of experiments is indicated in brackets.

The indacrinone molecule contains one assymetric carbon. The (-) enantiomer shows a much more pronounced diuretic effect than the (+) enantiomer. Interestingly, (-) indacrinone stimulates more markedly K fluxes than (+) indacrinone (see Table I).

Among the studied diuretics, a furopyridine: BN 50157 is the most potent activator of erythrocyte K fluxes that we have found (Table 1). The effect of this drug may be competitively antagonized by some other furopyridines. This result further suggests that the stimulated K fluxes are catalyzed by a K transport system with a specific binding site for some diuretic drugs.

Fig.2 shows that, for all tested furopyridines (see chemical structures in ref.1), the natriuretic activity is positively correlated with the stimulation of erythrocyte K fluxes.

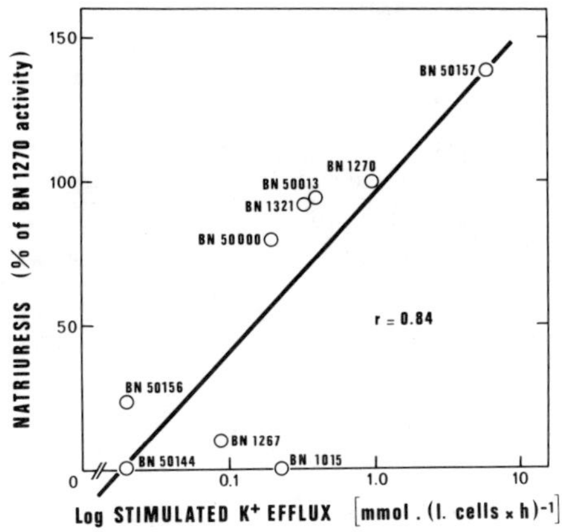

FIG. 2. Correlation between natriuretic activity and stimulation of erythrocyte K fluxes for natriuretic furopyridines.

DISCUSSION

The main result of this paper is that (Aryloxy)acetic acid diuretics and natriuretic furopyridines are able to stimulate K movements across human red cell membranes. The magnitude of this effect correlates with the intensity of the natriuretic effect.

The kinetic properties of the diuretic-stimulated,K-flux suggest that it is catalyzed by a specific K carrier (different from the Na,K-pump and Na,K cotransport system) with one or more receptor sites for the above molecules. In several kinds of cells, such as vascular smooth muscle cells,noradrenergic neurons and kidney cells, membrane potential is strongly dependent on K permeability. On the other hand, a change in membrane potential in different target cells modulates the secretion of natriuretic agents such as prostacyclin(3). This possible mechanism of action of furopyridine diuretics deserves further investigation.

REFERENCES

1. R.Garay,C.Nazaret,J.Diez et al. Biochim.Pharmacol. (in press).
2. D.Cusi and R.Garay. Mol.Pharmacol. 19, 438 (1981)
3. P.Braquet,C.Deby,R.Garay et.al. The Lancet i, 1218 (1983).

INSTANTANEOUS CLEARANCE: A NEW TOOL FOR THE CLINICAL PHARMACOLOGY OF DIURETICS

A. J. REYES,* AND W. P. LEARY**
*Departamento de Investigación Cardiovascular, Fundación Procardias, Montevideo, Uruguay; **Department of Clinical Pharmacology, University of Natal, Durban, South Africa

ABSTRACT

Instantaneous renal clearance is defined as the ratio between the urinary flow of any substance and its plasma concentration at any definite time. A mathematical model is presented that satisfactorily accounts for the continuous flow of any natural or artificial urinary solute, after the administration of placebo or any diuretic formulation to normal or diseased subjects, when urine is collected at various time intervals after dosing. The use of this model permits to evaluate the instantaneous renal clearance of the solutes studied.

INTRODUCTION

The current definition of renal clearance, CL, involves three variables that are functions of time

$$CL = U\dot{V}P^{-1}, \quad (1)$$

where U and P are the urinary and plasma concentrations of the considered substance and $\dot{V}$ is mean urine flow. P is measured in a blood sample and may be considered punctual in time, whereas U and $\dot{V}$ are derived from a urine sample produced during a certain time. Thus, (1) relates variables that have different time-dependencies. This fact may lead to erroneous inferences, especially when the effect of a diuretic causes rapid changes in U and $\dot{V}$.

The objective of this uptake is to present a new definition of CL, considering it a continuous function of time.

RATIONALE AND DEFINITION OF INSTANTANEOUS RENAL CLEARANCE

Let M be the mass of any urinary solute considered.

$$U = MV^{-1}, \quad (2)$$

where V is urine volume. Since $\dot{V} = Vt^{-1}$, where t is time, the product UV in (1) becomes

$$U\dot{V} = MV^{-1}Vt^{-1} = Mt^{-1} = \dot{M}, \quad (3)$$

where $\dot{M}$ is the mean urinary flow of the studied solute. From (3) and (1)

$$CL = \dot{M}P^{-1}. \quad (4)$$

Given that (4) is an alternative expression for (1) and that the instantaneous flow of any solute in urine may be defined as the first derivative of its mass with respect to time

Diuretics, Jules B. Puschett, Editor

$$CL_t = dM(dt)^{-1}P^{-1}, \tag{5}$$

where CL_t is instantaneous renal clearance, i.e., a continuous function of time derived from simultaneous events in urine and plasma.

The continuous measurement of a urinary solute flow would entail the continuous monitoring of urine flow and of the urinary concentration of the solute. However, ongoing research in the clinical pharmacology of diuretics uses an experimental design whereby, after voiding urine and single dosing with placebo or a diuretic formulation, urine is collected at definite times with the purpose of evaluating the time-courses of various renal excretions, in normal or diseased subjects.

A mathematical model has been described [1] that accounts for the amount of urine or of any substance in urine, M, accumulated as a continuous function of time (FIG. 1)

$$20M\,[\log(100-M)]^{-1} = \exp[2,3(t-t_1)(a+bt)^{-1}], \tag{6}$$

where $t_1 = t$ for $M = 0,1$, in the units used in calculations, and a (time) and b (dimensionless) are other parameters. With the object of evaluating the correlation coefficient and the a and b values through regression, the function (6) is thus linearised

$$(t-t_1)[\log 20\,M-\log\log(100-M)]^{-1} = a+bt. \tag{7}$$

For carrying out calculations, whenever necessary the experimental data should be multiplied by a possitive or negative power of 10, so as to allow the double logarithmation of 100-M.

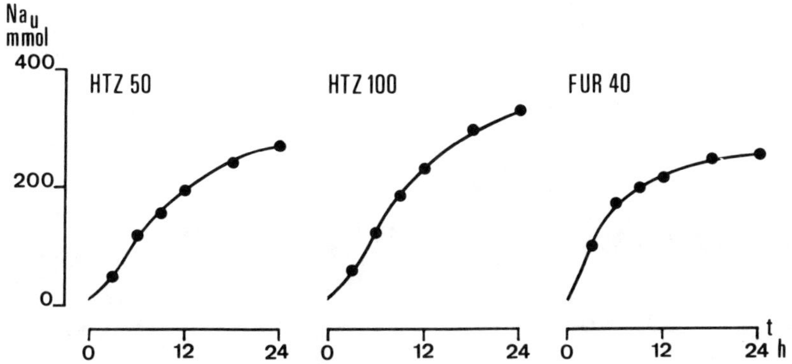

FIG. 1. Accumulated excretions of sodium in urine (Na_U) after the administration of hydrochlorothiazide 50 mg (HTZ 50), hydrochlorothiazide 100 mg (HTZ 100) or furosemide 40 mg (FUR 40) to eight normal volunteers at hour (h) 0. The mathematical model accounting for the function M(t), presented in equation (6), fitted the results satisfactorily ($r > 0,999$, $P < 0,001$ in all cases).

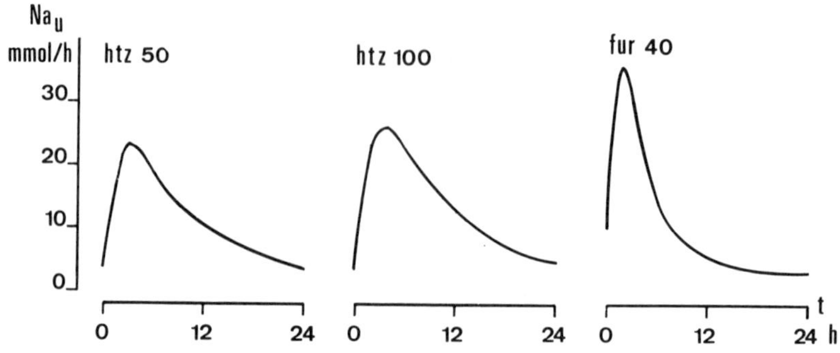

FIG. 2. Urinary sodium flows derived from the experimental accumulated excretions depicted in FIG. 1, as continuous functions of time, after single administration of various diuretic formulations to eight healthy volunteers at hour 0. Abbreviations are similar to those in FIG. 1.

Before proceeding to the statistical techniques, it is also necessary to evaluate t_1, which can be done with sufficient accuracy by linear extrapolation from 0 to the first experimental point.

After having evaluated a and b, the renal excretory flow as a function of time (FIG. 2) is thus derived

$$dM(dt)^{-1} = (a+bt)/(a+bt)^2[\![0.43^{-1}+0.43[(100-M)\log(100-M)]^{-1}]\!].(8)$$

Any $dM(dt)^{-1}$ value yields CL_t when multiplied by the P^{-1} value coinciding in time.

From (8), the time to maximal excretion after dosing can be assessed as the time at which $d^2M(dt)^{-2} = 0$.

APPLICATION AND DISCUSSION

The mathematical model for the flows of urine and urinary solutes fits the individual and the mean data on 10 natural urinary solutes, obtained by the authors in experiments comprising the administration of placebo and of 19 diuretic formulations to normal subjects. The model also holds for the data from all the pertinent literature indexed in Current Contents/ Life Sciences during 1981-3, including natural solutes, diuretics and their metabolites in urine. The r values were higher than 0,995 in all cases. The derived CL_t values sometimes differed significantly from their classical CL counterparts.

REFERENCE

1. A.J. Reyes, and W.P. Leary, Curr. Ther. Res. 30, 227-235 (1981).

EFFECTS OF DIFFERENT HIGH CEILING DIURETICS ON HUMAN ERYTHROCYTE NA^+, K^+, 2 CL^--COTRANSPORT.

BERNWARD GARTHOFF*, ANDREAS KNORR*, AXEL INGENDOH**, AND M.DE MENDONCA***
*Institute of Pharmacology and **Chemical Research Labs. Bayer AG. P.O.Box 101709, D 5600 Wuppertal 1, FRG; *** Hopital Necker, INSERM U 7, Paris, France

INTRODUCTION

The diuretic activity of high ceiling diuretics is thought to be characterized by their ability to inhibit the Na^+, K^+, 2 Cl^--cotransport system of the cell (1). The inhibitory activity of furosemide- and ethacrynic acid-analogs in red blood cells has been shown to correlate well with the natriuretic activity of these substances in man (2,3,4).

To clarify, whether the ability of a new diuretic substance to inhibit Na^+, K^+, 2 Cl^--cotransport in human erythrocytes is of additional value to predict relative potencies in humans, high ceiling diuretics of different structures were tested in this system. For comparison, their relative natriuretic potency was determined in a standard screening test in rats.

METHODS

Measurement of Red Cell Na^+-Transport

Na^+-transport was measured in human red cells which were previously loaded with Na^+ and depleted of K^+ by use of 0.02 mM PCMBS according to Garay and Dagher (5). Na^+ efflux from red cells was measured in a Na^+-free medium containing $MgCl_2$ (75 mM), sucrose (85 mM), MOPS-Tris (10 mM, pH 7.2 at 37° C), glucose (5 mM), and oubain (0.1 mM) at a hematocrit of 1.5%. Na^+-concentrations in the cells or in the supernatant were measured by flame photometry. Na^+-efflux rates were calculated by analysis of regression. Hematocrit and hemoglobin concentrations were determined in each sample and Na^+-efflux rates were related to cell volume.

Determination of Natriuretic Activity in Rats

Male Wistar rats were loaded with 10 ml/kg of tylose suspension, placed into metabolic cages and urinary Na^+-excretion was determined by flame photometry in the urine collected during 6 h. Diuretics were administered with the tylose suspension by gavage in a standard dose of 50 mg/kg.

RESULTS

Incubation of red blood cells with the diuretic substances expected from rat screening results to exert high ceiling activity resulted in half-maximal cotransport inhibitory concentrations (IC_{50}) of zero up to 2.1 µmol/l (see Tab. 1). Apparently, sulfamoyl diuretics furosemide, piretanide and bumetanide inhibited ouabain-insensitive Na^+-extrusion from human red blood cells within an acceptable concentration range, whereas the remaining agents were only of minor or of no efficacy in this system per se. Rat screening results did not correlate with IC_{50} values in human red blood cells; also the rank of efficacy of sulfamoyl diuretics was different in vivo (Pir > Fur > Bum) and in vitro (Bum > Pir > Fur).

Published 1984 by Elsevier Science Publishing Co., Inc.
Diuretics, Jules B. Puschett, Editor

TABLE I. Effect of high ceiling diuretics on ouabain-insensitive Na^+-extrusion from Na^+-loaded human red blood cells and on natriuresis in rats.

substance	cotransport inhibition IC_{50} (µmol/l)	natriuresis [a)] (mmol Na^+/kg/6 h)
muzolimine	984.0 (690.3 - 1714.9)	5.20 ± 0.29
furosemide	77.9 (56.8 - 102.1)	6.37 ± 0.31
piretanide	3.8 (1.4 - 7.4)	6.61 ± 0.19
bumetanide	2.1 (1.2 - 3.2	4.68 ± 0.20
indacrinone	530.8 (371.1 - 899.0)	2.13 ± 0.21
MK 447	Ø	10.27 ± 0.70
tizolemide	Ø	5.14 ± 0.41
7-chloro-1-propionyl-1,2,3,4.tetrahydroquinoline-4-one-oxime	606.4 (386.7 - 836.9)	10.16 ± 0.31

SUMMARY

Inhibition of cotransport in human red blood cells reflects the rank of efficacy of furosemide analogs in humans better than do rat screening results, as has previously been noted (4). However, high ceiling diuretics as effective as furosemide in rat and man, but having different structures and, therefore, probably acting by different mechanisms, cannot be determined using this system. On the other hand, such compounds might also become active in the cotransport system as metabolites or in the presence of cysteine (4).

REFERENCES

1. E.Schlatter, R.Greger, and C.Weidtke, Pflügers Arch. 396, 210-217 (1983).
2. B.A.Brooks, and A.F.Lant, Clin. Sci. Mol. Med. 54, 679-683 (1978).
3. H.C.Palfrey, P.W.Feit, and P.Greengard, Am. J. Physiol. 238 (Cell Physiol. 7), C 139-C 148 (1980).
4. J.C.Ellorey, and G.W.Stewart, Br. J. Pharmac. 75, 183-188 (1982).
5. R.P.Garay, and G.Dagher, Can. J. Biochem. 58, 1069-1074 (1980).

PHARMACODYNAMICS OF ACIDIC AND BASIC TRIAMTERENE ANALOGUES

HELMUT PRIEWER*, HEINRICH KNAUF** AND ERNST MUTSCHLER*
*Pharmacological Institute, University of Frankfurt, Frankfurt/West Germany, **Department of Internal Medicine, University of Freiburg, Freiburg/West Germany

INTRODUCTION

Due to its poor solubility in water it is difficult to prepare solutions of the potassium retaining diuretic triamterene for parenteral application. In previous investigations it was found by our group [1], that the phase-II-metabolite of triamterene, the p-hydroxy-triamterene sulfuric acid ester, has still a diuretic activity. We anticipated that other derivatives of 4-hydroxy-triamterene are effective as well. By introducing additional acidic or basic groups into such derivatives it should be possible to obtain better water soluble potassium retaining diuretics. Therefore, compounds of the following structure were synthesized [2,3]:

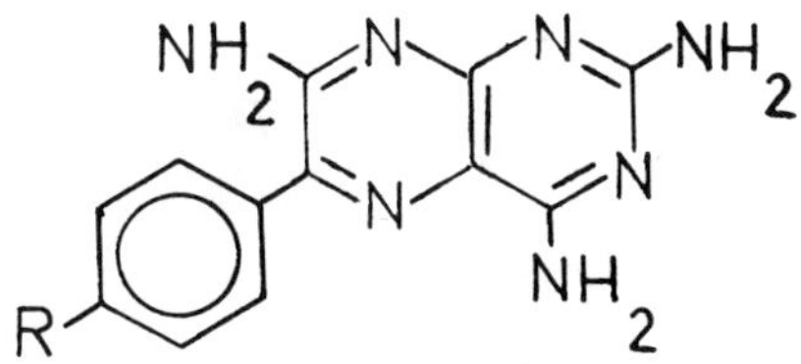

R = H TRIAMTERENE Tri

1. ACIDS

$R = O-(CH_2)_n-COOH$

n = 3	A3
n = 4	A4
n = 5	A5

2. BASES

$R = O-(CH_2)_n-N(CH_3)_2$

n = 2	B2
n = 3	B3

3. HYDROXY-BASES

$R = O-CH_2-CH(OH)-CH_2-N(R^1)_2$

$R^1 = CH_3$	H1
$R^1 = C_2H_5$	H2

METHODS

Male Wistar rats with a body weight of about 130 g were deprived of food for 18 hours. They received 2o ml/kg saline orally immediately before intravenous application of the compound to be tested. The i.v.-application was performed under light ether anaesthesia. Mostly, 6 animals per dose were used in a randomised fashion.

Urine samples were collected over a period of 150 min. Urine volume was measured and the concentrations of sodium, potassium, calcium and magnesium in urine were determined by flame photometry or atomic absorption spectrophotometry using a Zeiss apparatus FL 6.

Dose response curves were calculated by nonlinear regression analysis using the NONLIN computer program [4].

Diuretics, Jules B. Puschett, Editor

RESULTS

1. Acids

The natriuretic and potassium retaining effect of several acidic triamterene derivatives is illustrated in fig. 1. The most active compound is the carboxy-butoxy-triamterene (A4) which has a pronounced natriuretic activity whereas the antikaliuretic effect is reduced compared to triamterene.

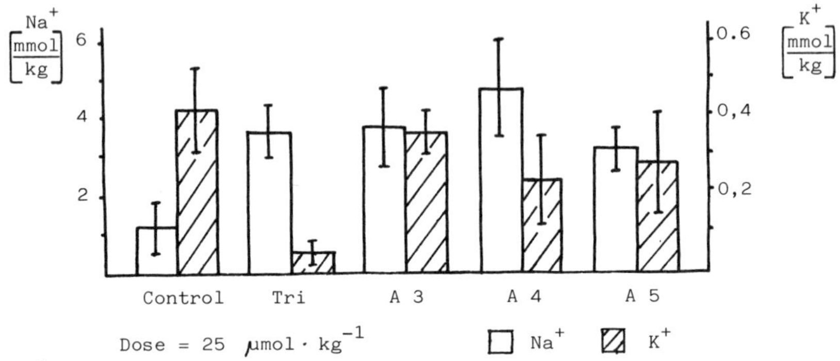

Fig. 1

2. Bases

The antikaliuretic potency of the basic compounds with two or three methylene groups in the side chain was not significantly different, but it is higher than that of triamterene. On the other hand there are nearly no differences in the natriuretic potencies of triamterene and the basic derivatives.

3. Hydroxy-bases

A further increase in potency was reached by introducing a hydroxyl group in the side chain of the bases. As far as the potassium-sparing effect is concerned these substances are effective at doses about ten times lower than triamterene (fig. 2).

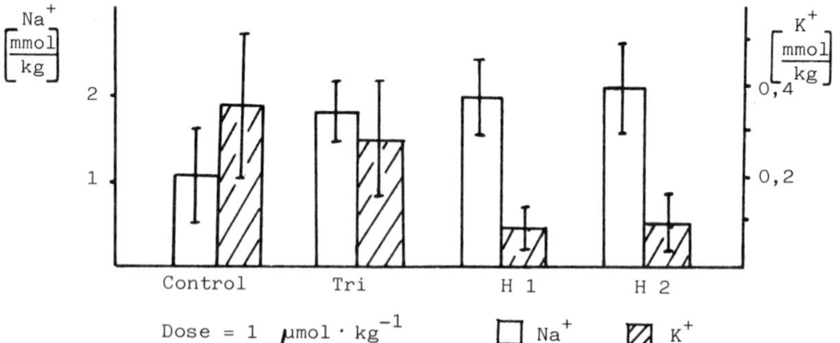

Fig. 2

4. Dose response curves

Tab. 1 shows the ED_{50} values of triamterene and the most promising acidic and basic derivatives.

COMPOUND	Na^+ (μmol kg^{-1})	K^+ (μmol kg^{-1})
CARBOXY-BUTOXY-TRIAMTERENE (A4)	5,86	20,63
TRIAMTERENE (Tri)	4,40	1,87
DIMETHYLAMINO-PROPOXY-TRIAMTERENE (B3)	5,53	0,54
(3-DIMETHYLAMINO-2-HYDROXY)-PROPOXY-TRIAMTERENE (H1)	9,36	0,24

Tab.1

DISCUSSION

The data clearly indicate that all the triamterene derivatives tested exhibit practically equal natriuretic potency, however, they differ significantly with respect to their potassium retaining effect. Whereas all acidic compounds are only weak antikaliuretics, the basic derivatives exhibit a much stronger potassium retaining potency. From these results we conclude that the charge of the side chain of the triamterene derivatives determines its K^+-retaining potency, the cationic compounds being the most effective antikaliuretics. Therefore, it can be postulated that the functional coupling of K^+ with Na^+ is obviously not a rigid one. A similar dissociation of the antikaliuretic from the natriuretic effect of triamterene has earlier been observed by Guignard [5].

SUMMARY

The acidic or basic derivatives of hydroxy-triamterene have natriuretic and antikaliuretic properties.In contrast to the natriuretic potency, which is nearly the same in all these groups of triamterene derivatives, there are great differences between the antikaliuretic potencies of the acids, bases and hydroxybases. Whereas the acidic derivatives have only a weak potassium retaining potency, the bases reduce the potassium excretion at a much lower dose. The potassium retaining effect is further enhanced by introducing a OH-group into the side chain of the bases.

REFERENCES

1. Knauf, H., Mutschler, E., Völger, K.-D., Wais, U., Arzneim.-Forsch./Drug Res. 28 (II), 1417-1420 (1978)
2. Vollmer, G., dissertation (Dep. of Pharmacol., Univ. Frankfurt) 1980
3. Wolf, E., dissertation (Dep. of Pharmacol., Univ. Frankfurt) 1981
4. Daniel, C., Wood, F.S., "Fitting Equations to Data" John Wiley & Sons, New York (1980)
5. Guignard, J.P., Peters, G., Europ. J. Pharmacol. 10 (2), 255-267 (1970)

PHARMACODYNAMICS AND KINETICS OF XIPAMIDE IN PATIENTS WITH KIDNEY AND LIVER DISEASE

HEINRICH KNAUF[*], HILDEGARD SPAHN[**] AND ERNST MUTSCHLER
[*]Department of Medicine, University of Freiburg, D-7800 Freiburg,
[**]Institute of Pharmacology, University of Frankfurt,
D-6000 Frankfurt/Main, W.-Germany

INTRODUCTION

Xipamide is a sulfonamide-type diuretic [1] which resembles closely to loop diuretics. Xipamide lacks the second sulfonamide group, which is typical for the benzothiadiazines. A criterion for the classification of xipamide is its pattern of electrolyte excretion, which reflects its site of action within the nephron.

METHODS

The studies were carried out on 21 informed healthy volunteers and patients, whose creatinine clearance ranged from 135 to 5 ml/min. Furthermore, 6 patients with hepatic cirrhosis with ascites were studied. The analyses of xipamide in serum, urine and ascites were performed using a densitometric method [2] .

RESULTS

Pharmacodynamics in Healthy Volunteers

A single oral dose of 40 mg xipamide (1 tablet Aquaphor[R]) causes a marked excretion of Na^+ and Cl^-, associated with a moderate kaliuresis [Fig. 1]. The excretion of Ca^{++} and Mg^{++} is also enhanced by the diuretic, the calciuresis being proportional to the natriuresis. This pattern agrees with that obtained by furosemide.

Saluretic Effects of Xipamide in Chronic Renal Failure

The xipamide-induced excretion of electrolytes is decreased according to the reduction of the creatinine clearance.
However, similar to furosemide, its saluretic efficacy is maintained down to end-stage renal failure. Thiazides are usually ineffective saluretics at a creatinine clearance $<$ 25 ml/min.

Efficacy of Xipamide in Patients with Hepatic Cirrhosis and Ascites

In most patients with ascites xipamide (40 mg) was able to reduce the intraabdominal fluid. In those patients in which xipamide was ineffective, other potent diuretics were no more effective either.

Pharmacokinetics

In healthy volunteers

Xipamide displays a high bioavailability, 73 % on average. About 40 % of xipamide are recovered as native drug in the urine, independent of the route of administration. The plasma level time curves could be described by a two compartment open model. C_{max} was determined to be 4.6 $\pm$ 1.3

Published 1984 by Elsevier Science Publishing Co., Inc.
Diuretics, Jules B. Puschett, Editor

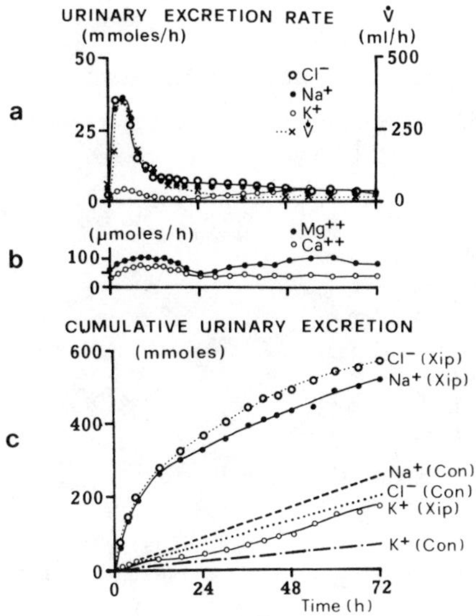

FIG. 1. Excretion rate of Cl^-, Na^+ and K^+ and urine flow (= $\dot{V}$) (a), excretion rate of Ca^{2+} and Mg^{2+} (b) and cumulative urinary excretion of electrolytes in comparison with the control period (c) induced by 40 mg xipamide.

μg/ml, $t_{1/2\beta}$ to be 7.0 ± 1.0 h ($\bar{x}$ ± SD), the renal clearance of the parent drug was 12 ± 2 ml/min [3].

In chronic renal failure

The elimination rate constant k of xipamide depends upon kidney function. However, in end-stage renal failure, the elimination half-life is only increased from 7 to 9 h. Thus, even in terminal renal failure, accumulation of native xipamide is moderate. This is explained by the elimination characteristics of the drug. The total plasma clearance as well as the renal clearance depend on the creatinine clearance [Fig. 2].

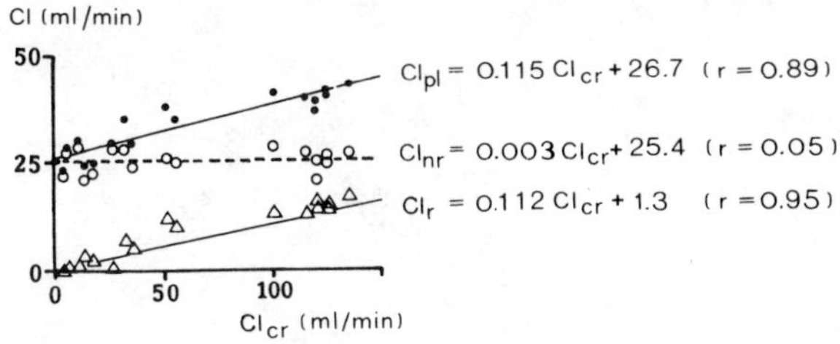

FIG. 2. Correlation between xipamide clearance Cl [total plasma clearance (•), nonrenal clearance (o) and renal clearance (Δ)] and creatinine clearance Cl_{cr}.

The nonrenal clearance is independent of kidney function and suffices to prevent clinically relevant accumulation of the parent drug in renal failure.

In patients with hepatic cirrhosis and ascites

In these patients C_{max} in plasma ranged from 4.6 - 10.1 µg/ml and $t_{1/2ß}$ was 7.1 ± 1.8 h. Xipamide enters the ascites, maximal concentrations ranging from 0.3 - 2.2 µg/ml [Fig. 3].

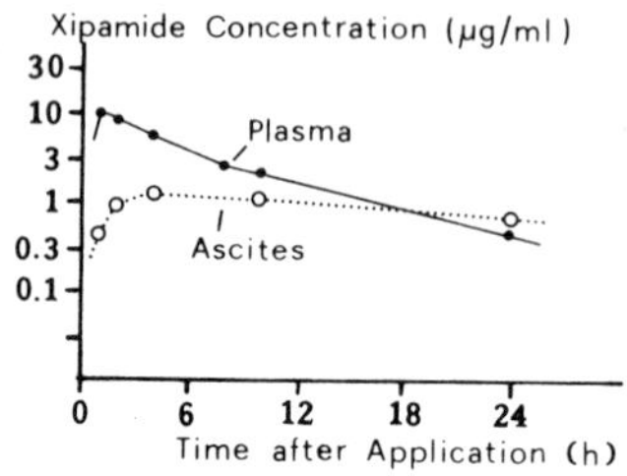

FIG. 3. Concentration time curve of xipamide in plasma and ascites of a patient following a single oral dose of 40 mg xipamide.

CONCLUSION

Xipamide is a long acting diuretic with pharmacodynamic characteristics similar to loop diuretics. It is effective and safe in chronic renal failure and hepatic cirrhosis with ascites. In these groups of patients the pharmacokinetic properties were not altered to a clinically relevant extent. The profile of action recommends the drug for long-term treatment.

SUMMARY

Xipamide closely resembles furosemide with respect to its saluretic properties. Its efficacy is also maintained down to end-stage renal failure and in patients with hepatic cirrhosis with ascites. In contrast to furosemide the duration of action of xipamide is almost 24 h, plasma half-life being 7 h in healthy volunteers and only 9 h in end-stage renal failure. Although xipamide enters the ascites, the plasma levels are not significantly altered.

REFERENCES

1. Liebenow, W., Leuschner, F., Drug Res. 25, 240-244 (1975)
2. Sobel, M., Mutschler, E., J. Chrom. Biomed. Appl., 183, 124-130 (1980)
3. Hempelmann, F.W., Dieker, P., Drug Res. 27, 2143-2151 (1977)

PHARMACODYNAMICS AND PHARMACOKINETICS OF A FUROSEMIDE-RETARD/ TRIAMTERENE COMBINATION

LOEW, D.*, E.H. GRAUL*, O. SCHUSTER*, E. MUTSCHLER**, M. SCHÄFER-KORTING**, P. SCHMIDT***

*Medicef-Institute, Intern. Center for Medical Environmental Sciences and Future Research, 3550 Marburg, Körnerstr. 36 W.-Germany; **Pharmacological Institute, University Frankfurt/ Main, W.-Germany; ***Department of Internal Medicine, University Vienna, Austria

ABSTRACT

The pharmacodynamics and pharmacokinetics of the combination furosemide-retard/ triamterene were investigated in 18 healthy volunteers and in 6 patients with nephrotic syndrome. In contrast to furosemide (30 mg) the combination showed a protracted course of effect without rebound phenomenon and was neutral to potassium and magnesium in healthy volunteers and in patients. The reasons for this are the adjusted half-life times and the synergism between the two substances. It could be shown by means of a remotely controlled release capsule that an absorption of approx. 20% occurred in the ileocecal region and of 3 % in the colon ascendens region.

INTRODUCTION

High ceiling diuretics such as furosemide have a greater reserve of performance than thiazides. The short duration of effect caused by the short half-life time of 1.3 – 1.5 h [1] and the increased excretion of potassium and magnesium are disadvantages, especially if the drug has to be administered chronically. These disadvantages should be reduced by the combination of a retard form of furosemide with the antikaliuretic triamterene.

The pharmacokinetics and pharmacodynamics of furosemide, furosemide-retard and the combination furosemide-retard/triamterene were investigated in 18 healthy male volunteers and 6 patients with nephrotic syndrome (proteinuria > 5 g daily).

RESULTS

Because of the retardation, lower maximum plasma levels of furosemide are reached after 3.4 – 4 h. The "apparent" $t_{1/2\,\lambda}$ is prolonged to 3.5 – 7 h (tab. 1).

furosemide

author	dose	t_{max} h	C_{max} ng/ml	$t_{1/2elim}$ h
RUPP (1980)	40	1,08	1672 – 2168	1,3 – 1,5
EBIHARA et al. (1983)	40	1,7	1220	2,4 (β)
BEERMANN (1982)	40	1,5	672	
LOEW/SCHUSTER (1984)	40	1,9	304 – 663	1,3

furosemide retard

author	dose	t_{max} h	C_{max} ng/ml	$t_{1/2elim}$ h
EBIHARA et al. (1983)	40	3.8	110	7.2
BEERMANN (1982)	60	4.0	107	
SCHUSTER/LOEW (1984)	30	3.4	62.3	3.5

Tab. 1
Important pharmacokinetic parameters of furosemide and furosemide-retard.

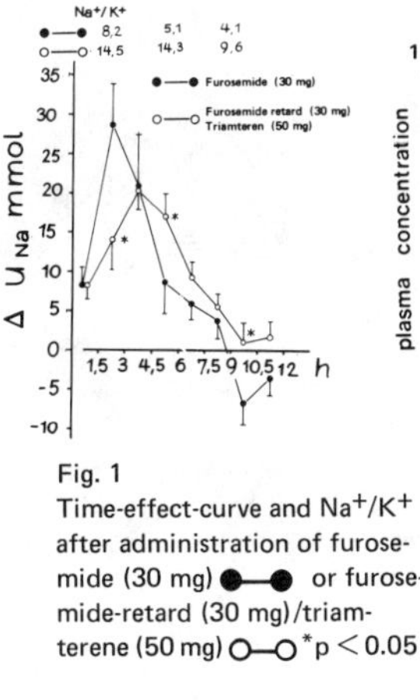

Fig. 1
Time-effect-curve and Na^+/K^+ after administration of furosemide (30 mg) ●—● or furosemide-retard (30 mg)/triamterene (50 mg) ○—○ *$p < 0.05$

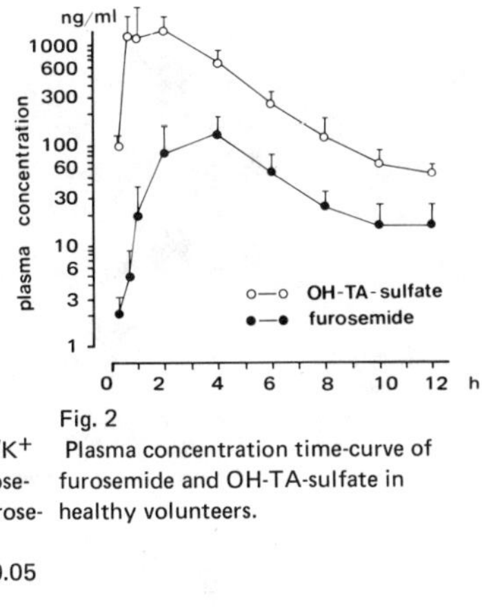

Fig. 2
Plasma concentration time-curve of furosemide and OH-TA-sulfate in healthy volunteers.

Diuretics, Jules B. Puschett, Editor

The combination furosemide-retard/triamterene in comparison with non-retarded furosemide produces not only a protracted diuresis without rebound phenomenon but also a significantly ($p \leqslant 0.01$) improved Na^+/K^+ (fig. 1). The plasma concentration time profile (fig. 2) of furosemide and OH-TA-sulfate in healthy volunteers after the administration of one capsule furosemide-retard/triamterene proved to be similar for both substances [4]. According to calculations of the pharmacokinetics of furosemide with a 2-compartment model with 2 inputs, the 2nd increase between 9 and 10.5 h corresponds to 20% of the total available dose of furosemide (fig. 3). To clarify this phenomenon the pharmacokinetics of furosemide in the gastrointestinal tract were investigated in a cross-over with 5 volunteers using a remotely controlled release capsule (fig. 4) placed in the region of the ileocecum of the colon ascendens. Based on the upper gastrointestinal tract, the relative bioavailability in the ileocecal region was approx. 20% and approx. 3% in the colon ascendens region.

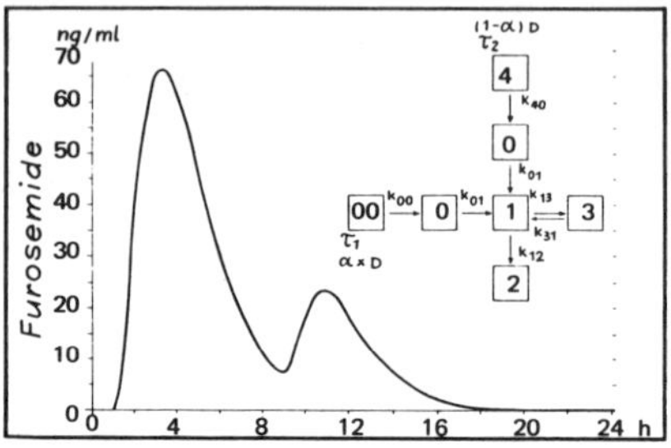

Fig. 3
Plasma concentration time-curve of furosemide after an oral dose of furosemide-retard (30 mg)/ triamterene (50 mg) administered to healthy volunteers fitted to 2-compartment model with 2 inputs.

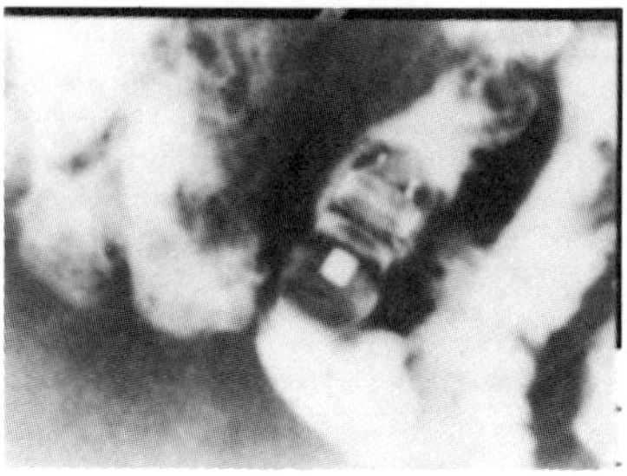

Fig. 4
The remotely controlled release capsule is situated in the ileum terminalis just before the valvula Bauhinii. The caecum is filled up with contrast.

The pharmacokinetics ($p \leqslant 0.05$) and pharmacodynamics of furosemide-retard and triamterene were investigated in 6 patients with nephrotic syndrome during a 5 day treatment. Fractionised and total excretion of urine sodium and chloride were significantly ($p \leqslant 0.05$) increased whereas potassium increase remained essentially unaltered (fig. 5). Maximum plasma levels of furosemide were observed between 4 - 6 h, the "apparent" $t_{1/2\lambda}$ for furosemide amounted to 6.5 h and for triamterene 3 h. No accumulation of furosemide, triamterene or OH-TA-sulfate was detected (fig. 6).

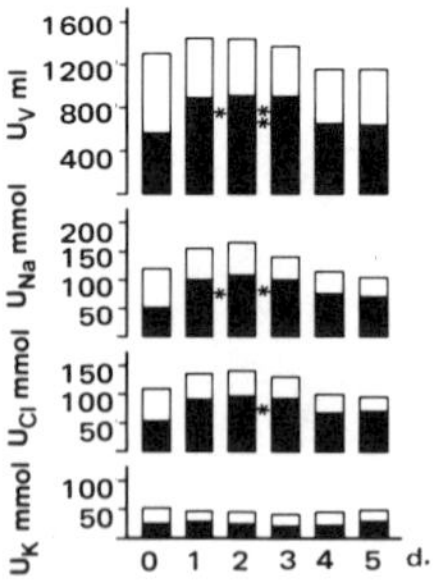

Fig. 5
Urine and electrolyte excretion in 6 patients with nephrotic syndrome before and after the daily administration of one capsule furosemide-retard (30 mg)/triamterene (50 mg).
Black part: excretion between 8 a.m. and 8 p.m.
Light part: excretion between 8 p.m. and 8 a.m.
*$p \leqslant 0.05$; **$p \leqslant 0.01$

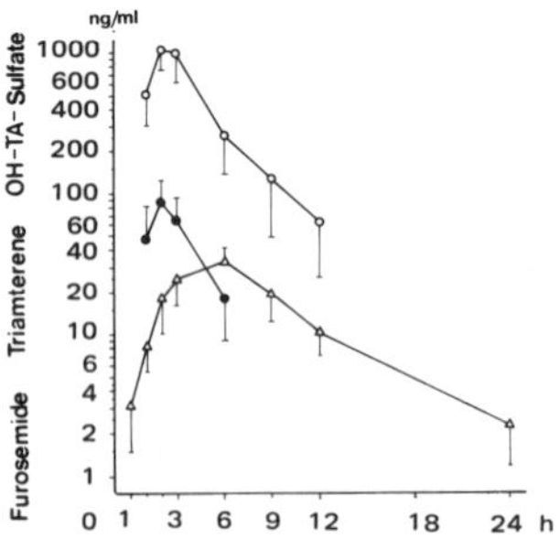

Fig. 6
Semi-logarithmic plot of the plasma concentration curves of furosemide, triamterene and OH-TA-sulfate in 6 patients with nephrotic syndrome.

CONCLUSION

Furosemide is pharmacodynamically characterised by a rapid onset of effect, a short duration of effect, a reserve of performance but also by an increased excretion of potassium and magnesium. The reasons for this profile of effect are the pharmacokinetic behaviour and the site of effect of furosemide. After oral administration maximum plasma levels are already reached after 1 – 1.9 h [1, 3, 5]. The elimination half life time is approx. 1.5 h. Some of these undesirable pharmacodynamic effects could be practically eliminated with the combination furosemide-retard/ triamterene. The apparent $t_{1/2\ \lambda}$ of 3.5 h for furosemide is well adjusted to those of triamterene and OH-TA-sulfate. As a consequence of the retardation of furosemide the effect lasts for approx. 10 h without rebound. In addition to being neutral to magnesium the present combination is characterised above all by being neutral to potassium. This synergistic effect has not only been able to be proved in the case of healthy volunteers but also in the case of patients with nephrotic syndrome and chronic cardiac insufficiency [2].

REFERENCES

1. B. Beermann, Clin. Pharmacol. Ther. 32, 584 - 591 (1982)
2. H. Burkhardt, E.H. Graul, R. Pfab, O. Schuster and D. Loew, Fortschritte der Medizin (1984) (in printing)
3. A. Ebihara, K. Tawara and T. Oka, Drug Res. 33, 163 - 166 (1983)
4. D. Loew, D. Barkow, O. Schuster and H.E. Knoell, Europ.J.Clin. Pharmacol. (1984) (in printing)
5. W. Rupp, Arch.int.Pharmacodyn.Ther. 245, 119 - 129 (1980)

Corresponding address:
Dr. Dr. med. D. Loew
Kuhloweg 37 - 39
5860 Iserlohn
West Germany

PHARMACOKINETICS OF HYDROCHLOTHIAZIDE

Y.ORITA, T.NAKANISHI, H.NAKAHAMA, Y.FUKUHARA, A.ANDO, H.ABE, M.YAMAZAKI°, S.ITOH°, Y.ITOH°, OSAKA UNIVERSITY, MEDICAL SCHOOL, FACULTY OF PHARMACEUTICAL SCIENCE°, OSAKA, JAPAN.

ABSTRACT

We found that the urinary excretion of hydrochlothiazide (hct) is a pharmacokinetic variable related to diuretic activity of hct. The results indicate that hct is a rather long acting diuretics and suggest that a device to increase urinary excretion of hct could contribute to the treatment of refractory edema.

INTRODUCTION

Hct is one of the most widely used diuretics. Attempts to find any relationship between pharmacokinetic variables of hct and diuretic activity have not been successful so far [1]. In the present study,HPLC was deviced by the authors [2], and concentrations of hct in body fluids were determined for 24 hrs.

MATERIALS AND METHODS

Nine healthy volunteers(in Tab.1) and twelve patients(in Tab.2) were chosen in the present study. The informed consent was obtained from each subject. Each subject was orally given 100 mg of hct at 9.00 a.m. after fasting overnight. Subjects were allowed to drink or eat ad lib after drug administration. Blood sampling and urine collection were done every one hour during the first 6 hrs, and thereafter at appropriate time interval.In cases of K.A. and H.K., bile was collected through a PTCD tube inserted into the common bile duct. Plasma,urinary and biliary concentrations of hct were determined by HPLC using Fine-SIL-5 column with extraction by ethylacetate and absorption by silica gel. The concentration in the blood cells was calculated by using hematocrit value. The plots of plasma concentration of hct versus time on semilogarithmic graph revealed to be linear till 10-12 hrs after administration. One compartment analysis was employed to obtain pharmacokinetic variables. The area under plasma concentration-time curve(AUC) was calculated by the trapezoidal rule. Creatinine clearance(Ccr) was determined as an index of renal function. Urinary excretion of sodium was also measured as a diuretic activity.

RESULTS AND DISCUSSION

Tabs.1 and 2 show pharmacokinetic variables. The time course of plasma and blood cell concentration of hct and cumulative urinary and biliary excretions of hct in patient K.A. are shown in Fig.1. Blood cell concentration of hct maximally elevated at 3-4 hrs after administration. Ratio of hct concentration of blood cells to that of plasma sustained 3-5 even at 24 hrs after administration. The daily biliary excretion of hct was 11.9 µg, which was only 0.02% of the urinary excretion of hct. A significant($P<0.01$) correlation between Ccr and 24 hrs urinary hct excretion was obtained and a significan inversed correlation between Ccr and AUC_{0-24} were observed. Renal

Diuretics, Jules B. Puschett, Editor

clearance of hct in most cases exceeded Ccr. The daily urinary excretion of hct has a significant correlation to diuretic activity($r=0.716, P<0.01$.Fig.2).

REFERENCES

1. B.Beermann and M.Groschinsky-Grind; Clin.Pharmacokinetics 5,221-245, 1980.
2. M.Yamazaki, Y.Itoh, Y.Takeda, H.Yaginuma, S.Itoh,A.Kamada, Y.Orita, A.Ando, T.Nakanishi, H,Nakahama; Chem.Pharm.Bull. in press.

TABLE 1 Normal Subjects (N = 9) Hydrochlorothiazide 100 mg P. O

	SEX	AGE (y)	HEIGHT (cm)	BW (kg)	Tmax (h)	Cmax (ng/ml)	AUC (0–6h) (ng·h/ml)	TOTAL URINARY EXCRETION (mg) (0–6h)	Ka	Ke	T½ (h)	RENAL CLEARANCE (ml/min)
A	M	25	170	59	2.0	540	2152	29.44	1.69	0.207	3.34	228.0
B	F	24	157	47	4.0	352	1133	37.24		0.183	3.78	547.8
C	M	24	170	60	3.0	463	2215	60.77	1.52	0.246	2.82	457.3
D	M	27	174	66	3.0	652	2335	44.40		0.219	3.16	317.0
E	M	23	160	54	4.0	584	2410	38.21		0.153	4.53	264.2
F	M	29	160	59	2.0	723	2994	50.58	2.19	0.211	3.28	281.6
G	M	30	169	56	2.0	499	2544	42.11	0.88	0.259	2.68	275.9
H	M	25	172	57	2.0	592.1	2523	48.15+α	2.041	0.173	4.00	
I	M	27	173	65	3.0	517.2	1981	37.16	0.582	0.166	4.17	312.6

TABLE 2 Patients (N=12) Hydrochlorothiazide 100mg P.O.

NAME	SEX	AGE (y)	DISEASE	EDEMA &/OR ASCITES	HEIGHT	BW	Ccr (ml/min)	Tmax	Cmax (ng/ml)	AUC (0–24h) (ng·h/ml)	TOTAL URINARY EXCRETION (0–24h) (mg)	Ka	Ke	T½ (h)	RENAL CLEARANCE (ml/min)
H. S.	M	53	NEPHROTIC SYNDROME	+	152	48	114	1.5	581.5	3107	62.91	1.952	0.274	2.53	337.5
S. K.	M	66	HEART FAILURE	±		55	67	3.0	1194.0	10470	19.36		0.073	9.49	105.7
R. S.	F	73	CHRONIC RENAL FAILURE	-	155	43	23	4.0	1169.1	10762	38.16		0.051	13.59	59.1
M. H.	F	46	IDIOPATHIC EDEMA	+	148	43	65	2.0	1016.0	9913	13.86	0.691	0.108	6.42	22.5
T. S.	M	34	HYPERTENSION	-	163	57	144	3.0	763.8	4923.3	75.62	0.407	0.113	6.13	256.0
A. H.	F	58	LUNG CANCER	-	-	-	75	3.0	729.4	6986.6	51.15	0.388	0.115	6.03	122.0
N. S.	F	27	CGN (MPGN)	±	150.5	45	66	2.0	791.2	4219.2	36.98	2.318	0.128	5.41	146.08
K. N.	M	48	DIABETIC NEPHROPATHY	±	167	54.5	45	2.0	917.9	8321.4	16.27	0.568	0.140	4.95	32.6
Y. K.	F	21	NEPHROTIC SYNDROME	±	150	49	117	2.0	597.0	3603.5	43.74	0.328	0.264	2.63	202.3
S. N.	M	69	NEPHROTIC SYNDROME	±	160.5	59	48	3.0	498.3	5849	21.71	0.101	0.072	9.63	61.9
K. A.	F	57	GALL STONE	-	150	47	53	2.0	929.8	5655.9	48.90	1.980	0.221	3.14	178.5
H. K.	M	69	GASTRIC CANCER	-	167	48	84	1.0	470.5		29.76		0.117	5.93	

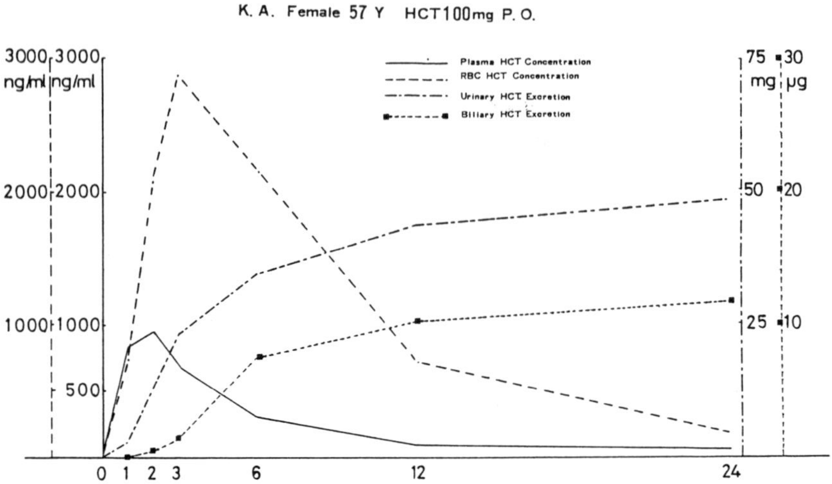

FIG.1 The time course of plasma and blood cell(RBC) HCTconcentration and cumulative urinary and biliary HCTexcretion in patient K. A.

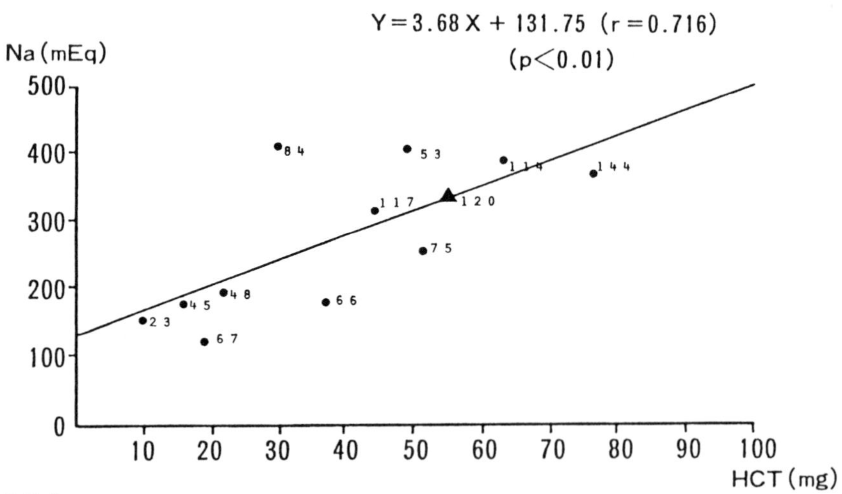

FIG.2

Correlation between total urinary HCT excretion (24hrs) and total urinary Na excretion (24hrs). (N=12)
Numerals indicate patients Ccr.

GASTRIC MOTILITY MODIFIES DIURETIC PROFILE OF LOOP DIURETIC PIRETANIDE

W. Rupp, M. Badian, H.-G. Grigoleit and V. Malerczyk
Clinical Research, Clinical Pharmacology, H 840, Hoechst AG, P.O.Box 800320, 6230 Frankfurt am Main 80, F.R.G.

INTRODUCTION

Within the frame of studies to measure the influence of gastrointestinal absorption of drugs on their pharmacodynamic effects the role of gastric motility on the absorption of piretanide, a new loop diuretic, was investigated in normal subjects.

STUDY DESIGN

In a double-blind, double-dummy crossover study 8 subjects received 6 mg of piretanide (1 tablet) immediately after either 40 mg of the spasmolytic hyoscin-N-butylamid (Buscopan^{R}) or isotonic saline intravenously. Food and fluid intake were standardized from 48 h before medication to 48 h thereafter.

KINETICS

As compared to the saline study, there were the following effects of the spasmolytic on the pharmacokinetic variables of piretanide (Fig. 1,2):

c_{max} 293 ± 71 ng/ml vs. 221 ± 68 ng/ml ($p < 0.05$)
t_{max} 0.81 ± 0.32 h vs. 1.88 ± 0.44 h ($p < 0.05$)
AUC (0-8h) 491 ± 98 $ng.ml^{-1}h$ vs. 452 ± 84 $ng.ml^{-1}h$ (NS)

DYNAMICS

According to the delay of absorption the pharmacodynamic variables were modified: Urine volume (0-2h) 1307 ± 282 ml vs. 718 ± 239 ml, urine volume (2-4h) 332 ± 228 ml vs. 781 ± 225 ml (Fig. 3,4)

Sodium excretion (0-2h) 174 ± 38 mmol. vs. 103 ± 25 mmol., sodium excretion (2-4h) 46 ± 30 mmol. vs. 106 ± 29 mmol.

Potassium excretion (0-2h) 18 ± 6 mmol. vs. 16 ± 3 mmol., potassium excretion (2-4h) 7 ± 3 mmol. vs. 12 ± 4 mmol.

There was no relevant difference in the accumulated excretion of urine, sodium and potassium from 4 h after medication onward.

CONCLUSION

It is concluded that the inhibition of gastric motility by the spasmolytic delays but does not impair the amount of absorption of piretanide. This is reflected accordingly by the pharmacodynamic variables.

Diuretics, Jules B. Puschett, Editor

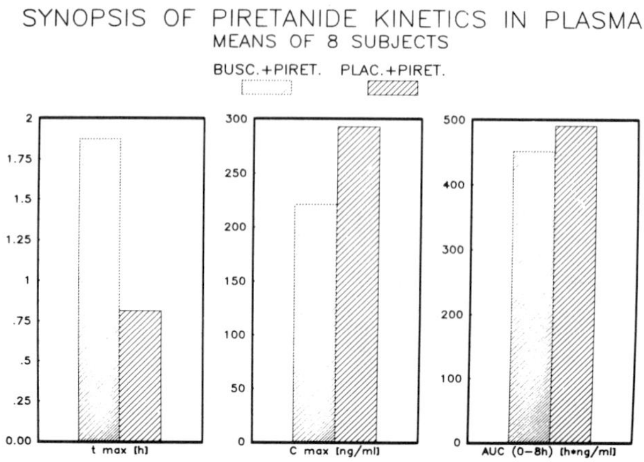

Synopsis of Piretanide Kinetics in Plasma. Means of 8 Subjects: t_{max}, c_{max}, AUC (0-8h).

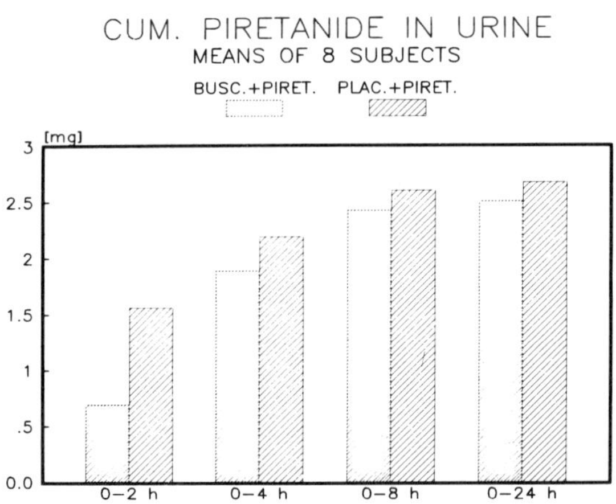

Cumulated renal excretion of Piretanide. Means of 8 Subjects: 0-2h, 0-4h, 0-8h, 0-24h.

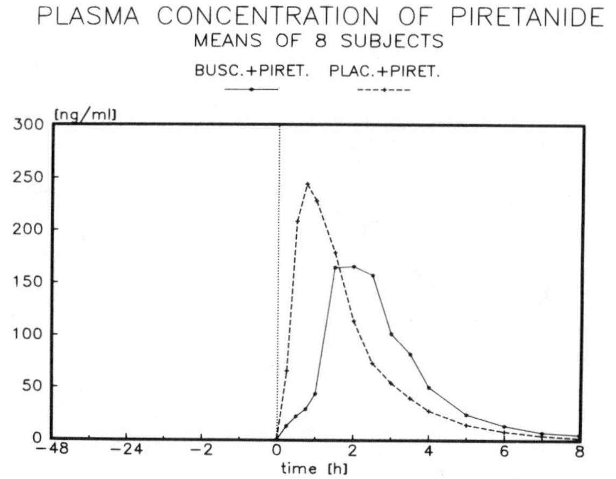

Time course of piretanide concentrations in plasma. Means of 8 Subjects.

——— BUSCOPAN$^{(R)}$ + PIRET.

------- PLACEBO + PIRET.

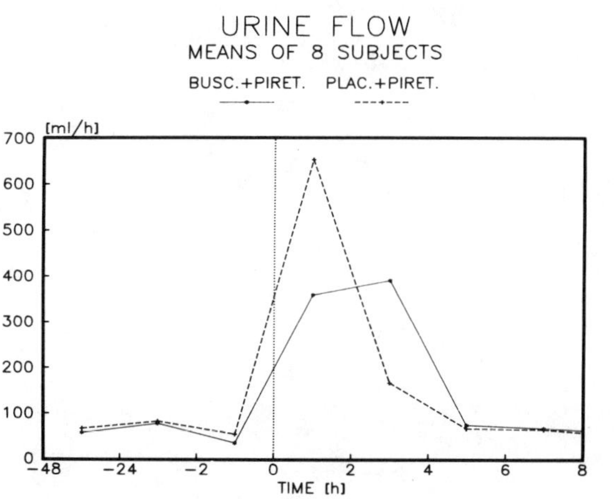

Profile of urine flow. Means of 8 Subjects.

——— BUSCOPAN$^{(R)}$ + PIRET.

-------- PLACEBO + PIRET.

SECTION XIII

CONCLUSION

THE FUTURE FOR DIURETIC THERAPY

Jules B. Puschett, M.D., Renal-Electrolyte Division, Department of Medicine, University of Pittsburgh School of Medicine, Pittsburgh, PA 15261 U.S.A.

My assignment in this discussion is to attempt to direct my remarks toward an analysis of the question "Where do we go from here with diuretic therapy?" I suppose another way of asking this question would be to phrase it "Are diuretics here to stay?" First, let me say that I undertake to answer these questions with some trepidation. Nevertheless, based on the data I have heard presented at this Conference, it seems to me that a pattern is beginning to emerge which may forecast the activity we can expect to see, both on the part of the pharmaceutical industry as well as the biological community, in the next few years. At the outset, it may be useful to consider the future of diuretic therapy in two major categories.

In general, diuretics are utilized for two broad classifications of patients, those with edema formation and those with hypertension. Indeed, it may be that volume overload is a factor in hypertension, but it is clear that this is not the only factor. Vasoconstriction appears to play an important role, as well. In fact, we have heard extensive discussions at this Conference about the renal blood flow effects of diuretics, as well as their extrarenal vascular actions. Nephrologists are especially aware of the significance of these vascular factors, since they have seen patients on dialysis, who are essentially anephric, who remain hypertensive despite the fact that it is possible to render their extracellular fluid volume normal or even slightly low. Furthermore, the hypertension may or may not be related to excessive activity of the renin-angiotensin system. Therefore, we need to recognize that it is necessary for us to think about diuretics in these two general categories, separately. Furthermore, it is important to realize that what may be a beneficial characteristic for drugs effective in one of these two types of disorder may not necessarily be desirable for the other. Let us proceed now to consider the features of a so-called ideal drug.

As with every other medication, we would like diuretics to be highly effective therapeutically while at the same time causing few, and hopefully only minor, side effects. At the first session of these meetings, we heard from Dr. Baer how the first really effective diuretic, chlorothiazide (Diuril) was developed. The fact that this agent and its congeners are still in widespread use despite a plethora of new drugs currently available, suggests to me that he and his colleagues succeeded admirably in developing an effective agent with few side effects. While the thiazides have certainly served their purpose, including helping to reduce the mortality and morbidity of hypertension, they, like all drugs, have their limitations. They are capable of producing only a moderate degree of natriuresis and they do not work in patients with glomerular filtration rates less than about 20-30 ml/min. However, fortunately, the discovery of furosemide was not too far off. Indeed, as we heard from Dr. Muschawek, we are in the 25th year of the development of this agent. With the availability of Lasix, we were able to cause the excretion of a much greater fraction of filtered sodium into the final urine. Thus, patients resistant to the thiazides, including those with reduced levels of GFR and with patho-physiological factors reducing sodium delivery to the distal nephron, could still be treated effectively. Indeed, the drug, given intravenously, has proved to be the mainstay of the therapy for acute pulmonary edema. Data presented to this meeting by Dr. Gensini documents the fact that both furosemide and bumetanide have beneficial effects on the circulation related to direct vascular actions as well as to reductions in extracellular fluid volume [1]. These findings reinforce our observations regarding the dual purposes for which diuretics are given.

Diuretics, Jules B. Puschett, Editor

Currently, diuretic complications and side effects are many (Table 1). Most of them represent an exaggeration of their beneficial qualities, whereas others reflect some unwanted effects on body metabolism and structure. Undoubtedly, one of the goals of new diuretic development should be the minimization or outright elimination of the toxic and metabolic effects. Of course, it is up to the physician, through intelligent use, to avoid volume depletion and azotemia. These complications arise from injudicious and overaggressive diuretic use.

TABLE 1. Diuretic complications and side effects.

1. Massive natriuresis → "pre-renal" azotemia → shock.
2. Hypokalemia.
3. Acid-base disturbances:
   a. Metabolic alkalosis - commonest.
   b. Metabolic acidosis - produced by the carbonic anhydrase inhibitors and "potassium-sparing" agents.
4. Ototoxicity.
5. Nephrotoxicity.
6. Hyponatremia.
7. Hyperuricemia.
8. Carbohydrate intolerance.

Based on this list of side effects, as well as the other limitations of diuretics with which we are all familiar, it is possible to compile a list of improvements to be desired in newly developed diuretic agents (Table 2).

TABLE 2. Improvements desired in new diuretic agents.

1. Act at more than one nephron site.
2. Long-acting.
3. Cause no increase in serum uric acid.
4. Do not result in activation of the renin-angiotensin system.
5. Have great natriuretic potency, minor kaliuretic tendencies.
6. Do not alter glucose metabolism.
7. Are well absorbed from the gastrointestinal tract, even in patients with anasarca.
8. Do not cause nephrotoxicity.
9. Do not cause ototoxicity.
10. Do not induce acid-base disturbances.
11. Do not reduce renal blood flow or glomerular filtration rate (even better, cause an increase in these functions).
12. Do not increase serum lipids.

Greater potency in diuretics is an attribute which is both to be desired and feared. On the one hand, we would like to have a drug which circumvents diuretic resistance by inhibiting sodium transport at more than one nephron site (see figure 1). Thus, for example, in patients who have severe reductions in glomerular filtration rate with an associated major increase in proximal tubule sodium reabsorption (site 1, figure 1), there will be a dramatic decrease in distal nephron sodium delivery. As a result, the thiazides will be ineffective for two reasons: First, they act at a site in the nephron, the early distal convolution (site 3, figure 1) which is very far downstream, and will be receiving dramatically reduced amounts of sodium for transport. Second, the quantity of sodium reabsorbed at this site is modest. It is of the order of 5-8% of filtered sodium. Third, because diuretics act at the luminal surface of the tubular epithelium, and because most drugs are secreted in the proximal nephron, reduced blood supply and lower GFR would make it difficult to get sufficient drug to the transport site in large enough amounts to be effective. In advanced renal insufficiency and/or when renal blood flow is reduced in a major way, even agents such as furosemide, ethacrynic acid and bumetanide would be rendered minimally effective since the majority of the sodium may be transported in the proximal nephron. Accordingly, agents which act at both sites 2 and 3 (figure 1) would be helpful, but a single agent which acts at sites 1, 2 <u>and</u> 3 would be especially nice to have for use in patients with serious functional and/or anatomical disorders of the kidney. At present, failing a single drug for this purpose, the members of my group have successfully utilized the combination of a loop of Henle agent, such as furosemide or bumetanide, to block site 2, along with metolazone, which blocks mainly at site 3, but also is effective in impairing sodium reabsorption in the proximal nephron, that is at site 1 (figure 1).

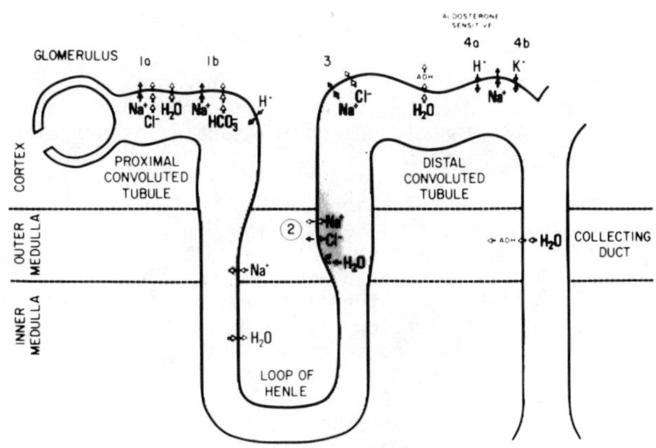

Figure 1. Major sites of ionic and water transport in the nephron. Solid arrows represent active and open arrows passive transport.

It would certainly be an advantage to have a drug which is long-acting. While the thiazides and metolazone have this characteristic, with demonstrable effectiveness for up to 48 hours in some cases, the loop of Henle agents are rapidly effective, but their effects are gone in 3-4 hours.

Responding to the contraction of the extracellular fluid volume induced by diuretics, the renin-angiotensin system is activated. This can have two effects: 1. Hypertension can occur or can be worsened, and 2. Secondary aldosteronism can occur. The latter can have a limiting effect on diuresis for reasons that are apparent on the basis of nephron physiology.

Located in the late distal nephron, and probably also in the collecting duct, are specialized transport sites at which sodium is reabsorbed in exchange for hydrogen and potassium (site 4, figure 1). Any agent that impairs sodium reabsorption proximal to this transport site will deliver to it increased amounts of sodium for reabsorption [2]. Furthermore, since transport at this site is regulated in part by the mineralocorticoids, (figure 1, site 4a), if hyperaldosteronism is induced, additional sodium will be reabsorbed, minimizing natriuretic effectiveness. It should be pointed out that every potent natriuretic agent, since it causes additional sodium to be delivered to this site and, therefore, to be exchanged for potassium, will also be a potent kaliuretic agent. Accordingly, I suggest to the chemists that when they design their new diuretic agents, they include a chemical grouping which interferes with the secretion of potassium into the tubular lumen. At present, attempts to accomplish this aim have centered upon administering loop of Henle agents along with drugs such as triamterene or amiloride which are effective at site 4b (figure 1).

Some progress has been made in avoiding hyperuricemia. Drugs such as indacrinone and indapamide as well as a new benzoxazole carboxylic acid, A-53385, are uricosuric [3]. Consequently, their use generally results in only minimal elevations in serum uric acid. Furthermore, we would very much like to avoid alterations caused by diuretics in carbohydrate metabolism, so that they could be used without concern in diabetic or pre-diabetic patients.

We always prefer to give medications orally rather than intravenously, both to reduce side effects and to lower the incidence of complications. Therefore, it would be helpful if most of the drug that is ingested were to become bioavailable. In addition, an absence of toxic effects on the kidney, and on both vestibular and auditory functions is much to be desired, as would be freedom from the introduction of acid-base disturbances. The most common of these is so-called contraction metabolic alkalosis of the hypokalemic variety.

Since renal blood flow and glomerular filtration rate (GFR) are frequently already reduced in our edematous patients, further reductions caused by diuretics would interfere with their natriuretic capabilities. In this regard, drugs such as SC-33643, the structure for which was presented by Dr. Weet, may provide an advantage, given its ability to vasodilate, elevating both renal blood flow and filtration rate [4]. Finally, and certainly of importance with regard to the pathogenesis of atherosclerosis, it would be helpful to have diuretics which did not elevate serum lipids. We have heard from Dr. Matsuda et al, that tripamide may represent such an agent [5]. Judging just by the number of new compounds that are being developed, one would have to come to the conclusion that the future for diuretic therapy is good.

TABLE 3. New diuretic agents.

Indapamide	HOE - 365
Tripamide	SC - 33643
Bumetanide	BN - 1270
Piretanide	A - 53385
Indacrinone (MK - 196)	(aryloxy) Acetic acid derivatives
Muzolamine	Dihydrofuropyridines
Xipamide	UP - 788-42

Table 3 provides an incomplete list of those agents which have either recently become available for commercial use, are in the investigational stage, or have just been synthesized. A number of these diuretics have already been mentioned. Piretnaide and muzolamine are new loop of Henle agents. Dr. Klaus and his co-workers report that in addition to its diuretic capability, piretanide has also been shown to have the capacity to interfere with norepinephrine-induced vasoconstriction [6]. This property may provide it with additional effectiveness as an antihypertensive agent. Muzolamine, Dr. Bartoli tells us, has prolonged activity over that seen with other loop diuretics [7], and Dr. Dal Canton and his colleagues have provided evidence that the mechanism of its antihypertensive effect is related only in part to its natriuretic activity [8]. Xipamide, a benzoic acid derivative, is reported by Dr. Knauf and Prof. Mutschler to be effective and safe in both chronic renal failure and chronic hepatic failure [9].

Newer agents, not mentioned earlier, include HOE-365, which Dr. Hropot and his colleagues, Drs. Englert and Lang, tell us is a hydroxyphenylsulfone that has both a potent saliuretic effect as well as an ability to inhibit vasoconstriction [10]. Dr. Pozet and his colleagues presented evidence for a thiazide-like effect of the drug BN 1270, which causes a prolonged natriuresis amounting to an increase of about 2% in filtered sodium excretion, comparable to the effect they noted with hydrochlorothiazide [11].

Dr. Plattner shared with us some structual and functional information on Abbott's new aminomethyl aryloxy acetic acid esters, which have high ceiling diuretic properties. Data on another new class of drugs, with neither sulfonamide nor carboxylic acid structure, were presented by Dr. Braquet's group from France. They are derivatives of dihydrofuropyridine, which have both antihypertensive and diuretic properties [12]. Finally, Dr. Cazes presented some observations on the new β-blocker, UP-788-42 [13]. Unlike other drugs of this class, not only does this agent not cause salt and water retention, but was actually diuretic and natriuretic in the rat and monkey. This effect, if demonstrable in humans, should provide an important improvement in β-blocker therapy.

In table 4 are listed some other agents not usually considered when one discusses diuretics. As reviewed above, there is the possibility that β-blockade may not be incontrovertibly associated with salt retention. For several years, the concept of the existence of a natriuretic humoral factor has been undergoing extensive investigation. While such a substance has not yet been isolated, it is my impression that the evidence for its existence is becoming more compelling. Whether such an agent is important pathogenetically either in antinatriuretic states such as cirrhosis of the liver, or, as Dr. de Wardener has suggested, in essential hypertension, remains to be determined [14].

TABLE 4. Some new and novel "diuretics."

1. Beta-blockers with diuretic properties.
2. Natriuretic hormone.
3. "Aquaretics."
4. Calcium channel blockers.

Drs. Kinter and Stassen provided us with an insight into a fascinating area of investigation, the development of agents which promote the excretion of solute-free water [15, 16]. Although they might not be especially helpful in salt-retaining states, they could represent a tremendous advance in the therapy of those patients with hyponatremia who have a persistent stimulus to ADH secretion or an ectopic source of its production.

We tend not to think of slow channel calcium blockers as agents which have renal effects. Presented in figure 2 is a study recently performed in my laboratory, in which a normal volunteer undergoing maximal steady state water diuresis was given 5 mg of a new calcium channel blocker, nitrendipine, by mouth. Within 30 minutes, the drug began to effect a natriuresis which eventually reached about 4% of filtered sodium load. That this was not the result of hemodynamic factors is verified by the following observations: First, there was no consistent change in glomerular filtration rate, determined as the clearance of inulin. Effective renal plasma flow, as estimated by the clearance of p-aminohippurate, did eventually rise, but the natriuresis began before that change in renal plasma flow occurred. Furthermore, phosphate excretion increased as did free water formation, suggesting that the drug had a direct effect to inhibit proximal tubular sodium and water (as well as phosphate) transport.

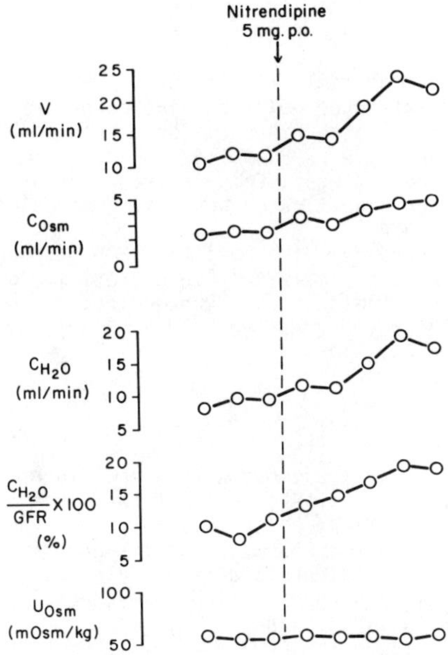

Figure 2. Effects of the administration of nitrendipine (given at the arrow) on urinary flow rate (V), solute clearance (Cosm), free water clearance (CH_2O), percentage free water clearance (CH_2O/GFR X 100), and urinary osmolality (Uosm) in a normal subject undergoing sustained maximal water diuresis. Urine collections were obtained approximately every thirty minutes.

Let me return for a moment to the second of the major uses of diuretics, that is, as antihypertensives. Will the β-blocking agents and slow channel calcium antagonists supplant the diuretics as first-step agents for hypertension? You have heard a very extensive and lucid discussion of the matter at this meeting by Drs. Materson and Peña [17]. Therefore, I need to add very little, except for my personal opinion. I think that diuretics will continue to be the mainstay of therapy for mild hypertension, because of their widespread use, reliability, effectiveness and minimal side effects. However, I believe that the newer drugs will have a significant impact, and that a group of patients, perhaps those who do not tolerate diuretic therapy, will be begun on these classes of newer drugs.

Finally, let me restate my original question: "What is the future for diuretic therapy?" It seems to me that the presence of so many people at this Conference from so many different countries strongly suggests that diuretics are here to stay. When I examine the newer compounds which have recently become available, as well as those in the developmental state, I have to conclude that diuretics will play a major role in our therapeutic armamentarium against edema states, hypertension and other disorders for some time to come.

REFERENCES

1. G. Gensini, Acute hemodynamic effects of intravenous bumetanide vs. furosemide in patients undergoing cardiac catheterization. In, Abstracts of the First International Conference on Diuretics, Miami Beach, Florida, March 5-9, 1984, p. 4.
2. J.B. Puschett and A. Rastegar, Comparative study of the effects of metolazone and other diuretics on potassium excretion. Clin. Pharm. Ther. 15:397-405, 1974.
3. P.R. Bunnell, Pharmacology of Abbott(A)-53385: A new high ceiling diuretic with uricosuric activity. In Diuretics: Chemistry, Pharmacology and Clinical Applications, Proceedings of the First International Conference on Diuretics, edited by J.B. Puschett, M.D., Elsevier Science Publishing Co., 1984, p. .
4. Ibid, J.F. Weet, p .
5. Ibid, Y. Matsuda, p .
6. Ibid, E. Klaus, p .
7. Ibid, E. Bartoli, p .
8. A. Dal Canton, One-year treatment with a new diuretic, muzolimine, in hypertensive patients. In, Abstracts of the First International Conference on Diuretics, Miami Beach, Florida, March 5-9, 1984, p. 31.
9. H. Knauf and E. Mutschler, Pharmacodynamics and kinetics of xipamide in chronic diseases of the kidney and liver. In, Diuretics: Chemistry, Pharmacology and Clinical Applications, Puschett, p .
10. Ibid, H.C. Englert and H.J. Lang, p .
11. Ibid, N. Pozet et al., p .
12. A. Esanu et al., Structure-activity relationship of a new series of diuretics: The dihydrofuropyridines. In, Abstracts of the First International Conference on Diuretics, Miami Beach, Florida, March 5-9, 1984, p. 33.
13. A. Cloarec, D. Cazes et al, UP 788-42, A new diuretic β-blocking agent. In, Diuretics: Chemistry, Pharmacology and Clinical Applications, Puschett, p .
14. H.E. De Wardener and G.A. MacGregor, The relation of a circulating sodium transport inhibitor (the natriuretic hormone?) to hypertension. Medicine 62:310-326, 1983.
15. F. Stassen, Molecular pharmacology and mechanisms of action of aquaretic agents. In, Diuretics: Chemistry, Pharmacology and Clinical Applications, Puschett, p .
16. Ibid, L. Kinter, p .
17. Ibid, B. Materson, p .